Natural, Alternative, and Complementary Health Care Practices

Natural, Alternative, and Complementary Health Care Practices

ROXANA HUEBSCHER, PhD, FNPC, HNC, CMT
Associate Professor, College of Nursing
University of Wisconsin Oshkosh
Oshkosh, Wisconsin

PAMELA A. SHULER, DNSc, CFNP, RN
Family Nurse Practitioner/Consultant
Sylva, North Carolina

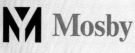

Mosby

An Affiliate of Elsevier Science

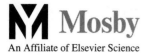
Mosby

An Affiliate of Elsevier Science

11830 Westline Industrial Drive
St. Louis, Missouri 63146

NATURAL, ALTERNATIVE, AND
COMPLEMENTARY HEALTH CARE PRACTICES
Copyright © 2004, Mosby, Inc. All rights reserved.   ISBN 0-323-01676-6

NOTICE

Pharmacology is an ever-changing field. Standard safety precautions must be followed, but as new research and clinical experience broaden our knowledge, changes in treatment and drug therapy may become necessary or appropriate. Readers are advised to check the most current product information provided by the manufacturer of each drug to be administered to verify the recommended dose, the method and duration of administration, and contraindications. It is the responsibility of the licensed health care provider, relying on experience and knowledge of the patient, to determine dosages and the best treatment for each individual patient. Neither the publisher nor the author assumes any liability for any injury and/or damage to persons or property arising from this publication.

International Standard Book Number 0-323-01676-6

Senior Editor: Michael Ledbetter
Senior Developmental Editor: Laurie K. Muench
Publishing Services Manager: Catherine Albright Jackson
Project Manager: Celeste Clingan
Designer: Teresa Breckwoldt

Printed in USA

Last digit is the print number: 9   8   7   6   5   4   3   2   1

Dedication

I dedicate this book to my colleagues and students at the University of Wisconsin Oshkosh College of Nursing who have kept my eyes open and my heart young; to the many, many patients who openly accept natural, alternative, and complementary health care practices; and to my family for being there for me through thick and thin.

RH

This book is dedicated to my husband, Keith, and my family. Their love, support, and encouragement through the years have given me the drive and stamina to pursue the dream the good Lord blessed me with—serving and loving others by striving to improve their health and well-being.

PAS

Contributors

Asha Kiran Anumolu, RN, MSN
Instructor
Georgia Southern University
Statesboro, Georgia

Diana W. Guthrie, PhD, FAAN, HTC, CHTP
Diabetes Nurse Specialist
Mid America Diabetes Associates;
Professor Emeritus, School of Medicine
University of Kansas
Wichita, Kansas

Helen Miller, RN, BSN, Dipl.Ac., C.A.
Acupuncturist
Jensen Health & Energy Center
Wauwatosa, Wisconsin

Wendy C. Noble, RN, MSN
Instructor, Associate Degree Nursing
Western Wisconsin Technical College
La Crosse, Wisconsin

Mercy Mammah Popoola, RN, CNS, PhD
Assistant Professor, School of Nursing
Georgia Southern University
Statesboro, Georgia

Louise Rauckhorst, BS, MSN, EdD, ANP
Professor and NP Track Coordinator
University of San Diego
San Diego, California

Alison M. Rushing, RN, MSN
Assistant Professor
Georgia Southern University
Statesboro, Georgia

Brenda Talley, PhD, RN, CNAA
Assistant Professor
Georgia Southern University
Statesboro, Georgia

Debra A. Bancroft, MSN, FNP, APNP
Rheumatology Nurse Practitioner
Rheumatic Disease Center
Milwaukee, Wisconsin

Linda Bergstrom, CNM, PhD
Nurse-Midwife
Rosebud Indian Health Service Hospital
Rosebud, South Dakota

Joan C. Engebretson, DrPH, HNC, RN
Associate Professor, School of Nursing
University of Texas Health Science Center
Houston, Texas

Judith Hallock, MSN, CFNP, RN
Family Nurse Practitioner
Sylva Family Practice
Sylva, North Carolina

Charon A. Pierson, PhD, APRN-BC, FAANP
Assistant Professor, School of Nursing and Dental Hygiene
University of Hawaii
Honolulu, Hawaii

Marilyn K. Shutte, RNC, MSN, APNP
Pulmonary/Adult Nurse Practitioner
Affinity Medical Group
Neenah, Wisconsin

Anne T. Thurston, ANP-C, MSN
Nurse Practitioner
Western Carolina Digestive Consultants
Sylva, North Carolina

We wrote this text with faith in a future balance of health care practices. We are frustrated by a system that gives drugs for every illness, symptom, and disease, and has no time to address concerns in-depth. Drugs are needed, of course, but using drugs for every problem takes away personal power, the power of knowing that there are many ways to take care of one's illnesses and one's health.

Many are writing about evidence-based medicine and ridiculing "opinion-based" health care. However, from our many years as nurse practitioners, we have come to believe that conventional health care practices are pretty much all opinion. We change our minds with each randomized double-blind placebo-controlled study; we are mutating our bacteria and viruses; and proclaiming for all who are depressed or anxious that we have quick-fix drugs. Yet there are no long-term studies on new medications; there also are drug recalls on a regular basis. In addition, there have been numerous changes in routine therapies over the years. For example, asthma, heart care, gastrointestinal therapy, arthritis treatment, low back pain, and numerous gynecologic treatments have been revisited on a regular basis. And each time we say, "this is it, the definitive treatment." The same health care system chastises those who do not follow the standard of care at the moment and often label as "off the wall," or some other derogatory term, those who seek deeper causes or choose unusual but possibly helpful treatments. Common, practical, and comforting therapies have fallen by the wayside. We do include herbs in the text because they are part of biologic-based alternatives, but in no detail. We advise readers to use an additional reputable resource if herbs are to be used as treatments because herbs are substances just as any other drug and need the same cautions with use.

It is time to give the care of the illness and choices back to the healee, the patient, the one who can be the most powerful in his or her own care. And it is way past time to give credence to a treatment "doctrine of reasonable certainty," (a phrase used by the German Commission E to explain how it bases its herbal recommendations on evidence from a long history of human use, combined with a moderate amount of scientific data).

This book is about comfort and care and doing no harm; it is about holistic healing, describing natural, alternative, and complementary therapies to use with, or instead of, drugs. We discuss things that have evidence and things that do not. The term *natural* in this text refers to practical health care routines and to solid nursing care, things that may have no evidence-based research because there is no way of measuring what is happening or simply because research has not been done. But the patient, the healee, feels *better*. There is much more to say. Heal on.

ACKNOWLEDGMENTS

We thank the faculty and staff of the University of Wisconsin Oshkosh College of Nursing for their open minds, good hearts, friendly spirits, and encouragement. We express our appreciation to Thomas C. Wilson, MD, MS, for believing in "whole person health care" and for providing Pam with the opportunity to practice "wholistic" health care. Dr. Wilson and his staff have been a constant source of encouragement and support. Also, Bill Morris, RPh, PA, CCN, Morris Compounding Pharmacy, and Mary A. Joyce, Kountry Kupboard Health Food Store, have been extremely supportive. We acknowledge the staff at the Great Smokies Diagnostic Laboratory for being a source of guidance, particularly in the area of hormone testing. We thank Laurie Muench, Senior Developmental Editor, for her gracious assistance during the entire process of writing and publishing this book. Finally, a special thanks to all our patients and their families. They bring joy and purpose to our lives.

Roxana Huebscher
Pamela A. Shuler

Table of Contents

Natural,
Alternative,
and
Complementary
Health Care
Practices

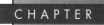

CHAPTER 1

INTRODUCTION TO NATURAL, ALTERNATIVE, AND COMPLEMENTARY HEALTH CARE PRACTICES

Roxana Huebscher ■ Pamela Shuler

HOW TO USE THIS TEXT

This text describes natural, alternative, and complementary (NAC) therapies and outlines NAC practices for common outpatient conditions. It is intended for use by health care providers (HCPs) who have knowledge of conventional therapies for the outlined disorders, yet have a desire to know the availability of other therapies. To use the text, HCPs need to have a working knowledge of allopathic information in order to integrate NAC therapies properly and they need to know when conventional treatment may be a better choice. Thus readers must be aware of conventional diagnoses and management to gain the most from this text.

If the reader has limited knowledge of NAC therapies, it may be helpful to read the second section first since this section defines NAC practices. Others will want to refer to the second section and appendixes as needed. Readers must have access to appropriate in-depth herbal resources to complement herbal content, keeping in mind that an herbal remedy is a substance just as is any drug. This text is not designed to be a protocol book, nor does it provide "recipes." Numerous suggestions for NAC treatments and parameters for NAC use are outlined using a system format with NAC categories.

The conventional or allopathic health care system has numerous diagnostic methods available, yet adequate and comfortable treatments have not kept pace with the ability to diagnose. If conventional HCPs discover a diagnosis or "cause" of signs and symptoms (and many times a cause is not found), conventional HCPs are often left with few treatment options other than pharmaceutical therapies or surgery. However, multiple treatment options are available for many illnesses. Patients often request treatments other than or in addition to drugs. Further, reliance on drugs and substances (legal and illegal) is a problem of epidemic proportion in the United States. Obviously, pharmaceutical treatments are needed. Drug treatment remains a mainstay of conventional therapy, and herbal therapies have existed for thousands of years. However, pharmaceutical treatments often lead to more problems. Antibiotic resistance, side effects, interactions, adverse effects, rebound signs and symptoms,

1

long-term sequelae, drug recalls, and iatrogenesis are processes familiar to the allopathic HCP (Huebscher, 1997). Approximately 10,000 prescription medications and 300,000 to 500,000 over-the-counter medications are currently available on the market. In addition, the Food and Drug Administration (FDA) approves approximately 20 to 30 new molecular entities each year (Huebscher, 1997); this growing number of drugs leads to an increased possibility of drug errors and interactions.

An additional concern exists with this expanding drug use, especially when few other interventions (including NAC care) are offered. What children see is often what they practice. Children may not understand the difference between taking a prescription or medicinal substance and using a recreational drug. Overreliance on pharmaceuticals may contribute to recreational drug use. Children and all health care consumers need to learn about the many self-care strategies and the alternatives to drugs that are available.

HCPs need to be aware of the many available NAC alternatives that provide therapeutic options that are safe, comforting, practical, and effective. Some of these therapies have a research base, but some do not. Evidence-based research, for the purposes of this text, includes not only double-blind placebo controlled studies, but it also includes patient-reported and clinician-observed evidence and knowledge, including a few anecdotal reports. Additionally, recognition of patient circumstances and preferences is important (Peters et al, 2002; Sackett, Rosenberg, 1995). Tables are provided in the following chapters, and references are listed at the end of every chapter for those who are interested in more in-depth reading.

Some argue that using NAC therapies may delay conventional treatment. More importantly, then, is the need for conventional HCPs to be aware of all available forms of care, including research (or lack of) and the risks and benefits of both kinds of therapies. This awareness will enable patients and HCPs to discuss openly the available choices and, within a treatment time frame, make appropriate care decisions. After HCPs obtain the history and conduct necessary examinations and diagnostic procedures, treatment from both the NAC and the conventional perspectives may proceed. Both types of care can be combined, and there is and always has been overlap.

Although a minimal research base exists for many NAC therapies, additional research is being funded and more information is becoming available. A lack of research does not mean a therapy is ineffective nor does misuse mean that a modality, properly used, has to be discarded. Most NAC therapies have few side effects or adverse sequelae. (The exception would be some herb or dietary supplement misuse and quality issues for any therapy). Additionally, many NAC therapies provide comfort, promote self-care, and give patients a sense of control over their health.

To make decisions with as much knowledge, wisdom, and compassion as possible, HCPs need to keep an open mind regarding NAC therapies. HCPs need to use both NAC and conventional care sensibly and always with the patient's knowledge, input, and consent. Sometimes, however, the patient's desire may not be what the HCP thinks is "right," yet holistic and ethical care requires that the "total" patient and all available therapies be considered.

DIFFERENTIATING HOLISTIC CARE FROM NAC CARE

Holism is a philosophy of care. Holism reflects the view that "an integrated whole has a reality independent of and greater than the sum of its parts" (Dossey et al, 1995, p. 6). Holism refers to caring for the mind-body-spirit—the whole person. Holistic care can be practiced in any setting, whether the setting is allopathic or NAC-oriented. NAC therapy refers to treatments, modalities, and processes, outside of conventional practice, any of which can be practiced holistically.

Any HCP can practice holistic care regardless of practice setting, and most NAC providers use a holistic approach and do not focus on systems, symptoms, diseases, or body parts of the patient. Rather, they consider and treat the whole physical, mental, emotional, spiritual, social, and environmental milieu. Nevertheless, out of necessity and convenience for the conventional health care model and how it works, these Chapters 2 to 10 are laid out in a systems-disease approach, because the allopathic practitioner must deal with the "chief complaint" and diagnosis. However, *and very importantly*, in an effort to avoid violating the principles of holistic practice, readers need to consider the whole body-mind-spirit with each of the concerns discussed.

SHULER'S PRACTICE MODEL

Shuler's (1991) practice model has been successfully used by HCPs who are interested in integrating the principles of holistic health care into allopathic and NAC-oriented settings (Shuler, Davis, 1993a; Shuler, Davis 1993b). The model considers the "whole" person as reflected throughout the provider-patient interaction. HCPs who use the model are encouraged to "regard the mind, body, spirit and environment as integrally entwined, while at the same time, realizing that it is possible and important to assess each dimension (physical, psychological, social, cultural, environmental, and spiritual) of a person's being individually. In addition, utilizing the wholistic model emphasizes the importance and influence of family, culture, and social interactions upon the patient's health and well-being" (Shuler, Huebscher, Hallock, 2001, p. 298).

Initially, the Shuler model serves as a guide for a two-phased wholistic assessment that includes the development of a wholistic patient database and the identification of the wholistic patient needs

(Shuler, 1991; Shuler, Huebscher, 1998). After the assessment phase, the model further directs the HCP in the development and implementation of the treatment plan and in the evaluation of patient outcomes (Shuler, Huebscher, 1998). (See Appendix A for model diagram and two model-based wholistic patient assessment forms to be used with comprehensive and episodic visits.) For a more complete description of the model and its application in practice, refer to the model references (Shuler, Davis, 1993a, 1993b; Shuler, Huebscher, Hallock, 2001; Shuler, Huebscher, 1998).

NAC DEFINITIONS AND TERMINOLOGY

Numerous definitions of NAC therapies are available. Eisenberg and colleagues (1993, 1998) define alternative and complementary therapies as "medical interventions not taught widely at U.S. medical schools or generally available at U.S. hospitals." Although this definition is rather narrow, the surveys in which this definition was used were landmark studies. In the two surveys by Eisenberg and colleagues, 34% (survey completed 1991, published 1993) and 42% (completed 1997, published 1998) of participants used at least one NAC therapy within the previous year. The cost of care for these alternative practices, extrapolated from the surveys, computed to billions of dollars, the majority of which was out of pocket (Eisenberg 1993, 1998).

Micozzi (1996) offers a more philosophic definition of NAC therapies:

> Complementary medical systems are characterized by a developed body of intellectual work that underlies the conceptualization of health and its precepts; that has been sustained over many generations by many practitioners in many communities; that represents an orderly, rational, conscious system of knowledge and thought about health and medicine; that relates more broadly to a way of life (or "lifestyle"); and that has been widely observed to have definable results as practiced. (p. 7)

More recently, Micozzi (2001) classified alternative practices as one of two types. The first type includes those practices that are old; they have many practitioners and patients with a well-developed clinical wisdom that is part of a belief system of a group or society. The second type includes recent practices with few practitioners in isolation from peers and without benefit of scientific testing or clinical studies.

A holistic nursing text by Dossey and colleagues (1995) defines alternative therapies as:

> Interventions that focus on body-mind-spirit integration and evoke healing by an individual, between two individuals, or healing at a dis-

tance (e.g., relaxation, imagery, biofeedback, prayer, psychic healing); may be used as complements to conventional medical treatments." (p. 6)

Dossey's nursing definition includes the more ethereal, as well as the usual NAC processes, and allows for the acceptance of spiritual and unknown factors. Although not included in their newer edition (Dossey et al, 2000), the earlier definition provides for more concepts than are usually considered in conventional views of healing. Such ethereal concepts need to be addressed when defining NAC practices.

Additionally, the term *natural* in this text refers to common self-care and nursing practices that may be neither alternative nor complementary yet may be an important aspect of therapy that becomes neglected in allopathic care. Natural modalities are practical and common sense therapies that provide comfort for everyday human miseries and complaints.

NAC CATEGORIES

With a few word changes, NAC categories in this text follow the format of the National Institutes of Health (NIH) National Center for Complementary and Alternative Medicine (NCCAM). NAC therapies in this text are the following:

- Alternative health care systems
- Mind-body-spirit interventions
- Biologic-based therapies
- Manipulative and body-based methods
- Energy therapies

The phrase *alternative health care systems* replaces the NCCAM phrase *alternative medical systems* because some of the systems in the NCCAM category are not covered under the practice of medicine in the United States. They are, however, considered complete systems of health care (e.g., homeopathy, naturopathy). *Mind-body-spirit interventions* is the phrase used instead of the NCCAM phrase *mind-body interventions* because the former incorporates the holistic aspect of NAC care, which includes the care of the spirit.

NAC PHILOSOPHICAL ISSUES

The philosophies of care and theoretical orientations of NAC practices may seem strange to conventional providers. NAC therapies have a different way of being and cannot evolve into a Western ("conventional") way of being. Some NAC practices are thousands of years old with beautiful philosophies and forms of care from which conventional HCPs could benefit (such as Ayurveda, Traditional Chinese Medicine, Native American traditions, and other cultural practices in the United States). (See Section 2 for health care practices of the Georgia Low Country, for example.) Other NAC care, such as homeopathy, has an unusual mode of action, yet some homeopathic remedies have shown efficacy in controlled trials, and homeopathy has been used for over 200 years.

Evidence for NAC Modalities

HCPs need to learn about the NAC modalities to understand how concepts of holism and NAC care differ from conventional therapies. HCPs may desire evidence from rigorous randomized placebo-controlled trials (RCTs)—the conventional "gold standard," however, many NAC modalities do not have such trials, although other types of study may be available. Thus HCPs need to consider other forms of evidence. Sackett (1995) says that evidence-based medicine has five ideas:

1. That our clinical and other health care decisions should be based on the best patient- and population-based as well as laboratory-based evidence,
2. That the problem determines the nature and source of evidence to be sought, rather than our habits, protocols, or traditions,
3. That identifying the best evidence calls for the integration of epidemiological and biostatistical ways of thinking with those derived from pathophysiology and our personal experience,
4. That the conclusions of this search and critical appraisal of evidence are worthwhile only if they are translated into actions that affect our patients,
5. That we should continuously evaluate our performance in applying these ideas (p. 332).

If we are to follow Sackett's ideas with NAC care, then all types of research and inquiry are needed. Furthermore, few other points about NAC evidence need to be considered.

First, for some NAC practices the available research may be a case study and worthy of reading. Even when one patient improves, HCPs need to gain understanding of why, because the HCP role is to assist in the healing process. Second, although RCT research usually is feasible for herbal and other supplemental therapies, many forms of NAC may not be conducive to this type of testing. To illustrate, consider that one of the common methods of study comparison with acupuncture is to perform "real" acupuncture on one group of research participants and "sham" acupuncture on a comparison group. Sometimes, improvement is observed in both groups; therefore the conclusion is that a placebo effect exists. In fact, acupuncture may be very regulating to the entire system and, in some conditions, points for acupuncture do not need to be as specific as in other cases. In one study of knee arthritic pain (Takeda, Wessel,

1994), the sham acupuncture points were, in fact, close to the real points. They could have been considered *ashi* or "ouch" points (tender points not on the specific meridian) that may actually be needled in a regular clinical situation to help the circulation in the painful area (Miller, 2001).

Third, for evidence the doctrine of "reasonable certainty" as used by the German Commission E could be used for NAC modalities as well as for herbs. Although RCTs may not be available, the Commission examines a variety of available evidence in consideration of herbal efficacy and safety:

> Unlike the United States Food and Drug Administration which evaluates drugs only in a passive manner based on data supplied by the manufacturer, Commission E actively checks so-called bibliographic data independently. Such data include information obtained from clinical trials, field studies, collections of single cases, scientific literature including facts published in the standard reference works, and expertise of medical associations. If controlled clinical data are lacking, safety and efficacy can still be determined on the basis of information in the literature, the presence of supplemental data supporting clinical results, and significant experimental studies supporting traditional use. Application of this kind of evaluation process results in the establishment of "reasonable certainty" of the safety and efficacy of the herb being evaluated. It is not the full equivalent of the "absolute certainty" required by the U.S. FDA for all drugs. However, it is much less costly than the $350 million expenditure required to prove the safety and efficacy of a new chemical entity in the United States. This is an important point. Expenditures of that magnitude will never be made for classic herbal remedies because patent protection is not ordinarily available for them and these exorbitant research costs cannot be recovered. Besides, the German experience has definitely shown that reasonable certainty of safety and efficacy is adequate for long-used remedies. (Blumenthal, 1998, pp. ix-x.)

Reasonable certainty of safety and efficacy, as well as "the combined results from clinically relevant research, clinical expertise, and patient preferences, produces the best evidence for ensuring effective, individualized patient care" (Mulhall, 1998; Rosswurm, Larrabee, 1999, p. 317). The more NAC knowledge that conventional HCPs have, the more likely they will accept the type of evidence that best fits an individual NAC modality. "The best research evidence is synthesized and combined with clinical judgment and contextual data" (Rosswurm, Larrabee, 1999, p. 319). The RCT is not the absolute evidence base for NAC care. For example, within the nursing profession, an effective argument can be posed that RCTs and intervention studies are relevant to only a small subset of nursing questions (Jennings, Loan, 2001, p. 126).

Assessing Quality

Assessing quality in NAC practices requires a systematic approach. Because regulation and credentials may be minimal for many NAC practices and providers and may vary from state to state, HCPs must avail themselves of background information for both the providers and the NAC practices.

Finding appropriate providers is an important element in NAC care. Misuse of a NAC modality or an improperly trained provider does not mean that a modality is ineffective or that the practice should be discarded in either NAC therapy or conventional practice. Consequently, finding qualified NAC providers is the seeker's (either the HCP or patient) responsibility, necessitating care and caution. Both the HCP and the care receiver or patient need to examine the quality issues. "We can expect ethical, caring, competent, confidential, and hygienic care from [NAC] practitioners. However, at this time, we cannot expect the same conventional theoretical orientation, rigorous research base, time frames for care, or legislative regulation" (Huebscher, 1997, p. 559). For example, chiropractic is

---

Box 1-1

NAC Quality Assessment Information

Definition of NAC practice
Philosophical base and history
Research base
  What research is available?
Clinical base: NAC practice application and use
  How and for what does it work?
Benefits and risks
Appropriate education for the practice
  How long? What are the credentials of the schools? What
  courses are required?
Common credential requirements for the NAC practice
State and local regulations
Usual cost of services
Time frames of care for usual treatments: what diagnoses or
symptoms are treated?
Education and credential requirements of particular NAC provider
Experience, general information, and background of NAC
provider
  What successes, reputation, and office practices (e.g.,
  scheduling, hygiene) are used?
Evaluation information for the NAC provider

licensed in every state in the United States; however, naturopathy is not recognized in some states, let alone licensed. A national certification examination for massage therapists is available, but states vary on regulation, and cities and counties in the same state may have differing stipulations for practice. Thus to assess the quality of a NAC practice, the HCP has to make a time commitment for investigation of the practice including validating regulation, securing credentials, practice standards, and obtaining information about the NAC practitioner's qualifications and experience.

Some quality issues are listed in Box 1-1. Because obtaining details on many practices may seem overwhelming, HCPs may want to begin a NAC knowledge base in one specific area of interest, invest in some personal NAC therapy for themselves, or become NAC practitioners in one area of interest.

REFERENCES

Blumenthal, M: *The complete German Commission E monographs*. Boston, 1998, Integrative Medicine Communications.

Dossey B et al: *Holistic nursing: a handbook for practice*, ed 3, Gaithersburg, Md, 2000, Aspen.

Dossey B et al: *Holistic nursing: a handbook for practice*, ed 2, Gaithersburg, Md, 1995, Aspen.

Eisenberg D et al: Trends in alternative medicine use in the United States, 1990-1997: results of a follow-up national survey, *JAMA* 280(18):1569, 1998.

Eisenberg D et al: Unconventional medicine in the United States. Prevalence, costs, and patterns of use, *N Engl J Med* 328(4):246, 1993.

Huebscher R: Improving quality in natural and alternative health care practice. In Meisenheimer C: *Improving quality: a guide to effective programs*, ed 2, Gaithersburg, Md, 1997, Aspen.

Huebscher R: Overdrugging and undertreatment in primary health care, *Nurs Outlook* 45:161, 1997.

Jennings B, Loan L: Misconceptions among nurses about evidence-based practice, *J Nurs Scholarship* 33(2):121, 2001.

Micozzi M: *Fundamentals of complementary & alternative medicine*, ed 2, New York, 2001, Churchill Livingstone.

Micozzi M: *Fundamentals of complementary & alternative medicine*, New York, 1996, Churchill Livingstone.

Miller H: *Personal communication*, 2001.

Mulhall A: EBN notebook: Nursing research and the evidence, *Evid Based Nurs* 1(1):4, 1998.

Peters D et al: *Integrating complementary therapies in primary care: a practical guide for health professionals*, Edinburgh, 2002, Churchill Livingstone.

Rosswurm M, Larrabee J: A model for change to evidence-based practice, *Image* 31(4):317, 1999.

Sackett DL, Rosenberg WM: On the need for evidence-based medicine, *J Public Health Med* 17(3):330, 1995.

Shuler PA: Homeless women's wholistic and family planning needs: an exposition and test of the Shuler nurse practitioner practice model. Doctoral dissertation,

University of California, 1991. Ann Arbor, Mich, University Microfilms International/Dissertation Information Service (order number 9126912).

Shuler PA, Davis J: The Shuler Nurse Practitioner Practice Model: a theoretical framework for nurse practitioner clinicians, educators and researchers, part 1, *J Am Acad Nurse Pract* 5(1):11, 1993a.

Shuler PA, Davis J: The Shuler Nurse Practitioner Practice Model: clinical application, part 2, *J Am Acad Nurse Pract* 5(2):73, 1993b.

Shuler PA, Huebscher R: Clarifying nurse practitioner's unique contributions: application of the Shuler Nurse Practitioner Practice Model, *J Am Acad Nurse Pract* 10:491, 1998.

Shuler PA, Huebscher R, Hallock J: Providing wholistic health care for the elderly: application of the Shuler Nurse Practitioner Practice Model, *J Am Acad Nurse Pract* 13:297, 2001.

Takeda W, Wessel J: Acupuncture for the treatment of pain of osteoarthritic knee, *Arthritis Care Res* 7(3):118, 1994.

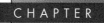

GENERAL WELL BEING

Wendy Noble ▪ Roxana Huebscher ▪ Helen Miller ▪ Louise Rauckhorst

WHAT IS WELL BEING?

Good health leads to an experience of "well-being, harmony, and unity" (AHNA), 2000; Dossey, 2001, p. 2). Well being, however, is more than simply a part of physical health. Well being is also life satisfaction, morale, self-esteem, a sense of mastery or control over life, and happiness (Antonovsky, 1987; Thoits, Hewitt, 2001). "Included under these rubrics are notions about life progress toward goals, transitory moods of gaiety, individual-environment fit, positive and negative affect, optimism, irritability, zest, apathy, fortitude, and satisfaction with one's attributes" (Antonovsky, 1987, p. 179).

To attain well being—health, life satisfaction, high morale, self-esteem, mastery, and happiness—the elements of daily life come into focus. These elements include, but are not limited to, nutrition, elimination, sleep, exercise-body movement, sexuality, relaxation, caring relationships, agreeable social activities, doing one's work in the world, contemplation, environmental harmony, spirituality, finding meaning, and recognizing and honoring the mystery elements of life. For purposes of this text, well being is a holistic process of feeling good in body, mind, emotion, and spirit, a process of "increasing awareness of reaching human potentials and the journey toward the transpersonal self (Dossey, Guzetta, 1995, p. 116). The chapter is necessarily lengthy because most all of these natural-alternative-complementary (NAC) treatments can be taken into all the other areas of the book.

Well-being strategies include therapies for sleep, anxiety, and depression, and include general stress management techniques. General nutrition, elimination, exercise and movement, and other strategies are discussed in each of the chapters as they relate to individual concerns. Detailed nutrition is beyond the scope of this text, and the reader is referred to conventional and alternative nutrition resources, although nutritional supplement information is covered in Section II. In addition, Section II has additional NAC information that is helpful for well being, including further information on mind-body-spirit interventions.

NAC THERAPIES FOR SLEEP

Sleep, as Shakespeare said, is the "balm of hurt minds, great nature's second course, chief nourisher in life's feast" (MacBeth, Act II).

Sleep, defined as periodic quiescence, has five different phases, Stages I through IV (from light to increasing deepness of sleep), and rapid eye movement (REM) sleep. Restful sleep, for many, is difficult:

> ...approximately 60 million Americans each year suffer from [insomnia], and the incidence increases with age (www.ninds.nih.gov, 2000). In addition, each year insomnia costs the [United States] about $100 billion in lost productivity and medical expenses. Insomnia also increases the risk of automobile accidents...about 100,000 car accidents and 1500 deaths annually are attributed to sleepiness. Experts believe that insomnia is as often to blame for car accidents as drunk driving. And some experts think chronic insomnia can cause poor health...depression, headaches, heart disease, and substance abuse (PL/PL, 2000, p. 13).

Most adults need approximately 7 to 8 hours of sleep a night, with a variation of from 5 to 10 hours (www.ninds.nih.gov, 2000). However, individual factors, including age and individual circadian rhythms, also play a part. In addition, shift work, travel across time zones, and ingested substances alter sleep.

Persons may have trouble falling asleep, staying asleep, or they may have problems with early awakening; some individuals may want to sleep too much. Health care providers (HCP) need to provide appropriate diagnosis of poor sleep complaints so that entities such as sleep apnea, depression, and other serious disorders are diagnosed and treated. Following appropriate diagnosis, the HCP can work with NAC sleep therapies before prescribing medications (e.g., benzodiazepines). Using NAC therapies with sleep concerns is an important step toward decreasing adverse drug events and enhancing self-care, especially in older adults. Box 2-1 describes general sleep aids.

ALTERNATIVE HEALTH CARE SYSTEMS FOR SLEEP CONCERNS

Traditional Chinese Medicine

Gach (1990) recommends acupressure points for insomnia. These points, listed in Table 2-1, can be self-administered or done by someone who knows how to use finger pressure. Appendix B lists the meridians and point locations.

Homeopathy

Section II of the text provides details about homeopathy. Because patients are able to self-remedy with homeopathy, HCPs need to be aware of various homeopathic principles and remedies. The remedies are highly dilute substances. One part remedy substance is diluted with varying diluent portions, anywhere from nine parts diluent (1X = 1 to 9), 99 parts diluent (1 C = 1 to 99), or more. Each subsequent dilution is made from one part of the preceding solution. For exam-

Box 2-1

General Sleep Aids

Comfortable, safe, quiet, and cool sleeping room
Comfortable bedclothes
Avoidance of daytime naps or take short "power" naps only
Bedtime ritual or presleep routine
Regular sleep schedule
Warm shower or bath
Pain relief measures
Sunlight during the day; light therapy; darkness for sleep
Exercise during the day but not within 2 hours of sleep
Work projects away from bedside
No activities in bed except sleep, intimacy, and "sleepy time" reading
Avoidance of shift work and travel that upsets sleep cycle

ple, one part of the one in 99 mixture is then added to 99 more parts diluent to make 2C. As with all homeopathic cases, remedies vary, depending on the type of signs and symptoms that accompany a concern (Cummings, Ullman, 1997; Skinner, 2001). For example, for sleeplessness, *coffea*, *arsenicum*, *nux vomica*, *pulsatilla*, *ignatia*, *chamomilla*, *passiflora*, and *arnica* each have different prerequisite insomnia symptoms. *Arnica* is helpful when the bed or pillow feels too hard, and the person is restless in bed, being unable to find a comfortable position (Cummings et al., 1997; Skinner, 2001). *Arsenicum* is helpful for sleeplessness that arises from anxiety, fears or being driven out of bed by anxiety, feeling anxious while sleeping, or being too tired to sleep (Cummings et al., 1997; Skinner, 2001). Skinner (2001) reports that:

> The treatment of insomnia with homeopathy is very difficult and reputedly has mixed results. However, acute episodes of insomnia that fit one of the two medicines that follow may gradually respond to one of the following medicines. The clinician should prescribe the medicine in the 30C potency: one dose in the morning for 3 days, then one dose a week for as long as it is needed. (p. 238)

Coffea cruda is used for sleeplessness after *good* news or fun when the thoughts are racing and when the patient is awakened by every sound. *Nux vomica* is taken by hard-driving people who are sleepless from a rush of ideas about *work, business, or projects*. "The patient awakens too early and cannot get back to sleep. He or she may weep and talk in his or her sleep, and be irritable and impatient during the

Table 2-1 Alternative Health Care Systems for Sleep

Intervention	Management	Treatment Regimen	Cautions, Precautions, Interactions	References
Homeopathy	Sleeplessness	Depends on accompanying history, signs, and symptoms *Coffea cruda; arsenicum; Nux vomica; lycopodium clavatum; pulsatilla; Ignatia amara; chamomilla; passiflora; arnica*	Each remedy has specific set of factors; need homeopathic education	Cummings, Ullman, 1997 LaValle et al, 2000 Skinner, 2001
Ayurveda yoga and breathing (Pranayama)	Insomnia	Postures: moon sequence, breath of arjuna, shoulder stand, fish	May not be appropriate for individuals with balance problems	Jones, 1998
Traditional Chinese medicine; acupressure	Insomnia	Points are practiced in this order: GV 16; GB 20s, B10s, B38s, H7 PC6; GV 24.5; CV 17, K6s, B62s (see Appendix B for point locations)	Tennis balls are placed between shoulder blades to press B38s if performing for self	Gach, 1990

CV, *conception vessel (Ren mo)*; B *or* UB, *urinary bladder*; K, *kidney*; PC, *pericardium*; GB, *gallbladder*; GV, *governing vessel (Du mo)*; H, *heart.*

day" (Skinner, 2001, p. 238). Thus a homeopathic practitioner needs education and homeopathic expertise, as well as the patient's background information before taking or prescribing homeopathic medications. Table 2-1 reviews some alternative health care systems for sleep.

MIND-BODY-SPIRIT INTERVENTIONS FOR SLEEP

Having a safe sleep environment should probably go without saying. However, HCPs may inadvertently overlook safety concerns. Safety problems may require involvement of social service or law enforcement agencies. Asking the question, "Are you safe at home?" may establish whether the reason for a sleep problem is from a dangerous situation (that may not benefit from "alternatives") or is from other causes.

Comfort and relief of pain are important. A cooler environment is more conducive to sleep than is a very warm one; bedclothes should be soft and nonrestrictive, and pain should be controlled with whatever measures are needed.

Discontinuing daytime naps or taking only short "power naps" may increase sleep at night. Also, the establishment of a nighttime ritual is important. This ritual might include things such as teeth brushing and other hygiene practices, as well as reading a devotional book or newspaper, saying a prayer, or any activity that can become a routine forerunner to sleeping.

Deep breathing, as another helpful sleep technique, helps the sleeper take the focus off "mind chatter" and come to deeper relaxation. Therapeutic breathing has several processes and techniques. The deep breathing instruction in Table 2-2 can be used to teach a simple slow, deep-breathing technique. Breathing processes are an important part of traditional health care practices. For example, practitioners of Ayurveda and yoga refer to the breath as Pranayama, meaning life force control; and breath work is a focus of meditative practices (Jones, 1998; Kornfield, 1996; Sharma, Clark, 2000).

Listening to music or imagery tapes may help some individuals fall asleep, as may praying or meditation (Naparstek, 2000; Miller, 1981). Also, research with progressive relaxation has shown improved sleep parameters (Johnson, 1991). Either passive or active relaxation strategies can be used.

A "worry list" at the bedside can help patients put their worries and thoughts to rest for the evening. Keeping pen and paper at the bedside, patients can jot down thoughts after getting into bed; this helps keep busy thoughts at bay. With their "stuff" written down, persons need not worry about forgetting what they have to do the next day. HCPs can tell patients to put their anxieties on the list also. The thoughts and anxieties will be there in the morning so the patient need not think about them during the night.

Table 2-2	Mind-Body-Spirit Interventions for Sleep			
Intervention	Management	Treatment Regimen	Cautions, Precautions, Interactions	References
Deep breathing	To help fall asleep or to fall back to sleep	Ten deep, very slow breaths (a deep breath is a breath that makes the abdomen move out when inhaling [i.e., taking "belly breaths"]); one slow breath is taken in for a count of five, held for a count of five, and let out for a count of five; patient should be aware of time between breath out and next breath in. Individual may fall asleep before	Hyperventilation may occur; important to take slow breaths. May be difficult for individuals with COPD	

		taking in 10 total breaths, or individual may have to take additional breaths before sleeping		
Exercise	Promotes healthy sleep Helps restless legs Helps relieve nocturnal leg cramps	For insomnia, exercise or walk during the day, 20-30 minutes most days of the week For leg cramps, stretch throughout the day, and exercise a few minutes before bedtime	Must be performed at least 2 hours before sleep if used to help relieve insomnia	www.ninds.nih.gov, 2002
Imagery	Promotes healthful sleep	Imagery tapes prerecorded or can make individual tape	No driving or operating equipment while listening to tapes	Emmett Miller, *Healing Journey* and *Easing Into Sleep* (1-800-52 TAPES) Naparstek, 2000 *Healthful Sleep* www.healthjourneys.com

Continued

Table 2-2 Mind-Body-Spirit Interventions for Sleep—cont'd

Intervention	Management	Treatment Regimen	Cautions, Precautions, Interactions	References
Meditation	Promotes healthful sleep Relieves insomnia	Mindfulness or transcendental meditation	No precautions or interactions	Kornfield, 1996
Prayer	Promotes healthful sleep Relieves insomnia	Inspirational reading or prayers of choice	Respect patient preference	
Relaxation	Promotes healthful sleep Relieves insomnia	Relaxation tapes, progressive relaxation	No driving or operating equipment while listening to tapes	Johnson, 1991
Sleep restriction therapy (decrease amount of time in bed)	Insomnia	If in bed 8 hours per night and only sleeping 5 hours per night, time in bed is decreased to 5 hours per night; to accomplish this, bedtime is altered, and rising time is kept constant	No precautions or interactions	National Heart Lung Blood Institute, American Academy of Sleep Medicine, 1998

		to maintain regular sleep-wake rhythm	
Worry list (putting worries aside for the night)	Insomnia	Bed time is decreased 15-30 minutes per night as sleep efficiency increases	No precautions or interactions
		Minimum amount of time in bed is 5 hours per night	
		Write down worries are recorded, and list is kept at bedside	
		Pen is handy to add to if individual has another worry	
		Some individuals, instead, throw their worries in the wastebasket	

COPD, *Chronic obstructive pulmonary disease.*

Exercise may have beneficial effects on sleep. However, the exercise needs to be completed at least 2 hours before retiring because the stimulation of exercise may "wake" persons up. Individuals who are bed- or wheelchair-bound can also participate in exercises such as range of motion of the joints, lifting soup cans or light weights, or stretching. Moderate exercises can be active or passive. Exercise and stretching the legs may also assist in decreasing restless leg syndrome or in nocturnal leg cramps.

On the other hand, keeping active stimulus away from the bedside may help promote sleep; work projects should be kept away from the nighttime routine. In addition, it is best to have no activities in bed other than sleep, intimacy, and "sleepy time" reading.

BIOLOGIC-BASED THERAPIES FOR SLEEP

Foods

Caffeine interferes with sleep. Even a small amount of caffeine, 200 mg in the morning, affects human sleep and should therefore be discontinued in persons with sleep disturbances (Landolt et al., 1995). Caffeine is an adenosine-receptor antagonist, and adenosine appears to be involved in the regulation of sleep. Thus avoiding caffeine is recommended for improved sleep.

A small snack may also be needed; although with some conditions (e.g., gastroesophageal reflux), food may need to be eaten a few hours before bedtime. A snack may be helpful to overcome any nighttime hypoglycemic problem and to help with sleep regulation substances. Especially good are snacks that contain tryptophan, an essential amino acid, and a precursor of serotonin (Peightel et al., 1999). Popular foods with tryptophan include milk and turkey. Box 2-2 describes some nutritional and substance hints for sleep.

Dietary Supplements

Nutrients, vitamins, and minerals L-tryptophan, 5-hydroxytryptophan (5-HTP), vitamin B6, niacin, and magnesium may be helpful for sleep (LaValle, 2000; Pizzorno et al., 2002; PL/PL, 2002). Serotonin is thought to be the initiator of sleep; tryptophan is a precursor of serotonin. Vitamin B6, niacin, and magnesium are conversion cofactors for tryptophan to serotonin; thus these supplements should be taken with the tryptophan (Murray, Pizzorno, 1999). 5-HTP is:

> one step closer to serotonin than L-tryptophan; not dependent on transport system for entry into brain; produces dramatically better results than L-tryptophan in promoting and maintaining sleep; increases REM sleep (by 25%) and increases deep sleep stages 3 and 4 without increasing total sleep time (Pizzorno et al., 2002, p. 280).

Thus the precursors of serotonin may be important in promoting sleep. Supplemental L-tryptophan is off the market in the United

Box 2-2

Nutritional-Substance Hints for Sleep

Eat evening small snack—glass of milk, turkey sandwich (tryptophan).
Avoid nicotine and alcohol.
Have pharmacist check medications for sleep effect or interference.
Melatonin may help patients wean from benzodiazepines.
Discontinue caffeine (at least temporarily); even a small amount of caffeine, (e.g., 200 mg in the morning) affects human sleep (Landolt et al, 1995).

6-Ounce Cup	*Caffeine Content*
Brewed coffee	80-140 mg
Instant coffee	60-100 mg
Decaffeinated coffee	1-6 mg
Black leaf tea	30-80 mg
Tea bag	25-75 mg
12-oz cola	30-65 mg

States because of contamination resulting in cases of *Eosinophilia myalgia*. However, tryptophan may be obtained from food.

Coenzyme Q10 has been recommended for the sleep problems that accompany heart failure. "Some of these patients have insomnia related to nocturnal dyspnea. Adjunctive use of coenzyme Q10 can decrease dyspnea and other symptoms and can help improve sleep" (PL/PL, 2000, p. 17; PL/PL, 2002). In addition, vitamin E is a suggestion for nocturnal leg cramps (Pizzorno et al., 2002), and iron, folate, and magnesium may help restless leg syndrome (NINDS. NIH.gov, 2002).

Herbs   Common herbals for sleep include German chamomile tea, used only if the patient is not allergic to the ragweed, chrysanthemum, daisy, or marigold family (Hoffmann, 1996; PL/PL, 2000, 2002). Valerian, which has a "dirty socks" smell, is also popular and the most researched herb for sleep (Blumenthal, 1998; PL/PL, 2002). Herbs that have little research but are known for their sedative properties include hops, lemon balm, lavender, and skullcap (Blumenthal, 1998, PL/PL, 2000). Hops along with other sedative herbs can be placed in a small pillow; this small pillow, in turn, is placed under the sleeper's regular pillow (McIntyre, 1994). Box 2-3 describes how to make a sleep pillow. Passionflower is approved in

Germany to treat nervousness and is found in sedative-hypnotic mixtures in other European countries (Fetrow, Avila, 1999).

Kava kava has been used for sleep (LaValle et al., 2000; PL/PL, 2000, 2002). Kava is an antianxiety herb and is meant for persons with anxiety who cannot sleep. Kava should not be used habitually and has been implicated in liver toxicity (PL/PL, 2000, 2002). Certain types of kava are off the market in some locations (www. herbalgram.org, accessed 5/12/2002). Kava has abuse potential, and quality guidelines for its use need to be followed.

Aromatherapy

Buckle (2001) recommends lavender and rose as aromatherapy sleep preparations. These essential oils can be placed on a tissue and inhaled, dispersed in the bath water, diluted in a carrier oil and used for massage, or placed in a diffuser or sleep pillow. Using pure, steam-distilled essential oils is important to reach the best effect. Oils can be expensive, and allergic reactions could be a problem in sensitive individuals.

Melatonin

Another sleep aid is melatonin, a hormone that comes from the pineal gland. The body synthesizes melatonin from tryptophan and serotonin (Lieberman, Bruning, 1997; PL/PH, 2002). Human melatonin levels rise in the evening. Melatonin supplementation only helps promote sleep if there are low levels of the substance in the

---

Box 2-3

Herb Sleep Pillow

Herb pillows are generally smaller than are regular bed pillows and are tucked under or laid along side the regular pillow. Plain cotton material, such as that used for regular pillow slips, encloses the dried herbs. The cotton pillow is covered with an attractive washable cover. An example of an herb sleep pillow follows. Dried herbs are mixed in the proportions shown.

1 cup lavender flowers
1 cup rose petals
1 cup hops
1 cup linden blossom
1 cup lemon balm
2 teaspoons orris root powder
3 drops oil of bergamot

McIntyre, 1994, p. 271.

body (Murray, Pizzorno, 1999; Pizzorno et al., 2002). A salivary test can be used to determine melatonin levels over a 24-hour period. Therefore, deficiencies in melatonin levels can be determined prior to use (Great Smokies Diagnostic Laboratory, 2001). Melatonin has a role in regulating:

> ...the body's circadian rhythm, endocrine secretions, and sleep patterns. Melatonin production is influenced by day/night cycles. Light inhibits melatonin secretion and darkness stimulates secretion (PL/PL, 2002, p. 877).

Melatonin may be a good substance for older adults who tend to have low levels of melatonin (Murray, Pizzorno, 1999; Eliopolous, 1999). Garfinkel and colleagues (1995) report that 2 mg per night for 3 weeks improved sleep when compared with placebo. Doses of 0.5 to 5 mg have been suggested for sleep (PL/PL, 2002).

In another study by Garfinkel and colleagues (1999), investigators used 2 mg of melatonin nightly for 6 weeks to help wean subjects (n = 34) off benzodiazepines. In the double-blind trial, 14 of the 18 melatonin subjects (78%) succeeded, whereas only 4 of the 16 controls (25%) succeeded. In addition, subjective sleep quality improved in the melatonin group. After this trial, investigators did a single-blind study giving all subjects melatonin for another 6 weeks; six additional subjects from the previous placebo group discontinued benzodiazepine use. Six months later, 79% of the 24 subjects who had discontinued benzodiazepine use were still off; they were continuing with the melatonin, and sleep quality scores were better than prestudy baseline. Not everyone agrees with the use of melatonin, however, because there are no long-term follow-up studies of its use (Butler, 1996). Table 2-3 outlines biologic-based therapies for sleep.

MANIPULATIVE AND BODY-BASED METHODS FOR SLEEP

Everything possible should be done to relieve pain before sleep. Measures may include warm packs, a warm bath or shower, massage, healing touch, rubs or liniments, or pain medication. Massage or a simple back rub may provide relaxation, help relieve pain, increase circulation, and produce sleep, including in critically ill patients (Bauer, Dracup, 1987; Buckle, 2000; Field et al., 1996; Richards, 1998). Various types of massage can be used from the simple gentle Swedish techniques to Shiatsu or reflexology. Table 2-4 provides an overview of body-based management.

ENERGY THERAPIES FOR SLEEP

Light, Sound, and Temperature

The appropriate light, sound, and temperature are imperative for good sleep. "Sleeping in too high a temperature (greater than 75° F) reduces quality of sleep because both slow wave and REM sleep are

Table 2-3 Biologic-Based Therapies for Sleep

Dosing varies with vitamins, minerals, amino acids, herbs, etc. depending on the type of preparation. A full-prescribing source should be consulted before using any herbs. Herbs can cause allergic reactions. Sedative herbs can cause drowsiness; thus no driving or operating machinery is recommended when taking herbs. Herbs should not be prescribed to children or to pregnant or lactating women unless an expert herbal source advises of their safety.

Intervention	Management	Treatment Regimen	Cautions, Precautions, Interactions	References
Nutrients				
Vitamin B3 (niacin)	Assists with sleep; provides conversion factor for tryptophan to serotonin	100 mg (or less if flushing occurs) Taken 45 min before bedtime Recommended UL: 35 mg/day	Doses as low as 30 mg associated with flushing Large doses have numerous side effects (e.g., hepatotoxicity) Recommended dose: higher than UL	Pizzorno et al., 2002; PL/PL, 2002; www.NAP.edu, 2002
Vitamin B6 (pyridoxine)	Assists with sleep; provides conversion factor for	25 mg bid Recommended UL: 100 mg/day	Can decrease folic acid concentrations and may interact with phenytoin,	LaValle et al, 2000 Murray, Pizzorno, 1999 Pizzorno et al, 2002

	tryptophan to serotonin		amiodarone, levodopa	
Folic acid	Helps relieve restless leg syndrome	Folic acid 5-10 mg qd; Recommended UL: 1000 μg/day	Recommended dose: higher than UL	Pizzorno et al, 2002
Vitamin E	Helps relieve nocturnal myoclonus, nighttime muscle cramps	400-800 IU qd Recommended UL: 1000 mg/day	Note: Vitamin E recommendations are IU or mg doses	Pizzorno et al, 2002; www.NAP.edu, 2002
Iron	Helps relieve restless leg syndrome	30 mg iron succinate or fumarate tid with meals (if serum ferritin is below 35 μg) Recommended UL: 45 mg/day	Rule out hemochromatosis or other iron overload before initiating iron therapy. Recommended dose is higher than UL.	Pizzorno et al, 2002; www.NAP.edu, 2002
Magnesium	Helps relieve insomnia, nocturnal myoclonus, muscle cramps at night; provides conversion	250-600 mg/day 250 mg at bedtime for nocturnal myoclonus Recommended	May cause diarrhea Use caution or do not use with renal impairment, or heart block	LaValle et al, 2000 Murray, Pizzorno, 1999 Pizzorno et al, 2002; www.NAP.edu, 2002

Continued

Table 2-3 Biologic-Based Therapies for Sleep—cont'd

Intervention	Management	Treatment Regimen	Cautions, Precautions, Interactions	References
Nutrients—cont'd				
Magnesium, cont'd	factor for tryptophan to serotonin	UL: 350 mg/day		
Coenzyme Q10	Is likely effective for insomnia related to CHF; decreases dyspnea and other Sx of CHF	100 mg/day divided into 2-3 doses	May interact with BP medications, chemotherapy, insulin, warfarin	PL/PL, 2002
L-tryptophan	Assists with sleep process	L-tryptophan foods before bedtime (e.g., turkey, milk) No supplement on market Obtain from food Clinical studies used 1.0-2.5 g	Contraindicated for those with eosinophilia Can interact with SSRIs and other sedative products (e.g., benzodiazepines) Taken off U.S. market because of contaminated	PL/PL, 2002

5-HTP	Assists with sleep	100-300 mg 30-45 min before sleep Start with lower dose and increase	supply and 1990 FDA recall Do not use with SSRIs	Pizzorno et al, 2002 PL/PL 2002
Herbs German chamomile *Matricaria recututa*	Provides sedative properties	Tea, capsules, liquid	*Caution:* Ragweed-daisy allergy may result because chamomile is in same family No driving or operating machinery after use	Fetrow, Avila 1999 Hoffmann, 1996 PL/PL, 2000
Hops *Humulus lupulos*	Provides sedative properties	Tea Sleep pillow Often used in combination with other herbs	No driving or operating machinery after use Not to be used by those with depression Anecdotal reports are available	Blumenthal, 1998 Fetrow, Avila, 1999 PL/PL, 2000

Continued

Table 2-3 Biologic-Based Therapies for Sleep—cont'd

Intervention	Management	Treatment Regimen	Cautions, Precautions, Interactions	References
Nutrients—cont'd				
Hops, cont'd			Not to be used habitually	
Kava kava *Piper methysticum*	Is possibly effective for anxiety, which can contribute to insomnia Is not effective for insomnia alone Not thought to affect benzodiazepine or GABA receptors; may affect limbic system	Kava extract standardized to 70% kava lactones Reports of severe liver toxicity	Contraindicated for those with endogenous depression or Parkinson's disease *Interactions:* ETOH, CNS depressants Not to be used habitually; has habituation-abuse potential Has possible liver toxicity Driving or operating machinery is not advisable after use	LaValle et al, 2000 PL/PL, 2000, 2002

Continued

Lemon balm Melissa officinalis	Has sedative properties Is used for tenseness and restlessness	Infusion and extract or part of sleep pillow	Also used to treat functional GI complaints and herpes cold sores Driving or operating machinery is not advisable after use	Blumenthal, 2000, 1998 LaValle, 2000
Passionflower Passiflora incarnata	Has sedative properties	Tea (dried herb), fluid extract, dry powder extract, tincture	May potentiate MAOIs; additive effects with CNS depressants, and anticoagulants Driving or operating machinery is not advisable after use When using with tryptophan or 5-HTP, additive effects may occur	Fetrow, Avila, 1999 LaValle et al, 2000 Pizzorno et al, 2002 PL/PL, 2000 PL/PL, 2002
Valerian Valeriana officinalis	Decreases sleep latency (time to sleep onset) and improving quality of sleep Relieves insomnia; increases GABA	Tea (dried root), tincture, fluid extract, dry powder extract	Has "dirty socks" smell SE: Headache, excitability, uneasiness, cardiac disturbances, impaired alertness	Blumenthal, 1998 LaValle et al, 2000 PL/PL, 2002

Table 2-3	Biologic-Based Therapies for Sleep—cont'd			
Intervention	Management	Treatment Regimen	Cautions, Precautions, Interactions	References
Nutrients—cont'd				
Valerian, cont'd	activity (i.e., has benzodiazepine-like effects)		Can show withdrawal after extended use Driving or operating machinery is not advisable after use Can potentiate effects of alcohol, barbiturates, and benzodiazepines (human trials have been conducted)	
Aromatherapy Lavender *Lavandula augustifolia*	Relieves insomnia; calms nervous tension	Topical in carrier as a massage or inhalation (e.g., lavender bath or few drops on tissue) 5-minute hand massage before	Has been used in traditional medicine for centuries Must be pure essential oils Must be diluted for topical use	Buckle, 2001 Fetrow, Avila, 1999

Rose *Rosa damascena*	Has sedative, antidepressant, antispasmodic effects	bed using 1% lavender Cotton ball with two drops under pillow Dried herb as part of sleep pillow Two drops on facial tissue inhaled four times/day	Need to find an agreeable scent Use rose otto (i.e., steam distilled), not rose absolute (i.e., extracted with petrochemicals)	Buckle, 2001
Hormone Melatonin (produced by pineal gland; *not* an herb)	Promotes sleep; helps relieve jet lag Has also been prescribed for patients with cancers	For sleep: dose range is 0.3-3.0 mg hs For jet lag: 5 mg hs beginning 3 days before travel and ending 3 days after travel	Driving or operating machinery is not advisable for 5 hours after taking melatonin No long-term human studies have been conducted *SE:* Sedation or drowsiness; headache, depressive Sx,	Fetrow, Avila, 1999 LaValle, 2000 PL/PL, 2002

Continued

| Table 2-3 | Biologic-Based Therapies for Sleep—cont'd |

Intervention	Management	Treatment Regimen	Cautions, Precautions, Interactions	References
Nutrients—cont'd				
Hormone Melatonin, cont'd			dizziness, cramps, irritability *Interactions:* Can worsen depression; increases seizure activity; is metabolized by liver Melatonin decreases effectiveness of nifedipine; increases heart rate and blood pressure	

bid, *Two times daily;* CHF, *congestive heart failure;* CNS, *central nervous system;* ETOH, *ethyl alcohol;* FDA, *U.S. Food and Drug Administration;* GABA, *γ-aminobutyric acid;* GI, *gastrointestinal;* HA, *headache;* hs, *at bedtime;* IU, *international units;* MAOIs, *monoamine oxidase inhibitors;* PL/PL, *Pharmacist's Letter/Prescriber's Letter;* qd, *every day;* SE, *side effects;* SSRIs, *selective serotonin reuptake inhibitors;* Sx, *symptoms;* tid, *three times daily;* UL, *tolerable upper limit (the maximum level of daily nutrient intake that is likely to pose no risk of adverse effects; usually represents total intake from food, water, and supplements)*

Table 2-4   Manipulative and Body-Based Methods for Sleep

Intervention	Management	Treatment Regimen	Cautions, Precautions, Interactions	References
Massage	Promotes relaxation, decreases pain, helps produce or increase sleep time	Gentle massage including effleurage, pétrissage, friction, vibration, range-of-motion exercises	Requires a provider Some do not like to be touched Foot or head massage may work for those who do not want or are not able to have back massaged	Bauer et al., 1987 Field, 2000 Field et al, 1996 Sunshine, 1996 Richards, 1998
"M" technique	Use with critically and terminally ill patients	Specific set of massage maneuvers for face, hands, feet Combined with aromatherapy	Training available	Buckle, 2000
Reflex Zone Therapy (reflexology)	Promotes relaxation and sedation	*Relaxation and sedation:* (1) Both extended palms are held against	Provider needed	Lett, 2000

Continued

Table 2-4 Manipulative and Body-Based Methods for Sleep—cont'd

Intervention	Management	Treatment Regimen	Cautions, Precautions, Interactions	References
Reflex Zone Therapy (reflexology), cont'd		the soles of feet; (2) Cupped palms are held over metatarsal phalangeal joint, one on top of foot with thumb under; (3) Palms held over medial heels; (4) One thumb is held over solar plexus zone on sole of foot (below 2nd and 3rd toes about 1-2 in and above arch of foot)		
Shiatsu (finger pressure therapy)	Promotes healthful sleep	Neck, back, thorax points	Points are close to carotid arteries; (so caution needed) skilled practitioner is needed Anecdotal reports available	Namikoshi, 1995

reduced. Cold temperatures produce frequent arousals and poor sleep and reportedly induces unpleasant and emotional aspects of dreams (Gordon, 1986, p. 141). Thus "coolness" is preferable for sleep. The optimal temperature has been calculated to be 68° F (Gordon, 1986). In addition, a quiet setting works best but if noise is a problem, ear plugs, "white noise," or music may help wash out background noise. Also, darkness at night and light exposure during the day is helpful for nighttime sleep.

Guilleminault and colleagues (1995) studied the use of different sleep hygiene strategies with 30 subjects who complained of less than 6 hours of sleep a night for at least 6-month's duration. The interventions were: (1) sleep strategies; (2) sleep strategies in addition to late afternoon exercise; (3) sleep strategies with early morning light therapy consisting of morning light therapy with 300 lux using a light box. The light was at 30 inches and exposure was for 45 minutes. All subjects showed a trend toward improvement, independent of the treatment received, but only the "structured sleep hygiene with light treatment" showed statistically significant improvement at the end of the trial (Guilleminault et al., 1995). Thus morning light therapy, in the form of sunshine or light boxes, may be helpful for improving sleep.

Healing Touch and Therapeutic Touch

Because healing touch (HT) and therapeutic touch (TT) may help relieve anxiety and reduce pain, these energy interventions may be helpful in sleep. The technique can be taught to household members or caretakers. Texts and classes are available (Krieger, 1993; Macrae, 1987). Table 2-5 describes energy therapies for restful sleep.

NAC THERAPIES FOR WELL BEING AND ANXIETY CONTROL

Self-awareness and stress management, or the ability to cope and react to the events of life, include various activities and processes that help a person find well being or a peaceful, productive, and sustainable life, in other words, ways of finding contentedness and happiness, an awareness of strengths, and deeper meaning in life. Some degree of stress is inevitable; however, finding ways to cope effectively, and finding purpose and meaning, are key aspects to overcoming the challenges of life.

Some patients have increased anxiety to the point that they are diagnosed with an anxiety disorder. Anxiety causes distress for patients and their families, interferes with the ability to focus, increases the perception of pain following surgery, and, in severe anxiety, patients exhibit a variety of physiologic changes. In anxiety, dysregulation of the hypothalamic-pituitary-adrenal (HPA) axis manifests as elevations in serum cortisol or in thyroid-stimulating hormone (also commonly seen in individuals with depression).

Table 2-5	Energy Therapies for Sleep			
Intervention	Management	Treatment Regimen	Cautions, Precautions, Interactions	References
Light therapy	Helps relieve insomnia	Exposure to morning sunshine Morning light therapy with 300-lux light box Light is distanced 30 in from individual and timed for 45 min	May cause eyestrain	Guilleminault et al, 1995
Appropriate temperature	Relieves insomnia	Temperature below 75° F probably best	Must not be too cold	Gordon, 1986 Hauri, 1982
Quiet	Relieves insomnia, promotes restful sleep	Use earplugs, move bedroom, use white noise	Earplugs or headphones may be dangerous (i.e., individual cannot hear smoke detectors, emergency signals)	
Therapeutic Touch	Promotes relaxation; decreases anxiety, pain	15-20 min session after individual is ready for bed	Needs trained practitioner and permission from participant	Braun et al, 1986

Treatment for anxiety disorders includes pharmacologic therapies, as well as modalities such as relaxation and cognitive approaches that assist the individual to modulate the activity of the autonomic nervous system. HCPs often find it difficult to work with anxious patients, believing that little can be offered other than pharmaceutical relief. However, if the HCP is able to convey a sense of calm presence and remain with the patient while offering simple interventions, there may be less need for antianxiety medications, and patients may regain a sense of control.

For some people, stress management and anxiety control interventions include prayer, meditation, or other spiritual outlets; for some, exercise, dance, or relaxation therapies, massage, or energy work such as HT or TT are effective; and for some, nature is the answer. Hobbies, pets, social support, and social activities are also important components. The HCP can provide a list of such modalities to patients so they may choose the options that are most appealing. Many of these processes are the "natural" part of NAC health care practices:

> There have been moments in your life when you were pure awareness. No concepts, no thoughts like "I am aware" or "That is a tree" or "Now I am meditating." Just pure awareness. Openness. A spacious quality in your existence. Perhaps it happened as you sat on a river bank and the sound of the river flowed through you. Or as you walked on the beach when the sound of the ocean washed away your thinking mind until all that remained was the walking, the feeling of your feet on the sand, the sound of the surf, the warmth of the sun on your head and shoulders, the breeze on your cheek, the sound of the seagull in the distance. For that moment your image of yourself was lost in the gestalt, in the totality of the moment. You were not clinging to anything. You were not holding on to the experience. It was flowing—through you, around you, by you, in you. At that moment you were the experience. You were the flow. There was no demarcation between you-sun-ocean-sand. You had transcended the separation that thought creates. You were the moment in all its fullness. Everyone has had such experiences. These moments are ones in which we have "lost ourselves," or been "taken out of ourselves," or "forgotten ourselves." They are moments in flow. It is in these moments of your life that there is no longer separation. There is peace, harmony, tranquility, the joy of being part of the process. In these moments the universe appears fresh; it is seen through innocent eyes. It all begins anew. (Ram Dass, 1978, pp. 1-2)

A holistic view of stress management and self awareness processes acknowledges life's mystery and embraces these transcendent moments leading to well being. Several of these processes are described here in the context of NAC categories.

ALTERNATIVE HEALTH CARE SYSTEMS FOR GENERAL WELL BEING AND ANXIETY CONTROL

Stress management and self-awareness cross cultures, socioeconomic status, and health care systems. For example, Roth and Creaser used mindfulness meditation with a bilingual (English- and Spanish-speaking) inner-city population. This study showed significant improvement in physical and psychologic health and self-esteem of the participants. Alternative health care systems have numerous therapies to enhance well being and help reduce stress. Given here are a few examples of anxiety relief and promotion of well being from the alternative health care system perspective.

Ayurveda

Ayurveda uses Pranayama, panchakarma treatments, meditation, and yoga, as well as diet and lifestyle modifications for well being and anxiety relief. *Pranayama* refers to regulating the breath and is done through specific exercises, including alternate nostril breathing. Pranayama is said to settle, balance, and refresh the whole body.

Panchakarma, meaning five actions, refers to several types of treatments. Treatments vary in length from 3 to 30 days. The purpose is to dislodge impurities from cells and flush the body. These therapies include forms of diet, purging, massage, heat, and elimination (Sharma, Clark, 2000).

In a metaanalysis, transcendental meditation (TM) has been effective for reducing stress (Eppley, 1989). During TM, the autonomic nervous system stabilizes, and the rate of respiration decreases. In addition, plasma lactate, a marker of metabolic activity, is decreased (Sharma, Clark, 2000).

Yoga and exercises are also important for stress relief. The sun salute *(Suryanamaskar)* integrates body, mind, and breath and strengthens muscles. There are 12 positions included in the sun salute yoga exercise (Sharma, Clark, 2000; Jones, 1998).

From the Ayurvedic perspective, anxiety is caused primarily by aggravation of vata dosha in the nervous system, which results in agitation of *prana* (the life force) and feelings of anxiety and fear and insomnia. Relief of anxiety thus involves balancing vata dosha with a vata-pacifying diet, calming herbal teas (valerian and musta), soaking in a warm bath with ginger and baking soda added to the water, warm almond milk, orange juice with 1 teaspoon of honey and pinch of nutmeg (to slow the heart rate), and acupressure to the middle of the palm, yoga (relaxation or corpse pose), and SoHum meditation while focusing attention to the top of the head (Lad, 1998).

Ayurvedic remedies may be sufficient to treat everyday worries and anxieties that are a normal part of life. However, if anxiety symptoms are severe and continuous and significantly interfere with social or work functioning, or if panic attacks occur, the individual should seek medical attention (Lad, 1998).

Traditional Chinese Medicine

Traditional Chinese Medicine (TCM) uses Tai Chi, Qi Gong (Novey, 2000; Ryu, 1996), Tuina, acupuncture, acupressure, herbs, and Feng Shui as forms of therapy. The way of viewing anxiety is quite different than that of a Western perspective.

Rather than the brain being the center of the mind as in Western thought, in TCM, each of the five internal Yin organs houses an aspect of the "soul" and has a corresponding mental faculty and emotion. Table 2-6 gives an overview of the Yin organs and describes the corresponding soul aspect, mental faculty, and emotion. This entire matrix is called the *Shen* and is considered to be a basic substance just as is Qi (live energy), Blood, and the body fluids. Anxiety is a symptom of Shen disturbance. In anxiety, the spirit does not feel settled and comfortable. The cause can be deficiency of Blood or Yin or the presence of a pathogenic factor influencing the spirit.

Mind and body are unified in TCM so that any emotional disturbance affects the physical state, and the physical condition in turn affects the emotions. If the Qi, Yin, and Blood are in harmony and the organs are functioning well, the positive aspects of the emotional correspondences will be active. For instance, when the Liver energy is functioning well, the demeanor will be alert, spontaneous, and relaxed, instead of anger. Anger will burst out when the energy feels restrained or stagnant. Physical symptoms of stagnant Qi include a feeling of a lump in the throat, tightness in the chest, and abdominal distention, along with the anger or irritability on a mental-emotional level (Maciocia, 1994).

Although each of the emotions corresponds to a particular organ, the Heart is involved in the mental and emotional balance of the entire system. The Heart is called the "emperor" of the organs, meaning that it is responsible for organizing and recognizing the functions of the other organs, particularly relating to the mind functions. When discussing anxiety, another very important concept exists in TCM. It is said that the Blood provides the material foundation for the mind and spirit. The Blood, as a Yin substance, anchors the mind, which is Yang in nature. The Yin or water component of the body is necessary to balance the Yang component in every respect. The Blood also has a special relationship to the Heart and Liver because the Heart circulates the Blood and the Liver stores the Blood. Box 2-4 gives examples of patterns of imbalance that manifest as anxiety. The treatment strategy for anxiety includes nourishing and supporting the Heart, calming the mind, and clearing pathogens. Treatment includes acupuncture, moxibustion, and herbs.

Table 2-6	Yin Organs and Respective Aspects of the Soul		
Organ	**Soul Aspect**	**Mental Faculty**	**Emotion**
Heart	Houses the mind (includes mental activity, memory, consciousness, thinking, sleep)	Overall consciousness, mental and emotional balance	Joy (excessive)
Liver	Ethereal soul (enters at birth; survives death)	Intuition, inspiration	Anger
Lung	Corporeal soul (allows sensation, hearing, feeling, sight; dies with body)	Meditation, inner calm	Sadness, grief
Spleen	Houses intellect (affects concentration, study)	Short-term memory, study	Worry
Kidney	Will power (includes mental drive and determination)	Long-term memory	Fear

(Maciocia, 1989; Maciocia, 1994)

Using the State-Trait Anxiety Inventory (STAI), a recent small blinded, randomized trial using auricular acupuncture showed a decline in anxiety. Three groups received auricular acupuncture using press tacks: group 1 (n = 22) received acupuncture at Shenmen ear point; group 2 (n = 15) received acupuncture at the relaxation ear point; group 3 (n = 18) received sham acupuncture. (See Appendix B for point locations.) Anxiety levels were taken just before treatment, at 30 minutes, 24 hours, and 48 hours using STAI. There was also a "Life Experiences" survey; and, in addition, arterial blood pressure, heart rate, and electrodermal activity were measured. Group 2 showed significantly less anxiety at 30 minutes and 24 hours compared with the other two groups as shown on the STAI rating. There were no significant changes in other parameters (Wang, Kain, 2001). Table 2-7 presents an overview of TCM anxiety treatment strategies, as well as other alternative health care system approaches.

Box 2-4

Examples of Patterns of Imbalance that Manifest as Anxiety

1. Heart Blood deficiency (often combined with other patterns):
   Symptoms:
   Pallor
   Dull eyes and complexion
   Mild anxiety
   Timidity or fearfulness
   Poor memory and concentration
   Palpitations
   Dizziness (Maciocia, 1994)

2. Stagnant Blood affecting the Heart, Liver, or both:
   Symptoms:
   Severe anxiety
   Feeling of oppression in the throat and chest
   Insomnia, often nightmares
   Restlessness, irritability
   Mood swings
   Palpitations
   If severe, this pattern can lead to psychosis or manic-depression (Maciocia, 1994).

3. Phlegm-fire obstructing the mind:
   Symptoms:
   Mental confusion
   Poor memory and concentration
   Feeling of heaviness of head and body
   Irritability, quick temper
   Poor appetite, nausea
   Obsessive behavior
   Dizziness
   Anxiety, restlessness (Hammer, 1990; Maciocia, 1994)

4. Kidney-heart Yin deficiency with heat:
   Symptoms:
   Insomnia
   Tinnitus
   Night sweats
   Anxiety, mental restlessness
   Backache
   Lack of will power (Hammer, 1990; Maciocia, 1994)

5. Liver Qi stagnation:
   Symptoms:
   Tightness in chest or ribs
   Irritability, moodiness
   Sighing, belching
   Mental confusion, anxiety
   Fatigue
   Premenstrual tension
   Abdominal distention (Maciocia, 1994)

Homeopathy

Homeopathic remedies are available for grief, anticipatory anxiety, business failure and financial loss, fears from a frightening event, insults, wounded honor, shame, embarrassment, ailments from bad news, emotional excitement, and mental exertion (Boericke, 2000; Skinner, 2001). As with all homeopathic treatment, a practitioner who is trained in homeopathy should evaluate and make a diagnosis based on a holistic case history. Remedies may be self prescribed for treatment of mild anxiety, but they are not a substitute for professional care in cases of severe or prolonged anxiety. The homeopathic approach is holistic, considering lifestyle factors such as diet, exercise, stress, environment, personality, temperament, and fears. The homeopathic practitioner may recommend lifestyle changes in addition to the remedies (Lockie, Geddes, 1995).

Lockie and Geddes (1995) recommend four homeopathic remedies for relief of anxiety. *Lycopodium* is recommended for anxiety associated with a lack of confidence and accompanied by insomnia, appetite disturbance, and cravings for sweets. For anxiety resulting from deep insecurity and accompanied by symptoms of rapid pulse, clammy skin, fatigue, and chills, the authors recommend *Arsenicum album*. Anxiety that is related to overwork and accompanied by symptoms of edginess, generalized fear, and desire for attention responds to *Phosphorus*. Anxiety that presents with symptoms of forgetfulness, obsession with work accompanied by fear of failure, and a preoccupation with physical ailments is treated with *Calcium carbonate*. These four remedies are among the key homeopathic remedies used most.

MIND-BODY-SPIRIT INTERVENTIONS FOR WELL BEING AND ANXIETY CONTROL

Expressive and Creative Arts

The arts can open new dimensions to persons caught up in unpleasantries, allowing freedom and creativity when other forms of therapy may not be working. The arts include activities such as sculpting, painting, writing a novel, acting, dancing, or playing a musical instrument, or the person may find healing more passively through seeing, sensing, watching, reading, or listening. In addition, art, dance, and music therapists use specific sessions geared to doing healing work.

Affirmations

Affirmations refer to strong, personal, positive, present-tense statements. Affirmations state a desire as if it is already happening.

Table 2-7   Alternative Health Care Systems for Well Being and Anxiety Control

Intervention	Management	Treatment Regimen	Cautions, Precautions, Interactions	References
Ayurveda	Promotes general well being; helps manage anxiety	Pranayama *Purification therapies:* Pancha karma, TM *Specific to anxiety:* Need to balance vata dosha (vata pacifying diet); herbal teas (valerian and musta); warm bath with ginger and baking soda added to water; drinking warm almond milk, orange juice with 1 tsp honey and pinch of nutmeg;	Pancha karma therapists are not available in all locations Requires trained yoga instructor Some postures may be difficult or not possible, especially with back disorders Participant should not hold breath if epilepsy or hypertension is present	Sharma, Clark, 2000 Jones, 1998 Lad, 1998

Continued

Table 2-7 Alternative Health Care Systems for Well Being and Anxiety Control—cont'd

Intervention	Management	Treatment Regimen	Cautions, Precautions, Interactions	References
Ayurveda, cont'd		acupressure to middle of palm; yoga for relaxation or corpse pose; So-Hum meditation while focusing attention to the top of head		
TCM; acupuncture	Supports and nourishes *Heart:* UB (14, 15, 44), Ren (14), Heart (7) *To open chest:* Pericardium (6), Ren (17) *To move and nourish Blood and Spleen:* Spleen (6, 10), UB (17, 20), Stomach (36)	1-2 times/wk for initial 4-8 wks of treatment, depending on response Once condition has stabilized, treatment is gradually decreased as needed See Appendix B for point location	Needles over chest and upper back are needled obliquely to avoid puncturing lungs Certain points are avoided if patient is pregnant With the first 2-3 sessions, fewer points may be used (e.g., 6-8	Deadman, 1995 Hammer, 1990 Maciocia, 1994

	To support Kidney: Kidney (3), UB (23), Ren (4) *To move Liver Qi:* UB (18), Liver (3, 14) *To resolve phlegm:* Stomach 25, 40 *To calm mind:* many of the above points, Du (18, 20), Gallbladder (12, 13), Pericardium (7)		needles compared with 12-14) to ensure stability of patients because their Shen is hypersensitive (author's personal note)	
Auricular acupuncture: microacupuncture system on ear can treat many conditions	*To calm anxiety:* relaxation point	One needle is used on each ear with body acupuncture treatment Sterile press tacks may be taped on ear for up to 1 wk	If press tacks are used, patient must be instructed on care and use of tacks and must watch for signs of infection	Wang, Kain, 2001
Moxibustion: a method of burning the mugwort herb over acupuncture	May be used over Ren 4 and UB 15 to support Kidney and Heart Qi	Use as needed. In more deficient or chronic conditions	Not to be used with heat conditions because use may aggravate symptoms	Maciocia, 1995

Continued

Table 2-7 Alternative Health Care Systems for Well Being and Anxiety Control—cont'd

Intervention	Management	Treatment Regimen	Cautions, Precautions, Interactions	References
points to improve Qi and blood supply and circulation		Patient may be taught to treat self at home	Must be used carefully to avoid burning skin	Bensky, Gamble, 1986 Fruehauf, 1995 Maciocia, 1994
Chinese herbal therapy: herbs are combined into a formula for best effect Other herbs are included to treat specific imbalances	*Examples of herbs to treat the Heart and Shen:* Suan Zao Ren (Semen Ziziphi Spinosa)—nourishes heart and calms spirit Yuan Zhi (Radix tenuifoliae)—calms Polygala spirit and clears phlegm Ren Shen (Radix ginseng)—benefits Heart Qi and calms spirit	Dose and length of treatment is dependent on individual If condition is chronic, herbal treatment will be taken for several months to 1-2 yrs	Experienced herbalist should be consulted to ensure accurate diagnosis and treatment Use of an inappropriate formula may exacerbate symptoms	

Long Gu (Os Draconis)—settles spirit and pacifies Liver

Qi Gong (active and passive, breath training)	Decrease stress	Relaxed practice 20 mins/day; best time is 11:00 PM to 1:00 AM or 5:00 AM to 7:00 AM Many exercises from which to pick and choose	Some moves may be difficult in pregnancy	Novey, 2000 Ryu et al, 1996 Kuhn, 1999
Homeopathy	Remedies relieve anxiety specific to signs and symptoms	Holistic assessment with attention to lifestyle, diet, exercise, stress, temperament, fears Symptoms matched to remedy: Lycopodium Arsenicum album Phosphorus Calcium carbonate	If chest pain or difficulty breathing accompanies anxiety, medical attention should be sought Homeopathic remedies should be avoided during pregnancy Remedies are safe for children and	Lockie, Geddes, 1995 Shealy, 1998

Continued

Table 2-7 Alternative Health Care Systems for Well Being and Anxiety Control—cont'd

Intervention	Management	Treatment Regimen	Cautions, Precautions, Interactions	References
Homeopathy, cont'd			older adults when doses are adjusted for age Remedies should not be taken within 30 minutes of eating Alcohol, tobacco, coffee and some essential oils (lavender, camphor, eucalyptus, thyme, peppermint). They may antidote remedies. Remedies should be stored in a cool dark place in a tightly closed container Spoon should be used to place remedy under tongue, avoiding touching with hands	

TCM, *Traditional Chinese Medicine*; TM, *transcendental meditation*; UB, *urinary bladder*.

Affirmations are positive self-talk. Examples include:
"Every day in every way I am better and better."
"I am strong, healthy, and confident."
"I am stress-free." (e.g., anxiety-free, acne-free, pain-free)
"My body is the perfect shape."
"I am prospering."
"I am doing well with my studies."
"I am a very good mother." (e.g., father, worker, nurse, friend)
Thus even though persons are not doing the activity at present, the affirmation is made in a positive present-tense mode as if they are. Note that there are only positive words in affirmations; "nots," "nos," or other negative words are avoided. For example, instead of saying I do *not* have pain (anxiety, fear), the patient says, "I am pain-free" (e.g., anxiety-free, free of fear).

Also to be avoided are words such as "try," "consider," "thinking about," "am going to," or "will." These words make the meaning a tentative or weak statement. Contrast the statements, "I will try to consider thinking about exercising" to "I am exercising three times a week." The theory behind affirmations is that persons are and do what they say they are. This concept is akin to Albert Ellis Rational Emotive Therapy (Ellis, 1975; Davis, 2000):

> Ellis' basic thesis is that emotions have nothing to do with actual events. Between the event and the emotion is realistic or unrealistic self-talk. The self-talk produces the emotions. Your own thoughts, directed and controlled by you, are what create anxiety, anger, and depression. (Davis, 2000, p. 108)

Thoughts can create positive manifestations as well. Between what is desired, or an event, and the outcomes of the desire or event are the cognitions, perceptions, emotions, thoughts, and interpretations of these thoughts and emotions. These interpretations are put forth in affirmative or negative ways. Being positive, or affirmative, is helpful to a productive outcome. To help with learning positive self-talk, Davis and colleagues (2000) include a beliefs inventory and homework sheets for refuting irrational ideas. There is also a rational emotive imagery technique provided and a way of developing alternative emotional responses. Along with learning to refute irrational ideas and to speak affirmatively comes the insight for change.

Take care with affirmations; they are powerful. What is asked for is received. Anecdotes abound on how persons have received what they asked for but not in the form they thought, such as the person who asked for money and received a large insurance check because they lost a limb, or another person who received money (insurance) because they were burglarized. Thus affirm in a way that is for the greatest good.

Thought Stopping

Thought stopping is closely aligned with both affirmation and assertiveness; to be positive, one must stop being negative. Thought stopping refers to the process of ridding the self of unwanted and unnecessary thoughts. Thought stopping involves concentrating on unwanted thoughts and, after a short time, suddenly stopping and ridding the thought from the mind. This process is done with the command "stop" or a loud noise. There are three explanations for the success of thought stopping: (1) the stop command is a punishment, and behavior then tends to be inhibited; (2) "stop" is a distracter; and (3) stopping is an assertive response. The person can then use thought substitutions of reassurance or self-acceptance (Davis et al., 2000). Box 2-5 covers thought-stopping instructions.

Assertiveness

Assertiveness refers to honest, direct, and respectful self-expression. Assertive behavior reflects both the content of a message and how the content is presented. With passive behavior, opinions, feelings, and wants may be withheld, expressed indirectly, or only partially expressed. Conversely, aggressive behavior often may result in a put-down. Thus you are assertive when you stand up for your rights in a way that does not violate another's rights (Alberti, Emmons, 1990; Davis et al, 2000).

Learning assertiveness and practicing the principles are important measures toward attaining less stress in life. Assertiveness training has been found "effective in dealing with depression, anger, resentment, and interpersonal anxiety, especially when these symptoms have been brought about by unfair circumstances" (Davis et al., 2000, p. 202). In addition, assertiveness may be an important factor in maintaining a healthy immune status. Dreher (1995) provides an overview of George Solomon's work; Solomon is considered the "father of psychoneuroimmunology" (PNI). Solomon and colleagues, including Temoshok (1987, 1991, 1993), studied long-term survivors of the human immunodeficiency virus (HIV). These researchers found that these persons shared several characteristics, including being able to assert themselves. One study was done in 1984, when long-term survival was rare, and included five HIV-positive persons who became "consultants" to their project:

> These five individuals were unique in their interests, life goals, and backgrounds. But they shared certain striking similarities in personality style and coping (Dreher, 1995, p. 170).

The following is an abbreviated list of shared traits as observed by Solomon and Temoshok:

Box 2-5

Thought-Stopping Instructions

Step 1. List your stressful thoughts
On a blank piece of paper, write down several distressing, irrational, useless thoughts that have become habits and are hard to stop. Ask yourself these questions about each of the stressful thoughts you have written down:
Is the thought unrealistic?
Is the thought counterproductive?
Is the thought self-defeating?
Is the thought hard to control?
Does it interfere with my concentration and what I really want to be doing?
Does it cause me a lot of discomfort?
Would I be a happier, more relaxed person without this thought?
  If you answered "Yes" to all of these questions for one of your distressing thoughts, thought stopping is likely to be a powerful technique for you. Thought stopping requires consistent motivation. Decide now if you really want to eliminate this stressful thought over the next week. Do not work on more than one stressful thought at a time.

Step 2. Imagine the thought
Close your eyes and bring into imagination a situation in which the stressful thought is likely to occur. Try to include normal as well as obsessive thinking. In this way, you can interrupt the stressful thoughts while allowing a continuing flow of healthy thinking.

Step 3. Thought interruption
Thought interruption can be accomplished initially by using one of two "startler" techniques:
  Set a stopwatch, egg timer, or alarm clock for 3 minutes. Look away, close your eyes, and ruminate on your stressful thought as described in Step 2. When you hear the ring, shout, "Stop!" You may also want to snap a rubber band you can wear loosely around your wrist, pinch yourself, or snap your fingers. Let your mind empty of all but the neutral and nonanxious thoughts. Set a goal of about 30 seconds after the stop, during which your mind remains blank. If the upsetting thought returns during that time, shout, "Stop!" again.
  Tape record yourself loudly exclaiming, "Stop!" at intermittent intervals (for example, 3 minutes, 2 minutes, 3 minutes, and 1 minute). You may find it useful to repeat the taped stop messages

Continued

Box 2-5

Thought-Stopping Instructions—cont'd

Step 3. Thought interruption—cont'd
several times at 5-second intervals. Proceed the same way as with the stopwatch, egg timer, or alarm clock. This tape recording shapes and strengthens your thought control.

Step 4. Unaided thought interruption
Now, take control of the thought-stopping cue without the timer or tape recorder. While ruminating on the unwanted thought, shout, "Stop!" and snap your rubber band or pinch yourself.

When you succeed in extinguishing the thought on several occasions with the shouted command, begin interrupting the thought with "Stop!" in a normal voice.

After succeeding in stopping the thought by using your normal speaking voice, start interrupting the thought with "Stop!" verbalized in a whisper.

When the whisper is sufficient to interrupt stressful thoughts, use the subvocal command. Imagine hearing "Stop!" shouted inside your mind. Tighten your vocal chords and move your tongue as if you were saying "Stop!" out loud. Success at this stage means that you can stop thoughts alone or in public, without making a sound or calling attention to yourself.

Step 5. Thought substitution
The last phase of thought stopping involves thought substitution. In place of the obsessive thought, make up some positive, assertive statements or images that are appropriate in the target situation. For example, if you are afraid of flying, you might say to yourself, "Flying commercial airlines is the safest mode of transportation. I can lean back and relax." Develop several alternative assertive statements to say to yourself, because the same response may lose its power through repetition. Imagine arriving at your destination and having a perfect vacation or productive business meeting.

Source: Davis M, Eshelman E, McKay M: The relaxation and stress reduction workbook, ed 5, Oakland, Calif, 2000, pp. 129-130, New Harbinger.

Active participation in their medical care and a sense of control over their health

Sense of meaningfulness and purpose in life

Being altruistically involved with other patients with acquired immunodeficiency syndrome (AIDS)

Acceptance of the reality of the AIDS diagnosis, alongside an adamant refusal to view the condition as a death sentence

Being assertive and having the ability to say "no"

Being sensitive to their bodies, their physical needs, and their needs for support (Dreher, 1995, p. 170).

In the formal study that followed, 18 survivors of AIDS presented the same personality patterns. The most striking finding in the formal study was a "yes" answer to the question, "Would you refuse to do a favor requested by a friend if you did not wish to?" The long survivors answered, "Yes"—they would absolutely refuse the favor. *That single trait was powerfully correlated with stronger, more active immune cells*" (Dreher, 1995, p. 171).

Practicing assertiveness means learning to avoid the compassion trap (Phelps, Austin, 1987). The compassion trap suggests that persons fall into a way of life in which they are not taking care of themselves, feeling that they exist to serve others, and that they always have to be compassionate (Phelps, Austin, 1987). This viewpoint can be especially true for women and probably anyone who is a nurturer, such as a nurse. The key here is in defining what compassion is and when to use it. However, terminology aside, assertive persons can retain their compassion while maintaining self-care, knowing when to say "No," and knowing when they are being "put down" without taking the "put-down" on as their own.

A second assertiveness point is learning the difference between traditional assumptions, (those things we may have been raised to believe as absolutes) versus legitimate rights. There are grey areas in many of these ideas, but they deserve thought. Examples of traditional assumptions include, "You should always try to accommodate others. If you don't, they won't be there when you need them." This concept is contrasted with, "You have a legitimate right to say 'no'" (Davis et al, 2000, p. 201). A second example: the traditional assumption of, "You should be flexible and adjust. Others have good reasons for their actions and it's not polite to question them" versus a legitimate right, such as, "You have a right to protest unfair treatment or criticism" (Davis et al, 2000, p. 200).

Learning assertiveness and teaching such techniques to patients can help relieve patient stress. Practicing assertiveness measures is good for both the health care provider and the care receiver.

Attitude and Personality Characteristics

Henry Dreher (1995) compiled other investigators' studies in his text, showing the health benefits of certain personality characteristics. Dreher (1995) describes persons who cope well with stress, viewing such persons as "immune power personalities." He defines such a personality as one "who is able to find joy and meaning, even health, when life offers up its most difficult challenges" (Dreher, 1996, p. 15). The term "power" refers to both strength and balance and not "sheer power" (Dreher, 1996). The seven investigators that Dreher describes defined and studied traits that seemed to help the immune system:

> Stress has been a buzzword since the 1960s when our culture began disseminating the notion that external pressures and upsetting events are key psychological factors in illness. Recent investigations have altered that view. They reveal that stress is an inevitable and sometimes even positive force in our lives. The pivotal psychological factor in illness is not stress, but rather, *how we cope with stress*. And how we cope depends, in large part, on our personalities (Dreher, 1996, p. 13).

The seven investigators and their categories of work are listed in Table 2-8.

Bibliotherapy, Journaling, Writing

Bibliotherapy refers to reading with the intention for healing. Reading materials need not be solely self-care literature but may also include other nonfiction or fiction, including short stories, works of literature, novels, or poetry. Health care providers can provide a reading list or keep a library shelf to lend out books or readings that may seem appropriate for a person.

Journaling is writing one's own personal narrative. "Journal writing is a creative intervention that requires active involvement by the client" (Snyder, 1998, p. 203). Journaling is not the same as keeping a diary, which is usually more time-structured. Keeping a journal can be clarifying and need not be done on a daily basis. To write concerns and problems, to develop solutions, and to reread one's thoughts may kindle introspection and meaning. The writing can take any form.

To begin journaling, the writer needs to purchase a book, tablet, loose leaf, or whatever "feels right." The next step is to sit down and write. There are several techniques of journaling. Free-flow journaling is writing down whatever comes to mind, similar to morning pages (Snyder, 1998; Cameron, 1992). Cameron discusses writing morning pages during which a person simply sits each morning, writing three pages a day, putting pen to paper (or pencil or keys). These writings, she says, help a person get rid of their "stuff" and get creative juices flowing for other creative endeavors.

Table 2-8	Attitude and Personality of Healthy Individuals
Investigator	**Theory and Overview**
Dreher, 1995; Weinberger et al., 1979	*ACE factor—attention, connection, expression.* Those who are tuned to mind-body signals of discomfort (e.g., pain, fatigue, distress, pleasure) cope better and have better immunity and better cardiovascular system.
Dreher, 1995; Pennebaker, 1990	*Capacity to confide.* Those who confide secrets, traumas, feelings to self and others have less illness, healthier psychologic profiles, and better immune responses.
Dreher, 1995; Kobasa (Ouellete) et al., 1985	*Hardiness—commitment, control, challenge.* Those who feel a sense of control over health-quality of life-social conditions; who have a commitment to what they do; and who view stress as a challenge have fewer chronic illnesses and symptoms—they are even better if they exercise. Hardier persons stayed healthier even if had family histories conducive to disease.
Dreher, 1995; Solomon et al., 1993, 1991, 1987	*Assertiveness.* Those who assert needs and feelings have better immune responses; they "...more readily resist and overcome a range of diseases associated with dysfunctional immunity—from rheumatoid arthritis to AIDS" (Dreher, 1996, p. 14).
Dreher, 1995; McClelland, 1989	*Affiliative trust—motive of unconditional love and a desire for positive, loving relationships based on trust and respect.* Those who form relationships based on unconditional love rather than power have better immune systems and a reduced incidence of illness.
Dreher, 1995; Luks, 1992; Thoits, Hewitt, 2001	*Healthy helping.* If individuals help others, they can get a physical, mental, and spiritual "helper's high." They will have fewer illnesses.
Dreher, 1995; Linville, 1985	*Self-complexity—"the healthy hydra."* Those who are capable of exploring their "self aspects" or their many personality facets have strengths on which to rely when another part is hurt; they are less prone to stress, depression, and illness.

Adapted from Dreher H, The immune power personality, New York, 1995, Dutton.

A second form of journaling is intensive journaling, which is a more systematic method, aimed at "enabling persons to reflect upon their lives and to grow" (Snyder, 1998, p. 205). Progoff (1975) suggests sections in the journal that can be divided into several dimensions: life or time dimensions, dialogue, and depth. The life or time dimension is writing a life history, steppingstones, intersections, roads taken and not taken, and "now." Dialogue dimensions include dialoguing with persons, work, society, events, and the body; and the depth dimension includes a dream log, dream enlargement, twilight imagery log, imagery extensions, and inner wisdom dialogue. Day (2001) describes the technique of an "Alpha Poem" in which the alphabet is written vertically down the left side of the page and then each successive line begins with the letter. Lines can be words or whole phrases. Day also discusses writing "Lists of 100," such as 100 ways to nurture the self. She suggests character sketches as a "written portrait of another person or a part of the self" (p. 137); unsent letters; and writing with the nondominant hand.

HCPs and patients can use journals to write affirmations, obtain a clearer sense of self, uncover feelings, clarify intuitions, gain insight, uncover hidden resources, hash out hurts, work through problems and illnesses, or to express beauty and joy (Snyder, 1998).

Relaxation

Relaxation exercises are commonly used interventions for anxious patients. The relaxation exercises have many forms, including progressive muscle relaxation or autogenics. Most relaxation exercises include a breathing exercise. Examples of breathing exercises include diaphragmatic breathing or chakra breathing.

Diaphragmatic breathing   Diaphragmatic breathing stimulates the parasympathetic nervous system and reduces the physiologic symptoms of anxiety: rapid pulse, hyperventilation, and elevated blood pressure. The patient breathes in slowly through the nose, allowing the abdomen to gently rise on the inhalation. Then, with the lips softly pursed, he or she exhales slowly, allowing the abdomen to fall. The exhalation should be slower than was the inhalation, slowly counting to three on the in breath and to four on the out breath. The patient can hold one hand over the abdomen, feeling the difference between a deep abdominal breath and shallow chest breathing. The HCP can count slowly for the patient. If the patient is very anxious, he or she may not be able to focus on the breathing without external direction. If the patient is exhibiting tension in the arms or shoulders or sitting with crossed legs or arms, suggest that he or she relax the shoulders and allow legs and arms to be limp. As always, the HCP's calm presence and manner are important in creating a relaxing environment. Slow, deep breathing is also useful when patients are too anxious to attend to instructions or use imagery or visualization.

Chakra breathing   Gerber (2000) describes a variant of diaphragmatic breathing and visualization that uses the chakras, moving through the colors of the chakra system. Chakras are energy centers in the human body. Chakra is a Sanskrit word meaning "wheel," referring to "wheels of energy." Chakras have been a part of Hindu and yogic traditions for many centuries. Each chakra has a specific vibrational speed and an associated color corresponding to the colors of the rainbow. The charkas are red of the root chakra at the base of the spine, orange at the lower abdomen, yellow at the solar plexus, green at the heart, blue at the throat, indigo at the forehead, and ending with violet-white at the top of the head (Brennan, 1988). Liberman (1991) discusses the effect of the color blue, citing a study designed to measure physiologic responses to colors (Gerard, 1958). Twenty-four male subjects responded to the color red with increased anxiety and hostility, whereas blue produced relaxation, a decrease in blood pressure and respiratory rate, and decreased arousal.

To practice the chakra visualization, patients begin by sitting in a straight-backed chair with both feet flat on the floor. As the patient begins to focus on breathing, he or she visualizes each of the charkas, starting with the root chakra. The patient is instructed to visualize a red rose for the root chakra. Then, the patient visualizes the red color arising in streams from the earth and flowing through the soles of the feet and up to the root chakra. This image is held through three breath cycles, and then the patient releases the color into the energy field surrounding their body. Next, the patient visualizes an orange flower and breathes in orange light through the feet and into the sacral chakra, just below the navel. On the third exhalation, the patient visualizes releasing the orange light and being surrounded by its warm healing energy. This cycle is repeated with a flower or plant of the color corresponding to each chakra. The third chakra is the solar chakra, located just under the diaphragm, and its color is yellow. The fourth chakra, the heart chakra, is located over the heart, and its color is green. When the patient reaches the throat, the fifth chakra, he or she can visualize a blue light coming in through the crown of the head and filling the area around the throat. On the third breath, the blue light is sent out through the crown, and the patient is bathed in the light. The brow chakra, sometimes called "the third eye," is the sixth chakra and is located in the center of the forehead; its color is indigo. This color should also be breathed in and out through the crown. The seventh chakra, the crown chakra, is located at the top of the skull and is associated with the color violet or white. When the chakra system is completed, the patient imagines all the colors swirling around and through his or her body.

Then, on inhalation, instruct the patient to raise his or her arms slowly above the head, and slowly lower them on exhalation. This entire cycle can be repeated several times for maximal benefit (Gerber 2000). Another example is simple color breathing for anxiety. Because blue exerts a calming effect, Gerber suggests breathing in the color blue and allowing it to permeate the body, inducing a sense of calm and relaxation.

Progressive muscle relaxation In progressive muscle relaxation, the HCP guides the patient to tense and relax each muscle group. HCPs can start with the toes and move up the body; or with the face and head, moving downward; or with the hands and arms, tensing and relaxing, then moving to the face and head, and then moving down the body, progressively tensing and relaxing each muscle group. Bourne (1990) recommends starting with three deep abdominal breaths, then clenching the fists for 7 to 10 seconds, then releasing for 15 to 20 seconds. The patient holds the tension long enough and releases it slowly to notice the difference when the muscles are relaxed. Then, the patient tenses and releases each muscle group moving in the following order: biceps, triceps, facial muscles, the muscles in the back of the neck, shoulders, chest, stomach, lower back, buttocks, thighs, calves, feet, and toes. The HCP can help the patient count and reminds the patient to completely relax one muscle group before moving on to the next. Progressive muscle relaxation may be helpful for patients who are having difficulty relaxing before sleep or who have chronic anxiety.

Other relaxation processes Researchers at the Mind-Body Institute have examined physiologic changes associated with different forms of relaxation, including Transcendental Meditation, Zen, yoga, autogenic training, progressive relaxation, and hypnosis with suggested relaxation. The physiologic changes noted included decreases in oxygen consumption, respiratory rate, heart rate, blood pressure, and muscle tension, as well as increases in alpha waves (Benson, 1993). Other research findings suggest that relaxation therapy induces a response in opioid receptors and helps strengthen immune function (Freeman, Lawlis, 2001).

Relaxation exercises are effective for patients with mild-to-moderate anxiety and may help reduce severe anxiety in patients who are motivated to practice regularly. However, patients who hyperventilate or who have panic attacks may not benefit from these exercises.

Imagery

Achterberg, Dossey, and Kolkmeier (1994) have several guided imagery scripts for anxiety and panic attacks. One of the scripts involves visualizing the physiologic changes that occur with anxiety and with relaxation. Other scripts focus on creating an inner sense of calm and safety. One simple exercise for people with anxiety is to imagine a special place where they feel safe, protected, and peaceful. Box 2-6 features a script with elements of a "favorite place." Because anxious or depressed people often feel a sense of disconnection with their bodies and senses, this imagery encourages the participant to activate all of the senses. This exercise encourages these patients to reconnect with that awareness, and feel more fully alive. In addition, patients with chronic anxiety believe that they have little control over their thoughts and emotions and may benefit from realizing that their thoughts carry only the power attributed to them. Imagery encourages the patient to view intrusive thoughts with an air of detachment, recognizing that they are simply thoughts that can be released.

Box 2-6

Guided Imagery for Relaxation

Begin by closing your eyes and making yourself comfortable. Loosen any restrictive clothing, uncross your arms and legs, and allow yourself to sink into the surface of the floor or the chair. Take a deep breath in, allowing your abdomen to rise gently, and slowly exhale, relaxing the muscles of your neck...your shoulders...your arms...your back...your legs. Continue to take slow deep breaths as you fully relax and feel your body becoming heavy and limp. *(Pause)* Now, allow your mind to wander to a place that feels very safe, very comforting, and very peaceful to you. It might be a familiar place that has special meaning to you; it might be a place you have never seen before.... It might be in the mountains...near the ocean...in a lush green forest...you decide where it is. *(Pause)* When you arrive in this place, take a moment to be aware of it with all your senses. *(Pause)* Do bright sunshine or darkness and moonlight surround you? What season is it? What are the colors of this season? What is in front of you? What is behind you? Can you see the sky? What does it look like? What is under your feet? What do you see in the distance? Slowly look around you and take in everything you see in this place. *(Pause)* What do you hear? Are there sounds of nature, of trees blowing in the wind or water rushing nearby? Are there any sounds of...birds, frogs, crickets...? What sounds do your feet make as you slowly walk around? Be aware of the silent sound of your own breathing...breathing in and out, in harmony with the rhythms around you. Take a moment to be aware of all the sounds in this special peaceful place. *(Pause)*

Continued

Box 2-6

Guided Imagery for Relaxation—cont'd

What do you touch? What does the air feel like? Do you feel warm sunshine on your face...a cool breeze...the heat of a crackling campfire...? Feel the air in this place. *(Pause)* What do your feet feel under them? It may be shifting sand; it may be wet leaves, or rocks. Be aware of the sensations of your feet. What do you smell? Do you smell damp autumn leaves...hot dry mountain air...salty ocean air...? Take a moment to be aware of the smells of the earth and the air in this place. *(Pause)*

Now, allow yourself to be fully relaxed and comfortable in this place. As you look around and note how peaceful and safe you feel, release any tension or worry that you may have brought with you. Visualize your worry or fear in front of you...separate from you. Observe it for a moment, and then simply release it, as if it were a balloon floating off into the air. If you have another worry or fear, bring it to your vision, note it, and then release it. Do this with any thoughts or emotions that you want to release. As you release your negative thoughts or emotions, feel yourself becoming more calm...more confident. Know that you have within you the answers to your questions and worries...and that when you are quiet and still, you will receive them. Allow your mind to be calm, quiet, and still as you feel the peaceful energy of this special place. Be open to its healing presence. *(Pause)* When you are ready, take three more slow deep breaths and slowly open your eyes. Remember the sensations of being in that special place. Know that the peaceful quiet place is within you, and you can return there any time.

Noble, 2002

Most patients with anxiety can benefit from guided imagery, although imagery takes practice and use of the imagination. Very anxious patients may have difficulty focusing on directions or concentrating on the imagery, and patients who have a history of abuse or trauma and who are subject to disturbing intrusive thoughts are not good candidates for imagery. Also, patients who have psychotic disorders and are paranoid or delusional should not be treated with guided imagery. However, patients who are interested in gaining tools that they can use to decrease their anxiety may be receptive to guided imagery.

HCPs who use guided imagery in their practice should develop and become familiar with a repertoire of exercises. Guided imagery training programs are available for nurses and other HCPs, including the Nurses Certificate Program in Imagery (www.imageryrn.com) and the Academy for Guided Imagery (www.interactiveimagery.com).

Prayer

Personal prayer may be effective in reducing feelings of anxiety. Meisenhelder and Chandler (2000) examined the relationship between prayer and physical and mental health using a survey of church members. Findings indicated a positive association between frequency of prayer and level of mental health. People who prayed more often had higher mental health scores than did participants who prayed less frequently. Shuler and colleagues (1994) also found a positive relationship between prayer and psychologic well being. Among inner-city homeless women, those who reported prayer as an effective coping mechanism indicated fewer worries and concerns when compared with women who did not use prayer in coping.

Hebert and colleagues (2001) at Johns Hopkin's University School of Medicine, conducted focus group discussions with patients who had recently had a life-threatening illness. Study findings indicated that patients want HCPs to inquire about personal coping and support mechanisms. If the patient discloses the importance of spirituality in their lives, they do not expect the provider to discuss their spiritual beliefs, however, they would like for their beliefs to be respected and incorporated into their plan of care as appropriate (Hebert et al., 2001).

Some HCPs may find it a little uncomfortable exploring spiritual coping mechanisms with their patients. Anandarajah and Hight (2001) suggest use of the "HOPE" questions as a tool for assessment. Concepts covered with patients include: H, sources of hope, strength, and love; O, role of organized religion; P, personal spiritual practices; and E, effects of spirituality on medical care and end of life decisions (Anandarajah, Hight, 2001). Another form of spiritual support for patients is intercessory prayer, or another person praying for them. Byrd's (1988) notable study suggests the beneficial therapeutic effects of intercessory prayer on patients in the coronary care unit. Harris and colleagues (1999) supported Byrd's findings in a recent study. When Harris and colleagues (1999) replicated the Byrd study, they similarly found an association with improved patient health outcomes and intercessory prayer.

Social Support and Social Activity

Social support and social activities include friends, family, work, play, hobbies, pets, gardening and plants, even objects or security blankets. Social support and social activities are a major joy of life, assisting an individual in coping with stressful events and in maintaining health. Individuals who are exposed to stressful life events and subsequently do not become ill may have coping and social resources different from those who do become ill (Hogue, 1977; Kinney et al., 1992). The magnitude of importance of social support is appreciated when viewed from studies that span birth to death. For example, the length of labor is shorter with social support (Sosa et al., 1980); and support has a positive influence on pregnancy and parenting. An Israeli study of 10,000 married men showed that love and support from a wife reduces risk for angina pectoris, even in the presence of high-risk factors (Medalie, Goldbourt, 1976). In a Harvard, Yale, and Rush Institute for Healthy Aging study of over 2700 subjects, all over the age of 65 (Glass et al., 1999), social, productive, and physical activity were independently associated with survival. The social and productive activities were just as important as were physical activity. In addition, social support for persons with early-stage Alzheimer's provides emotional support, modeling, and enhanced coping ability (Luskin et al., 1999; Davies et al., 1995).

Social support also includes support groups such as 12-step programs, grief support groups, or other community or private groups of like-minded individuals who offer encouragement, empathy, and hope. Because 12-step programs are anonymous, they are not as well understood and probably play a larger role in helping people cope than is known via research.

The HCP can compile a resource manual of groups and agencies for referral purposes. Religious, prayer, or meditation groups, community organizations, hobby groups, family services, respite and day care services, and volunteer opportunities all need to be included in such reference manuals. In addition, self-care processes need to be taught to persons who may need these skills. Table 2-9 lists mind-body-spirit interventions for anxiety.

BIOLOGIC-BASED THERAPIES FOR WELL BEING AND ANXIETY CONTROL

Numerous studies have been conducted relating psychologic well being to nutrients. The total scope of nutrition discussion is beyond this text, however, in general, a good diet means clean, whole foods, minimal processing, no additives, eating the foods that are in season for the climate, a regular eating pattern, and appropriate nutrients, including the food pyramid components with enough fruits and vegetables, low fat, fiber, water, and vitamins, minerals, and essential amino and fatty acids. In addition, alcohol should be minimized, and caffeine and simple sugars should be cut down or discontinued. Chapter 13 provides an overview of the recently revised vitamin and mineral recommendations.

Diet Therapy

The understanding of the connection between nutrients and neurotransmitters may lead to greater understanding of how foods influ-

Table 2-9   Mind-Body-Spirit Interventions for Well Being and Anxiety Control

Intervention	Management	Treatment Regimen	Cautions, Precautions, Interactions	References
Affirmation	General well being, anxiety	Personal, positive, present-tense statements. Examples: "I love and approve of myself, and I trust the process of life. I am safe" (p. 14); "I love and accept myself at every age. Each moment of life is perfect" (p. 11)	No precautions or interactions	Hay, 2000
Assertiveness	General well being; relationship and work negotiations	Assertiveness training	No precautions or interactions	Alberti and Emmons, 1990 Davis et al., 2000 Phelps, Austin, 1987
Attitude	General well being; possible improved immune status	Develop or cultivate attitude and immune power personality traits (see Table 2-8)	No precautions or interactions	Dreher, 1995, 1996 who gives an overview of Linville, 1985 Luks, 1992 McClelland, 1989

Continued

Table 2-9 Mind-Body-Spirit Interventions for Well Being and Anxiety Control—cont'd

Intervention	Management	Treatment Regimen	Cautions, Precautions, Interactions	References
Attitude, cont'd				Kobasa, 1985 Pennebaker, 1990 Schwartz, in Dreher, 1995 Thoits, Hewitt, 2001 Day, 2001 Snyder, 1998
Bibliotherapy, journaling, writing	Reading or writing	Choose reading or writing materials (or both) of personal preference	No precautions or interactions	
Biofeedback		Several sessions needed to develop	Trained HCP needed who is skilled with biofeedback	Peters, Chaitow et al, 2002
Breathing techniques	Promote a sense of calm Slow breathing reduces anxiety Activate parasympathetic nervous system	Diaphragm breathing Chakra breathing Color breathing Quiet room with no interruption Assist patient by verbally guiding	Not recommended for patients with severe anxiety or panic attacks if a history of hyperventilation is present	Gerber, 2000 Peters et al, 2002

	them through the exercises	Patients with neuromuscular disorders may not be able to complete the progressive muscle relaxation	
Hobby	Promotes relaxation and general well being, distraction Allays anxiety, helps with addiction release	*Personal preference:* musical instrument, sewing, knitting, carving, building, collecting, creative arts, reading, writing, puzzles, crafts	No precautions or interactions
Imagery	Assists patient to use suggestion to induce feeling of calm and security Promotes sense of control over emotions	Quiet room, free of distractions May use own recorded script or HCP-read script or commercial tapes or CDs Participant follows script and accesses imagination to promote sense of calmness	Not suggested for those with intrusive memories, history of trauma or abuse Not advised for patients with psychoses Do not drive or operate machinery while listening to imagery tapes/ CDs	Achterberg et al., 1994 Emmett Miller tapes @ 800-52tapes Naparstek tapes and CDs @ www. healthjourneys.com

Continued

Table 2-9 Mind-Body-Spirit Interventions for Well Being and Anxiety Control—cont'd

Intervention	Management	Treatment Regimen	Cautions, Precautions, Interactions	References
Meditation	Promotes relaxation, relieves stress, decreases respiration, promotes growth, and insight	A simple meditation to repeat to self over and over while sitting in a quiet comfortable place: "May I be filled with loving-kindness"; "May I be well"; "May I be peaceful and at ease"; "May I be happy" When you can do this well with yourself, include others in the meditation, e.g. "May_be well." Spend 5-30 min/day focusing on the breath Be mindful in activities	Driving or operating machinery is not recommended	Kornfield, 1996 Pettinati, 2001
Music	Promotes general well being, for	Personal preference HCP can compile	No precautions or interactions	Aldridge, 1994 White, 2001;

	those with Alzheimer's disease or dementia Decreases anxiety and pain Decreases nausea Increases oxygen saturation in infants Reduces respiratory rate	library of music (e.g., classical, light jazz, new age, spiritual, light rock, easy listening, country) Instrumental music recommended with 20-min recordings Limit extraneous noise, and get comfortable Personal preference		www.musictherapy.org
Pet therapy	Improves well being Provides social support, companionship Become stimulus for exercise Reduces anxiety Promotes physical contact and comfort Service animal programs		Pets require care, love, and attention Some living situations do not allow pets Pets may exacerbate allergies	Huebscher, 2000 Raina, 1999 Paws with a cause, www.pawscause.org Guide Dog Foundation, www.guidedog.org Canine Companions for Independence, www.caninecompanions.org Helping Hands, www.helpinghandsmonkeys.org Delta Society, www.DeltaSociety.org

Continued

Table 2-9   Mind-Body-Spirit Interventions for Well Being and Anxiety Control—cont'd

Intervention	Management	Treatment Regimen	Cautions, Precautions, Interactions	References
Prayer and spiritual support	Promotes positive coping, support Reduces worries, concerns; Improves mental health	Respect spiritual beliefs and practices Incorporate personal prayer as appropriate Ask HOPE questions: H, sources of hope strength, love; O, role of organized religion P, personal spiritual practices E, effects of spirituality on medical care and end of life decisions	No precautions or interactions	Anandarajah and Hight, 2001 Meisenhelder et al., 2000 Shuler et al, 1994
Relaxation	Increases general well being Reduces muscle tension Promote relaxation	Privacy Autogenics Progressive muscle relaxation Quiet room free of interruption Teach steps of exercise and prompt patient	Not recommended for those with neuromuscular disorders	Bourne, 1990 Davis et al., 1998, 2002

Social support	Promotes general well being May improve health status	Friends, family, pets, hobby and church groups, volunteering, parent groups, 12-step programs, social programs, senior groups	No precautions or interactions
			Davis et al., 1998, 2000
Thought stopping	Promotes general well being Reduces anxiety, phobias, obsessive thoughts	1. Explore (list) stressful thoughts 2. Imagine the thought 3. Thought interruption 4. Unaided thought interruption 5. Thought substitution; practice conscientiously throughout the day for 3-7 days	See Box 2-5 for details

HCP, *Health care provider.*

ence moods and emotions (Miller, 1996). Miller (1998) cites a case study in which the subject was able to recover from years of drug and alcohol addiction and psychologic problems by adopting a diet that limited caffeine and simple carbohydrates.

Dietary suggestions for patients with anxiety are similar to those for many other conditions: limit or eliminate caffeine, limit consumption of simple carbohydrates, eliminate or restrict intake of alcohol, and increase intake of whole grain and natural foods. Murray and Pizzorno (1998) recommend a high-potency vitamin and mineral formula to ensure adequate B and C vitamins.

Herbal Therapy

Kava kava Kava kava (*Piper methysticum*) is an herbal remedy recommended for anxiety and for sedation as well (Facts and Comparisons, 2001; Fetrow, Avila, 1999; Pittler et al., 2000). Kava, native to the Pacific Islands, has been used for years on social and ceremonial occasions, similar to other cultures' social use of alcohol. Kava is effective for reducing anxiety, yet does not have the sedative properties of conventional anxiolytics (e.g., benzodiazepines).

Using the Hamilton Anxiety Scale and other self-reports, researchers from a German placebo-controlled, double-blind study found that anxious subjects reported a significant decrease in their symptoms after 25 weeks on kava kava (Volz, Kieser, 1997). In another study, over a period of 5 days, subjects received placebo, oxazepam, or kava, and were then given a memory and word recognition test. The event-related potentials in electroencephalographic (EEG) readings were evaluated while the subjects attempted to discriminate between words that had been previously seen and new words. Oxazepam inhibited the recognition of both the old and the new words, whereas the subjects who received kava had increased word recognition and greater evoked response potential differences between old and new words (Munte et al., 1993).

Doses of kava vary depending on type of herb used, such as dried extract or kava pyrone content (Fetrow, Avila, 1999). Although kava may have psychologic dependence, it is not physically addicting and it is nonhypnotic. However, cautions do exist. In large daily doses or with long-term use, patients can develop dermatitis. Kava should not be mixed with alcohol, benzodiazepines, barbiturates, or other CNS depressants. The potential for abuse of kava is a concern because of its mood-altering properties. The safety of kava in children and in pregnant and lactating women has not been established. Patients with Parkinson's disease should be advised to avoid kava because it can interfere with dopamine production, worsening the symptoms of Parkinson's, and kava interacts with levodopa (Fetrow and Avila, 1999). Recently, the American Botanical Council (ABC) issued safety information concerning possible liver problems with kava. Several cases of adverse events, including liver toxicity and death, have been reported. In most of the cases, other medications with potential liver toxicity were also being taken. Persons with liver problems or those taking other substances known to affect the liver should not take kava. In addition, kava should not be taken in increased doses or on a regular basis and not for longer than 3 to 4 weeks (ABC release on Kava Safety, www.herbalgram.org, 2001; PL/PL, 2002).

Valerian   Valerian is an herb that promotes relaxation and sleep. Valerian, widely used in Europe, has had several large German open-label studies and a few randomized controlled studies (Barrett et al., 1999). Three small randomized controlled studies showed significant improvement in the quality of sleep and decreased sleep latency with the use of valerian (Leathwood et al., 1982, 1985; Lindahl et al., 1989; Blumenthal, 2000). In another study of 100 patients with anxiety, a combination of valerian and St. John's wort was compared with diazepam. The improvement in measures of anxiety was significantly greater among the subjects taking the herbal combination than it was among the diazepam group (Barrett 1999; Schulz et al., 1994).

Aromatherapy

Aromatherapy, through the sense of smell and combined with massage, has many applications for anxiety and other strong emotions. Box 2-7 describes some of the essential oils that are recommended to help patients feel more calm, focused, and relaxed. For most anxious patients, aromatherapy is delivered through massage, combining the benefits of touch, massage, and aromatherapy in one treatment. There are some cautions when using aromatherapy. Oils should never be ingested internally and are not applied full strength to the skin. Before application to the skin, essential oils are diluted in a carrier oil, such as almond oil, using about 15 drops of essential oil to 1 ounce of carrier oil or lotion. For bathing, oils are dispersed in bath water so the skin does not contact the concentrated oil. Contraindications include allergy, skin sensitivities, and caution is necessary if the patient has asthma or other respiratory conditions, epilepsy, or hypertension. Many people are sensitive to scents and may develop allergic reactions to essential oils. Avoid any aromatherapy in early pregnancy, and keep oils away from children. Consult a practitioner who has training and experience with aromatherapy if any concerns about its safe use occur. Photosensitivity may develop in some patients (Buckle, 1997; Shealy 1998). Robins (1999) cites several studies reporting contact dermatitis from essential oils. One study with 585 subjects found that 3% reported either transient burning (peppermint oil) or adverse reaction to the odor

Box 2-7

Aromatherapy for Anxiety

Bergamot
Bergamot balances and instills a sense of calm. It has a light, citruslike floral scent and is widely used in perfumes. Most bergamot contains bergapten, which causes photosensitivity, although bergapten-free preparations are available. HCPs should advise patients to avoid using bergamot before sunlight exposure.

Cedarwood
Cedarwood is grounding, calming, and stabilizing. The scent is sweet and woody. Do not use during pregnancy.

Chamomile
Chamomile helps relieve nervous tension and release built-up feelings of frustration. The scent is sweet and warm.

Geranium
Geranium helps calm the mind and relieve agitation. Geranium has balancing properties that help connect to intuition and inner wisdom. The scent is sweet and floral.

Lavender
Lavender is useful in a variety of conditions. The emotional effect is described as healing and soothing the heart and opening the heart to forgiveness and compassion. The scent is floral and mild.

Neroli
Neroli has soothing and calming properties that are especially useful in acute states of anxiety. Neroli has a delicate floral scent.

Sandalwood
Sandalwood is described as having a gentle sedative effect with calming and balancing properties. Associated with the third chakra, sandalwood is often used in meditation. Sandalwood has a warm woody scent.

Shealy (1998) and Fischer-Rizzi (1990)

(clary sage). The author notes that well-constructed controlled studies of aromatherapy are few, and that most data are based on subjective responses rather than physiologic measurement. Table 2-10 lists biologic-based therapies for anxiety.

Table 2-10   Biologic-Based Therapies for Well Being and Anxiety Control

Intervention	Management	Treatment Regimen	Cautions, Precautions, Interactions	References
Diet, dietary supplements	Promotes general well being May reduce anxiety	Good diet; individual assessment for nutritional deficits, including vitamins, minerals Possible vitamin-mineral supplements Combination of vitamins and minerals are often required Find motivating factors to assist patients in making change (e.g., How can you include more fruits and vegetables in your meals or snacks?) Limit caffeine, alcohol, simple carbohydrates	Diet diary and vitamin and mineral evaluation may help define deficiencies	Miller, 1996, 1998 Murray, Pizzorno, 1998 (see also conventional and alternative nutrition information)

Continued

Table 2-10	Biologic-Based Therapies for Well Being and Anxiety Control—cont'd			
Intervention	*Management*	*Treatment Regimen*	*Cautions, Precautions, Interactions*	*References*
Herbal therapy	May reduce anxiety Promotes sleep and relaxation	Kava-kava: varying doses, depending on preparation Valerian: drink tea or decoction 30-45 mins before bedtime; there is also a tincture and standardized extract	Not for habitual use Kava kava is contraindicated for those with Parkinson's disease Kava kava should not be combined with other CNS depressants Potential for abuse exists Warning: possible liver toxicity Valerian should not be combined with sedatives Driving and operating machinery is to be avoided	Barrett, 1999 Blumenthal, 2000 Fetrow, Avila, 1999 Leathwood et al., 1985 Murray, 1994 Murray, Pizzorno, 1998 Shealy, 1998

| Aromatherapy | Promotes calm and relaxation | Must be pure essential oils
Oils are selected for their properties: *bergamot*, lavender, rose have calming effects. Others include: *Cedarwood, chamomile, geranium, lavender, neroli, sandalwood.* Dilute 12 to 15 gtts of essential oil with 1 oz carrier oil (e.g., almond oil) or lotion
Use with massage, bath, or room diffuser | Can be expensive
Must be diluted
Do not apply directly to skin
Caution with allergy, asthma, respiratory conditions, allergies, sensitive skin, epilepsy, hypertension
Photosensitivity may develop with *bergamot*
Avoid use for those who are pregnant
Never take essential oils internally
Disperse thoroughly in bath water to avoid direct contact with oil | Buckle 1993, 1997, 2001
Gottlieb, 1995
Robins, 1999
Shealy, 1998

Limit sunlight exposure |

Lavender, the first oil studied by Gattefosse, the chemist credited with discovering the healing properties of essential oils, is described as the "rescue remedy" of essential oils and is often recommended as the oil that has the most uses. Gottlieb (1995) recommends lavender, geranium, melissa, ylang ylang, and bergamot for relief of anxiety. Essential oils are usually applied through massage, a diffuser, or by adding 10 to 15 drops to bath water. Some people add 10 or 12 drops of oil to their shampoo or conditioner. Adding five drops of oil to a bowl of warm water and then using a washcloth as a compress can relieve muscle tension, as well as deliver the aromatherapy.

MANIPULATIVE AND BODY-BASED METHODS: MASSAGE

Various types of massage provide general relaxation and tension release. Massage decreases pain during labor and the length of labor, as well as decreasing anxiety (Field et al., 1997). Massage has been used to decrease agitation in persons with dementia (Snyder et al., 1995), including foot massage (Snyder, Cheng, 1998). A 6-minute back massage helps decrease pain in the intensive care unit (Richards, 1998), and massage postoperatively helps decrease pain (Nixon et al., 1997).

Field (2000) has compiled a text of massage research. Almost all of the studies, although small, show positive results. Included were massage studies on persons with asthma, cystic fibrosis, attention deficit hyperactivity disorder, depression, anxiety, anorexia and bulimia, atopic dermatitis, diabetes, premenstrual syndrome, migraine headaches, fibromyalgia, and rheumatoid arthritis.

Massage can be an effective way to promote relaxation in anxious patients. In a study of 113 hospitalized patients who received massages during their hospital stay, 98% reported feeling more relaxed, 93% reported feeling a sense of well being, and 88% reported a positive mood change (Smith et al., 1999). In the outpatient setting, patients can be referred to qualified massage therapists. In the inpatient setting, offering a simple back massage, using the long strokes of effleurage, and alternating with pétrissage can help patients who are anxious and tense. Oil or lotion reduces friction. Ask patients if they have any fragrance allergies, sensitive areas, or any skin sensitivities before starting, and use fragrance-free oil or lotion whenever possible. Provide a quiet private place for massage and be sure the patient is draped appropriately and has proper support with bolsters or pillows. For patients who are not candidates for back massage, a simple hand or foot massage may be calming. Use lotion instead of oil for hands and feet. Avoid massaging masses, fractures, injuries, skin lesions, varicosities or thrombophlebitis. Vigorous massage is contraindicated in patients with high fever. Discuss with the patient's HCP or oncologist before initiating regular massage with patients with cancer.

ENERGY THERAPIES FOR WELL BEING AND ANXIETY CONTROL

HT, TT, and Reiki may help reduce anxiety and promote relaxation in both adults and children, including in cardiovascular patients (Heidt, 1981; Quinn, 1984), oncology patients on chemotherapy (Guerrero, 1986), hospitalized psychiatric patients (Gagne, Toy, 1994; Hughes et al., 1996), and hospitalized children (Kramer, 1990). Krieger (1993) notes that patients with anxiety are sensitive to TT, suggesting the practitioner start with a few moments of unruffling the energy field, then stabilizing the solar plexus chakra and the heart chakra. The author recommends stabilizing the throat chakra and interspersing the chakra work with gentle unruffling, moving toward the feet to keep the energy flowing down and outward. Before initiating TT or HT, the HCP prepares by centering and setting the intention for the highest good.

Studies of TT were conducted in which anxiety levels were not decreased (Egan, 1998; Parkes, 1985: Hale, 1986; Quinn, 1989; Randolph, 1984). Quinn (1988) provides several possible explanations for these inconsistencies, including the practitioner's expertise level (or lack of), TT treatment time period, small sample sizes, and whether stress or anxiety might be normal for some situations and a protection from threat; thus TT (or any relaxation) should not be applied to such situations. In addition, practitioners need expertise and to spend enough treatment time, probably at least 15 to 20 minutes. Table 2-11 provides treatment regimen suggestions for manipulative and body-based methods and for energy therapies for general well being and for anxiety control.

NAC PRACTICES FOR DEPRESSION

Major depression is the most common psychiatric disorder in the United States. Approximately one out of eight adults will experience an episode of depression in their lifetime (Stuart, Laraia, 2001). The cause is unknown, but most theories suggest an interaction of genetic, biologic, environmental, and personality factors. Certain personality traits such as pessimism, learned helplessness, and poor self-esteem seem to predispose individuals to depression (Frisch, Frisch, 1998; Stuart, Laraia 2001). Patients with major depression have a persistent depressed mood that is different from their usual functioning and that interferes with social and occupational functioning. Patients often experience a profound sense of hopelessness and worthlessness and may also have accompanying physiologic signs and symptoms in sleep cycles, appetite, and energy level. In addition to major depression, there are variants of depression such as postpartum depression, seasonal affective disorder, bipolar disorder, and dysthymic disorder.

In many primary care settings, the use of selective serotonin reuptake inhibitors (SSRIs) as a treatment for depression has become

Table 2-11 Manipulative and Body-Based Methods and Energy Therapies for Well Being and Anxiety Control

Intervention	Management	Treatment Regimen	Cautions, Precautions, Interactions	References
Massage therapy	Promotes general relaxation and well being, increase circulation Promotes relaxation for hospice patients Decreases agitation in patient's with Alzheimer's disease or dementia Decreases labor pain, length of labor, anxiety; symptoms of asthma, cystic fibrosis, atopic dermatitis, diabetes, migraine headaches, fibromyalgia, rheumatoid arthritis;	Assess patient's skin Fragrance-free oil or lotion is used Lotions for hands and feet are used; oil for back Privacy is provided Effleurage, pétrissage, tapotement, friction is provided Hand or foot massage is provided as appropriate Feet are washed first Various modalities, (Swedish massage, etc) are used for relaxation Deep tissue and neuromuscular work	Patient needs to feel comfortable with therapist Areas of skin breakdown should be avoided Massage is not performed over varicosities, masses, injuries, open wounds, athlete's foot, fractures, or on legs if a risk of clots exists No massage is recommended for those with fever Caution is recommended in patients with cancer	Field, 2000, 1996, 1997 Meek, 1993 Rowe et al., 1999 Snyder et al., 1995 Snyder, Cheng, 1998

				References
		burn débridement improves	is used to reduce specific tension or painful areas	
Aromatherapy massage	Promotes calming effects		Lavender, rose (see Table 2-10 and Box 2-7)	May cause allergic reaction Use pure essential oils Must be diluted Can be expensive	Buckle, 2001
Shiatsu	Relieves fatigue Develops stamina and fighting spirit		Various Shiatsu regimens	Requires skilled practitioner	Namikoshi, 1995
TT, Reiki; HT	Promotes general well being Decreases anxiety Promote sense of calm and relaxation through balancing energy		HCP centers self, set intention; assesses energy field; unruffles; modulates energy; know when to stop Stabilize throat, solar plexus, and heart chakras	Trained practitioner needed Permission from patient must always be obtained Minimum of 15-20-min sessions	Easter, 1997 Krieger, 1993 Heidt, 1981 Kramer, 1900 Quinn, 1984, 1988, 1989

HCP, *Health care provider*; HT, *healing touch*; TT, *therapeutic touch*.

commonplace. For some patients, short-term use of SSRIs, along with counseling, is appropriate; however, a word of warning is warranted. Glenmullen (2000), a clinical instructor of psychiatry at Harvard Medical School, notes dangerous side-effects with long-term use of Prozac-type drugs. In his book, *Prozac Backlash*, he portrays an alarming picture of the numerous neurologic side effects that can occur as the brain reacts over time to artificially elevated levels of serotonin. Glenmullen (2000) suggests that HCPs avoid exposing patients to SSRIs, unless moderate-to-severe depression is diagnosed. The author argues that no more than 25% of patients who are currently taking such drugs should be taking them. Glenmullen (2000) supports the use of alternative therapies in the treatment of mild-to-moderate depression and includes a discussion of therapies that he deems effective.

NAC practices are commonly used for depression (Ernst, Rand, Stevenson, 1998). However, the foundation for any intervention with depressed patients is to establish a sense of therapeutic presence. Presence is creating a sacred space in which HCPs remain nonjudgmental and establish a healing connection with patients (Freeman, Lawlis, 2001). In this sacred space, HCPs listen to the stories of their patients and participate with their patients in the healing process. In listening to patients and exploring the personal meaning of these stories with them, HCPs connect with their patients and help them access their own inner healing resources (Dossey, 1999). Dossey describes the process of "being with" and "being there" in nursing practice. HCPs can develop this sense of presence by centering, by setting their intention to be fully present in the moment, and by shifting their focus from "doing" to "being." The patient who is depressed often feels alone, hopeless, and worthless. In being fully present and open to the experience of the patient, the HCP establishes a healing relationship that validates the worth of the patient.

ALTERNATIVE HEALTH CARE SYSTEMS FOR DEPRESSION

Ayurveda

From the Ayurvedic perspective, depression can result from an imbalance in any of the doshas. Excessive vata, pitta, or kapha dosha may lodge in the nervous system, interfere with the normal functioning of the mind and cause depression. Although each of these three types of depression is treated in different ways, the first step is to modify the diet so as to correct the doshic imbalance. Mild depression can sometimes be successfully treated with Ayurvedic remedies. Ayurvedic treatments may lessen the need for prescription antidepressants; however, they are not a substitute for having a psychiatric HCP monitor the individual's progress.

Vata-type depression is usually associated with fear, anxiety, nervousness, and insomnia. Ayurvedic treatment of vata-type depression includes dashamoola, ashwagandha, and brahmi, or holy basil and sage tea, warm sesame oil nose drops (nasya), massaging the top of the head and soles of the feet with sesame oil, and spending more time relating to people (Lad, 1998).

Pitta-type depression is associated with anger or fear of failure, of losing control, or of making mistakes. Although a mild pitta depression is possible, this type of depression often involves suicidal thoughts, thus the individual should consult a mental health practitioner. Pitta (fire principle) types are the most vulnerable to seasonal affective disorder during the winter months. Treatment of pitta-type depression includes scalp and sole of foot massage with coconut or sunflower oil, brahmi-jatamamsi-shatavari tea, brahmi ghee nose drops (nasya), and meditation (Lad, 1998).

Kapha depression is characterized by mental heaviness, excess sleep, weight gain, lethargy, and drowsiness. Treatment includes fasting for 3 to 4 days on apple juice, increasing the amount of physical exercise, ginger tea, punanarva ghee nose drops (nasya), yoga (sun salutation 12 times a day, and shoulder stand, plow poses), Ujjayi Pranayama (breathing exercise) (Lad, 1998).

Homeopathy

Section II gives detailed information on homeopathy. Extensive case taking is the foundation of homeopathic treatment. The practitioner identifies the objective and subjective symptoms and gathers information about the nature, quality, and duration of each symptom. Careful assessment of symptoms and identification of the remedy that most closely matches the symptoms is extremely important. The treatment for the depressed patient will vary greatly, depending on the nature of the presenting symptoms.

Few studies have been conducted regarding homeopathic remedies in psychiatric disorders. Davidson (1997) describes a study of 10 women and 2 men with diagnoses of depression, social phobia, panic disorder, or any combination, who were not responding to conventional therapies. Each subject was treated concurrently with an individualized remedy and conventional therapy. The response rates on standardized self-reports indicated that some subjects with these conditions were responsive to the homeopathic remedies.

Traditional Chinese Medicine

Acupuncture   Acupuncture may have some benefits as a treatment; the National Institutes of Health (NIH) has funded a 5-year study of the use of acupuncture to treat depression. Ross (1995) states that either stagnant or deficient Qi causes depression and that the effectiveness of treatment is based on accurate Qi diagnosis. The author identifies 15 depression syndromes that have corresponding acupuncture points. Specific patterns of acupuncture points correspond to the presenting symptoms of depression. Allen, Schneyer, and Hitt (1998) compared using specific versus nonspecific acupuncture points for the treatment of depression. The nonspecific acupuncture points were those that might be used to treat headache or back pain. The authors assigned 38 women to one of three groups: depression-specific acupuncture treatment, nonspecific acupuncture, or a wait group without treatment. At the end of 8 weeks, the women who received depression-specific acupuncture treatment had greater improvement in symptoms than did the women who received nonspecific treatment. At the end of the study, when all groups of women had received the depression-specific acupuncture, 64% of the subjects were in clinical remission.

Acupressure Acupressure points correspond to acupuncture points but are stimulated with finger pressure instead of needles. Patients can be taught how to find and stimulate their own acupressure points to provide relief of symptoms. Gach (1990) suggests stimulating the bladder (B or UB) 38 points for depression. This process can be done by lying on the floor on the back, and placing two tennis balls under the muscles between the shoulder blades. While applying the pressure of the tennis balls, the patient should breathe slowly and deeply and relax the muscles of the back and neck.

Other pressure points that may be useful in depression are gallbladder (GB) 20, B 10, and governing vessel (GV or Du mo) 19, 20 and 21. GB 20 is found in two indentations at the base of the skull between the two large neck muscles, 2 to 3 inches apart. B or UB 10 is located ½ inch below the base of the skull on both sides of the muscles of the neck. GV (Du mo) 19, 20, and 21 are located at the crown of the skull. GV (Du mo) 20 is located by placing the index finger behind the right ear and left ear and then slowly moving the fingers up until they reach the small indentation toward the back of the top of the head. GV (Du mo) 19 is about 1 inch in back of GV 20, and GV 21 is 1 inch in front of GV 20. Appendix B demonstrates the locations of meridians for these acupressure points. Table 2-12 provides an alternative health care systems approach to depression.

MIND-BODY-SPIRIT INTERVENTIONS FOR DEPRESSION

Cognitive-Behavioral Therapy

Cognitive-behavioral therapy (CBT), a commonly used approach in psychiatric treatment, is an effective intervention for depression. The goals of CBT are to help the patient substitute more positive attributions for negative ones, to recognize and change cognitive distortions, and to develop more adaptive coping strategies (Stuart, Laraia 2001). Examples of cognitive approaches are thought stopping, reframing, and "decatastrophising."

Table 2-12	Alternative Health Care Systems for Depression			
Intervention	**Management**	**Treatment Regimen**	**Cautions, Precautions, Interactions**	**References**
Ayurveda	Treats vata-type depression	Dashamoola, ashwagandha, and brahmi, or holy basil and sage tea, warm sesame oil nose drops (nasya), massaging the top of the head and soles of the feet with sesame oil, spending more time relating to people	Qualified psychologic assessment and care are needed	Lad, 1998
	Treats pitta-type depression	Scalp and sole of feet are massaged with coconut or sunflower oil; Brahmi-jatamamsi-shatavari teas, brahmi ghee nose drops, and meditation	Pitta-type depression may have suicidal thoughts; must have qualified psychologic care	Lad, 1998

Continued

Table 2-12 Alternative Health Care Systems for Depression—cont'd

Intervention	Management	Treatment Regimen	Cautions, Precautions, Interactions	References
Ayurveda, cont'd	Treats kapha-type depression	Fasting for 3-4 days on apple juice, increasing physical exercise, ginger tea, punanarva ghee nose drops, yoga Sun salutation 12 times per day, shoulder stand, plow poses Ujjayi Pranayama (breathing exercises)	Qualified psychologic assessment and care needed Some patients may not be able to perform yoga postures	Lad, 1998
Homeopathy	Remedy that most closely matches depression symptoms is used (e.g., *Arsenicum album* for anxious, restless, and obsessively neat; *Ignatia* for depression that follows deep grief;	Match symptoms to remedy through full-case history taking (e.g., *Arsenicum alba*, 6 c q2h for up to 10 doses); See Section II for homeopathic information. Examples: *Ignatia*, 6 c q2h for up to 10 doses, then tid for	Avoid skin contact with remedies Store away from light and heat Skilled homeopathic practitioner is needed	McCabe, 2000 Boericke, 2000 Lockie, Geddes, 1995

	Pulsatilla for tearfulness, emotional lability, and emotional attention-seeking, or for depression associated with hormonal changes in women	up to 14 days; *Pulsatilla*, 6 c tid for up to 14 days Take remedies on empty stomach Assess response-stop if no effect		Ross, 1995 Allen et al., 1998
Acupuncture	Decreases symptoms of depression	Skilled practitioner needed	Caution is recommended in clotting disorders Safety is not established for children Trained practitioner	Freeman, Lawlis, 2001
Acupressure	May decrease symptoms of depression	Points: B (UB) 38; GB 20; B 10; GV (Du mo) 19, 20, 21	No precautions or interactions	Gach, 1990

B (UB), *Bladder*; GB, *gallbladder*; GV (*Du mo*), *governing vessel*; tid, *three times daily.*

In thought stopping, the individual loudly says, "Stop!" when a pattern of negative thinking is noted, thus interrupting the pattern. See Box 2-5 for thought-stopping instructions.

In reframing, the individual is encouraged to "frame" a thought or an event in a more positive way and to recognize that the meaning attributed to events has a significant impact on coping. For instance, the patient who loses a job may "frame" that event in terms of failure, confirmation of worthlessness, and despair; or, he or she may reframe the event in terms of opportunity to learn a new trade, return to school, or pursue other interests, all perspectives that promote an active coping response to a potential threat.

Decatastrophising is an approach for patients who are easily overwhelmed and who dwell on the worst possible interpretation of events. In treatment, the patient is encouraged to appraise his or her situation realistically and to consider the worst possible consequence or outcome of that situation. Usually, patients realize that even the worst possible actual outcome is not devastating or life threatening. Patients can then move toward more adaptive coping.

In both adults and adolescents, CBT is used both as an adjunct to pharmacologic interventions and as a primary treatment of mood disorders. Reinecke and colleagues (1998) published a review and meta-analysis of CBT studies done with depressed adolescents. The authors found decreases in negative self-attributions (self-blame and self-criticism) and cognitive distortions among the adolescent subjects treated with CBT.

Clarke and colleagues (1999) compared results in adolescents who received "booster sessions" of CBT after initial treatment. The subjects who received the booster sessions were reported as 100% recovered at 12-month follow up, compared with 50% of the assessment-only subjects. The mean time of recovery for the booster group was 23.5 weeks, whereas the assessment-only group mean recovery time was 67.05 weeks. Casteleman (1996) discusses a University of British Columbia analysis of 28 separate studies comparing CBT with other forms of treatment. The subjects who learned to use CBT did better than did subjects with no treatment, with medication, and those treated with psychotherapy.

HCPs who use CBT can help their patients recognize the impact of their cognitive distortions by focusing on the ABCs of therapy. "A" is the actual event or antecedent, without any interpretation or judgment (e.g., the patient receives a poor job review). "B" is the patient's beliefs or behaviors in response to "A." ("I'll never be good at this. This proves that I'm a loser. Maybe I should just quit." versus "This is a new job and I've been under a lot of stress at home. I need to learn more about my job so I feel more confident. I've been successful before and I can learn how to do this.") The HCP helps the patient challenge the cognitive distortions, pointing out facts that contradict the distortions or demonstrate the fallacy of the belief. "C" is the consequence of the actions in "B." (The patient has low self-esteem, quits the job, or adopts a strategy for success.) The HCP helps the patient recognize how the response to the actual event can result in very different outcomes and works with the patient to rehearse more realistic and positive responses.

The disadvantages of CBT are that effective treatment is intensive and lengthy, requiring training on the part of the practitioner and a significant commitment on the part of the patient. Nonetheless, HCPs can teach patients self-talk strategies and introduce the basic concepts of cognitive restructuring in brief sessions. This treatment can be a therapeutic intervention that is part of an overall treatment approach for depression.

Journaling

Journaling is an approach that encourages the patient to explore his or her feelings and inner-healing resources. The patient with depression may find that journaling provides access to emotions that are difficult to identify and express through verbal interaction. Baldwin (1990) writes of returning from despair with a deepened sense of discovery and connection. The author notes that the spiritual journey often takes us through darkness, and that through the process of surrender, we may emerge changed and strengthened. Persons who suffer from depression often feel as though their world has lost its order and predictability and that nothing will ever be the same. Baldwin (1990) suggests that persons who experience this type of despair write in their journals about what is happening. These persons might answer the following questions: (1) "What do I know intuitively about this time in my life?" (2) "What assumptions am I letting go of?" and (3) "What is despair teaching me to pay attention to?" (Baldwin, 1990, pp. 97-99).

As a form of release and self-exploration for persons with mood disorders, Copeland (1999) recommends journaling. Persons with depression and bipolar disorder commented on how they had found journaling to be therapeutic. Benefits include keeping a chronology of the illness, releasing emotions, tracking progress, freeing up feelings, thus making it easier to talk about them in therapy, and avoiding internalizing negative thoughts. Box 2-8 gives suggestions that may be helpful for journal writing. See also the section on anxiety for journaling information.

Guided Imagery

Guided imagery has benefits for individuals with mood disorders. If the patient is severely depressed, concentrating on the guided imagery may be difficult. However, if the patient is able to focus, guided imagery may facilitate an awareness of feelings. (See Box 2-6

Box 2-8

Suggestions for Journaling

1. Rule one is that there are no rules. The journal is whatever you want it to be and can include anything you choose to put in it. Poetry, drawings, scribbles, bad grammar, profanity, and prayer are all acceptable in journal entries. The journal is not meant to meet anyone else's approval.
2. Select journal materials to which you feel connected. Some people choose journals with covers that have symbolic meaning or special beauty. Some people prefer to use simple notebooks or tablets. Some people use the computer; others prefer paper and pencil. The main point is to use materials with which you are comfortable and will be drawn to use.
3. Consider what your intent is in journaling. Setting a conscious intention sometimes helps access deeper levels of awareness. If this idea seems too intimidating or your intention is unclear, simply allow whatever evolves to unfold.
4. Do not feel obligated to journal every day. You may find that you use your journal more when you need to process life changes or emotions and less during more stable periods.
5. Do not edit your journal entries. The value of the entries is in their uncensored content, even if they provoke discomfort.

Noble, 2002.

---

for a guided imagery script example for relaxation.) Naparstek (1994) includes a script for depression in her book *Staying Well with Guided Imagery*, as well as audiotapes that focus on bringing emotions into awareness (www.healthjourneys.com). Because depressed people often experience a detachment from their feelings, guided imagery can be a means of unblocking energy and gaining access to emotions.

Guided imagery exercises are intended to promote a sense of calm and an opportunity to focus on pleasant images. Initially, most patients benefit from someone actually guiding them through the process rather than simply listening to a recording. After they have practiced and are comfortable with the imagery process, patients may find recordings helpful. When guiding patients in imagery the HCP should be familiar with the selected script and be able to read it in a calm unhurried manner. The presence of the HCP provides reassurance and support, while allowing an opportunity to evaluate the patient's response.

Before beginning, patients should have physical needs met, thus avoiding distractions. In addition, a room in which no interruptions will occur, assuring privacy and quiet, is important. Most scripts are approximately 10 minutes. Ambient gentle music may facilitate the imagery and may help create a relaxing environment. After the session is done, patients are given a few minutes to remain with the experience and note any reactions. Patients maintain control over the imagery and can choose to create whatever images they find healing. Guided imagery has few complications or risks. However, patients who are psychotic and vulnerable to auditory or visual hallucinations may not be able to control the content of the images and are not good candidates for imagery.

Music

Music is a complementary intervention that can be used alone or combined with guided imagery. Campbell (1997) describes clinical applications for music, including for depression. Bonney (1990), a psychologist and music therapist, has combined music and guided imagery in her healing work and named her approach, "Guided Imagery and Music" (GIM). Conducting research on the healing effects of music since the 1970s, Bonney's organization, the Bonney Foundation, now trains people to use guided imagery and music in the context of healing.

Gardner (1990), a musician-researcher who has used various forms of music, includes chanting and droning in her healing work. The author contends that music has great healing potential. According to Gardner, music that is created with the deliberate intention of providing emotional or spiritual peace will have a more profound effect on people than will secular or popular music that is written without a particular intention. For example, Gardner has a musical composition for patients with AIDS that is centered on the tones of F-sharp, the key that resonates most with the heart-thymus-lung area. Gardner focused on this area because of the power of the heart chakra in healing, the significance of the thymus in immune function, and the diseases of the lungs associated with AIDS. Gardner selected instruments that would evoke a sense of despair (bassoon and contrabassoon) and then raises the listener out of despair into hope (flute, harp, and vibraphone). When creating healing music, Gardner considers the frequencies of the instruments, the correspondences of the tones with the chakras, and the proportions of the music. Two of Gardner's healing pieces are "A Rainbow Path" (1984) and "Viriditas" (1989). Other recommended contemporary healing music composers include Constance Demby, Steven Halpern, George Deuter, and Georgia Kelly (Gardner, 1990).

Two studies of effects of music therapy with depressed adolescents include one by Field (1998) who examined shifts in right frontal EEG activity and cortisol levels. Field studied depressed teens who listened to selected pieces of both rock and classical music. Although the teens did not self-report significant changes in their moods, shifts in EEGs occurred toward frontal symmetry and salivary cortisol levels were reduced, both findings that may be consistent with a decrease in depression. Both the rock music and the classical music were calming for the teens, although three subjects preferred only the classical music. In Guerra's (1998) study of teens who were depressed resulting from grief issues, subjects were randomly assigned to either a conventional therapy group or a music therapy group. In the music therapy group, the teens shared music they had selected, played instruments as a means of self-expression, and wrote their own songs. The teens in the music therapy group showed significantly greater improvement on depression inventories than the control group.

Considering the musical tastes of patients is important when selecting music. Even though a piece may be designed to promote a certain effect, the response may be negative if the music is too different from the listener's taste. If possible, music that has a rhythm of 60 to 70 beats per minute should be included so that the body can entrain itself to this rhythm, simulating a resting heart rate. Patients may not react to any music if it is listened to continuously; thus listening times should be scheduled at intervals.

Bonney (1990) suggests that sedating music may be appropriate for some situations, although stimulating music is better for others. Some music, including New Age music, may be too unfocused and dreamy for the depressed patient, who may prefer music that is more energetic. Thompson (1993) has composed a series of compositions entitled *Brainwave Suite* that is intended to stimulate desired brain wave patterns, producing alpha, beta, theta, and delta patterns.

Exercise

Exercise may be an effective antidepressant therapy for many people, and strength training may be as effective as is aerobic exercise. Exercise raises the levels of serotonin and norepinephrine metabolites, raises levels of endorphins, and releases opioid peptides. Exercise also increases oxygen flow to the brain. The psychologic benefits of exercise include a sense of well being and control. A review of 14 clinical studies by Tkachuk and Martin (1999) found significant benefits of aerobic exercise for depressed patients and improvement in mood after implementation of a regular exercise program.

Blumenthal and colleagues (1999) studied 156 older adults who were assigned to one of three regimens: (1) 30 minutes of exercise three times a week, (2) the antidepressant sertraline (Zoloft), or (3) both exercise and Zoloft. After 6 months, the group who exercised had more positive outcomes than did the other two groups. The researchers suggested that the subjects who just exercised might have had a greater sense of control over the outcomes than did the groups who took medication.

Before suggesting an exercise program for depressed patients, HCPs should follow some of the suggestions made by Sime (1996):

1. Advise patients over age 50 or with preexisting medical conditions to have a physical examination before beginning any exercise program.
2. Explore the patient's exercise history to develop a plan consistent with the patient's interests and abilities.
3. Educate the patient about the potential benefits of exercise to promote commitment.
4. Take advantage of the patient's environment (e.g., lakes, walking paths, fitness trails).
5. Help the patient develop the program from a broad spectrum of activities.
6. Encourage exercise with others to promote socialization and increase motivation.

Prayer and Spiritual Support

Distress of the human spirit is an appropriate diagnosis for patients who are struggling with the pain of depression. Patients who are in the deep despair of depression often feel that they have lost their sense of purpose and connection. Styron (1992) describes depression as the loss of faith that life will ever be restored to normal. The author writes about his experiences with depression in terms of going from pain to pain, rather than from one daily event to another. Dossey (1999a) notes that the most significant difference between alternative and conventional medicine is the alternative practitioner's acceptance of the role of spirituality in healing. In addition, some research supports the role of spirituality. Shuler and colleagues (1994) looked at the effects of spiritual or religious practices on psychologic well being among inner-city homeless women. Women who perceived prayer as an effective coping mechanism reported significantly fewer worries and depressive symptoms. Furthermore, the use of prayer was significantly related to less use of alcohol, street drugs, or both (Shuler et al., 1994). Baetz and colleagues (2002) reported similar findings among a group of patients in a Canadian tertiary care psychiatry inpatient unit. Findings from their study indicated an association between the use of private spirituality, which included prayer, and lower depressive symptoms, as well as less current alcohol use.

In *Healing Words* (1993), Dossey lists studies in which prayer had a healing effect. Mackenzie and colleagues (2000) found significant relationships in elderly patients between religious or spiritual health and the ability to cope with negative life events. Studies have demonstrated that patients who score high on measures of religiosity or spirituality have more rapid remissions from depression than do those with lower scores (Mackenzie et al., 2000). Luckoff (2000), a psychologist who focuses on spiritual aspects of mental health and illness, points out that many mind-body interventions are grounded in religious traditions and that many mental illnesses are more appropriately characterized as "spiritual emergencies."

The participants in Mackenzie's study (2000) did not want HCPs to participate actively in their religious practices with them (preferring to leave that to clergy). However, patients want to have their spiritual concerns addressed during illness. HCPs can assist patients in several ways. Assessing spiritual needs is a starting point. HCPs often address spirituality in the form of a question such as, "Do you go to church?" However, this question does not touch on the essence of spirituality. Spirituality is a part of a person whether or not they attend a house of religious practice or subscribe to a religious doctrine. Because a difference exists between spirituality and religious practice, a more pertinent area of questioning is asking what a person's spiritual practices are, what gives a sense of meaning and purpose, and how that spirituality is expressed in their lives.

If the patient wishes to have spiritual or religious connection, the HCP can refer to clergy or to a spiritual counselor or incorporate a form of prayer as part of care. Dossey (1999b) discusses prayer as intention *plus* love, noting that some people would also add a term for "the absolute." A way HCPs can incorporate prayer for themselves and their patients in a general meaningful way is by letting go of attachment to outcomes, asking for the greatest good, and setting healing intention with loving kindness and care. In addition, intercessory prayer (being prayed for by others) may be helpful (Byrd, 1988; Harris, 1999).

Another way of maintaining spiritual connection during times of crisis is that of ritual. HCPs should create a respectful and private space for patients in residential or institutional settings in order to engage in spiritual or religious ritual. Prayer and meditation can be part of the healing environment, and HCPs need to consider ways that these practices can be incorporated without personal bias or judgment (inpatient and outpatient). Setting aside private time, using music and books or materials that are sacred or have special meaning, and finding a sense of sacred space through intention and respect are suggestions to promote ritual.

HCPs often identify their interventions in terms of what they *do* for their patients. Taylor (2002) suggests that spiritual care relies more on "being" than on doing, based on the presence of a healing relationship between HCP and patient. Thus if HCPs engage in centering and mindfulness, and focus their work on caring intention, spiritual presence is developed through the reverence for healing, rather than through actual spoken words. By being fully present, listening with an open heart, and accepting the experiences of the patient without need to "fix" or change things, HCPs create an environment in which patients feel comfortable addressing the spiritual aspects of depression. Table 2-13 lists mind-body-spirit interventions for depression.

BIOLOGIC-BASED THERAPIES FOR DEPRESSION

Dietary Supplements

Despite studies showing benefits from dietary changes and vitamin supplements, skepticism exists among mainstream psychiatrists about nutritional theories of mental illness. The lack of education about nutrition in most medical schools may be a factor (Miller, 1996). A number of studies suggest that the symptoms of major psychiatric disorders may be related to subclinical deficiencies of vitamins, particularly B vitamins and folic acid. Miller (1996) notes that a deficiency of thiamine causes symptoms of depression, anxiety, neurologic impairment, and mental confusion, and that a deficiency of niacin causes symptoms that closely resemble psychosis. In addition, depressed patients may have anorexia and eat sporadically, focusing on carbohydrates.

Murray (1999), a naturopathic physician (ND), makes specific dietary recommendations for individuals suffering from depression. These include eliminating caffeine, reducing fat intake, including at least five servings of fruits and vegetables per day, a moderate protein intake, and increasing the amounts of whole grains and complex carbohydrates in the diet. Murray also recommends vitamin and mineral supplements in the treatment of depression. Murray believes that deficiencies in Vitamins B6 and B8, folate, Vitamin B12, magnesium, and zinc can lead to depression, particularly in women (Horrigan, 1999). Weil (1995) recommends reducing the intake of protein and fat and increasing the intake of fresh fruits and vegetables, as well as a daily regimen of supplements.

Amino Acids   Because depletion of the neurotransmitters norepinephrine and serotonin appears to be a factor in depression, dietary supplementation with their precursor amino acids may be helpful. The timing and choices of food intake affect the conversion of tryptophan and tyrosine into serotonin (Miller, 1996). Miller (1996) cites a number of controlled studies investigating possible therapeutic uses of amino acid precursors, particularly tryptophan and tyrosine. The FDA removed L-tryptophan from the market in 1989 after at least 37 deaths and over 1500 incidents of eosinophilia myalgia syndrome, attributed to a contaminated supply of L-tryptophan. In the United States and Canada, L-tryptophan now is available only by prescription. The FDA issued a cautionary statement that advises consumers to avoid L-tryptophan because of continued concerns about the

Table 2-13 Mind-Body-Spirit Interventions Depression Intervention

Intervention	Management	Treatment Regimen	Cautions, Precautions, Interactions	References
Affirmations	Reduces depression, anger the patient feels he or she does not have a right to have or for hopelessness	Affirm "I now go beyond other people's fears and limitations. I create my life" (Hay, 2000, p. 28) (Positive statements, personal, present tense)	No precautions or interactions	Hay, 2000
CBT	Decreases negative thought patterns associated with depression	Teach strategies of thought stopping, reframing, decatastrophising Rehearse with patient Provide guidelines See Box 2-8	No precautions or interactions Evaluate response	Castelman, 1996 Reinecke et al., 1998 Clarke et al., 1999
Journaling	Helps express thoughts and feelings Facilitates self-reflection and exploration		No precautions or interactions	Baldwin, 1990 Copeland, 1999
Guided imagery	Promotes exploration of feelings Calms and relaxes	Quiet environment Structured time Tapes or CDs: Miller's	Not recommended for patients with psychotic depression	Miller, 1980, 1981, 1989; Naparstak, 1991, 1993,

		Healing Journey, I Can, or *Easing into Sleep;* Naparstek: *Healing Trauma, Depression, Grief, Stress I* and *Stress II* or *Affirmations, Relationships I* and *II, Self-Confidence and Peak Performance, Alcohol and Drug Recovery, General Wellness* or *Healthful Sleep*	while symptoms are present Assess response May "unlock" emotions from which patient is detached	1994, 1995, 1999, 2000
Music therapy	Offers nonverbal form of expression Calms and relaxes	Involve patient in music selection Structured time Quiet environment	No precautions or interactions	Campbell, 1997 Gardner, 1990 Guerra, 1998
Exercise	Improves mood Promotes sense of active control	Involve patient in planning activities Select exercise that will interest patient	Recommend physical examination if participant is over age 50 or has medical conditions Consider age, physical health of patient	Tkachuk, Martin, 1999 Freeman, Lawlis, 2001 Sime, 1996

Continued

Table 2-13 Mind-Body-Spirit Interventions Depression Intervention—cont'd

Intervention	Management	Treatment Regimen	Cautions, Precautions, Interactions	References
Exercise, cont'd			Encourage proper attire and safety equipment	
Prayer and spiritual support	Provides positive coping, support, and guidance	Assess needs Respect spiritual beliefs, practices Incorporate personal and intercessory prayer as appropriate Offer support and referrals as appropriate Provide privacy, space for ritual Set intention for highest good	No precautions or interactions	Anandarajah et al., 2001 Baetz et al., 2002 Byrd, 1988 Dossey, 1995, 1999a, 1999b Harris et al., 1999 Hebert et al., 2001 Luckoff, 2000; Mackenzie et al., 2000 Shuler et al., 1994 Styron, 1992

CBT, *Cognitive-behavioral therapy*

safety of the supply. However, patients can still get L-tryptophan benefits from dietary sources such as milk, chicken and turkey, beans, nuts, and soy products.

L-tryptophan is converted to 5-HTP, which can then be converted to serotonin. Murray (1994) discusses the efficacy of tryptophan, L-tyrosine, and 5-HTP in the treatment of depression. Murray states that 70% of 5-HTP is converted to serotonin, compared with only 3% of L-tryptophan, therefore exerting a much stronger antidepressant effect. A Swiss 1991 double-blind study comparing 5-HTP (100 mg two to three times daily between meals) to fluvoxamine (Luvox) showed a decrease in symptoms on the Hamilton Depression Scale with both treatments, but the percentage of decrease was slightly higher in the 5-HTP group (60.7% versus 56.1%). In addition, the 5-HTP group reported significantly fewer side effects than did the fluvoxamine group (Poldinger et al.,1986). Patients need to combine 5-HTP with adequate B vitamins, because B vitamins, especially vitamin B6, are necessary for the absorption of amino acids. Murray recommends dosages of 100 mg to 200 mg of 5-HTP three times a day. Safety during pregnancy and with children has not been established. Individuals with bipolar disorder, or those who are taking another antidepressant, should not take 5-HTP without medical supervision. 5-HTP may exacerbate manic states and may produce a synergistic serotonin syndrome if combined with other serotonin-enhancing drugs (Murray, 1996).

S-adenosyl-L-methionine   S-adenosyl-L-methionine (SAM-e) is another supplement that is possibly effective for depressed patients. SAM-e is distributed in "virtually all tissues and fluids" and "contributes to the synthesis, activation and/or metabolism of hormones, neurotransmitters, nucleic acids, proteins, phospholipids, and some drugs" (PL/PL, 2002, p. 1111). The dose is from 400 to 1600 mg/day (1600 mg/day most commonly used in clinical trials). SAM-e can cause GI upset, thus it should be increased gradually and as tolerated. Murray (1996) recommends gradually increasing the daily dose over 20 days up to a maintenance dose of 400 mg qid. Patients with bipolar disorder should not take SAMe, because it may produce or exacerbate manic episode.

Fatty acids   Pizzorno and Murray (1998) suggest that because the brain is rich in fatty acids, and fatty acids are responsible for maintaining the fluidity of nerve cell membranes, fatty acids may influence the transmission of the neurotransmitters norepinephrine and serotonin. An association has been established between depression and low-fat diets, and researchers suspect deficiency of omega-3 fatty acids (Wells et al., 1998; Hibeln, Salem, 1995). Weil (1999) recommends eating salmon, sardines, and other fish high in omega-3 fatty acids several times a week, or sprinkling ground flaxseed on soup and cereal. In a 4-month double-blind study in 30 patients with bipolar disorder, comparing omega-3 fatty acids to placebo, the omega-3 group had significantly longer periods of remission and better control of symptoms than did the placebo group (Stoll et al., 1999). The authors of the study suggest that omega-3 fatty acids inhibit neuronal activity in a manner similar to lithium carbonate and valproate.

Herbal therapy St. John's wort (*Hypericum perforatum*) has been used for years in Europe as an effective treatment for mild-to-moderate depression and for other psychologic conditions. St. John's wort appears to block the reuptake of serotonin, and to a lesser extent, may block the reuptake of norepinephrine and dopamine. Murray and Pizzorno (1998) cite 25 double-blind controlled studies in which St. John's wort was more effective than was either placebo or conventional antidepressants and had fewer side effects than did the antidepressants. Linde and colleagues (1996) report the findings of a metaanalysis of 23 randomized trials of St. John's wort, most of which were done in Germany. The authors found that the results showed that St. John's wort is as effective as is standard antidepressant therapy but with fewer reported side effects. Some studies have found that St. John's wort is slightly less effective than is tricyclic antidepressants (TCAs), although more effective compared with placebo (Gaster, Holyrod, 2000).

HCPs who suggest St. John's wort to patients should be aware of certain cautions. Any significant severe depression, especially when accompanied by suicidality, should be evaluated by a psychiatrist, psychologist, or mental health practitioner. St John's wort may decrease the effectiveness of indinavir and other protease inhibitors, thus it is not advised for patients with AIDS. Because of the mild monoamine oxidase inhibitory effect, patients should be advised to follow a low-tyramine diet, avoiding sources that are especially high in tyramine: aged, smoked, pickled and fermented foods and beverages such as wine and over the counter antihistamines and cold remedies. St. John's wort can reduce the effectives of digoxin, theophylline, warfarin, and oral hormonal contraceptives. St. John's wort can also interfere with the effectiveness of immunosuppressants such as cyclosporin, thus it should not be advised for transplant patients. Use with triptans (5-HT1 agonists) may increase the risk of serotonergic adverse effects and possibly serotonin syndrome (PL/PL, 2002). Finally, St. John's wort should not be combined with other antidepressants because of the risk of serotonin syndrome (PL/PL, 2000).

The recommended dose for St, John's wort is commonly 300 mg three times a day (PL/PL, 2002). Occasional side effects include GI irritation and photosensitivity. As with all herbal medications, it is important for HCPs to remind patients to include St. John's wort in any list of medications they report. Table 2-14 lists biologic-based therapies for depression.

MANIPULATIVE AND BODY-BASED AND ENERGY THERAPY FOR DEPRESSION

Massage
In a small study, Field (2000) describes positive results on depression with massage. The author studied 32 depressed adolescent mothers and compared massage with relaxation therapy. The massage group showed reduced stress and depression across the course of the study.

Light Therapy
Depression that occurs during the winter months and improves as the hours of daylight lengthen in spring is termed *seasonal affective disorder* (SAD). An estimated 25 million people in the United States suffer from SAD (Liberman, 1991). SAD is viewed as a dysregulation of the pineal gland resulting from lack of sunlight. As patients spend an increasing number of hours indoors exposed to artificial light, they are deprived of the benefits of full-spectrum light. The pineal gland regulates the secretion of hormones in circadian rhythms and synchronizes them with the external environment. The pineal gland secretes melatonin throughout the 24-hour cycle, peaking during the early hours of the night and decreasing during daylight (Liberman, 1991). Lewy and colleagues (1980) are credited with discovering that bright artificial light may suppress melatonin secretion.

The SAD form of depression differs from other forms of depression in that the patient's appetite increases and there is a tendency to sleep for long stretches of time. Many patients describe SAD as similar to wanting to hibernate after storing up calories for the long winter.

A double-blind study, with one group exposed to dim yellow light and the other group exposed to full-spectrum light, found dramatic improvement with the full-spectrum light and no improvement noted with the yellow light (Rosenthal et al., 1984). The subjects exposed to the full-spectrum light self-reported having increased energy, feeling "wonderful," feeling productive and being able to return to normal activities. This study established light therapy as a viable treatment for SAD (Liberman, 1991). The patients who had the best response were those whose symptoms included carbohydrate craving, hypersomnia, afternoon and evening lethargy, and worsening of symptoms in the evening. Nonresponders, by comparison, were more seriously ill and more likely to show vegetative symptoms,

Table 2-14 Biologic-Based Therapies for Depression (see complete prescribing and precaution information before using the following products)

Intervention	Management	Treatment Regimen	Cautions, Precautions, Interactions	References
Diet, 5-HTP, vitamins, SAM-e, Omega-3 fatty acids	May decrease symptoms of mild-to-moderate depression	Eliminate caffeine, reduce fat and protein intake Include at least five servings of fruits and vegetables every day Increase intake of whole grains and omega-3s, Dl-phenylalanine, B complex Folic acid, vitamin B6, inositol (B8), vitamin B12; vitamin C; vitamin E; 5-HTP 150-300 mg qd	Do not combine 5-HTP with antidepressants (TCAs, SSRIs, MAOIs) 5-HTP and SAM-e are contraindicated for those with bipolar disorders 5-HTP may cause seizures in some patients with Down syndrome SAM-e may cause GI upset Safety of 5-HTP and SAM-e are not established for use by children and pregnant women	Hibbeln et al., 1995 Miller, 1996 Murray, 1994 PL/PL, 2002 Stoll et al., 1999 Weil, 1998, 1999 Wells et al., 1998

| St. John's wort (Hypericum perforatum) | Decreases symptoms of mild-to-moderate depression | SAM-e: start with 200-400 mg bid; on day 10, take 400 mg tid; at 3 weeks, start maintenance dose of 400 mg qid

300 mg tid extract standardized to 0.3% hypericin was usual dose in trials; other doses depend on type of preparation | Do not take over-the-counter cold medications with St. John's wort

Follow low-tyramine diet

St. John's wort may interfere with oral contraceptives, digoxin, certain immunosuppressants, protease inhibitors, triptans, theophylline, warfarin (decreases protime) | Gaster, Holyrod, 2000
Murray, Pizzorno, 1998
Murray, 1996
PL/PL, 2002 |

Continued

Table 2-14 Biologic-Based Therapies for Depression (see complete prescribing and precaution information before using the following products)—cont'd

Intervention	Management	Treatment Regimen	Cautions, Precautions, Interactions	References
St. John's wort (Hypericum perforatum), cont'd			St. John's wort may cause photosensitivity Do not combine St. John's wort with other antidepressants May induce psychosis in those with Alzheimer's dementia	

bid, *Twice daily*; GI, *gastrointestinal*; 5-HTP, *5-hydroxytryptophan*; MAOIs, *monoamine oxidase inhibitors*; qd, *every day*; qid, *four times daily*; SAM-e, *S-adenosyl-L-methionine*; SSRIs, *selective serotonin reuptake inhibitors*; TCAs, *tricyclic antidepressants*; tid, *three times daily*.

suicidality, guilt, and worsening of symptoms in the morning (Terman, 1996; Stuart and Laraia, 2001).

Liberman (1991) recommends six 40-watt full-spectrum fluorescent tubes the equivalent of 2500 lux, although new light sources provide as much as 10,000 lux. The length of time the patient sits in front of the lights may range from 30 minutes to 4 hours, depending on the brightness of the lights, the amount of normal sunlight exposure, and the patient response. Most patients report better effects with morning rather than evening exposure.

Drawbacks to this therapy include the time involved and the cost of the lights. Some patients have reported eyestrain, nausea, irritability, and headache (Stuart, Laraia, 2001). Increasing the distance the patient sits from the lights and avoiding looking directly into the light can usually address these effects. Patients can use lights as an adjunct to antidepressant therapy with minimal adverse effects (Castleman, 1996).

Other Energy Work

HT, TT, Shen, and Reiki may promote a sense of relaxation and well being and can be effective caring interventions for patients with depression. HT or TT sessions start with setting the intention to provide the highest good for the receiver, and this intention is communicated in the caring nature of the treatment. Easter (1997) reviewed the current nursing literature on HT to evaluate the quality of research. Several of the studies demonstrated benefits of decreased anxiety and increased sense of well being. Hughes (1996) studied the effects with seven psychiatric inpatient adolescents who received TT over a 2-week period. The responses included feeling relaxed, feeling less angry, having more energy, and being better able to express their feelings appropriately. One subject described the treatment: "It feels like you're in a shield and it takes you to a faraway place" (Hughes 1996, p. 15).

When using TT with depressed patients, Krieger (1993) suggests focusing on the spleen and liver. Krieger also advises focusing on the kidney adrenal area over the solar plexus chakra. The movements should be slow, gentle, and rhythmic. The nurse should use unruffling throughout the treatment to facilitate movement of energy to and through the foot chakras. Simply unruffling the energy field may be helpful for people who feel "blocked" or tense. TT or HT can be effective interventions for patients who are uncomfortable with physical touch. The patient must always give consent for the treatment. Any actual physical contact must be used cautiously with psychiatric patients, particularly those with a history of abuse or sexual trauma. Table 2-15 lists energy therapies for depression.

Table 2-15 Manipulative and Body-Based and Energy Therapies for Depression

Intervention	Management	Treatment Regimen	Cautions, Precautions, Interactions	References
Massage therapy	Relieves depression	30 min/day on 2 consecutive days for 5 wks was used in study of depressed adolescent mothers	Check for allergy to lotion or oil Some patients may not be comfortable with massage	Field, 2000
Light therapy	Reduces symptoms SAD	Patient sits in front of 10,000 lux, full-spectrum lights for 30 mins/day Better response reported when used early in the day Length of time depends on amount of normal sunlight exposure and patient response	Some reports of eyestrain, nausea, irritability, headache Do not look directly into light	Lewy et al., 1980; Rosenthal et al., 1984 Liberman, 1991 Castleman, 1996

HT and TT	Promote relaxation	HCP centers and sets intention	Obtain permission	Easter, 1997
	Reduce anxiety	Quiet calm environment	Assess patient tolerance for physical contact (especially if patient is paranoid or has history of sexual abuse)	Hughes, 1996
	Help access emotions	Preparation of patient		Krieger, 1993

HCP, *Health care provider;* HT, *healing touch;* SAD, *seasonal affective disorder;* TT, *therapeutic touch,*

REFERENCES

Achterberg J, Dossey B, Kolkmeier L: *Rituals of healing: using imagery for health and wellness*, New York, 1994, Bantam Books.

Alberti R, Emmons M: *Your perfect right*, San Luis Obispo, Calif, 1990, Impact.

Aldridge D: Alzheimer's disease: rhythm, timing and music as therapy, *Biomed Pharmacother* 48:275, 1994.

Allen J, Schneyer R, Hitt S: The efficacy of acupuncture in the treatment of major depression in women, *Psychol Sci* 5:397, 1998.

American Holistic Nurses Association: *AHNA standards of holistic nursing practice*, Flagstaff, Ariz, 2000, The Association.

Anandarajah G, Hight E: Spirituality and medical practice: using the HOPE questions as a practical tool for spiritual assessment, *Am Fam Phys* 63(1):81, 2001.

Antonovsky A: *Unraveling the mystery of health*, San Francisco, 1987, Jossey-Bass.

Baetz M et al: Canadian psychiatric inpatient religious commitment: an association with mental health, *Can Psychiatr Assoc J* 47(2):159, 2002.

Baldwin C: *Life's companion: journal writing as a spiritual quest*, New York, 1990, Bantam Books.

Barrett B, Kiefer D, Rabago D: Assessing the risks and benefits of herbal medicine: an overview of scientific evidence, *Altern Ther Health Med* 5(4):40, 1999.

Bauer W, Dracup K: Physiologic effects of back massage in patients with acute myocardial infarction, *Focus Crit Care* 14(6):42, 1987.

Bensky D, Gamble A: *Chinese herbal medicine materia medica*, Seattle, 1986, Eastland Press.

Benson H: The relaxation response. In Goleman D, Gurin J, editors: *Mind body medicine: how to use your mind for better health*, Yonkers, NY, 1993, Consumer Report Books.

Blumenthal J et al: Effects of exercise training on older patients with major depression, *Arch Intern Med* 19:2349, 1999.

Blumenthal M, Goldberg A, Brinckman J: *Herbal medicine: expanded Commission E monographs*, Newton, Mass, 2000, American Botanical Council.

Blumenthal M, senior ed: *The complete German Commission E monographs: therapeutic guide to herbal medicines*, Newton, Mass, 1998, American Botanical Council.

Boericke W: *New manual of homoeopathic materia medica and repertory*, New Delhi, 2000, B. Jain Publishers.

Bonney H, Savory L: *Music and your mind*, Barrytown, NY, 1990, Station Hill Press.

Bourne E: *The anxiety and phobia workbook*, Oakland, Calif, 1990, New Harbinger.

Braun C, Layton J, Braun J: Therapeutic touch improves residents' sleep, *Am Health Care Assoc J* 12(1):48, 1986.

Buckle J: The role of aromatherapy in nursing care, *Nurs Clin North Am* 36(1):57, 2001.

Buckle J: The 'M' technique, *Massage and Bodywork* 15(1):52, 2000.

Buckle J: *Clinical aromatherapy in nursing*, San Diego, Calif, 1997, Singular.

Buckle J: Aromatherapy: does it matter which lavender essential oil is used? *Nurs Times* 89:32, 1993.

Butler R: Warnings about melatonin, *Geriatrics* 51(2):16, 1996.

Byrd RC: Positive therapeutic effects of intercessory prayer in a coronary care unit population, *South Med J* 81:826, 1988.

Cameron J: *The artist's way*, New York, 1992, Putnam.

Campbell D: *The Mozart effect: tapping the power of music to heal the body, strengthen the mind, and unlock the creative spirit*, New York, 1997, Avon Books.

Castleman M: *Nature's cures*, Emmaus, Penn, 1996, Rodale Press.

Clarke G et al: Cognitive-behavioral therapy of adolescent depression: efficacy of acute group treatment and booster sessions, *J Am Acad Child Adolesc Psychiatry* 38:272, 1999.

Copeland M: *Living without depression and manic depression: a workbook for maintaining mood stability*, Oakland, Calif, 1999, New Harbinger Publications.

Cummings S, Ullman D: *Everybody's guide to homeopathic medicine*, New York, 1996, Tarcher Putnam.

Davidson J et al: Homeopathic treatment of depression and anxiety, *Altern Ther Health Med* 3:46, 1997.

Davies H, Robinson D: Supportive group experiences for patients with early-stage Alzheimer's disease, *J Am Geriatr Soc* 43(9):1068, 1995.

Davis M, Eshelman E, McKay M: *The relaxation and stress reduction workbook*, Oakland, Calif, 2000, New Harbinger Publications.

Davis M, Eshelman E, McKay M: *The relaxation and stress workbook*, Oakland, Calif, 1998, New Harbinger Publications.

Deadman P, Al-Khafaji M: The treatment of psycho-emotional disturbance by acupuncture with particular reference to the Du Mai, *J Chin Med* 47:30, 1995.

der Marderosian A: *The review of natural products*, St Louis, 2001, Facts and Comparisons.

Ellis A: *A new guide to rational living*, North Hollywood, Calif, 1975, Wilshire Books.

Dossey B: Holistic nursing: taking your practice to the next level, *Nurs Clin North Am* 36(1):1, 2001.

Dossey B: On holistic nursing, Florence Nightingale and healing rituals, *Altern Ther Health Med* 5(1):78, 1999.

Dossey B, Guzzetta C: Exploring the process of change. In Dossey B, editor: *Holistic nursing: a handbook for practice*, ed 2, Gaithersburg, MD, 1995, Aspen.

Dossey L: You people: intolerance and alternative medicine, *Altern Ther Health Med* 5(2):12, 109, 1999a.

Dossey L: Healing and the non-local mind, *Altern Ther Health Med* 5(6):4, 1999b.

Dossey L: *Healing words*, San Francisco, 1993, Harper.

Dreher H: Immune power personality, *Noetic Sci Rev*, Autumn:13, 36, 1996.

Dreher H: *The immune power personality: 7 traits you can develop to stay healthy*, New York, 1995, Dutton.

Easter A: The state of research on the effects of therapeutic touch, *J Holistic Nurs* 2:158, 1997.

Egan E: Therapeutic touch. In Snyder M, Lindquist R, editors: *Complementary/alternative therapies in nursing*, New York, 1998, Springer.

Eliopoulos C: Sleep and rest. *Integrating conventional and alternative therapies*, St Louis, 1999, Mosby.

Ernst E, Rand J, Stevinson C: Complementary therapies for depression: an overview, *Arch Gen Psychiatr* 55:1026, 1998.

Facts and Comparisons: *The review of natural products*, St Louis, 2001, Facts and Comparisons.

Fetrow C, Avila J: *Complementary and alternative medicines*, Springhouse, Penn, 1999, Springhouse.

Field T: *Touch therapy*, Philadelphia, 2000, Churchill Livingstone.

Field T: Music shifts frontal EEG in depressed adolescents, electronic version, *Adolescence*, 1998. Retrieved 5/27/2001 from the World Wide Web: http://www.bedfordmartins.com/online/cite6.html.

Field T et al: Labor pain is reduced by massage therapy, *J Psychosom Obstet Gynaecol* 18:286, 1997.

Field T et al: Massage and relaxation therapies' effects on depressed adolescent mothers, *Adolescence* 31:903, 1996.

Fischer-Rizzi S: *Complete aromatherapy handbook: essential oils for radiant health*, New York, 1990, Sterling Publishing.

Freeman L, Lawlis F: *Complementary and alternative medicine: a research based approach*, St Louis, 2001, Mosby.

Frisch N, Frisch L: *Psychiatric mental health nursing*, Albany, NY, 1998, Delmar.

Froehle RM: Ear infection: a retrospective study examining improvement from chiropractic care and analyzing for influencing factors, *J Manipulative Physiol Ther* 19(3):169, 1996.

Fruehauf H: Commonly used Chinese herb formulas for the treatment of mental disorders, *J Chin Med* 48:21, 1995.

Gach M: *Acupressure's potent points*, New York, 1990, Bantam.

Gagne D, Toye RC: The effects of therapeutic touch and relaxation therapy in reducing anxiety, *Arch Psychiatr Nurs* 8:184, 1994.

Gardner K: *Sounding the inner landscape: music as medicine*, Stonington, Maine, 1990, Caduceus.

Gardner K: *A rainbow path*, LR 103, LP, cassette and CD, Durham, NC, 1984, Ladyslipper Records.

Gardner K: *Garden of ecstasy*, LR 197, cassette and CD, Durham NC, 1989, Ladyslipper Records.

Garfinkel D et al: Facilitation of benzodiazepine discontinuation by melatonin, *Arch Intern Med* 159:2456, 1999.

Garfinkel D et al: Improvement of sleep quality in elderly people by controlled-release melatonin, *Lancet* 346:541, 1995.

Gaster B, Holyrod J: St. John's wort for depression: a systematic review, *Arch Intern Med* 160:152, 2000.

Gerard RM: "Differential Effects of Colored Lights on Psychophysiological Functions," PhD dissertation, UCLA, 1958.

Gerber R: *Vibrational medicine for the 21st century*, New York, 2000, Harper Collins.

Glass TA et al: Population based study of social and productive activities as predictors of survival among elderly Americans, *BMJ* 319:478, 1999.

Glenmullen J: *Prozac backlash*, New York, 2000, Simon and Schuster.

Gordon W: *Sleep: A guide for health professionals*, Stanford, Calif, 1986, Cortex Research and Development.

Great Smokies Diagnostic Laboratory: *Functional assessment resource manual*, Asheville, NC, 1999, The Laboratory.

Guerra P: *Team of researchers reach depressed youth through music therapy*, 1998. Retrieved 5/27/2001 from the World Wide Web: http://www.counseling.org/ctonline/archives/ct0598/music.htm.

Guerrero M: The effects of therapeutic touch on state-trait anxiety level of oncology patients, *Masters Abstracts International* 24(3):252, 1986. (University Microfilms No 1326756.)

Guilleminault C et al: Nondrug treatment trials in psychophysiologic insomnia, *Arch Intern Med* 155:838, 1995.

Hale E: A study of the relationship between therapeutic touch and the anxiety levels of hospitalized adults, *Dissertation Abstracts International* 47:1928B, 1986. (University Microfilms No. ADG86—18897.)

Hammer L: *Dragon rises, red bird flies: psychology and Chinese medicine*, New York, 1990, Station Hill Press.

Harris WS et al: A randomized, controlled trial of the effects of remote, intercessory prayer on outcomes in patients admitted to the coronary care unit, *Arch Intern Med* 159:2273, 1999.

Hauri P: *Current concepts: the sleep disorders*, Kalamazoo, Mich, 1982, Upjohn.

Hebert RS et al: Patient perspectives on spirituality and the patient-physician relationship, *Gen Intern Med* 16(10):685, 2001.

Heidt P: Effect of therapeutic touch on anxiety level of hospitalized patients, *Nurs Res* 30:32, 1981.

www.herbalgram.org (2002), ABC release on kava safety.

Hibeln JR, Salem N: Dietary polyunsaturated fatty acids and depression: when cholesterol does not satisfy, *Am J Clin Nutr* 1:1, 1995.

Hoffmann D: *The complete illustrated holistic herbal*, Rockport, Mass, 1996, Element.

Horrigan B: Michael Murray ND: a natural approach to health, *Altern Ther Health Med* 5(2):76, 1999.

Huebscher R: Pets and animal-assisted therapy, *Nurse Pract Forum* 11(1):1, 2000.

Hughes P, Meize-Grochowski R, Harris C: Therapeutic touch with adolescent psychiatric patients, *J Holistic Nurs* 14(1):6, 1996.

Jones A: *Yoga: a step-by-step guide*, Boston, 1998, Element.

Johnson J: Progressive relaxation and the sleep of older noninstitutionalized women, *Appl Nurs Res* 4(4):165, 1991.

Johnston J: Sleep problems in the elderly, *J Am Acad Nurse Pract* 6(4):161, 1994.

Kobasa S et al: Effectiveness of hardiness, exercise, and social support as resources against illness, *J Pschosom Res* 29:525, 1985.

Kornfield J: *The inner art of meditation*, 1996, videotape. Boulder, Colo, Sounds True.

Kramer NA: Comparison of therapeutic touch and casual touch in stress reduction of hospitalized children, *Pediatr Nurs* 16:483, 1990.

Krieger D: *Accepting your power to heal*, Santa Fe, NM, 1993, Bear and Co.

Kuhn M: *Complementary therapies for health care providers*, Philadelphia, 1999, Lippincott.

Lad V: The complete book of Ayurvedic home remedies, New York, 1998, Three Rivers Press.

Landolt H et al: Caffeine intake (200 mg) in the morning affects human sleep and EEG power spectra at night, *Brain Res* 675:67, 1995.

LaValle J et al: *Natural therapeutics pocket guide*, Hudson, Ohio, 2000, Lexi-Comp.

Lett A: *Reflex zone therapy for health professionals*, Edinburgh, 2000, Churchill Livingstone.

Lewy A, Wehr TA, Goodwin FK: Light suppresses melatonin secretion in humans, *Science* 210:1267, 1980.

Leathwood PD et al: Aqueous extract of valerian root (*Valeriana officinalis L*) improves sleep quality in man, *Pharmacol Biochem Behav* 17(1):65, 1982.

Leathwood PD, Chauffard F: Aqueous extract of valerian reduces latency to fall asleep in man, *Planta Med* 51(2):144, 1985.

Liberman J: *Light: medicine of the future*, Santa Fe, NM, 1991, Bear and Co.

Lieberman S, Bruning N: *The real vitamin and mineral book*, Garden City Park, NY, 1997, Avery.

Lindahl O, Lindwall L: Double blind study of a valerian preparation, *Pharmacol Biochem Behav* 32(4):1065, 1989.

Linde K et al: Saint John's wort for depression–an overview and meta-analysis of randomized clinical trials, *BMJ* 313:253, 1996.

Linville P: Self-complexity and affective extremity: don't put all your eggs in one cognitive basket, *Social Cognition* 3(1):94, 1985.

Lockie A, Geddes N: *Homeopathy: the principles and practice of treatment*, London, 1995, Dorling Kindersley Limited.

Loo M: Complementary/alternative therapies in select populations: children. In Spencer J, Jacobs J, editors: *Complementary/alternative medicine: an evidence-based approach*. Edinburgh, 1999, Churchill Livingstone.

Luckoff D: The importance of spirituality in mental health, *Altern Ther Health Med* 6:80, 2000.

Luks A: *The healing power of doing good*, New York, 1992, Fawcett Columbine.

Luskin F et al: Complementary/alternative therapies in select populations: elderly persons. In Spencer J, Jacobs J, editors: *Complementary/alternative medicine: an evidence-based approach*, Edinburgh, 1999, Churchill Livingstone.

Maciocia G: *The foundations of Chinese medicine*, New York, 1989, Churchill Livingstone.

Maciocia G: *The practice of Chinese medicine*, New York, 1994, Churchill Livingstone.

Mackenzie E et al: Spiritual support and psychological well-being: older adults' perceptions of the religion and health connection, *Altern Ther Health Med* 6:37, 2000.

Macrae J: *Therapeutic touch: a practical guide*, New York, 1987, Knopf.

McCabe V: *Practical homeopathy*, New York, 2000, St. Martin's Griffin.

McClelland D: Motivational factors in health and disease, *Am Psychol* 44(4):675, 1989.

McIntyre A: *The complete woman's herbal*, New York, 1994, Henry Holt.

Medalie JH, Goldbourt U: Angina pectoris among 10,000 men: psychosocial and other risk factors, *Am J Med* 60:910, 1976.

Meek S: Effect of slow stroke back massage on relaxation in hospice clients, *Image* 25(1):17, 1993.

Meisenhelder JB, Chandler EN: Prayer and health outcomes in church members, *Altern Ther Health Med* 6:56, 2000.

Miller E: "Healing Journey" and other stress relief tapes. 1-800-52-TAPES.

Miller M: Diet and psychological health, *Altern Ther Health Med* 2(5):40, 1996.

Miller M: Diet and psychological health: a case study, *Altern Ther Health Med* 4:54, 1998.

Munte TF: Effects of oxazepam and an extract of kava roots (*Piper methysticum*) on event-related potentials in a word recognition task, *Neuropsychobiology* 27:46, 1993.

Murray M: A natural approach to health, *Altern Ther Health Med* 2:76,1999.

Murray M: *Natural alternatives to prozac*, New York, 1996, William Morrow.

Murray M: *Natural alternatives to over-the-counter drugs*, New York, 1994, William Morrow.

Murray M, Pizzorno J: Insomnia. In Pizzorno J, Murray M, editors: *Textbook of natural medicine*, vol 2, Edinburgh, 1999, Churchill Livingstone.

Murray M, Pizzorno J: *Encyclopedia of natural medicine*, ed 2, Rocklin, Calif, 1998, Prima Publishing.

Namikoshi T: *Shiatsu: Japanese finger pressure therapy*, New York, 1995, Japan Publications.

Naparstek B: *Healthful sleep*, Akron, Ohio, 2000, Image Paths.

Naparstek B: www.healthjourneys.com. Numerous CDs and tapes available.

Naparstek B: *Staying well with guided imagery*, New York, 1994, Warner Books.

NCCAM web site: http://www.nccam.nih.gov/fi/concepts/rfa/at-00-003.html

Nixon M et al: Expanding the nursing repertoire: the effect of massage on post-operative pain, *Aust J Adv Nurs* 14:21, 1997.

Novey D: *Clinician's complete reference to complementary and alternative medicine,* St Louis, 2000, Mosby.

Parkes B: Therapeutic touch as an intervention to reduce anxiety in elderly hospitalized patients, *Dissertation Abstracts International* 47:573B, 1985. (University microfilms No 8609563.)

Peightel J, Hardie T, Baron D: Complementary/alternative therapies in the treatment of psychiatric illnesses. In Spencer J, Jacobs L, editors: *Complementary/alternative medicine,* St Louis, 1999, Mosby.

Pennebaker JW: *Opening up: the healing power of confiding in others,* New York, 1990, William Morrow.

Peters D, Chaitow L, Harris G, Morrison S: Integrating complementary therapies in primary care. Edinburgh, 2002, Churchill Livingstone.

Pettinati P: Meditation, yoga and guided imagery, *Nurs Clin North Am* 36(1):47, 2001.

Pharmacists' Letter/Prescriber's Letter: *Natural medicines comprehensive database,* ed 4, Stockton, Calif, 2002, Therapeutic Research Faculty.

Pharmacists' Letter/Prescriber's Letter: Insomnia. In natural medicines in clinical management, Stockton, Calif, 2002, Continuing Education Booklet.

Phelps S, Austin N: *The assertive woman,* San Luis Obispo, Calif, 1987, Impact.

Pittler M, Ernst E: Efficacy of kava extract for treating anxiety: systematic review and meta-analysis, *J Clin Psychopharmacol* 1:84, 2000.

Pizzorno J, Murray M, Joiner-Bey H: *The clinician's handbook of natural medicine,* Edinburgh, 2002, Churchill Livingstone.

Poldinger W, Calanchini B, Schwarz W: A functional-dimensional approach to depression: serotonin deficiency as a target syndrome in a comparison of 5-Hydroxytryptophan and fluvoxamine, *Psychopathol* 24:53, 1991.

Quinn J: Therapeutic touch as energy exchange: replication and extension, *Nurs Sci Q* 2(2):79, 1989.

Quinn J: Building a body of knowledge: research on therapeutic touch 1974-1986, *J Holistic Nurs* 6(1):37, 1988.

Quinn J: Therapeutic touch as energy exchange: testing the theory, *Adv Nurs Sci* 6(2):42, 1984.

Raina P, et al: Influence of companion animals on the physical and psychological health of older people: An analysis of a one-year longitudinal study, *J Am Geriatric Soc* 43(3):323, 1999.

Ram Dass: *Journey of awakening: a meditator's guidebook,* New York, 1978, Bantam.

Randolph G: Therapeutic and physical touch: physiological response to stressful stimuli, *Nurs Res* 33:33, 1984.

Reinecke M, Ryan N, DuBois D: Cognitive behavioral therapy of depression and depressive symptoms during adolescence: a review and meta-analysis, *J Am Acad Child Adolesc Psychiatr* 37:26, 1998.

Richards KC: Effect of a back massage and relaxation intervention on sleep in critically ill patients, *Am J Crit Care* 7:288, 1998.

Robins J: The science and art of aromatherapy, *J Holist Nurs* 17(1):5, 1999.

Rosenthal N: *Seasons of the mind,* New York, 1989, Bantam.

Rosenthal N et al: Seasonal affective disorder: A description of the syndrome and preliminary findings with light therapy, *Arch Gen Psych* 41:72, 1984.

Ross J: *Acupuncture point combinations: the key to clinical success,* Dallas, 1995, Churchill Livingstone.

Roth B, Creaser T: Mindfulness meditation-based stress reduction: experience with a bilingual inner-city program, *Nurse Pract* 22(3):150, 1997.

Rowe M, Alfred D: Effectiveness of slow-stroke massage in diffusing agitated behavior in individuals with Alzheimer's disease, *J Gerontol Nurs* 25(6):22, 1999.

Russek L, Schwartz G: Narrative descriptions of parental love and caring predict health status in midlife: a 35-year follow-up of the Harvard mastery of stress study, *Altern Ther Health Med* 2(6):55, 1997.

Ryu H et al: Acute effect of Qi gong training on stress hormonal levels in man, *Am J Chin Med* 24(2):193, 1996.

Schulz J et al: Glutathione, oxidative stress and neurodegeneration, *Eur J Biochem* 16:4904, 2000.

Sharma H, Clark C: *Contemporary ayurveda*, Philadelphia, 2000, Churchill Livingstone.

Shealy CN: *The illustrated encyclopedia of healing remedies*, Boston, 1998, Element Books Limited.

Shuler PA et al: The effects of spiritual/religious practices on psychological well-being among inner city homeless women, *Nurs Pract Forum* 5:106, 1994.

Sime WE: Guidelines for clinical applications of exercise therapy for mental health. In Van Raalte JL, Brewer BW, editors: *Exploring sport and exercise physiology*, Washington, DC, 1996, American Psychological Association.

Sime WE: Exercise in the prevention and treatment of depression. In Morgan WP, Goldston SE, editors: *Exercise and mental health*, Washington, DC, 1987, Hemisphere.

Skinner S: *An Introduction to homeopathic medicine in primary care*, Gaithersburg, MD, 2001, Aspen.

Smith M et al: Benefits of massage therapy for hospitalized patients: a descriptive and qualitative evaluation, *Altern Ther Health Med* 5:64, 1999.

Snyder M: Journal writing. In Snyder M et al, editors: *Complementary/alternative therapies in nursing*, New York, 1998, Springer.

Snyder M, Cheng W: *Complementary/alternative therapies in nursing*, New York, 1998, Springer.

Snyder M, Egan E, Burns K: Efficacy of hand massage in decreasing agitation behaviors associated with care activities in persons with dementia, *Geriatr Nurs* 16(2):60, 1995.

Solomon GF et al: Prolonged asymptomatic stats in HIV seropositive persons with fewer than 50 CD4+ T-cells/mm3: preliminary psychoimmunologic findings, *J AIDS* 6(10):1173, 1993.

Solomon GF, Kemeny ME, Temoshok L: Psychoneuroimmunologic aspects of human immunodeficiency virus infection. In Ader R, Felton DL, Cohen N, editors: *Psychoneuroimmunology II*, New York, 1991, Academic Press.

Solomon GF et al: An intensive psychoimmunologic study of long-surviving persons with AIDS, *Ann N Y Acad Sci* 496:647, 1987.

Sosa et al: The effect of a supportive companion on perinatal problems, length of labor, and mother-infant interaction, *N Eng J Med* 303:597, 1980.

Stoll A et al: *Study results omega-3 fatty acids in bipolar disorder*, 1999, Department of Psychiatry, Harvard Medical School. Retrieved 2/16/2001 from the World Wide Web: http://www.ncbi.nlm.nih.gov/entrez/query.

Stuart G, Laraia M: *Principles and practice of psychiatric nursing*, ed 7, St Louis, 2001, Mosby.

Styron W: *Darkness visible: a memoir of madness*, New York, 1992, Vintage.

Sunshine W et al: Fibromyalgia benefits from massage therapy and transcutaneous electrical stimulation, *J Clin Rheumatol* 2(1):18, 1996.

Tavola T et al: Traditional Chinese acupuncture in tension-type headache: a controlled study, *Pain* 48:325, 1992.

Taylor E: *Spiritual care: nursing theory, research and practice*, Upper Saddle River, N.J., 2002, Prentice Hall.

Terman M, Terman JS, Williams D: Seasonal affective disorder and its treatments, *J Pract Psychiatr Behav Health* 5:287, 1998.

Thoits P, Hewitt L: Volunteer work and well-being, *J Health Social Behav* 42:115, 2001.

Thompson J: *Brainwave suite*, Roslyn, NY, 1993, Relaxation Company.

Tkachuk G, Martin G: Exercise therapy for patients with psychiatric disorders: research and clinical implications, *Prof Psychol Res Pract* 30:275, 1999.

Volz HP, Kieser M: Kava-kava extract WS 1490 versus placebo in anxiety disorders–a randomized placebo-controlled twenty-five week outpatient trial, *Pharmacopsychiatry* 1:1, 1997.

Wang S, Kain Z: Auricular acupuncture: a potential treatment for anxiety, *Anesth Analg* 92(2):548, 2001.

Weil A: Natural help for depression, *Self Healing* (newsletter), p. 1, September 1999.

Weil A: *Spontaneous healing*, New York, 1995, Alfred Knopf.

Weinberger DA, Schwartz G, Davidson RJ: Low-anxious, high-anxious, and repressive coping styles: psychometric patterns and behavioral and physiological responses to stress, *J Abnorm Psychol* 88:369, 1979.

Wells AS et al: Alterations in mood after changing to a low fat diet, *Brit J Nutr* 1:23, 1998.

White J: Music as intervention, *Nurs Clin North Am* 36(1):83, 2001.

www.ninds.nih.gov/health_and_medical/pubs.sleep and restless leg syndrome (2002) accessed Dec 19, 2002.

CHAPTER 3

RESPIRATORY CONCERNS

Roxana Huebscher ▪ Helen Miller ▪ Louise Rauckhorst

NAC THERAPIES FOR RESPIRATORY CONCERNS

This chapter outlines NAC therapies for common outpatient respiratory concerns, including upper respiratory infection (URI), sinusitis, otitis media (OM), pharyngitis, influenza, asthma, and allergy, as well as discussing a few NAC therapies for less common conditions, such as cystic fibrosis and tuberculosis. Depending on diagnosis, a variety of treatments are available for respiratory concerns. However, most people with respiratory complaints can also benefit from routine "natural" respiratory care. For example, recommended treatment for acute bronchitis, in otherwise healthy adults, is now symptomatic therapy rather than antibiotics (Gilbert et al, 2001; WARN, 2000). Some sinusitis and otitis media have the same recommendations, although children under age 2 are treated with antibiotics for otitis media (Berman et al, 2001; Gilbert et al, 2001). Thus health care practitioners need to know comfort measures and symptomatic therapies as part of natural-alternative-complementary (NAC) routine care. Box 3-1 outlines routine therapies that are useful with many respiratory conditions. Box 3-2 is a honey and lemon cough syrup recipe, and Box 3-3 is a recommended nasal wash for sinusitis. In addition to the ways that the National Jewish Hospital recommends for the sinus wash in Box 3-3, a netti pot can be used to administer the solution. A netti pot is a small glass pot that looks similar to an Aladdin's lamp. The thin spout can be fit into the nostril while the head is held parallel to the floor. The saline is poured into one nostril until it runs out the other nostril; then the other side is done.

ALTERNATIVE HEALTH CARE SYSTEMS FOR COMMON RESPIRATORY CONCERNS

Ayurveda
For the common cold, one herb that may be useful, if started within 48 to 72 hours of symptoms, is *andrographis:* "Although [*andrographis*] is used for a wide variety of indications in Ayurvedic and herbal medicine, clinical evidence of effectiveness in humans is limited to the common cold" (PL/PL, 2002, p. 69-70). However, people also use the herb for influenza, pharyngitis, allergies, and sinusitis. The

Box 3-1

Routine Natural Respiratory Care

Increased fluids
Frequent hand washing
Rest
Honey and lemon cough syrup (NO HONEY SHOULD BE GIVEN TO CHILDREN UNDER 2 YEARS OF AGE)
Saline gargles for sore throat
Saline nasal spray for nasal congestion and saline nasal washes for sinus congestion
New toothbrush now and when symptoms are gone
Warm packs to ears or sinuses for pain
A few drops of warm (not hot) oil (e.g., olive) into ear canals for pain (only if the eardrum is not perforated)
Chicken soup
Vitamin C, approximately 500-2000 mg/day
Zinc gluconate or acetate lozenges within 24 hours of onset of common cold symptoms

Box 3-2

Honey and Lemon Cough Syrup Recipe: An Old Home Remedy

Mix one part honey to nine parts lemon juice (an adequate portion is 1 teaspoon of honey to 9 teaspoons of lemon juice). Lemon juice can be from a natural lemon or the bottled concentration of pure juice. Heat the mixture just long enough to blend. The mixture will be thin. Place in a clean small bottle or glass with cover. Take 1 teaspoon as needed for cough. No specific interval is needed between doses. Make fresh daily. NO HONEY SHOULD BE GIVEN TO CHILDREN UNDER 2 YEARS OF AGE.

(Huebscher, 2002)

herb is thought to have immunostimulant properties; it may increase antibodies and phagocytosis by macrophages. Theoretically, andrographis may interfere with immunosuppressants (PL/PL, 2002).

Traditional Chinese Medicine
Astragalus, a traditional Chinese herb, seems to affect the immune system and has been used for cold and influenza; evidence at this time

Box 3-3

Nasal Wash Treatments for Adults

1. Wash hands.
2. Make nasal wash solution.
Mix:
    ½ tsp uniodized salt (Iodized salt can cause irritation if used over a long period.)
    8-oz glass of warm water
    A pinch of baking soda (a small amount that you can pick up between two fingers)
    After you are finished with wash, discard what is not used; make solution fresh daily.
3. Perform nasal wash. For extreme congestion, use the full 8 ounces; otherwise, 4 ounces is usually enough. Lean far over the sink with head down when ready to do nasal wash.
Method I—Use a large ear (bulb) syringe, which can be purchased at most drug stores. Fill syringe with saltwater. Insert the tip just inside the nostril and pinch nostril around tip of the bulb syringe to keep the solution from running out of the nose. Gently squeeze the bulb to swish the solution around in the nose; then blow nose lightly. Repeat in other nostril.
Method II—Use a Water Pik with a Grossan Nasal Irrigator Tip. Pour the saltwater into the water reservoir, and set the Water Pik at the lowest possible pressure. Insert the tip just inside the nostril and allow the fluid to run out of the mouth or other nostril. Blow nose lightly. Repeat in other nostril.
Method III—Wash hands. Pour some saltwater into palm, then sniff the liquid up the nose, one nostril at a time. Blow nose lightly. This technique may not be as effective compared with other methods.
4. Thoroughly clean equipment *after each use* to prevent the growth of bacteria. Nasal washes may be performed several times a day. Fill the bulb with hot water; swish the water around, and empty completely. Suspend the bulb with the syringe tip down in a clean glass to allow the bulb to drain completely. Do not allow the bulb tip to sit in a puddle of water. Once a day, rinse out the syringe with 70% isopropyl alcohol; draw alcohol into syringe, swish, and empty completely. Again, suspend the bulb with tip down in a clean glass.
    For the Grossan nasal adaptor, wipe with a clean, wet cloth after each use; and once a week, flush it through with a weak chlorine solution (one part bleach to nine parts water). Rinse thoroughly with two to three cycles of fresh water.

Adapted from National Jewish Medical and Research Center: Medfacts. Nasal wash treatment, *2000, Patient Information Sheet.*

in support of this herb is weak: "Population studies show that people consuming astragalus tend to have a lower occurrence of the common cold. But there are no clinical studies showing it works" (PL/PL, 2000, p. 4). Lower doses seem to stimulate the immune system, whereas higher doses (greater than 28 grams per day) seem to suppress the immune system. Astragalus may possibly interact with acyclovir, immunosuppressants, or cylclophosphamide (PL/PL, 2000).

Large Intestine 4 and 20, and the extra bitong point (along the edge of the nasal bone in the groove along the nose), are accupressure points for URI and sinus conditions. Stomach 2, a small notch in line with the pupil below the eye, is used if tenderness is present at this area. Appendix B lists the locations of the accupressure meridians and points.

Homeopathy

Homeopathic treatments are available for OM, otitis externa, sore throats, colds, coughs, sinus problems, and bronchitis, as well as asthma and allergy (Boericke, 2000; Cummings, Ullman, 1997; Skinner, 2001). A trained homeopathic practitioner needs to assess the condition for appropriate treatment because accompanying symptoms help to determine which homeopathic remedy to use.

Otitis media

OM in children has shown improvement with homeopathic treatment (Friese in Loo, 1999):

> In a prospective clinical study of children between 1 and 11 years of age, homeopathic treatment of 103 children was compared with conventional treatment of 28 children. Homeopathic remedies were found to be more effective in reducing pain and preventing relapses. (Friese in Loo, 1999, p. 374)

Numerous homeopathic remedies are available for respiratory conditions. Some of the common treatments for OM are *Apis mellifica, Belladonna, Chamomilla, Ferrum phosphoricum, Hepar sulphuris calcareum,* and *Pulsatilla.* Less commonly indicated homeopathic treatments for OM include *Calcarea carbonica, Capsicum annuum, Gelsemium sempervirens, Kali bichromicum, Lachesis mutus, Lycopodium clavatum, Mercurius vivus or solubilis, Tuberculinum,* or *Tuberculinum aviare.* Again, these treatments have symptomologic indications for use. Accompanying symptoms determine which treatment to use (Skinner, 2001). For example, *Apis mellifica* is used when there is a red, inflamed external ear that is sore with "stinging pain," whereas *Belladonna* is used when "the tympanic membrane is very red and bulging, often associated with reddened throat, cold extremities, and pounding throbbing pain in the ear," and it is commonly a "right-sided otitis that comes on suddenly" accompanied by "high fever with bright red face and glassy appearance of the eyes; diminished thirst; sensitive to being jiggled and jarred, may occur with difficult dentition" (Skinner, 2001, p. 188). *Chamomilla* is used when the pain from the earache makes the child scream, cry, or produce an irritable whine, and relief comes when the child is carried around, becoming angry if put down, which can be from teething. The "child asks for various things that are rejected when offered." There may be thirst, clear nasal discharge, green stool, one red and one pale cheek. (Skinner, 2001, p. 189).

Sinusitis

Similarly, sinusitis homeopathic remedies vary with symptoms. The most commonly indicated medicines are *Hepar sulphuris calcareum*, *Kali bichromicum*, *Mercurius vivus* or *Mercurius solubilis*, *Pulsatilla*, and *Silice*. Less commonly indicated medicines for sinusitis are *Bovista*, *Hydrastis canadensis*, *Mercurius sulphuratus ruber*, *Sticta pulmonaria*, and *sulphur*.

For example, *Hepar sulphuris calcareum* is used when there is soreness at root of nose, painful obstruction in the nose, and "thick, offensive nasal discharge smelling like old cheese." The patient is chilled and "sensitive to drafts." There may also be "pharyngitis that extends to ears with swallowing." *Mercurius vivus* or *Mercurius solubilis* is used when there is green or yellow discharge, a "metallic taste, offensive perspiration and breath. Alternately chilly and warm; tongue holds indentations from teeth" (Skinner, 2001, p. 212-213).

Pharyngitis and tonsillitis

Skinner (2001) states that the homeopathic treatment for pharyngitis depends on the quality and distribution of the pain, tonsillar swelling, alleviation or aggravation by cold or warm drinks, whether swallowing is painful with or without food, and other distinct symptoms. The most commonly indicated remedies are *Arsenicum album*, *Hepar sulphuris, calcareum*, *Lachesis mutus*, *Lycopodium clavatum*, and *Mercurius vivus* or *Mercurius solubilis*.

A trained homeopathic practitioner is needed to determine the appropriate remedy. See Section II for an overview of homeopathy and the philosophy of care regarding the Law of Similars and remedy usage, remembering that homeopathic remedies are highly dilute. Table 3-1 covers alternative health care systems for a few respiratory concerns.

MIND-BODY-SPIRIT INTERVENTIONS FOR RESPIRATORY CONCERNS

Ivker (2000), a Doctor of Osteopathy, who himself once suffered from chronic sinusitis, developed and recommends regimens for both prevention and treatment of sinusitis, allergies, and asthma, as well as other common respiratory symptoms. Ivker's regimens consist of biologic-based therapies (Table 3-2), manipulative and body-based methods and energy therapies (negative-ion generators, acupressure, reflexology), and various mind-body-spirit techniques. Ivker's

Table 3-1 Alternative Health Care Systems for Respiratory Concerns

Intervention	Management	Treatment Regimen	Cautions, Precautions, Interactions	References
Ayurveda herbals (Rasayanas)	Prevention and treatment of colds and influenza. Thought to have immuno-stimulant properties. Possibly increases antibody activity and phagocytosis by macrophages.	Andrographis (Andrographis paniculata). Start within 48-72 hrs of Sx. Most trials used dried extract standardized to contain 4.0-5.6 mg andrographolide. For decreasing cold symptoms, a dose of 400 mg tid has been used in clinical trials. For cold prevention, 200 mg daily for 5 days each week, was used in clinical trials.	SE: GI distress, anorexia. May inhibit fertility. Interactions: theoretical interactions with anticoagulant-antiplatelet drugs, antihypertensives, immunosuppressants. Contraindicated in pregnancy and lactation. Abortifacient effects.	PL/PL, 2002

Continued

Table 3-1 Alternative Health Care Systems for Respiratory Concerns—cont'd

Intervention	Management	Treatment Regimen	Cautions, Precautions, Interactions	References
Traditional Chinese Medicine	Colds, influenza	Herbal—*Astragalus membranaceus* powder, 1-30 g/day is typically used. "Doses greater than 28 g might cause immunosuppressions" (p. 104)	Lower doses seem to stimulate the immune system, whereas higher doses seem to suppress. Some evidence suggests that long-term ingestion can decrease chance of developing URI.	PL/PL, 2002
	URI and sinus concerns	Acupressure—Large Intestine 4 and 20 (beside nose at mid-point of its widest part); the extra bitong point (along edge of the nasal bone in groove along nose); Stomach 2 (small notch in line with pupil below eye, used if pain at this area).	Appendix B lists the locations of the meridians and points.	Ivker, 2000

| Homeopathy | OM | *Apis mellifica; Belladonna; Chamomilla; Ferrum phosphoricum; Hepar sulphuris calcareum; and Pulsatilla.* Less commonly indicated homeopathic treatments for OM include *Calcarea carbonica; Capsicum annuum; Gelsemium sempervirens; Kali bichromicum; Lachesis mutus; Lycopodium clavatum; Mercurius vivus or solubilis; Tuberculinum or Tuberculinum aviare.* | Qualified homeopathic practitioner needs to do case finding. Each remedy is based on numerous signs and symptoms and not merely on the diagnosis of OM. | Skinner, 2001 |
| | Pharyngitis | *Arsenicum album; Hepar sulphuris calcareum; Lachesis mutus; Lycopodium* | Qualified homeopathic practitioner needs to do case finding. Each remedy is | Skinner, 2001 |

Continued

Table 3-1 Alternative Health Care Systems for Respiratory Concerns—cont'd

Intervention	Management	Treatment Regimen	Cautions, Precautions, Interactions	References
Homeopathy, cont'd		clavatum; Mercurius vivus or Mercurius solubilis	based on numerous signs and symptoms and not merely on the diagnosis of pharyngitis.	
	Sinusitis	Hepar sulphuris calcareum; Kali bichromicum; Mercurius vivus or Mercurius solubilis, Pulsatilla; Silice. Less commonly indicated medicines for sinusitis are Bovista; Hydrastis canadensis; Mercurius sulphuratus ruber; Sticta pulmonaria; and sulphur.	Qualified homeopathic practitioner needs to do case finding. Each remedy is based on numerous signs and symptoms and not merely on the diagnosis of sinusitis	Skinner, 2001

GI, Gastrointestinal; OM, otitis media; PL/PL, Pharmacist's Letter/Prescriber's Letter; SE, side effects; Sx, symptoms; tid, three times a day; URI, upper respiratory infection.

Table 3-2 Biologic-Based Therapies for Respiratory Concerns

A complete prescribing source should be consulted before using biologic therapies. Vitamin and mineral dosing is often higher compared with the recommended upper limit. At times of illness or deficiency, people may need more of such supplements. However, caution should be used because of little study. Any herb can cause an allergic reaction. Herbs are generally contraindicated in pregnancy and lactation and with children unless research data or a long history of safe use has been established.

Intervention	Management	Treatment Regimen	Cautions, Precautions, Interactions	References
Foods	Improve respiratory symptoms; sinusitis	Onions, garlic, ginger, hot peppers. Garlic 1 or 2 cloves/day or 1200-2000 mg tid.	An old therapy. SE: breath odor; GI upset; may not be for everyone.	www.askdrweil.com, 2001; Ivker, 2000; Murray, Pizzorno, 1999; Pizzorno et al, 2002; Rakel, 2003
	Chronic sinusitis	Omega-3 fatty acids; fish oil, cold-water fish, or flaxseed or 2 tbsp flaxseed oil/day.	Cold-water fish, including salmon, tuna, mackerel, sardines	Ivker, 2000; Rakel 2003
Elimination of certain foods	Cold, URI; chronic sinusitis	Eliminate concentrated sweets, dairy products, wheat, eggs, citrus, corn, peanut butter, and known food allergens.	Ensure adequate diet through alternate sources.	Ivker, 2000; Pizzorno et al, 2002

Continued

123

Table 3-2 Biologic-Based Therapies for Respiratory Concerns—cont'd

Intervention	Management	Treatment Regimen	Cautions, Precautions, Interactions	References
Candida-elimination diet and program	Chronic sinusitis, allergies	For people who have tried a respiratory treatment program at least 4-8 wks and have not noticed a change. Consists of assessment including history and laboratory tests. Can then use a score sheet to see possibility of *Candida* based on symptoms, signs, and laboratory work. (See Box 3-4 for sample program.)	Program may use conventional medications as well. Numerous recipe books available to ensure adequate alternate foods.	Crook, 1986; Ivker, 2000
Water	URI, acute and chronic sinusitis, bronchitis, pneumonia	1/2-2/3 oz of water/lb of body weight		Ivker, 2000

Remedy	Condition	Instructions	Comments	References
Honey and lemon cough syrup	Cough	(See Box 3-2 for one recipe.) Take 1 tsp as needed. Also can use 1:1 ratio with a pinch of cayenne pepper.	Anecdotal, old home remedy. Not for infants or young children because of honey content and possible botulism spores. May cause allergy from pollens. Has been used for asthma.	DerMarderosian, 2001; Ivker, 2000; Rakel, 2003
Saline throat gargles	Pharyngitis, laryngitis, tonsillitis	Gargle and spit with warmest water possible. (¼ tsp in ½ to 1 cup.)	Old home remedy. Do not swallow.	Rakel, 2003
Saline nasal spray Saline nasal washes	Common cold Sinusitis	Up to hourly. (See Box 3-3 for instruction.) Can also use netti pot.	Ensure clean solution. Takes practice and motivation on part of the patient. Ensure clean solution.	Ivker, 2000 National Jewish Hospital
Beta carotene or vitamin A	Sinusitis, chronic sinusitis	Adult: beta carotene 25,000 IU qd or 5000 IU of vitamin A.	Recommended adult vitamin A UL is 3000 µg/day. Limit vit A to 9000-10,000 IU upper limit daily in childbearing age. Advise smokers not to use beta carotene supplements. Caution: vitamin A is a fat-soluble vitamin.	Ivker, 2000; NAP, 2001; Pizzorno et al, 2002; PL/PL, 2002

Continued

Table 3-2 Biologic-Based Therapies for Respiratory Concerns—cont'd

Intervention	Management	Treatment Regimen	Cautions, Precautions, Interactions	References
Vitamin B6	Sinusitis, chronic sinusitis	200 mg bid with sinusitis; 50 mg bid with chronic.	Adult recommended UL is 100 mg/day. Long-term use (greater than 2 mon) of high doses can lead to sensory neuropathy.	Ivker, 2000; PL/PL, 2002
Vitamin C	Viral URI, sinusitis; chronic sinusitis. Decreases duration, severity of common cold; is a natural antihistamine.	Adult sinusitis treatment: 3000-5000 mg tid (Ivker) or 500 mg q2h (Pizzorno et al); Prevent URI: 2000 mg tid (Weil); chronic sinusitis or allergy preventive maintenance: 1000 to 2000 mg qd to tid.	Large doses can cause diarrhea. Recommended UL is 2000 mg, but bowel tolerance may vary and many recommend more to prevent or treat URI and other respiratory ailments.	Baker et al, 1995; Cohen et al, 1997; Hemila, 1997; Ivker, 2000; PL/PL, 2000; LaValle, 2000; NAP, 1999; Pelton, 2001; Pizzorno et al, 2002; www.askdrweil.com, 2001; PL/PL, 2002.

Supplement	Indication	Dosage	Notes	References
Vitamin D (also known as calciferol)	May increase resistance to and improve course of tuberculosis.	400 units/day	Adult recommended UL is 50 µg /day. (1 µg of calciferol = 40 IU of vitamin D). Fat-soluble. Stay within UL.	Fuller and Casparian, 2001; NAP, 2001; PL/PL, 2002.
Vitamin E	Sinusitis, antioxidant	Adult, 400 IU bid. Children over age 3 years, 200 IU bid.	Adult recommended UL is 1000 mg/day. Fat-soluble. Stay within UL.	Ivker, 2000; NAP, 2001
Calcium (citrate)	Sinusitis, chronic sinusitis	1000-1500 mg/day.	Recommended adult UL is 2500 mg/day	Ivker, 2000; NAP, 2001
Chromium picolinate	Chronic sinusitis; helps decrease sugar cravings when on Candida diet.	Adult: 200 µg/day. Start 6 wks into Ivker, program.	No UL set but recommended adult adequate intake set, depending on age, at 20 to 35 µg/day.	Ivker, 2000; NAP, 2001
Magnesium (citrate, aspartate, or glycinate)	Chronic sinusitis	Adult: 500 mg/day	Adult recommended UL is 350 mg/day.	Ivker, 2000; NAP, 1997
Selenium	Acute and chronic sinusitis	100-200 µg/day	Adult recommended UL is 400 µg/day.	Ivker, 2000; NAP, 2001
Zinc picolinate	Sinusitis and chronic sinusitis	Adult: 20-60 mg/day. Child over age 3 years: 10 mg bid.	Recommended adult UL is 40 mg/day. See SE below for zinc. UL for children: age 4-8 yrs, 12 mg; 9-13 yrs, 23 mg; 14-18 yrs, 34 mg.	Ivker, 2000; NAP, 2001; Pizzorno et al, 2002

Continued

Table 3-2	Biologic-Based Therapies for Respiratory Concerns—cont'd			
Intervention	Management	Treatment Regimen	Cautions, Precautions, Interactions	References
Zinc lozenges	Viral URI, allergy	For URI at beginning Sx and later Sx, dissolve lozenge in mouth made from zinc acetate or zinc gluconate-glycine (minimum dose 13 mg zinc per lozenge); every 2 hrs while awake. Lozenge must not have additives (e.g., citric acid, mannitol, or sorbitol) that decrease absorption of the zinc.	Recommended UL is 40 mg/day. SE: bad taste, nausea; renal impairment; interferes with copper absorption if taken in large amounts; unsafe in large amounts. Contraindicated for treating HIV. Zinc absorption is reduced in rheumatoid arthritis. Avoid use with glaucoma. Must have adequate zinc/copper ratio. Interactions with some tetracyclines, fluoroquinolones, potassium-sparing and thiazide diuretics.	Al-Nakib et al, 1987; Eby et al, 1984; Godfrey et al,1996; Ivker, 2000; Mossad et al, 1996; PL/PL, 2000

Agent	Use/Action	Dose	Cautions	References
Bee propolis	Acute sinusitis	Adult, 500 mg tid; children, 500 mg one time/day.	May worsen asthma due to possible allergens.	Ivker, 2000; PL/PL, 2002.
Echinacea *Echinacea purpurea* (also is *Echinacea pallida* and *Echinacea angustifolia*)	Possibly effective for . treatment of colds and influenza; PL/PL says not effective for prevention although is used for this and for acute and chronic sinusitis, allergy	Doses vary depending on form of mixture (tincture, juice, crude extract in tablets, tea). Start when Sx first appear and use for 7-10 days. Sinusitis treatment 200 mg tid or 25 gtts qid, 5 times/day.	Not for long-term use. Caution with ragweed allergy. Contraindicated in persons with HIV, collagen disorders, tuberculosis, multiple sclerosis, autoimmune disorders. May inhibit fertilization and alter sperm DNA. Which formulation or species is most beneficial is unclear.	Ivker, 2000; PL/PL, 2000, 2002
Elderberry *Sambucus nigra*	Influenza treatment—inhibits hemagglutinin activity and replication of several strains of influenza viruses A and B. Contain flavonoids and tannins.	Cooked berry juice. Adult: 4 tbsp/day for 3 days of elderberry juice-containing syrup. Child, 2 tbsp/day for 3 days. (Brand name Sambucol, JB Harris was used in study.)	Read cautions. Berries must be cooked. Raw berries can cause nausea, vomiting, severe diarrhea. Interactions: caution with diuretics.	Fetrow and Avila, 1999; LaValle, 2000; PL/PL, 2000; Zakay-Rones et al, 1995

Continued

Table 3-2 Biologic-Based Therapies for Respiratory Concerns—cont'd

Intervention	Management	Treatment Regimen	Cautions, Precautions, Interactions	References
Ginger root tea	URI symptoms	Grate 1 inch of peeled ginger root, boil with 2 cups of cold water, simmer 5 minutes. Add ½ tsp cayenne pepper and simmer 1 minute more. Remove from heat and add 2 tbsp fresh lemon juice, honey to taste and one or two cloves of mashed garlic. Cool; strain if desired (Weil).	Allergy to any ingredients. No honey to infants or young children.	www.askdrweil. com, 2001; Ivker, 2000
Goldenseal *Hydrastis canadensis*	Acute sinusitis	Dosage based on berberine content. Try standardized extract. Dried root or as infusion (tea): simmer 0.5-1.0 gram dried root or rhizome in 150 ml of boiling water for 5-10	Use short term only. Likely unsafe when used long term or high doses. Theoretical drug interactions. May decrease B-vitamin absorption with	Ivker, 2000; Pizzorno et al, 2002; PL/PL, 2002

		minutes, then strain (tid). Also is tincture, fluidextract, solid extract.	prolonged use. Has vasoconstrictive action; may interfere with blood pressure medications. SE: GI irritation and not to be taken with infectious or inflammatory GI conditions.	
Grape seed extract (Proanthocyanidin)	Sinusitis	Adult, 100 mg tid on empty stomach. Child over age 3 years, 100 mg qd.	Theoretically, because of tocopherol content, may increase effect of warfarin.	Ivker, 2000
Grapefruit seed extract	Sinusitis	Adult, 100 mg tid or 10 gtts in water. Children over age 3, 4 gtts in water bid.	Must be a preservative-free product (free of benzethonium chloride). When preservative-containing product used, can cause vomiting, collapse, convulsions, coma. Interacts with several drugs.	Ivker, 2000; PL/PL, 2002

Continued

131

Table 3-2 Biologic-Based Therapies for Respiratory Concerns—cont'd

Intervention	Management	Treatment Regimen	Cautions, Precautions, Interactions	References
Aroma-therapy	Respiratory symptoms such as cough, bronchitis, croup.	Anise, camphor, eucalyptus, menthol, peppermint, spike lavender, rosemary, clary sage, menthol. Few drops in hot bath or as inhalation (steam, on tissue)	Avoid use of undiluted essential oil. Eucalyptus has been used for tuberculosis.	Buckle, 2001; 2002; Ivker, 2000; PL/PL, 2000

bid, Twice a day; DNA, deoxyribonucleic acid; gtts, drops; HIV, human immunodeficiency virus; IU, international units; NAP, National Academy Press; PL/PL, Pharmacist's Letter/Prescriber's Letter; qd, daily; qid, four times a day; SE, side effects; Sx, symptoms; tid, three times a day; UL, upper limits—the maximum level of daily nutrient that is likely to pose no risk of adverse effects. Includes intake from food, water, and supplements; URI, upper respiratory infection.

program is set up in stages with specific steps to follow, giving some "quick fixes" for respiratory symptoms as well. Ivker's mind-body-spirit interventions include things such as air cleaners, exercise, and expression of emotion, including anger release and acknowledging, accepting, and dealing with sad, mad, and fearful emotions. "The more you allow yourself to accept, embrace, and feel both joy and pain, the greater will be your sense of emotional health" (p. 280). Ivker advocates meditation, prayer, gratitude, and intuition.

BIOLOGIC-BASED THERAPIES FOR RESPIRATORY CONCERNS

Nutritional Supplements for Upper Respiratory Infections

Numerous dietary practices, as well as supplements, including vitamins, minerals, and herbs, have been suggested for respiratory concerns such as sore throat, colds, sinusitis, and influenza. Some recommended foods and nutrients include garlic, onions, hot peppers, flaxseed or fish oil, and honey and lemon for cough, as well as increasing fluid intake. In addition, staying away from simple sugar and dairy products is also a recommendation (Ivker, 2000; Murray, Pizzorno, 1999; Pizzorno et al, 2002; PL/PL, 2002; Weil, 1999).

Zinc and vitamin C show benefit for the common cold (Godfrey et al, 1996; Hirt et al, 2000; Hemila 1997; Mossad et al, 1996; PL/PL, 2002). For example, in a randomized, double-blind, placebo-controlled study, 100 employees of the Cleveland Clinic who had developed cold symptoms in the prior 24 hours took either zinc gluconate with glycine lozenges (with 13.3 mg zinc) or a placebo calcium lozenge. The treatment group had decreased duration of colds by almost one half (median was 4.4 days for zinc and 7.6 days for placebo). Zinc participants reported fewer days of cough, headache, hoarseness, nasal congestion, nasal drainage, and sore throat, but no differences were seen in length of time they had fever, or the level of muscle aches, or scratchy throat and sneezing that they experienced. One participant dropped out of the zinc group because of side effects. The zinc group also had more side effects, including nausea and bad taste (Mossad et al, 1996). Some researchers who criticized the study believe that because zinc lozenges often have a bad taste, the participants may have known the difference between the supplement and placebo, a factor that may have compromised the study.

In addition a few other zinc lozenge studies have shown no benefit. However, these studies used different forms of zinc or had additives that decreased the absorption of the zinc. Godfrey, Godfrey, and Novick (1996) reviewed the zinc clinical trials from 1984 to 1996 and elaborated on the chemical components used in the zinc products. For example, Douglas and colleagues (1987) used a zinc preparation that was made effervescent by adding tartaric acid and sodium bicarbonate; and Farr and colleagues (1987) used citric acid to help with the taste problem. These combinations with zinc complexed the zinc in saliva, and thus essentially *no* zinc ion was available in the mouth (Godfrey et al, 1996). Using zinc gluconate or acetate without flavoring agents, citric acid, mannitol, or sorbitol is probably best (PL/PL, 2000), although without flavoring, the unpleasant zinc side effect of nausea may be more prominent.

Vitamin C appears to decrease the duration and intensity of colds (Hemila, 1997; PL/PL, 2000; Pelton et al, 2001). The exact amount to take is not known because varying amounts were used in the studies, and the individual necessary amount varies depending on usual dietary intake and individual needs. The recommended adult tolerable upper limit of vitamin C is 2000 mg per day (NAP, 2001; Pelton et al, 2001). However, some people take vitamin C until they reach bowel tolerance (since diarrhea is a side effect of excess vitamin C). Furthermore, the individual tolerable upper limit probably depends on plasma vitamin C status. In a study of college students, from 12% to 16% had marginal plasma status, and 1% to 2% had a vitamin-C deficiency; the marginal status was even more pronounced in smokers (Johnston et al, 1998). Since adequate intake and upper limit doses can vary based on individual needs and illness status, vitamin C probably can benefit students and other persons during respiratory infection.

Andrew Weil (1999), a physician and NAC advocate, recommends several nutrients and herbs for the common cold, what he calls his "home remedies." These items include vitamin C (2000 mg three times a day) to prevent colds; two cloves of raw chopped garlic mixed with food, as soon as person feel symptoms; *Echinacea purpurea* tincture in warm water or tea four times a day at the first sign of cold or influenza; zinc gluconate or zinc acetate lozenges; and ginger root tea.

Ivker (2000, 2001) has numerous biologic-based therapies for respiratory concerns, including for chronic sinusitis. Therapies include diet, vitamins, minerals, and herbs, as well as steam inhalations, nasal irrigations, and other hydrotherapy (alternate hot and cold showers, hot compresses). Ivker suggests a program of specific therapies for people who have chronic sinusitis and acute flare-ups. The biologic component includes starting with vitamins C and E, grape seed extract, a multivitamin, garlic, Echinacea, and grapefruit seed extract. Three weeks (or sooner) into the program, the patient adds beta carotene, selenium, zinc picolinate, magnesium, calcium, and goldenseal. Six weeks (or sooner) into the program, Ivker suggests vitamin B6, chromium picolinate, bee propolis, and omega-3 fatty acids. Ivker suggests time frames so patients do not become overwhelmed. If the sinus program is not working after approximately 4 weeks, Ivker suggests Candida elimination based on Crook's (1986) work. Box 3-4 provides an overview of a sample Candida-elimination

Box 3-4

General Guidelines for Candida Elimination

Phase I: Eliminate the overgrowth of Candida
Allopathic medications are used by some for this purpose.
If allopathic medications are not desired, homeopathic remedies
can be tried (e.g., Aqua Flora, Candida-Away, Myocan Combo).
Other products include Flora Balance or Latero-Flora (a strain of
bacteria bacillus laterosporus), or Candida-free (a blend of
essential aromatic oils).
A trained colon hydrotherapist can administer colonic treatments
to cleanse bowel.
Candida-control diet works more slowly and consists of increased
water and natural agents such as psyllium to eliminate colon toxicity.

Phase II: Eliminate the "fuel" for Candida through diet
Candida and hypoallergenic diet. Minimum time frame for diet is
3 to 6 months. The first 21 days, avoid starch and high-sugar
foods, including fruit.
1. Diet consists of protein and fresh organic vegetables, a limited
   amount of complex carbohydrates and fat-containing foods,
   and a small amount of fresh fruit.
   Protein: no less than 60 g/day (note: this is greater than the
   RDA for anyone under 150 lb); antibiotic- and hormone-free;
   fish, canned fish, turkey, chicken, lamb, wild game, Cornish
   hens, eggs, seeds, and nuts.
   Organic vegetables: 50% to 60% of total diet; green leafy, low
   and moderately low starch.
   Complex carbohydrates: enough to maintain energy; starchy
   vegetables (potatoes, sweet potatoes, yams, winter squash,
   pumpkin); legumes (after 21 days), whole grains (non-gluten
   grains include brown rice, millet, quinoa, amaranth); whole
   grains in limited amounts are barley, spelt, wild rice, corn,
   buckwheat, oats, cornmeal, bulgur, couscous; no wheat and
   rye the first 3 weeks; and always restrictions for food
   allergies, which can be determined with rotation diet.
   Oils: flaxseed oil 1-2 tbsp/day; extra virgin olive, canola, walnut,
   sesame oils, cold-pressed and used within 6 weeks of opening.
   Fruits: introduced after 21 days; limit to one serving per day
   until known that symptoms do not get worse.
   Yeast and mold-containing foods (fermented): introduced
   gradually (once every 3 to 4 days) after 21 days on diet and
   only if not allergic; yogurt, kefir, buttermilk, low-fat cottage
   cheese, sour cream, tofu, tempeh, miso, soy sauce, raw almond
   butter, raw sesame tahini. Dairy is discouraged, however.
2. Avoidance of sugar and concentrated sweets and sweet
   products: cakes, cookies, candy, donuts, pastries, ice cream,
   puddings, soft drinks, pies, and anything containing sucrose,
   fructose, maltose, lactose, glucose, dextrose, corn sweetener,
   corn syrup, sorbitol, manitol, honey, molasses, maple syrup,

Continued

Box 3-4

General Guidelines for Candida Elimination—cont'd

date sugar, barley malt, rice syrup, NutraSweet, saccharine, other artificial sweeteners, and table salt (if it contains sugar). To diminish sugar cravings, supplement with chromium picolinate, biotin, and a yeast-free B complex.

3. Avoidance of milk and dairy products: includes cheese, as well as rice milk (rice milk has high carbohydrate content); unsweetened soymilk is permitted; and small amount of butter is permitted.

4. Avoidance of bread and yeast-raised items, mushrooms, alcohol, white or refined flour products, processed-refined foods, and preservatives.

5. Avoidance of beef, pork, caffeine (herbal and green tea ok), fried foods, fast foods, sausage, hot dogs, vinegar, mustard, catsup, sauerkraut, olives, and pickles.

6. Avoidance of hydrogenated oils and margarine.

7. Avoidance of grapes, plums, bananas, dried fruit, and canned fruit and canned vegetables.

8. Rotate the acceptable foods; do not eat a particular food more than once every 3 to 4 days (especially grains). Freeze leftovers and use at a later date.

Phase III: Restore normal intestinal flora
Use Lactobacilus acidophilus and bifidus products. Begin after Phase I and during Phase II (about 6 weeks into program).
To ensure potency, buy only refrigerated brands with expiration date between one and 10 months from date of purchase.
Buy liquid cultures (such as yogurt culture) or powdered forms containing whey (dairy) or nondairy varieties. Buy the plain kind with no sweeteners or additives. People who are sensitive to dairy should not use yogurt as consistent source of the friendly bacteria.

Phase IV: Strengthen the immune system
Use vitamin, mineral, and herbal regimen (see Table 3-2) and biotin; other essential fatty acids such as primrose or black currant oil, amino acid supplements, adrenal-enhancing supplement.
For complete details, see the sources below.

Sources: Ivker R: Sinus survival, New York, 2000, Tarcher Putnam. Ivker R, Nelson T: Asthma survival, New York, 2001, Tarcher Putnam. Crook W: The yeast connection, New York, 1986, Vintage. The yeast connection cookbook. Rakel D: Integrative medicine, Philadelphia, 2003, WB Saunders.

diet. Some of Ivker's supplemental therapies for sinusitis treatment are included in Table 3-2. Ivker adds that if the routine is followed and problems remain, several other diagnoses need to be ruled out, including food or inhalant allergy, leaky gut syndrome, parasites, hypochlorhydria, pancreatic enzyme deficiency, *Helicobacter pylori*, hypothyroidism, and heavy metal poisoning (e.g., mercury).

Nutritional Supplements for Influenza and Tuberculosis

"Adequate levels of vitamin D may confer resistance to tuberculosis, and individuals who receive vitamin D supplements have been shown to have an improved course of the disease" (Fuller, Casparian, 2001, p. 3). Eucalyptus has been used orally for tuberculosis (Buckle, 2001; PL/PL, 2002). In addition, Echinacea and elderberry are recommended for influenza having been studied with influenza A and B (PL/PL, 2000; 2002; Zakay-Rones et al, 1995).

Aromatherapy

Although support for essential oils is sparse, anise, camphor, clary sage, eucalyptus, rosemary, spike lavender, menthol, and peppermint oil are used for cough, sinusitis, and nasal congestion (PL/PL, 2000; Buckle, 2001, 2002). These oils are for use diluted, as steam inhalation, or topical use. Table 3-2 outlines some biologic-based therapies for respiratory concerns.

MANIPULATIVE AND BODY-BASED METHODS FOR RESPIRATORY CONCERNS

Chiropractic for Otitis Media

Chiropractic has been used for OM. "A retrospective nonrandomized study of 46 children under 5 years of age receiving treatment from a single chiropractor reported decrease in otitis symptoms" (Loo, 1999, p. 374; Froehle, 1996). Because there is normally a spontaneous resolution with many of the common bacteria that cause OM, including 90% with *Moraxella catarrhalis*, 50% with *Haemophilus influenzae*, and 10% with *Streptococcus pneumoniae* (Gilbert et al, 2002), randomization and a control group would strengthen the chiropractic finding. Whether chiropractic or the natural course of the disease is at play could then be determined.

Massage for Cystic Fibrosis

Field (2000) researched 20 children with cystic fibrosis in a randomized study in which the parents were trained to do massage. A parent gave a 20-minute massage each evening at bedtime (n = 10) for 30 days. Box 3-5 outlines the massage technique used. The control group (n = 10) had a parent read to them for 20 minutes each evening. The 10 children who received massage had a significant decrease in anxiety, significant improvement in mood, and significant increase in

Box 3-5

Massage Technique for Children with Cystic Fibrosis

Starting with the child on his or her back and sitting at a 45-degree angle, the massage begins by stroking with flats of fingers.
1. Face and head area:
   a. Strokes to forehead starting from the middle with both hands and then moving toward side of face
   b. Strokes under cheekbones, using fingertips from nose to jaw (under cheekbones) and back
   c. Strokes upward from middle of jaw to sides of face
   d. Massage to outer ears, bottom to top
   e. Small circles with fingers over entire scalp
2. Neck: fingertips and flats of fingers in upward strokes from base of neck to base of skull
3. Chest:
   a. Smooth strokes along the sternum and upper ribs, using flats of fingers and palms
   b. Strokes from waist to shoulder along the side of body
4. Abdomen: following the colon
   a. Circular, clockwise strokes over the abdomen
   b. Flat, gliding clockwise strokes over the abdomen
   c. Strokes to the sides of the trunk, from waist up to the shoulder
5. Arms:
   a. Short and long strokes with thumbs to top of hand and then to palm
   b. Long, gliding strokes from wrist to shoulder
   c. Rolling arm from wrist to shoulder, using flats of hands
6. Front of legs:
   a. Long strokes from ankle, to outside at hip and back down to foot, first using one hand and then using both hands to deliver strokes
   b. Small circles over the knee
7. Foot:
   a. Strokes, using thumbs, to work top of foot from ankle to toes
   b. Circles and criss-cross strokes, using thumb, to bottom of foot
   c. Squeezes and light pulls to each toe
With the child face down:
8. Back:
   a. Criss-cross strokes, with flats of hands, from waist to neck
   b. Small circles, using fingertips, along side of spine from neck to waist

Box 3-5

Massage Technique for Children with Cystic
Fibrosis—cont'd

   c. Strokes with flats of hands from spine to side, starting at
      waist and moving up to neck and back down
   d. Strokes down back from neck to waist using flats of hands
9. Back of Legs:
   a. Strokes on outside of legs from ankle to hip
   b. Circular movements, using thumbs, to back of knee
   c. Large circles over back of calf muscle, moving from ankle to
      knee, and then flat strokes moving back and forth to ankle
   d. Continuous circles around the ankles
   e. Large circles over bottom of foot, using thumbs
   f. Shaking, rocking of leg

From: Field T: Touch therapy, *Philadelphia, 2000, Churchill Livingstone.*

peak flow readings for both the first day and the last day of massage. A depression scale was also checked; none of the children were depressed at the beginning of the study, and no changes were noted on the depression scale at the end of the study. In addition,

"parents who massaged their children also experienced reduced anxiety. Also, because parents can be easily taught to massage their children on a daily basis, this form of therapy can be considered a cost-effective method." (Field, 2000, p. 192)

ASTHMA AND ALLERGIES

Asthma morbidity and mortality has increased dramatically in the last decade, affecting 3% to 5% of the U.S. population (Slovis, Brigham, 2001). Because asthma can be a life-threatening condition, allopathic remedies are often necessary lifesavers. In addition, NAC strategies may help prevent serious events. Allergic rhinitis, or hay fever, one of several allergic conditions (along with eczema, urticaria, angioedema, and anaphylasis), is also a common human affliction. Allergy recognition and environmental control are imperative and part of natural therapy for both allergic conditions and asthma. Air pollution, dust, mold, dander, and mite and roach debris play a role in asthma occurrence and allergy exacerbations. Several NAC modalities can help those with allergy and asthma. In addition, self-care in asthma is extremely important.

Asthma is defined as "a chronic inflammatory disorder of the airways in which many cells and cellular elements play a role, in particular, mast cells, eosinophils, T lymphocytes, neutrophils, and epithelial cells" (NIH-NHLBI, 1997, p. 1), producing multiple soluble mediators such as cytokines, leukotrienes, and bradykinins (Slovis, Brigham, 2001). Diagnosis is based on clinical data and diagnostic testing, including pulmonary function studies. Making the correct diagnosis is extremely important because conditions that mimic asthma may occur; and wheezing, or lack of wheezing, neither confirms nor rules out the diagnosis.

Allergic rhinitis is associated with asthma. Up to 80% of patients with asthma also have allergic rhinitis; up to 38% of patients with allergic rhinitis have asthma; and up to 70% of children with abnormal sinus x-rays also have allergic rhinitis. Further, many individuals with chronic sinusitis have allergy as an underlying factor, and approximately 50% of children with allergic rhinitis have at least one episode of sinusitis in a 12-month period (Corren, Storms, 1998). In patients with asthma, "chronic sinus disease is directly related to severity of lower airway disease" (Byrd et al, 2000, p. 37).

Individuals with asthma may exhibit symptoms that include wheezing, breathlessness, chest tightness, and cough, especially at night or in the early morning. These symptoms are usually associated with reversible airflow obstruction (spontaneous or treated); the inflammation causes hyperresponsiveness to a variety of stimuli (NIH, 1997). Classifications of asthma include mild intermittent, mild persistent, moderate persistent, and severe persistent. In addition, certain conditions contribute to asthma, such as rhinitis, sinusitis, gastroesophageal reflux, some medications, and viral respiratory infections (NIH, 1997).

> Although allergic rhinitis presents as a localized disorder, with itching and irritation of the nose, watery nasal discharge, nasal congestion, and paroxysmal sneezing, the condition is actually a systemic IgE-mediated inflammatory disease, and more generalized symptoms, including fatigue and malaise, frequently accompany it. (Corren, Storms, 1998, p. 2)

ALTERNATIVE HEALTH CARE SYSTEMS FOR ASTHMA AND ALLERGIES

Ayurveda for Asthma

From the Ayurvedic perspective, an excess of kapha dosha in the stomach moves upward to the lungs and airways, creating spasm and blocking air movement. This condition results in asthma symptoms such as wheezing. The goal of treatment is to bring the excess kapha that is lodged in the lungs back to the stomach, from which it can be eliminated (Lad, 1998). Tirtha (1998) distinguishes three dosha-specific constellations of asthma symptoms. Dry cough and wheezing, anxiety, and timing of attacks at dawn or dusk characterize vata-type asthmatic episodes. Pitta-type asthmatic episodes are typically demonstrated with wheezing accompanied by coughing, production of yellow phlegm, irritability, and timing of attacks around midday or midnight. Kapha-type asthmatic episodes, in contrast, are characterized by wheezing accompanied by coughing with production of clear white phlegm, fluid in the lungs, and the timing of attacks mainly in the midmorning or evening. Tirtha (1998) also states that bronchial asthma "may be healed if treated when it first arises, otherwise it is only controllable" (p. 412). Janssen (1989) applied a Maharishi Ayurveda program in the treatment of 10 chronic diseases, including asthma. There were 126 patients in the uncontrolled pilot study. Improvements were seen in asthma, eczema, and chronic sinusitis as well as other conditions (Sharma et al, 1991).

Ayurvedic herbs include *Tylophora asthmatica (indica)*, a standard remedy for asthma and other respiratory tract disorders, in which mucus accumulation occurs (Hackman et al, 1999; Murray and Pizzorno, 1999). In addition, for long-term prevention, cinnamon, trikatu (an herbal formula of black pepper, pippali, and dry ginger), ginger, licorice, bay leaf, spinach juice, and pippali are recommended. To strengthen lungs, tonic herbs such as Ashwagandha, Country mallow (Bala), Chyavan Prash, Haritaki are recommended. For immediate asthma relief, Ephedra or Lobelia has been used, as well as Sitopaldi, Punarnava, pippali-pepper, onion juice, and brown mustard seed oil or paste (Frawley, Lad, 1998; Frawley, 2000; Lad, 1998; PL/PL, 2002).

Yoga, using both the breathing exercises (pranayama) and the postures (asanas), is a recommendation for asthma. Yoga has been studied and shown to produce a significant reduction in asthma medication use and number of asthma attacks and an increase in peak flow rate when compared with controls (Nagarathna, Nagendra, 1985). Mental improvements were noted in two other studies, although no improvement in lung function was noted (Ernst, 2001; Fluge et al, 1994; Vedanthan et al, 1998).

Ayurveda for Allergies

From the Ayurvedic perspective, a healthy immune system is one that is continually evolving and integrating its experiences into meaningful responses of the individual's body-mind-spirit continuum. When the relationships among body, mind, and spirit are harmonious and integrated, the immune cells are able to unerringly discriminate potential sources of nourishment from sources of toxicity. When basic harmony and integration are lacking (e.g., a doshic imbalance), the immune system may either become too aggressive or fail to perform its defensive functions. Overactive immune responses to external provocations result in autoimmune disorders (Simon, 1997).

According to Ayurvedic pathogenesis, allergies are a doshic (i.e., individual constitutional) reaction to a specific allergen (Lad, 1998). Vata-type allergies are characterized by gastric discomfort, bloating, intestinal colic, or any combination and may lead to sudden sneezing, wheezing, headache, ringing in the ears, or insomnia. Pitta-type allergic reactions result in rashes and itching, including hives, urticaria, eczema, or other allergic dermatoses. In contrast, kapha-type allergies are most often experienced in spring when environmental pollen counts increase and result in the symptoms of hay fever, colds, sinusitis, asthma, or any combination.

For effective Ayurvedic treatment of allergies, it is necessary to determine whether the allergy symptoms are of the vata, pitta, or kapha type, and then develop the treatment plan accordingly. A correspondence usually exists between the individual's basic constitution and the way allergies are demonstrated, especially if the individual's current state shows an imbalance in the same dosha that predominates in his or her basic constitution. For example, if a person whose basic constitution is highly pitta in nature is also in a state of pitta imbalance or aggravation, the individual's response to allergenic challenges would tend toward the development of a skin rash, whereas a person with a highly pitta constitution and currently aggravated kapha would be more likely to respond to allergenic challenges by developing hay fever (Lad, 1998).

Traditional Chinese Medicine for Asthma

In Oriental medicine, asthma is directly related to a deficiency of defensive energy that is based in the Lungs and Kidneys. The Spleen is also part of the imbalance because it needs to process fluids properly. (See Appendix B for location of the organ system meridians.)

The energy, or Qi (pronounced *chee*), of the Lungs is blocked by the invasion of pathogens into the Lungs. These pathogens can be allergens, viruses or bacteria, or a host of other initiating factors, including diet, exercise, or constitutional deficiencies. When the Qi is unable to move normally, the airways cannot move air. Phlegm may build up and contribute to the blockage (Maciocia, 1994).

Excess and deficiency conditions

Asthma is differentiated into excess and deficiency conditions. Excess conditions are acute and occur with sudden onset. The symptoms, including chills, aching, and dilute white sputum, resemble the onset of the common cold. The difference between a cold and asthma is that the symptoms do not resolve, and thus become internal and chronic. This condition wears down the normal Qi of the body and inhibits the body's ability to repair itself. As Lung function is impaired, breathing becomes rough and labored; coughing and wheezing result, and the phlegm becomes thicker. The phlegm may remain white, or it may become yellow and sticky, indicating that heat has become a factor. Other signs of heat are thirst, sweating, and restlessness (Maciocia, 1994).

Deficiency conditions are more chronic by comparison and are a sign that the Qi is weakened. Often in asthma, signs of both excess and deficiency will be present because the breathlessness that occurs is acute, but it stems from the inability of the Lungs, Kidneys, or Spleen (or any combination) to function normally (Deadman, 1982).

In children, the Spleen is naturally weak, so phlegm buildup and frequent exposure to viruses affect Lung function. Because children are usually able to recover from acute illnesses fairly easily, asthma is a sign that constitutional weakness may be very significant. Constitutional weakness means that a genetic predisposition is present.

In young and middle-aged adults, many factors contribute to asthma. The health care practitioner needs to assess diet, digestion, lifestyle, sleep habits, and the patient's specific symptoms to differentiate treatment.

In older adults, the Kidney energy naturally declines and may be more of a factor in addition to those previously listed. In any age group, allergies are a concern, as well as emotional triggers (Maciocia, 1994).

Traditional Chinese Medicine research

Table 3-3 lists several research studies using acupuncture for the treatment of asthma. In two of the studies, all of the measured lung function studies did not significantly improve (Biernacki and Peake, 1998; Yu and Lee, 1976), even though symptoms or well being did improve. This result may be an indication that the overall system was functioning better and the subjects felt a change in their anxiety around the breathing process because acupuncture can be regulating to the entire system. The patients may be able to rally their own resources more effectively to deal with stimuli affecting breathing, as was shown by a decrease in bronchodilator use.

Table 3-3   Research on Acupuncture for the Treatment of Asthma

Study	Type	Number	Measure	Outcome
Biernacki and Peake, 1998	Double-blind real vs. sham acupuncture with cross-over	23 patients	Respiratory function tests and Asthma Quality Life Questionnaire (AQLQ) within 1 hr and after 2 wks with each course of treatment	No difference in respiratory function with either treatment. Significant improvement in AQLQ in both groups and reduction in use of bronchodilators in both groups.
Christensen et al, 1984	Real vs. sham acupuncture	Total 17 patients. Group A = real acupuncture, 8 patients; Group B = sham acupuncture, 9 patients.	Patient diary recording morning peak flow rate (M-PEFR), evening peak flow rate (E-PEFR), number of puffs (NOP) of inhaler medication needed per day, and rating of severity of asthma symptoms. Blood samples at wk 2, 7, and 11.	M-PEFR, E-PEFR, and NOP: significant increase ($P < 0.05$) in Group A after 2 wks compared with Group B in M-PEFR and E-PEFR. No significant differences noted after that. Real acupuncture group improved significantly throughout the study. Group A decrease in med use.
Jobst et al, 1986	Real vs. sham acupuncture	24 patients total; 12 matched pairs	Patient rating of general well being, level of breathlessness, oxygen cost of exercise. Timed 6-minute walk and peak	Real acupuncture group showed improvement in all subjective ratings and 6-minute walk ($p < 0.01$). Lung function unchanged in

...either group.

Fung et al, 1986	Real vs. sham acupuncture in pediatric patients	19 patients, randomized treatment, 20 mins before exercise	expiratory flow rate (PEFR). Lung function tests during acupuncture and after exercise. Room temperature, humidity, and barometric pressure were stable.	Both real and sham acupuncture showed improvement; real acupuncture provided better protection than did sham ($p < 0.05$).
Kleijnen et al, 1991	Literature review of controlled research trials	13 trials reviewed	18 predefined methodologic criteria	Quality of studies mediocre. Results contradictory.
Tashkin et al, 1985	Real vs. sham acupuncture with cross-over	25 patients	Lung function tests and patient diary of symptoms and medication use	No significant benefit after treatment for either group.
Yu and Lee, 1976	Real vs. sham acupuncture in acute asthma attack	20 patients divided equally	Lung function tests and patient report of subjective improvement	Subjective improvement in all patients with real acupuncture. Significant increase in two of three lung function tests with real acupuncture.

Traditional Chinese Medicine treatment for asthma

The treatment strategy for asthma is to resolve phlegm, open the Lungs, and support the function of the Lungs and Spleen so as to normalize air movement. Treatment is always focused on regulating Lung Qi and stabilizing breathing. Any underlying deficiency must be supported (Scott, 1990).

In addition, acupressure can be used to treat allergies. Points include Large Intestine 4 and 20, and the extra bitong point (along the edge of the nasal bone in the groove along the nose). Stomach 2, a small notch in line with the pupil below the eye, is used if tenderness is present at this area (Ivker, 2000). Appendix B lists the locations of the meridians and points.

Homeopathy for Allergic Rhinitis

Homeopathy has been researched for perennial allergic rhinitis (Taylor et al, 2000). Fifty patients were given an oral 30 C (homeopathic doses can be X, C, or M, depending on dilution) homeopathic preparation of principal inhalant allergen or placebo. The participants receiving the homeopathic solution had significant improvement in nasal inspiratory peak flow when compared with the placebo group. The authors concluded that the "addition of these results to those of three previous trials (n = 253) showed a mean symptom reduction on visual analogue scores of 28% (10.9 mm) for homeopathy compared with 3% (1.1mm) for placebo with a 95% confidence interval (p = 0.0007)" (Taylor et al, 2000, p. 471).

Skinner (2001) lists numerous remedies for allergic rhinitis and seasonal allergies. Several treatments have to do with the eye symptoms. *Allium cepa* is for streaming eyes and nose with irritative nasal discharge, but the lacrimal discharge is not irritative, and symptoms are worse in spring and in August. *Ambrosia artemesiaefolia* is used for severe itching of the eyelids, and *Apis mellifica* is for swollen red eyelids with red conjunctiva and symptom alleviation with cool compresses. Other remedies include *Aralia racemosa*, *Arsenicum album*, *Arsenicum iodatum*, *Arum triphyllum*, *Arundo mauritanica*, *Bromium*, *Carbo vegetabilis*, *Dulcamara*, *Histaminum hydrochloricum*, *Nuxs vomica*, *Pulsatilla*, *Wyethia helenioides*. Each substance has typical symptomologic features (Skinner 2001; Fleisher, 2002).

Homeopathy for Asthma

Homeopathic remedies are available for asthma:

> One derivative version of homeopathy is "isopathy," which involves high dilutions of a preparation of the allergen(s) to which the individual is sensitive. Isopathic treatment was superior to placebo in improving symptom scores of 28 adults over 21 days in one rigorous study, though the clinical implications of this were far from certain in

view of the short duration, small sample and small effect on lung function. (Ernst, 2001, p. 214; Reilly, 1994)

Skinner (2001) lists various types of asthma and several remedies, including asthma attacks from molds and damp environments (*Blatta orientalis, Natrum sulphuricum*), asthma with nausea (*Ipecacuanha, Lobelia inflata*), and asthma with perspiration (*Sambucus nigra, Silicea, sulphur*). A trained homeopathic practitioner is essential for working with allergy and asthma. Table 3-4 lists alternative health care system treatments for asthma and allergy.

MIND-BODY-SPIRIT INTERVENTIONS FOR ASTHMA AND ALLERGIES

Having maximal environmental controls to prevent or minimize reactions is important to persons with asthma. In addition, several other mind-body-spirit interventions may be useful with asthma, including affirmations, autogenic training (AT), biofeedback, breathing techniques, hypnotherapy, imagery, journaling, meditation, prayer, and relaxation. Exercise, enough sleep, and a positive attitude also can help heal.

Environmental Controls

Numerous environmental controls are needed for asthma. The patient should identify the source of air pollution, allergens, and triggers. In addition to routine asthma work-up, Ivker and Nelson (2001) recommend a panel of tests to find sources for symptoms. These tests include a comprehensive digestive stool analysis with three ova and parasite examinations; an adrenal stress index test (saliva); food allergy testing, liver detoxification panel; intestinal permeability; and red blood cell magnesium. These tests are called *functional* laboratory tests and are different than the usual conventional lab tests.

A major factor in escalating asthma symptoms is increased sensitization to indoor allergens. Thus decreasing dust mites is important, as well as knowing other environmental triggers. To help determine allergen causes for a severe asthmatic, a home visit may be necessary (Marilyn Shutte, respiratory NP specialist, personal communication-class lecture, 3/01). "The majority [of sensitivity] is derived from cats, molds, cockroaches, and dust mites" (Brunton, Saphir, 1999, p. 67). Dust mites proliferate indoors where warm air and high humidity are present (70% to 90%), whereas in cool dry areas, such as the Rocky Mountains, the indoor allergens are more likely to be dogs, cats, and cockroaches.

Decreasing dust-mite density can decrease the expression of some asthma symptoms and nonspecific bronchial hyperreactivity but has little or no effect on symptom severity. Duration and severity of asthmatic attacks seem to depend on conditions such as a recent

Table 3-4 Alternative Health Care Systems for the treatment of Asthma and Allergies

Intervention	Management	Treatment Regimen	Cautions, Precautions, Interactions	References
Ayurveda				
Diet	Follow appropriate diet for individual's predominant dosha(s).	Avoid most dairy products, especially all cheeses, fermented and salty foods, nuts, yeast, and mushrooms.	Ascertain dosha.	Tirtha, 1998; Lad, 1998
Herbs	For asthma. Possibly effective when used by inhalation. Inhibits histamine release from mast cells in addition to other actions.	*Coleus forskohli:* 10 mg forskolin powder, using a Spinhaler inhalator, has been used.	May alter platelet aggregation. May interact with NSAIDs, antihistamines, decongestants, anticoagulants, antihypertensives. Discontinue before surgery.	LaValle, 1999; PL/PL, 2002
	Long-term asthma prevention, allergies. Possible suppression of inflammatory responses	*Tylophora indica* 250 mg qd to tid	May interact with other asthma medications. Contraindicated in serious infection, organ transplant, major	Hackman et al, 1999; LaValle, 1999; Murray and Pizzorno,

		systemic disease, recent major surgery.	1999; Gupta, 1979
Long-term prevention	Cinnamon 1 tsp and Trikatu ½ tsp. Mix with 1 cup boiling water. Take bid.		Lad, 1998
	Ginger and licorice, equal parts. Mix ½ tsp of herb mix in 1 cup water. Take bid.	Licorice contraindicated if edema, hypertension, heart failure, osteoporosis.	Frawley and Lad, 1998
	Ground bay leaf ½ tsp and ½ tsp pippali (long pepper). Mix in 1 tsp honey.	No honey to children under age 2 yr	
	Spinach juice ⅓ cup and pinch of pippali. Drink bid.		
	Ground mustard seed ½ tsp and pippali (or black pepper) ½ tsp. Steep in 1 cup hot water for 10 mins; add 1-2 tsp honey; drink bid or tid. Sip q15 min through day for better results.		

Continued

Table 3-4 Alternative Health Care Systems for the Treatment of Asthma and Allergies—cont'd

Intervention	Management	Treatment Regimen	Cautions, Precautions, Interactions	References
Ayurveda—cont'd				
Herbs, cont'd	To strengthen lungs, tonic herbs	Chyavan Prash 5 g powder or 1 tsp jelly in warm water or milk (bid).		Frawley and Lad, 1998; Tirtha, 1998; PL/PL, 2002.
		Ashwagandha 1-6 g daily in capsule or tea form	GI upset	
		Country mallow (Bala) 250 mg– 1 g/bid	Country mallow contains ephedrine and it is most concentrated in the seeds.	
		Haritaki 250-500 mg powder. Insert seven cloves in peeled banana. Keep overnight and eat the next morning. Do not eat for next hour, then drink 1 cup hot water with 1 tsp honey.	No honey to children under age 2 yr	Lad, 1998
	To dilate bronchi and reduce kapha	Low dose Ephedra CAUTION Lobelia CAUTION	READ ALL CAUTIONS. Short-term use only. Ephedra contraindicated	Frawley and Lad, 1998

	if hypertension, heart problems; both ephedra and Lobelia can immediately weaken vata, and long-term use depletes pitta and kapha	
Immediate symptom relief—general	Sitopaldi ½ tsp, Punarnava ½ tsp, pinch Pippali and abrak bhasma. Mix with several tsp honey and take entire amount a little at a time. Onion juice ½ cup and black pepper ⅛ tsp. Mix with 1 tsp honey and take at first Sx. Brown mustard seed oil or paste. Rub a little onto chest; healing to lungs. Especially good for kapha-type asthma.	If Sx severe or these treatments not working, or any Sx of heart problems, individual needs to seek immediate medical attention. Conventional asthma treatment must be available.	Lad, 1998
Breathing exercises (prana-yama)	Slow, deep, rhythmic abdominal breathing for 5 to 15 mins, bid to qid.		Castleman, 2000; Singh, 1990

Continued

Table 3-4 Alternative Health Care Systems for the Treatment of Asthma and Allergies—cont'd

Intervention	Management	Treatment Regimen	Cautions, Precautions, Interactions	References
Ayurveda—cont'd				
Yoga	For asthma: to help prevent breathing difficulties; improved respiratory function, lower respiratory rate, increased chest expansion during inspiration, increased vital capacity, and increased breath holding.	Breathing exercises (prana yama): slow, deep, rhythmic abdominal breathing for 5-10 mins tid to qid. Postures (asanas): The Bow, Cobra, and Vajrasana (sit on heels) poses and inverted poses such as Shoulder Stand and Plow.	Regimen should be developed with approval of primary care provider and supervised by an experienced yoga teacher. Perform as tolerated. Some postures may be difficult if balance is poor or if musculoskeletal problems are present.	Nagarathana, Nagendra, 1986, 1985; Sharma, Clark, 2000; Jones, 1998; Lad, 1998; Kuhn, 1999; Vedanthan, 1998
Traditional Chinese Medicine				
Acupuncture	For improving lung function: selection of points depends on the specific combination of symptoms and on the severity of	Treat daily during acute attack. When beginning treatment to stabilize chronic asthma, treat one to two times/wk for 6-8 wks, then individualize	Acupuncture points on the chest and upper back must be needled obliquely to avoid puncturing lungs.	Maciocia, 1994; Chen, Chen, 1999; Deadman, 1982; O'Connor,

	symptoms when the patient presents for treatment.	according to patient's response and needs. See Appendix B for the following points Lung 1 and 7, Urinary Bladder (UB) 13 and 43, Dingchuan. To resolve phlegm: Stomach 40, Spleen 6. To support kidney Qi: Kidney 6, UB 23. For lung heat: Large Intestine 4, Lung 5. For cough: Ren 17 and 22, Lung 6. To open chest and calm anxiety: Pericardium 6.	Bensky, 1981
Acupressure	Can assist energy of lungs and chest. Use of touch may also be calming during more acute symptoms.	Use upper back points listed above and points on chest and sternum.	Be sure emergency asthma or allergy treatment is available and used as needed.	Scott, 1990
	Allergy	Large Intestine 4 and 20, and the extra bitong point (along the edge of the nasal bone in the groove along the nose).	Ivker, 2000

Continued

Table 3-4 Alternative Health Care Systems for the Treatment of Asthma and Allergies—cont'd

Intervention	Management	Treatment Regimen	Cautions, Precautions, Interactions	References
Traditional Chinese Medicine—cont'd				
Acupressure, cont'd		Stomach 2, a small notch in line with the pupil below the eye, is used if tenderness is present at this area.		
Chinese herbal therapy is prescribed for each patient according to specific needs. Many herbs besides those listed are considered. Support for kidney, spleen, and liver may be	Examples of common herbs for asthma are: 1. Ma Huang (Herba ephedrae): opens lungs and stops wheezing. 2. Hou Po (Cortex Magnoliae Officinalis): moves phlegm and stagnation in chest. 3. Jie Geng (Radix Platycodi Grandiflori): circulates lung Qi, expels phlegm and helps	Dose will depend on patient's weight. Formulas for acute attack of asthma may be taken only until Sx stabilize; then a formula is given to ease the lungs and correct underlying pathologic condition. This formula or variation of it may be taken for 6 mos.	An experienced herbalist must be consulted to prescribe herbal formulas accurately and safely. Taking an inappropriate formula may worsen Sx. Note on ma huang: this herb is a powerful stimulant to be used cautiously, especially in sensitive or weak patients. Patients with cardio-vascular disorders such as in hypertension	Bensky, Gamble, 1986; Chen, Chen, 1999; Maciocia, 1994

needed depending on the other imbalances present.	cough. Directs herbs to lungs. 4. Sang Bai Pi (Cortex Mori Albae radicis): alleviates wheezing and cools heat in lungs.		should be monitored closely or do not use at all. Only used in combination with other herbs. Ma huang has abuse potential.	
Homeopathy	Allergy; asthma	Numerous remedies depending on all symptoms presented and not just the conventional diagnostic category. Asthma examples: Arsenicum album—asthma with restlessness and anxiety. Ipecac—chest constriction and cough Pulsatilla—chest pressure and air hunger Sambuscus—asthma sx that awaken one at night	Seek a qualified practitioner so patient can have symptom pattern assessed.	Freeman, Lawlis, 2001; Loo, 1999; Mark, 2003

bid, *twice a day*; NSAIDs, *nonsteroidal antiinflammatory drugs*; PL/PL, *Pharmacist's Letter/Prescriber's Letter*; qd, *daily*; qid, *four times a day*; Sx, *symptoms*; tid, *three times a day*.

rhinovirus infection or prolonged use of a beta-2 agonist. Endotoxin and ozone exposure also may enhance the late response to bronchial allergen challenge (Brunton, Saphir, 1999). The following NAC methods can be offered as part of self-care and to complement conventional therapy for allergy and asthma. Conventional therapy must always be available to persons with asthma. In addition, Box 3-6 lists management strategies and environmental controls for allergy and asthma.

Autogenic Training

In a study of 24 adults with moderate-to-severe asthma, significant improvement in lung function was shown using autogenic training (AT) (Henry et al, 1993 in Ernst, 2001). In a study of 38 adults using AT, improvement in anxiety but no change in lung function occurred (Speiss et al, 1988 in Ernst, 2001); and in another study of 31 adults, sympathomimetic use was decreased but there was no change in symptoms or airway resistance (Deter, Albert, 1983 in Ernst, 2001).

Autogenics includes standard exercises. Suggestions include heaviness and warmth of arms and legs; cardiac regulation; respiration awareness; abdominal warmth; and cooling of the forehead. First, the heaviness and warmth are used with arms and legs. The sequence is right arm, left arm (or left first if person is left-handed), both arms, right leg, left leg, both legs, then arms and legs (Lichstein, 1988). This sequence is followed by the other exercise suggestions. Section II gives detail on autogenics.

Biofeedback

Ernst (2001) reports that two biofeedback studies showed promise in affecting asthma. "There were significant improvements in lung function and symptom scores in 33 children given biofeedback over 5 months, whereas those randomized to placebo biofeedback showed improvement in symptom scores only" (Ernst, 2001, p. 212; Kotses et al, 1991). In another randomized controlled trial with 20 adolescents (Coen et al, 1996), an improvement in symptoms occurred compared with a no-treatment control group, although no changes in lung function occurred.

Breathing Exercises

Several breathing exercises have been used in asthma: Buteyko breathing technique (BBT), physiotherapy, yoga breathing, concentrating on the out breath, and "belly breathing" (Bowler et al, 1998; Chaitow et al, 2002; Ernst, 2001; Ivker, 2001). Ernst (2001) states, "breathing exercises appear promising but [have] insufficient evidence to make firm judgments" (p. 213). One Buteyko study showed a significant reduction in beta-2 agonist use, plus a trend toward improvement in quality of life and in decreased inhaled steroid use

Box 3-6

Management Strategies and Environmental Controls for
Allergy and Asthma: Body, Bugs, Bedding, and Surroundings

Body
Perform allergy testing and immunotherapy
Elimination diet
Vitamin C
Avoid scents and allergen fabrics (wool, mixed fabrics).
Know how to use your peak flow meter and know what your
action plan is for problems.

Bugs
Eliminate cockroaches and cockroach debris. Scrub surfaces.
Keep food put away.
Move to a dry climate with low levels of dust-mite allergens (often
not practical).
Follow household instructions to keep dust mites down.
To avoid mold, keep things dry.

Bedding, bedroom
Encase mattresses, box springs, and pillows in allergy-proof
covers.
Use cotton blankets (no wool or down).
Wash bed linens weekly in hot (> 55° Celsius) water.
Wash rest of bedding every 2 weeks.
Dry clean or wash pillows regularly.
Remove draperies or blinds in bedroom; shades are preferable (if
you have curtains, wash weekly).
Remove carpeting in bedroom (hardwood or vinyl only); it is best
to have no carpet in house.
Remove all stuffed animals and other dust-catching items in
bedroom.

Surroundings
Use wood, plastic, leather, or vinyl furniture or encase stuffed
furniture.
Noncarpeted floors are best; if must have carpet, low-pile type is
best.
Every 3 months, carpeting should be sprayed with 3% solution of
tannic acid (denaturing agent) or acaricidal benzyl benzoate
spray or powder; this can be an irritant; consequently, it is not
recommended for frequent use.
Cover hot air vents with filter; change or clean regularly.

Continued

Box 3-6

Management Strategies and Environmental Controls for
Allergy and Asthma: Body, Bugs, Bedding, and
Surroundings —cont'd

Change furnace filter regularly.
Use air conditioners and dehumidifiers.
Maintain relative humidity at 35% to 55% (use humidifier as
needed, keep meticulously clean).
Immediately repair any plumbing or basement leaks.
Keep rain gutters, drains, and roof well drained.
Maintain clean and appropriately sealed windows.
Use air filter and negative ion generator.
Limit number of houseplants because they gather dust.
Regularly clean tub or shower-bath, closets, kitchen, and basement
with diluted bleach or cleaning agents.
Use exhaust fan to ventilate bathrooms.
Ask someone other than the person with the allergy to do the
cleaning.
Vacuum at least twice weekly. A central vacuum is best, or use a
vacuum cleaner with double-walled bag and high-efficiency
particulate air (HEPA) filters. HEPA filters should meet minimum
filtration efficiency of 99.97% for particles of 0.3 microns.
Dust with a dust attracting–type cloth rather than damp dust.
Wear HEPA mask that seals nose and mouth as needed.
No pets is best; but if you have furry pets, ask someone other than
the person with the allergy to brush the pet regularly and to do so
away from the person with the allergy.
Wash the pet once a week.
Keep pet out of the bedroom.
Make bedroom the most allergy-proof room in the house. Take
everything out of this room and clean it thoroughly; return minimal
number of clean furnishings.

*(Brunton, Saphir, 1999; Codina, Lockey, 2000; Ivker, Nelson, 2001; Marilyn
Shutte, 2000.)*

over controls, however, no significant differences were found in lung
function tests (Bowler et al, 1998; Chaitow et al, 2002; Ernst, 2001).
In this study, participants with asthma decreased bronchodilator use
by 90% and steroids by 40% after 3 months (Courtney, 2000). The
Buteyko therapist spent more time with the study subjects than they
did with the control group, however. Thus time spent may also have
been a factor in the improvement.

The Buteyko technique is based on the view that "people with asthma are under stress and therefore breathe too rapidly and too deeply...Buteyko training involves learning to make breathing shallow and slow" (Ernst, 2001, p. 212). Buteyko breathing is in contrast to the usual deep-belly breathing that is taught for relaxation. Buteyko, after whom the treatment is named, was the former head of the Laboratory of Functional Diagnostics in the Siberian Soviet Academy of Sciences and believed that asthma is a defense mechanism that the body produces against the loss of carbon dioxide (CO_2).

> Low levels of CO_2 are known to produce bronchospasm and asthmatics are known to have low levels of CO_2 in the lungs and blood during mild and moderate asthma attacks. [CO_2] has been shown to be a bronchodilator, so increasing local levels in the lungs during an attack can relieve spasm of the bronchi. (Courtney, 2000, p. 20)

Buteyko believed that CO_2, as a chemical regulator, was essential for the regulation of the cell and that by teaching patients "techniques of slow, periodic underbreathing" he could reduce asthma symptoms in 90% of his patients and control alveolar hyperventilation (Chaitow et al, 2002; Ivker, Nelson, 2001). Study on BBT is minimal. Information is printed here and is also available through the Eucapnic breathing web site (www.breatingCO2.com). Since patients may be using the technique or want information, health care providers need to be informed.

BBT consists of:

> Encouraging shallow breathing (hypoventilation) so that the individual becomes accustomed to a sense of slight "lack of air."
>
> Use of a "control pause" as an exercise, in which normal exhalation is held until a "distinct sensation" of "slight lack of air" is experienced, at which time breathing recommences, *without loss of control of the shallow rhythm* (i.e., the control pause is not followed by a deep breath.
>
> The control pause is practiced a number of times daily to encourage an increase in CO_2 tolerance.
>
> "First aid" use of a "maximum pause" is suggested, in which the exhaled breath is held until moderate discomfort is experienced, at which time breathing recommences, *without loss of control of the shallow rhythm* (i.e., the maximum pause is not followed by a deep breath). The maximum pause is used to relieve the symptoms of hyperventilation (similar to rebreathing CO_2 from a paper bag).
>
> CAUTION: Buteyko instructors suggest that caution should be used regarding use of the maximum pause in the case of patients with cardiovascular or kidney disease, hypertension, epilepsy, or diabetes. (Chaitow et al, 2002, p. 224-225)

Another form of breathwork is Eucapnic breathing. Eucapnic breathing incorporates the Buteyko method (Courtney, 2000). Eucapnia refers to "balanced levels of carbon dioxide" and the training includes other information and teachings on forms of breathing, the role of diet and food, the impact of stress and anxiety and how to overcome this impact, the role of muscles of respiration and freeing up these muscles, the role of breathing in exercise, and how to optimize one's breathing for any level of exercise (www.breathingco2.com).

Still another breathing technique is concentrating on the out breath while breathing slowly through the nose and doing basic belly breathing that emphasizes more time with the out breath than the in breath. Ivker (2001) suggests breathing out long and slowly for 4 to 5 seconds and breathing in for 1 to 3 seconds with a goal of breathing out for 8 to 12 seconds and in for 2 to 4 seconds. This type of breathing can be done while lying, sitting, or walking. Any breathing exercise should be stopped if it exacerbates asthma symptoms.

Hypnosis

Hackman and colleagues (1999) compiled a critical review of the use of hypnosis with asthma. Ernst (2001) reports on three hypnosis studies, each with a control group, showing symptomatic improvement or lung function improvement. Temes (1999) suggests that hypnosis can help a patient with breath retraining via posthypnotic suggestion and that it may help ease an asthma attack, cautioning that "suggestions may alter perception but not necessarily actual physiological change" (p. 122). Ernst (2001) cautions that patients may become less aware of bronchoconstriction with hypnosis and thus may undertreat an acute attack. Although hypnosis alone is not to be used during acute attacks, a patient who is well trained in self-hypnosis may be able to use it as an adjunct while emergency measures are in process. This use may help alleviate panic and fear (Heap, Aravind, 2002). Methods include a "technique with an image of drawing all the tension from the chest" (Heap, Aravind, 2002, p. 338). Relaxed breathing and control of hyperventilation may also be part of hypnosis therapy.

Imagery and Relaxation

Relaxation techniques have been used with asthma and chronic obstructive pulmonary disease (COPD) (Freedberg et al, 1987; Gift et al, 1992; Renfroe, 1988). Studies have shown mixed results (Ernst, 2001). However, relaxation techniques are a general comfort measure, can lend to a feeling of well being, and can provide a way to control tension and anxiety. (Snyder, 1998)

Naparstek (1994) states that imagery can complement other efforts at allergy treatment (the best of which is avoidance of allergens). She provides an allergy imagery script. The allergy imagery script is best used with early symptoms. The author uses cellular-physiologic imagery for the respiratory, digestive, and dermatologic systems, thus the imagery may also do well for asthma. Box 3-7 gives an imagery script for allergy. In addition, Naparstek has an audiotape for relieving asthma (Naparstek, 1992).

Journaling

Smyth and colleagues (1999) studied the effect of journaling on people with asthma. Subjects were asked to write 20 minutes a day for 3 days. The subjects either journaled on a stressful event (the treatment group) or on inconsequential events (the control group). Even though this study was only 3 days long, the patients with asthma improved lung function by 19%.

Day (2001), in a general discussion on journaling, says that this type of writing can facilitate healing through catharsis and insight, by observing cycles and patterns, getting to know different parts of the self, strengthening intuition and guidance, feeling self-empowerment and self-esteem, releasing past hurts and judgments, and witnessing the journey of healing. In this respect, journaling may help people with asthma. In addition, Day (2001) describes a method of journaling in which the individuals write down the dialogue between other people or themselves and their illness, sometimes called voice dialogue. This technique may be helpful for individuals with asthma and allergy as well, and they may speak to their lungs or immune system through journaling.

Meditation and Prayer

As for any chronic condition, these types of mind-body-spirit interventions can bring comfort. Meditation may help with breathing techniques, and meditation-prayer may bring inner strength, wisdom, and solace. Ernst (2001) reports on an asthma meditation study that was complicated by the treatment group continuing to meditate after they were crossed over into the control group status. In the first phase, however, the patients who meditated experienced a significant decrease in airway resistance, a good reason to continue to meditate (Wilson et al, 1975). Similarly, prayer may induce calming feelings, thereby reducing anxiety, promoting relaxation, and enhancing breathing.

Other Interventions

Ivker and colleagues (2001) in their book, *Asthma Survival*, discuss various ways of healing the mind, including many of the techniques previously listed. In addition, the authors discuss dealing with anger,

Box 3-7

Imagery for Allergies

(approximately 8 minutes) See if you can position yourself as comfortably as you can...shifting your weight so that you're allowing your body to be fully supported...checking to see that your head, neck, and spine are straight...and just taking a moment to feel the support underneath you...(pause)...

And gently allowing your eyes to close...and imagining that from somewhere above you...a cone of powerful white light is softly and steadily moving down...forming a tent of vibrant, tingling energy all around you...surrounding and protecting you...keeping out anything that might harm or irritate you...so you can be safe and comfortable...relaxed and easy...as you watch the light illuminate everything it touches with exquisite brightness...highlit definition...vibrating color...giving everything it shines on a fresh, new beauty...

You can feel the air around you intensifying, glowing, dancing with sparkling energy...and with a sense of gentle wonder for such stunning beauty...you can feel the tingling energy of the light moving down into your body...softly entering your head and neck...moving into your shoulders and chest...

Feeling the gentle, persistent warmth penetrating into any tightness in the neck and shoulders...in the chest...slowly, easily loosening, massaging, and opening...kneading and softening...and continuing down the spine...filling your back and torso...reaching into every organ...into the layers of tissue...deeper and deeper...

Sending a warm, vibrating softness into any discomfort in the belly...gently massaging and opening...filling it with powerful, reassuring warmth...

And moving down into your legs...and filling your feet...all the way to the tips of your toes...

So just letting yourself feel the vibrant, healing energy of the light...working its magic deep inside your body...moving with deliberate intelligence to places that feel congested, irritated, or uncomfortable...and softly infusing those places with soothing, healing comfort...

Feeling it soak into places that are swollen and sore...and sensing them begin to shrink back to normal size...perhaps opening passageways for breathing...gently warming and loosening and widening the airways in the head, neck, and chest...softly relaxing tense muscle bands around the tubes...and feeling the new space as it opens up...making even more room for the gentle flow of sweet, vital air...soft and slow and easy...

Box 3-7

Imagery for Allergies—cont'd

Or perhaps sensing a shift in the swollen feeling in the belly as everything settles back down...feeling a warm concentration of the remarkable light soaking directly into any inflamed places in the lining of the stomach or intestines...gently shrinking them back to normal size...leaching out unneeded fluid and particles... smoothing and calming irritated membrane...and sensing the linings beginning to subside back to their original shape and form...allowing nourishment to again move freely into every part of your body with speed and efficiency...

Or perhaps sensing the healing power of the light soothing and calming irritated skin...softly returning any reactive patches to their original soft, smooth, pliable texture...so that red, scaly, or swollen places are quickly sloughed off...and replaced by calm, healthy, new cells...growing smooth, soft, healthy skin...

And seeing the light...like a flare...highlighting and magnifying the cells that are accustomed to reacting quickly to irritation...and sending them a clear, calming message to settle down...and save their energy for the real enemies of the body...not these neutral particles that mean no harm...and just sensing this reassuring message going directly into the guardian cells of the lungs, the intestines, or the skin...wherever it is needed...telling them that all is well...they can stay ready, but calm and easy...able to exercise wisdom and discrimination...and able to save their strength for those things that truly harm the body...

And understanding that it is not just the cells that are being shown this...but that you, too, are settling down...developing a balanced sense of calm...less reactive to the environment...able to save your energy for the real battles...more safe and sure, steady, balanced, and strong...safely protected in your skin and in the cushion of energy surrounding you...attuned to the peaceful stillness at your center...stronger and more resilient than you have ever been...

And so...feeling peaceful and easy...relaxed and safe and comfortable...infused with light, and feeling all through your body the penetrating warmth and power of this awareness...you watch as the light slowly begins to withdraw...returning to wherever it came from...until it is gone altogether for now...knowing it is yours to call forth again...whenever you wish...

And so...feeling yourself sitting in your chair...or lying down...breathing in and out...very rhythmically and easily...gently and with soft eyes...coming back into the room whenever you are ready...knowing you are better for this...

And so you are...

(From Naparstek B: Staying well with guided imagery, New York, 1994, Warner.)

including writing an angry letter (then burning or tearing it up), punching a pillow, and screaming in a private place. In addition, the authors mention dream work, optimism, and humor. Music has been used for dyspnea and anxiety in patients with COPD with some immediate relief (but not over a 5-week period) and may be helpful in asthma also (McBride et al, 1999). Table 3-5 lists mind-body-spirit interventions for asthma and allergies.

BIOLOGIC-BASED THERAPIES FOR ASTHMA AND ALLERGIES

Dietary Measures: Foods and Elimination Diets

Weil, on his popular web site (www.askdrweil.com, 2001), recommends the liberal use of onions, garlic, and hot peppers as allergy control because these foods help inhibit inflammation. Weil also recommends sparse use of milk and meat products. Murray and Pizzorno (1999), both Naturopaths, suggest liberal amounts of garlic and onions (*Allium* family) and green tea (*Camellia sinensis*) because it has antioxidant components and also has methylxanthine. Murray and Pizzorno (1999) recommend eliminating food allergens, additives, and bananas (if they aggravate). The authors also recommend trying a vegan diet for a minimum of 4 months. The exception to the vegan diet is the addition of cold-water fish; children who eat fish more than once a week "have one-third the risk for asthma of children who do not eat fish regularly" (Murray, Pizzorno, 1999, p. 1099; Hodge et al, 1996). In addition, Murray and Pizzorno recommend the practice of the 4-day rotation diet for people with many food allergies.

Because 2% to 6% of patients with asthma are hypersensitive to food (Monteleone, Sherman, 1997; Ernst, 2001), food allergy should not be ignored; foods that are suspect should be eliminated for at least a 2-week period (authors suggest varying time frames). Patients need to keep diaries and observe changes in symptoms. Several foods may need to be eliminated all at once because symptoms may not change unless all allergens are eliminated. Hackman and colleagues (1999) report a study from India (Lal et al, 1995) in which 83% of parents whose children had asthma believed certain foods precipitated asthmatic attacks; this contrasts to the estimated 8.5% of the general population who have true allergic reactions to food (Moneret-Vautrin et al, 1996 in Hackman et al, 1999). Elimination and rotation diets are beneficial for persons who have numerous food allergies or difficulty controlling symptoms (Rockwell, 1999) and may be more beneficial than conventional providers think.

Vitamins, Minerals, and Antioxidants

Vitamin C seems to have a protective effect against exercise-induced asthma and asthma symptoms (Cohen et al, 1997; Baker et al, 1995,

Table 3-5 Mind-Body-Spirit Interventions for the Treatment of Asthma and Allergies

Intervention	Management	Treatment Regimen	Cautions, Precautions, Interactions	References
Affirmations	Asthma preventive maintenance	"It is safe now for me to take charge of my own life. I choose to be free." For babies and children: "This child is safe and loved. This child is welcomed and cherished" (Hay, 2000, p. 15). "I love and approve of myself," and "I am always doing the best I can" (Ivker et al, p. 215). "My lungs are strong and healthy. I can breathe freely." "My lungs are free of congestion." "The universe is providing me with the ability to breathe abundantly" (Fradet, p. 218).	Repeat affirmations 10-20 times/day. Affirmations need to be positive, personal, present-tense statements.	Hay, 2000; Fradet et al, 1995; Ivker, Nelson, 2001

Continued

165

Intervention	Management	Treatment Regimen	Cautions, Precautions, Interactions	References
Autogenics	Asthma: improvement in lung function or anxiety; decreased medication use.	Freeman and Lawlis (p. 253) give example: My arm is very heavy (muscular relaxation). My arm is very warm (vascular dilation). My heartbeat is very regular (stabilization of heart function). It breathes me (regulation of breath). Warmth is radiating over my stomach (regulation of visceral organs). There is a cool breeze across my forehead (regulation of blood flow in the head).	See Section II, Chapter 12 for details on mind-body-spirit and autogenics.	Deter, Albert, 1983; Ernst, 2001; Freeman, Lawlis, 2001; Henry et al, 1993; Speiss et al, 1988
Biofeedback or combined with breathing	Asthma: improvement in lung function or symptom scores (or both)	Several sessions are usually required.	Requires a trained technician.	Coen et al, 1996; Ernst, 2001; Freeman, Lawlis, 2001; Kotses

Breathing techniques	Increase individual's tolerance for CO_2. For asthma: To help decrease hyperventilation and anxiety.	BBT, Eucapnic breathing, yoga breathing, belly breathing slowly with concentration on the out breath. Practice for 5 to 10 mins tid.	Requires a skilled practitioner to teach the technique.	et al, 1991; Rogers, 2001 in Micozzi, 2001 Bowler et al, 1998; Chaitow et al, 2002; Courtney, 2000; Ernst, 2001; Ivker, Nelson, 2001; Sharma, Clark, 2000
Hypnosis	For asthma: To improve symptoms or lung function.	Several sessions may be needed: weekly, then monthly with probable improvements observed between seventh and twelfth hypnotic sessions. Clenched-fist technique with image of drawing all the tension out of chest.	Requires trained therapist aware of the patho-physiologic aspects involved. Hypnosis alone, not to be initiated at time of acute attack, but well-trained patient may use self-hypnosis when needed.	Ernst, 2001; Ewer, Stewart, 1986; Freeman, Lawlis, 2001; Heap, Aravind, 2002; Morrison, 1988; Maher-Laughnan et al, 1962; Research Comm of BTA, 1968; Temes, 1999
Journaling	Asthma, allergy for insight, improved lung function	Many types of journaling; can dialog between illness and self or between two persons; alpha poem. (See Chapters 2 and 12.)		Day, 2001; Smyth et al, 1999

Continued

Table 3-5 Mind-Body-Spirit Interventions for the Treatment of Asthma and Allergies—cont'd

Intervention	Management	Treatment Regimen	Cautions, Precautions, Interactions	References
Imagery, guided imagery	Asthma, allergy to help relieve symptoms; strengthen immune system.	See narrative in this chapter for a discussion on allergy-guided imagery. Also, listen to tapes or compact disks (CDs) at least once daily for 3-4 wks.	No driving or operating machinery while listening to tapes or CDs.	Naparstek, 1994, 1992 (audiotape—A Meditation to Help Relieve Asthma)
Meditation	Asthma and allergy for: relaxation, general well being; insight; help with breathing technique; strength for the journey; hope and faith.	Mindfulness meditation or transcendental meditation; daily or twice daily for 20-30 mins.	One study showed decreased airway resistance with meditation.	Kornfield, 1996 (videotape—The Inner Art of Meditation) Thich Nhat Hanh, 1997 (The Blooming of a Lotus: Guided Meditation Exercises for Healing and Transformation) Ernst, 2001

Prayer	Stress relief, improves quality of life; improves optimism; provides positive form of coping; enhances psychologic well being.	Prayer can be said at anytime, anywhere. Individual preference		Ai et al, 2002; Dunn, Horgas, 2000; Flannelly, Inouye, 2001; Meisenhelder, Chandler, 2000; Shuler et al, 1994
Relaxation, Progressive muscle relaxation	Use for asthma and allergy to control tension and anxiety.	Regular practice. "Tense" and "relax" techniques used. Tension is held for 7 seconds, then relaxed. Attention called to the difference between the two. Specific muscle groups used. Tense, then relaxation follows tension. Make a fist and hold it. Push elbow down on chair. (Then perform on nondominant side.) Lift eyebrows. Squint eyes and wrinkle nose. Clench	Some relaxation may potentiate the effect of some medications; lower doses may be needed (e.g., insulin); hypotension.	Ernst, 2001; Snyder, 1998; Snyder et al, 2002

Continued

Table 3-5	Mind-Body-Spirit Interventions for the Treatment of Asthma and Allergies—cont'd			
Intervention	Management	Treatment Regimen	Cautions, Precautions, Interactions	References
Relaxation, Progressive muscle relaxation, cont'd		teeth. Widen mouth. Pull chin to chest. Take deep breath, hold, and pull shoulder blades back. Pull stomach in. Lift leg and hold straight out. Point toes to ceiling. (Then perform on nondominant side.)		

BBT, *Buteyko breathing technique;* CO$_2$, *carbon dioxide;* tid, *three times a day.*

170

Pelton et al, 2001) and, in the National Health and Nutrition Examination Survey (NHANES II), low dietary levels of ascorbic acid have been associated with asthma, bronchitis, and wheezing (Hackman et al, 1999; Schwartz and Weiss, 1990). Two grams of ascorbic acid was found to improve forced expiratory volume (FEV1) over a placebo (Hackman et al, 1999; Bucca et al, 1990).

> Vitamin C functions as both a very mild antihistamine (it inhibits the release and enhances the degradation of histamine) and as a phosphodiesterase inhibitor (the same action as some asthma medications). Vitamin C reduces the frequency and intensity of bronchial spasms in asthmatics. (Pelton et al, 2001, p. 362)

Vitamins A and E, magnesium, and selenium may also be useful nutrients for asthma (Baker et al, 1995; Hackman, 1994; Murray, Pizzorno, 1999). Similarly, lycopenes have shown benefit. Subjects were given 30 mg of lycopene every day for 1 week; after 1 week, 55% of the patients on lycopene experienced significant improvement of FEV1, whereas those in the control group had a drop of more than 15% of their FEV1 (Neuman et al, 2000). The B vitamins and omega-3 fatty acids (found in deep-water fish such as salmon, tuna, and mackerel) may also play a role in the immune system (Gamble, 1995; Murray, Pizzorno, 1999).

For allergy problems, Weil (www.askdrweil.com, 2001) suggests the use of quercitin, a bioflavenoid from buckwheat and citrus. Quercitin "stabilizes the membranes of mast cells which release histamine, the body chemical that mediates many allergic reactions" (p. 1). Weil recommends 400 mg twice daily between meals and says it has to be taken regularly because it works with allergy prevention rather than symptom relief; quercitin takes up to 8 weeks to show effects.

Zinc has also been implicated in asthma and allergy (Hackman et al, 1999) either with deficiency (Spector, 1990; Keen, Gershwin, 1990) or excess zinc from occupational exposure (Malo et al, 1993).

Herbs

Herbs such as stinging nettle leaf (*Urtica dioica*) have been used for allergic rhinitis; at least one published study with its use has been conducted (Mittman, 1990; LaValle et al, 2000), although little research has been done the only proven pharmacologic action, according to Fetrow and Avila (1999) is as a diuretic. Weil (www.askdrweil.com, 2001) suggests one or two capsules of the freeze-dried stinging nettles extract (leaf) to relieve immediate allergy symptoms, every 2 to 4 hours as needed. LaValle and colleagues (2000) suggest 300 to 1200 mg of freeze-dried leaf two to four times a day as needed.

Ma huang (*Ephedra sinica*) has been used for many years for bronchial asthma and the effectiveness is well known (PL/PL,

3/15/2000). Ma huang is ephedra and has the same therapeutic and adverse effects that go along with synthetic epinephrine. However, ma huang has a more profound central nervous system effect. The recommendation is for "no more than 8 mg total ephedra alkaloids per dose or no more than 24 mg total ephedra alkaloids per 24 hours" (LaValle et al, 2000, p. 429). Although ma huang has a well-known history of effectiveness, it has been an herb of abuse (including for weight loss and body-building). A reminder of the side effect profile:

> Chronic use of ma huang can cause rapid development of tolerance and dependence. Use of ma huang is contraindicated in anxiety, anorexia, bulimia, hypertension, glaucoma, cerebral insufficiency, urinary retention due to prostate enlargement, pheochromocytoma, thyrotoxicosis, heart disease, and diabetes. (PL/PL, 3/15/2000, p. 23)

In addition, people on antihypertensives and antidepressants should not take ma huang. Numerous drug-drug interactions have been cited, including with beta blockers, monoamine oxidase inhibitors (MAOIs), phenothiazines, and theophylline (Fetrow, Avila, 1999). "Avoid confusion with Mormon tea (*American ephedra, Ephedra nevadensis*). Mormon tea is alkaloid-free and lacks both the therapeutic effects and toxicity of ephedrine" (PL/PL, 3/15/2000, p. 24).

For asthma, Murray and Pizzorno (1999) recommend herbal expectorants in combination with *Ephedra sinensis. Glycyrrhiza glabra* (licorice), an expectorant and a demulcent (i.e., produces soothing effects) is one of the herbals. *Glycyrrhiza glabra* has a long history of being antiinflammatory and antiallergic. Other herbs include *Ginkgo biloba* with action probably resulting from the ginkgolides that "antagonize platelet-activating factor (PAF), a key chemical mediator in asthma, inflammation, and allergies" (p. 1102). An Ayurvedic herb, *Coleus forskolii*, is recommended for asthma (Murray, Pizzorno, 1999; LaValle et al, 2000). Forskolin inhibits histamine release from mast cells in addition to other actions. Forskolin is:

> believed to activate adenylate cyclase, increasing intracellular c-AMP [cyclic adenosine monophosphate] concentrations and activation of a number of key enzymatic pathways...may act through direct binding to PAF receptors. This binding may inhibit platelet aggregation in addition to blocking inflammatory reactions mediated by platelet-derived products. (LaValle et al, 2000, p. 413-414)

This herb may cause hypotension and alter platelet aggregation and thus may interact with numerous other medications.

In a systematic review of Chinese, East Indian, Japanese, and other herbs (Huntley, Ernst, 2000), some promising evidence was found in single studies with *Picrorrhiza kurroa, Solanum* spp, *Boswellia serrata*, Saibuko-to, marijuana, and dried ivy extract, but evidence was "insufficient to make firm judgements" (Ernst, 2001, p. 213).

Ivker and Nelson (2001) have an *Asthma Survival Program* for preventing and treating asthma. Therapies include environmental strategies, as well as biologic-based therapies. Ivker and Nelson provide recommendations and dosages and supplements for adults and children. Box 3-8 lists the adult supplements recommended for preventive maintenance and for treating asthma. The authors suggest beginning several of the supplements, then adding more 3 weeks later and still a few more 6 weeks from the start of the program. This progression helps the patient feel less overwhelmed by the amount of supplements. See the Ivker text for complete information and guidelines. Not all of the suggestions are validated with studies; however, a healthful diet with adequate intake from food and supplements is a common sense approach to a chronic condition such as asthma.

Immunotherapy

Immunotherapy (allergy shots) may be helpful for some allergy sufferers (Durham et al, 1999; Adkinson, 1999).

> Immunotherapy is directed at treating underlying allergies when there is a clear demonstration of IgE-mediated allergy and avoidance of the allergen is not possible. Indications for this treatment include severe symptoms, poor response to medications, long-term need for medication, presence of secondary complications, and/or inability or reluctance to follow environmental control measures. Its long-term efficacy depends on an optimal maintenance dose of allergen injected subcutaneously every 2 to 4 weeks for 3 to 5 years. Because of the risk of anaphylaxis, immunotherapy should be administered by a health care professional experienced in its administration. (Corren, Storms, 1998, p. 7)

In a study of 32 participants with hay fever, all 32 had received immunotherapy for 3 years and were then separated into the placebo injection or grass-pollen injection for another 3 years. The symptoms remained diminished in both the placebo injection group and the grass-pollen vaccine group as well. Both of these groups had fewer symptoms than did a separate group (the control group). The 15 subjects in the control group had never received injections; this control group used more rescue antiallergy medication and had more allergy symptoms over the 3-year period (Dunham et al, 1999). This study shows the benefit of 3 years of injections. An intervening factor in this study may be a provider visit effect for the group receiving the placebo injection.

A longer study was a retrospective study with asthma patients who were allergic to house-dust mite (HDM) or to HDM and grass pollen and who had been treated with specific immunotherapy (SIT) in childhood. After having been off the SIT for about 9 years, they were reevaluated in adulthood:

Box 3-8

Program for Preventive Maintenance and Treating Asthma with Supplements

For Both Preventive Maintenance and Treating Asthma of Adults

Multivitamin
Vitamins B6 and B12
Vitamin C
Vitamin E
Proanthocyanidin
Omega-3 fatty acids
N-acetylcysteine
Garlic
Acidophilus
Magnesium (glycinate, arginate, or aspartate)
Selenium
Start the following after 3 weeks with the above program (or earlier if patient chooses):
  Beta carotene
  Calcium (citrate or hydroxyapatite)
  Zinc
Start the following after 6 weeks into the program (or sooner if patient comfortable doing so):
  Chromium
  Pantothenic acid
  Folic Acid
  Whole adrenal extract (only if fatigue is a significant symptom or with a history of long-term steroid use)

For Preventive Maintenance Only

Bromelain
Candida-free
  If Candida is suspected, take no longer than 2 months without supervision
Hydrochloric acid
  After protein meals
  Start after 6 weeks into program (or sooner if comfortable with doing so)
  Only if no gastroesophageal reflux disease (GERD) or gastric symptoms

Box 3-8

Program for Preventive Maintenance and Treating Asthma
with Supplements—cont'd

For Treating Asthma Only (Not for Preventive Maintenance)
Quercetin
Lobelia
Ephedra (only if wheezing is a primary symptom, but not with
high blood pressure; see cautions)
Ginkgo biloba
Coleus forskohlii
For Complete program, see the following source.

(*From Ivker R, Nelson T*: Asthma survival, *New York, 2001, Tarcher
Putnam.*)

The results were compared with those of a control group of patients
with asthma with comparable asthma features who were treated with
appropriate antiasthmatic drugs during childhood but who never
received SIT. At re-evaluation, the risk for frequent asthmatic symptoms was three times higher in the control group than in the SIT-
treated group. The frequent use of antiasthmatic medication was also
more pronounced in the control group, although the difference statistically was not significant. Lung-function parameters and results of
SIT with HDM were comparable in both groups. It is concluded that
SIT has long-term effects on curbing asthmatic symptoms in young
adults. (Cools et al, 2000 in Keegan, 2001, p. 77)

Table 3-6 lists the biologic-based therapies for asthma and allergy.

Preventing Bee and Other Stings

Another aspect of allergy for many individuals is hypersensitivity to
stings. Allergic individuals should wear medic-alert identification and
carry a prescription anaphylaxis kit. Stings usually occur in self-
defense. Bees leave a stinger and are attracted by flower and perfume
fragrance, bright colors, smooth water, and even some house paint.
Wasps can sting repeatedly, do not leave a stinger, and are attracted by
odors such as perspiration, fruit juices, leather, bright colors, spoiling
food, and a water supply. Yellow jackets nest in the ground, and paper
hornets may be close to the ground, making them hazardous to feet
and ankles. Desensitization is available. Honey bees, wasps, hornets,
and yellow jackets (i.e., *Hymenoptera*) have common antigens in their
venom (Battan, Dart, 2001). Box 3-9 gives suggestions for avoiding
stings. Treatment for sting without allergy can be ice, cold compresses,
and topical applications of soothing substances such as baking soda.

Table 3-6 Biologic-Based Therapies for Asthma and Allergy

A complete prescribing source should be consulted before using biologic therapies. Vitamin and mineral dosing often is higher compared with the recommended upper limit. At times of illness or deficiency, persons may need more of such supplements. However, caution should be used because of the lack of study. Any herb can cause an allergic reaction. Herbs are generally contraindicated in pregnancy and lactation and with children unless research data or a long history of safe use has been established.

Intervention	Management	Treatment Regimen	Cautions, Precautions, Interactions	References
Onions, garlic, hot peppers	Improve respiratory symptoms for allergy. Garlic for asthma preventive maintenance and treatment.	As tolerated. Garlic 1200 mg/day for asthma maintenance and 1200-2000 mg tid for treatment.	An old therapy; breath odor; GI upset; may not be for everyone.	www.askdr.weil.com, 2001; Ivker, Nelson, 2001; Murray, Pizzorno, 1999; PL/PL, 2002
Omega-3 essential fatty acids	Asthma preventive maintenance and treatment	Flaxseed oil, flaxseed, cold-water fish (salmon, sardines, herring, mackerel, tuna). Adult dose: EPA 400-600 mg/tid. DHA 300-500 mg/day. EPA and DHA are used in combination in fish oil preparations	Americans tend to have much more omega-6 fatty acids than omega-3. Avoid or decrease saturated and transfatty acids. Fish oil may give fishy taste and have GI side effects	Gamble, 1995; Hodge et al, 1996; Ivker, Nelson, 2001; Mark, 2003; Murray, Pizzorno, 1999; PL/PL, 2002

N-acetyl cysteine	Derivative of the amino acid L-cysteine. Stimulate glutathione synthesis and act as antioxidant and free-radical scavenger.	By inhalation is a mucolytic agent for chronic lung disorders. Orally, seems to decrease risk of chronic bronchitis. 500 mg/day asthma maintenance; 500 mg tid for asthma treatment.	Unpleasant odor. Use straw to take.	Ivker, Nelson, 2001; PL/PL, 2002
Vegan diet	Asthma, allergy; improvement in symptoms, possibly pulmonary function.	Whole grains, legumes, fruits, vegetables, omega-3s	To ensure adequate intake of nutrients, care must be taken. May need to eliminate milk and milk products. Calcium intake is needed.	Murray, Pizzorno, 1999
Avoidance diet, elimination diet, or rotation diet	Asthma, allergy	Avoid common allergens such as milk (dairy), wheat (or gluten, which includes rye, oats, and barley), corn, citrus, peanuts, chocolate, eggs. Eliminate specific food products for a minimum of 2 wks; rotate foods back one at a time every 4-6 days to see symptom effects. Keep symptom	Also need to eliminate additives, food coloring, MSG, sulfites. Allergy testing may be done to clarify food allergies. There also are special elimination diets with different formats. See Box 3-4 for sample Candida-elimination diet.	Mark, 2003; Murray, 1998; Murray, Pizzorno, 1999; Ivker, 2000; Ivker, Nelson 2001

Continued

Table 3-6 Biologic-Based Therapies for Asthma and Allergy—cont'd

Intervention	Management	Treatment Regimen	Cautions, Precautions, Interactions	References
Avoidance diet, elimination diet, or rotation diet, cont'd		checklist; if have symptoms in 24-72 hrs, may be reacting to the added food.		
Honey and lemon cough syrup	Cough, bronchitis	See Box 3-2 for one recipe; take 1 tsp as needed.	Anecdotal, old home remedy. Has been used for asthma. Honey not recommended for infants or young children because of possible botulism spores. May cause allergy resulting from pollens.	DerMarderosian, 2001; Ivker, 2000
HCL acid	Asthma and food allergy are associated with low gastric acid levels. HCL improves digestion.	10-20 grains after protein meals for asthma maintenance. Murray suggests starting with one capsule of 10 grains (600 mg) at large meal. If no aggravation, take capsules with large meals until feeling warmth in stomach or reach seven	To be used only if hypochlorhydria is a problem. Not for persons with GERD	Ivker, Nelson, 2001; Murray, 1998

| | | capsules, whichever is first. When taking several, take capsules throughout meal. Continue capsules with meals and when Sx of warmth occur, decrease dosing. Every 3 days decrease by 1 capsule or more. | |
| Vitamin A | Vitamin A deficiency results in increased susceptibility to respiratory conditions; use for preventive maintenance and treatment of asthma, allergy. | Dietary intake: 700-900 µg/day. Dark colored fruits and vegetables—carrots, sweet potatoes, broccoli. Beta carotene 25,000 IU qd for asthma maintenance and tid for treating asthma | Recommended adult Vitamin A UL is 3000 µg/day. Large doses of vitamin E can interfere with vitamin A. Vitamin A antagonizes action of vitamin D. Vitamin A is fat-soluble thus has potential for toxicity. Takes more of a food source to obtain recommended intake than previously thought. CAUTION: tid 25,000 IU dose is for 1 month maximal use. Women of childbearing age must not overdose. | Ivker, Nelson, 2001; McDowell, 1995; Murray, Pizzorno, 1999; www.nap.gov, 2002 |

Continued

Table 3-6 Biologic-Based Therapies for Asthma and Allergy—cont'd

Intervention	Management	Treatment Regimen	Cautions, Precautions, Interactions	References
Pantothenic acid (also called Vitamin B5)	Asthma preventive maintenance and treatment; allergy; coenzyme in fatty acid metabolism	Maintenance 250 mg/day. Treatment 500 mg qd to tid after meals. If for allergy, start 4-5 days after begin allergy therapy and still have Sx.	Adult recommended UL not determined but RDA is 4 to 5 mg/day. Dose recommended for respiratory complaints is very high. Large amount of pantothenic acid causes diarrhea. One case of eosinophilic pleuropericardial effusion on 300 mg/day reported. Can interact with medications.	Ivker, 2000; Ivker, Nelson, 2001; NAP, 2001; PL/PL, 2002
Vitamin B6 (pyridoxine)	Asthma preventive maintenance and treatment; vitamin B6 deficiency can decrease antibody production and suppress immune response.	50 mg/day to bid (adult suggested dose). For treating adult asthma, 200 mg bid.	Recommended adult UL is 100 mg/day. Asthmatic children on theophylline may have decreased vitamin B6. Best taken with other B vitamins to maintain balance in a B25 or B50 preparation. Toxicity can occur; sensory neuropathy is Sx.	Gamble, 1995; Ivker, Nelson, 2001; NAP, 2001

Supplement	Indication	Dosage	Comments	References
Vitamin B12	Asthma preventive maintenance and treatment.	Maintenance: 500 μg/day sublingual; treatment: 1000 μg/day sublingual.	Recommended adult UL not determined but RDA is 2.4 μg/day.	Ivker, Nelson, 2001
Folic acid	Asthma preventive maintenance and treatment.	Maintenance 800 μg/day. If on steroids, add 1 to 5 mg/day for treatment of asthma.	Recommended adult UL is 1000 μg (1 mg). Can mask neurologic complications in persons with vitamin B12 deficiency.	Ivker, Nelson, 2001; NAP, 2001
Vitamin C	Asthma, protect against exercise induced asthma, improve respiratory function, allergy.	1000 mg/day for URI; 2000 mg improved FEV in study. 1000-2000 mg qd tid for preventive maintenance of asthma.	Recommended adult UL is 2000 mg/day. Large doses can cause diarrhea. UL may vary depending on individual status or illness.	Baker et al, 1995; Cohen et al, 1997; Hemila, 1997; PL/PL, 2000, 2002; LaValle, 1999; NAP, 2001; Pelton et al, 2001
Vitamin E— natural d-alpha mixed tocopherols	Asthma preventive maintenance or treatment, allergy.	400 IU qd to bid	2000 RDA for vitamin E is 15 mg (22 IU based on the alpha tocopherol form); the tolerable UL is 1000 mg (1500 IU).	Gamble, 1995; Ivker, Nelson, 2001; Murray, Pizzorno, 1999

Continued

181

Table 3-6   Biologic-Based Therapies for Asthma and Allergy—cont'd

Intervention	Management	Treatment Regimen	Cautions, Precautions, Interactions	References
Vitamin E— natural d-alpha mixed toco- pherols, cont'd			Has drug interactions. Iron can bind and inactivate vitamin E. The RDA is quite low compared with usual dosing.	www.askdrweil.com, 2001; Ivker, Nelson, 2001; PL/PL, 2000, 2002
Flavonoids (polyphenolic antioxidants that occur in fruits such as apples, vegetables, onion, tea, red wine). Quercetin is a flavonoid.	Asthma, allergy; antioxidant, antiinflammatory	Increase consumption of foods highest in flavonoid: onion, kale, French bean, broccoli, endive, celery, cranberry. Others: lettuce, tomato, red pepper, broad bean, strawberry, apple, grape, red wine, tea tomato juice. For allergy, 400 mg bid between meals. Treating asthma 1000 mg tid.	Concurrent use of vitamin C enhances antioxidant activity of quercetin, and concurrent use with bromelain might increase GI absorption of quercetin. Quercetin can cause headache and tingling of extremities.	

Glutathione	Asthma treatment; glutathione deficiency associated with lung disease.	100 mg tid	However, PL/PL says likely ineffective when taken orally because it is not absorbed. Is usually used IV for treating chemotherapy toxicity.	Ivker, Nelson, 2001; PL/PL, 2002
Lycopenes	Protect against exercise induced asthma symptoms	Increase lycopene foods: tomatoes (raw, cooked, or in tomato products, such as sauces and ketchup), grapefruit, watermelon. Heat releases high concentrations of free lycopene, thus cooked tomatoes may be better than raw.		Neuman et al, 2000
Calcium (citrate)	Asthma preventive maintenance and treatment	1000 to 1500 mg/day	Recommended adult UL is 2500 mg/day	Ivker, 2000; NAP, 2001
Chromium picolinate	Asthma preventive maintenance and treatment	200 µg/day	Adult recommended UL is not determined, but adequate intake set at 20-35 µg depending on age.	Ivker, Nelson, 2001; NAP, 2001

Continued

183

Table 3-6 Biologic-Based Therapies for Asthma and Allergy—cont'd

Intervention	Management	Treatment Regimen	Cautions, Precautions, Interactions	References
Magnesium (glycinate, arginate, or aspartate)	Asthma preventive maintenance and treatment, allergy. Magnesium chelate or aspartate may stop the severe asthmatic episode (Gamble). Opens constricted bronchial tubes.	Gamble recommends 500-750 mg/day for asthma. Ivker recommends 500 mg/day prevention and bid for treatment.	Adult recommended UL is 350 mg. May cause diarrhea; caution with renal impairment. Drugs that can cause depletion of magnesium: oral contraceptives, estrogens, loop diuretics, thiazides, digoxin, tetracycline.	Gamble, 1995; Ivker, Nelson, 2001; LaValle et al, 1999; NAP, www.nap.gov 2001; Murray, Pizzorno, 1999;
Selenium	Asthma preventive maintenance and treatment; and allergies, antioxidant, supports immune system. Regulation of reduction and oxidation status of vitamin C. May help prevent incidence of lung cancer.	200 µg/day for treatment and 100-200 µg/day for maintenance. Crab, fish, poultry, wheat, Brazil nuts are good selenium sources.	RDA: 55 µg/day; recommended adult UL, 400 µg. Toxicity can occur with large doses, including loss of hair and nails, skin lesions, digestive dysfunction, nervous system abnormalities.	Ivker, Nelson, 2001; LaValle, 2000; NAP, 2001; PL/PL, 2002

Zinc	Asthma preventive maintenance and treatment, and allergies. Essential trace element. Cofactor in many processes including DNA, RNA, and protein synthesis. Nearly 100 specific enzymes depend on zinc as a catalyst. May increase immune response.	20-40 mg/day for maintenance and 40-60 mg/day for treatment.	Recommended adult UL, 40 mg. SE: bad taste, nausea; renal impairment; interferes with copper absorption if taken in large amounts; unsafe in large amounts. Contraindicated in HIV. Zinc absorption is reduced in rheumatoid arthritis. Avoid in glaucoma. Must have adequate zinc/copper ratio. Interactions with some tetracyclines, fluoroquinolones, potassium-sparing and thiazide diuretics and others.	Al-Nakib et al, 1987; Eby et al, 1984; Godfrey et al, 1996; Ivker, Nelson et al, 2001; Mossad et al, 1996; PL/PL, 2000, 2002
Herbs				
Bromelain (pineapple, *ananas comosus* or *sativus*)	Asthma preventive maintenance; for swelling especially nasal and paranasal sinuses.	1000 mg on empty stomach or 80 to 320 mg in two or three doses/day for 8-10 days.	Potato protein and soybean inhibits bromelain activity. Zinc inhibits bromelain activity. Magnesium activates	Ivker, Nelson, 2001; PL/PL, 2002

Continued

185

Table 3-6 Biologic-Based Therapies for Asthma and Allergy—cont'd

Intervention	Management	Treatment Regimen	Cautions, Precautions, Interactions	References
Herbs—cont'd				
Bromelain (pineapple, *ananas comosus or sativus*), cont'd			bromelain. May increase risk of bleeding. Bromelain use increases tetracycline levels. Cross allergenicity between wheat flour and bromelain.	Murray, Pizzorno, 1999; Ivker, Nelson, 2001; LaValle et al, 2000; PL/PL, 2002
Coleus forskolii	Inhibits histamine release from mast cells in addition to other actions.	Standardized extract of 10 mg of forskolin powder using a spinhaler inhaler has been used.	Hypotension; alters platelet aggregation. May interact with cardiovascular disease.	Ivker, 2000
Echinacea Ephedra and *ma huang* (contains ephedrine)	Allergy Chinese herb used for asthma, respiratory symptoms.	See Table 3-2. Formulations vary. Not recommended but has history of use for asthma	Not for long term use. READ ALL CAUTIONS. CNS STIMULANT. Abuse potential. Contraindicated in anxiety, anorexia, bulimia, diabetes, hypertension, glaucoma,	DerMarderosian, 2001; PL/PL, 3/15/2000, 2002

Herb	Uses	Dosage	Comments	References
Grape seed extract (proanthocyanidin)	Asthma preventive maintenance and treatment.	Adult: preventive maintenance, 100 mg qd to bid on empty stomach. Treating asthma, 200 mg tid on empty stomach. Child over age 3 yrs, 100 mg once/day.	cerebral insufficiency, urinary retention caused by prostate enlargement, pheochromocytoma, thyrotoxicosis, heart disease, and diabetes. Theoretically, may increase effect of warfarin because of tocopherol content.	Ivker, 2000; PL/PL, 2002
Grapefruit seed extract	Asthma treatment	Adult, 100 mg tid or 10 gtts in water. Children over age 3, 4 gtts in water bid.	Must be a preservative-free product (free of benzethonium chloride). When preservative-containing product used, can cause vomiting, collapse, convulsions, coma. Interacts with several drugs.	Ivker, Nelson, 2001; PL/PL, 2002
Ginkgo biloba	Asthma treatment; allergies. Antioxidant	120 to 240 mg/day of standardized extract	Allergy. Has drug interactions, including	Gamble, 1995; Ivker, Nelson, 2001;

Continued

Table 3-6	Biologic-Based Therapies for Asthma and Allergy—cont'd			
Intervention	Management	Treatment Regimen	Cautions, Precautions, Interactions	References
Herbs—cont'd				
Ginkgo biloba, cont'd	properties; thought to reduce inflammation via inhibiting platelet-activating factor		with antiplatelet and anticoagulant medications—can increase risk of bleeding. Can increase blood pressure when given with thiazides.	PL/PL, 2000, 2002
Ginseng (*Panax ginseng*) also called Asian ginseng	Constituents may stimulate natural killer cell activity and other immune system activity. Possibly effective for preventing cold and influenza when used in combination with an influenza vaccine	100 mg qd or bid of standardized extract of 4% ginsenosides. Ginseng is started 4 wks before immunization.	SE: insomnia, and other. Not to be used long term; possibly safe if used appropriately for less than 3 months. Insufficient data for longer use. NOT RECOMMENDED FOR USE WITH CHILDREN; likely unsafe.	Blumenthal, 2000; PL/PL, 2000, 2002
Licorice (*Glycyrrhiza glabra*)	Expectorant and a demulcent; being investigated	1-4 g of powdered root or 1 cup of tea tid after meals. Simmer the	Do not over consume; not for more than 4-6 wks use without supervision.	Blumenthal, 2000; Murray, Pizzorno, 1999; PL/PL, 2002

	as an anti-inflammatory.	1-4 g of powdered root in 150 ml water 5-10 mins. Strain.	Large-dose toxicity Sx include lethargy, hypertension, hypokalemia, paralysis. Has interactions with antihypertensives, steroids, insulin, others. Contraindicated in diabetes, heart failure, hypertension, hypokalemia (licorice can cause hypokalemia), kidney insufficiency, liver disease, hypertonia.	
Lobelia (*Lobelia inflata*)	Asthma symptoms	Tincture: 25 gtts in mint tea q3-4h. 0.6 to 2.0 ml of the tincture	READ ALL CAUTIONS. SE: nausea, vomiting, diarrhea, dizziness, tremors. Dose-dependent cardiac activity. Overdose can cause death (0.6 to 1.0 g is toxic).	Ivker, Nelson, 2001; PL/PL, 2002

Continued

Table 3-6   Biologic-Based Therapies for Asthma and Allergy—cont'd

Intervention	Management	Treatment Regimen	Cautions, Precautions, Interactions	References
Herbs—cont'd				
Stinging nettles (*urtica dioica*) (above-ground parts)	Allergic rhinitis, allergies	Weil suggests one or two capsules of the freeze-dried stinging nettles extract (leaf) for immediate allergy symptoms q2-4h prn. LaValle suggests 300 to 1200 mg of freeze-dried leaf bid to qid prn. PL/PL suggests 300 mg tid.	Allergy. SE: diarrhea. Some drug interactions: antidiabetic drugs (increase glucose); antihypertensive medications (lower blood pressure), anticoagulants (decrease drug effects), CNS depressants (additive effects).	Fetrow, Avila, 1999; LaValle et al, 2000; www.askdrweil.com, 2001; PL/PL, 2002

Other

Acidophilus	Asthma preventive maintenance and treatment; improve GI flora.	Lactobacillus and bifidus. Use dairy-free acidophilus and bifidus morning and evening on empty stomach for 3 wks at a time, following antibiotics or every few months as Candida preventative. Strength of lactobacillus quantified by number of organisms. Typical dose ranges from 1-10 billion organisms daily in 3-4 divided doses.	SE: flatulence usually subsides with continuing use.	Ivker, Nelson, 2001; PL/PL, 2002
Immunotherapy	For allergy; may help decrease symptoms for long periods	Testing and series of injections	Costly, time-consuming, possibility of allergic reaction to product.	Cools et al, 2000; Keegan, 2001

bid, Twice a day; CNS, central nervous system; DHA, docosahexanoic acid; DNA, deoxyribonucleic acid; EPA, eicosapentaenoic acid; FEV, forced expiratory volume; GERD, gastroesophageal reflux disease; GI, gastrointestinal; gtts, drops; HIV, human immunodeficiency virus; IU, International Units; IV, intravenous; MSG, monosodium glutamate; NAP, National Academy Press; PL/PL, Pharmacist's Letter/Prescriber's Letter; prn, as needed; qd, daily; qid, four times a day; RDA, recommended daily allowance; RNA, ribonucleic acid; SE, side effects; Sx, symptoms; tid, three times a day; UL, upper limits—the maximum level of daily nutrient that is likely to pose no risk of adverse effects. Includes intake from food, water, and supplements; URI, upper respiratory infection.

Box 3-9

Avoiding Stings

Wear light-colored clothes, and tie hair up to avoid entanglement.

Avoid perfumes, fragrances, hairspray, and bright colors.

If a stinging insect approaches, stay still or move very slowly; never slap or brush at insect; they sting when frightened or antagonized.

Take care when picking up clothing that has been laying outdoors.

Avoid orchards and fields in bloom.

Running, riding horses, swimming, bicycles and motorcycles, and convertibles are especially dangerous because colliding insects can cause stings.

Ask someone who is not allergic to mow lawn, trim hedges, and prune trees during the dangerous season.

Keep a bee cloth or paper cup with small piece of cardboard for a lid in car to trap frightened insects.

In early spring, ask someone who is not allergic to inspect your property for nests and stinging insects.

Destroy yellow jacket nests at night, or use an exterminator. Bee handlers may take a hive of bees for you.

(Miles Laboratory, 1986)

MANIPULATIVE AND BODY-BASED METHODS FOR ASTHMA AND ALLERGIES

Chiropractic

Ernst (2001) reports that chiropractic aims to improve "the function of the lungs by reducing any restricted movement of the ribs and treating muscle tension in the intercostal muscles" (p. 215). Ernst states that the two most rigorous randomized controlled trials found no differences between chiropractic and sham chiropractic manipulation (Balon et al, 1998; Nielson et al, 1995).

In the Nielson study, the 31 subjects received treatment twice weekly for only 4 weeks. Subjects were between the ages of 18 and 34. Symptoms and bronchial hyperreactivity from baseline were significantly reduced in both the sham and the treatment group (Freeman, Lawlis, 2001). Some benefit was received from these chiropractor visits; thus what movements were used with the sham treatment as well as the routine chiropractic needs further study.

Massage

Massage is comforting, can increase circulation, and can possibly help movement of the diaphragm. Field (2000) studied massage therapy with children who had asthma. A significant improvement was found in children who had a 20-minute massage at bedtime nightly for 30 days. The massage was given to the child by a trained parent. In the young children (ages 4 to 8 years), peak flow increased, as well as all pulmonary function tests, and anxiety decreased. In addition, the children's salivary cortisol levels dropped.

In older children (ages 9 to 14 years), anxiety levels were lower on the first day only, and improvement on one peak flow measure (the average flow rate) that increased by 52%. In addition, the 9- to 14-year olds' salivary cortisol levels were in the normal range, thus having less room for decrease (Field, 2000).

Massage may also be useful for adults. Courtney (2000) recommends musculoskeletal therapy to "allow the lungs to carry out the function of breathing" (p. 20) in combination with Eucapnic Breathing Retraining. Courtney believes this combination helps restore lung function.

> By working on the muscles of breathing to normalize their function, one can enhance the effectiveness of Eucapnic Breathing Retraining, achieving faster and longer lasting results. Habitual incorrect use of respiratory muscles tends to reinforce incorrect breathing. A commonality I've found is that after working on a client to release dysfunction in primary and accessory muscles of breathing, several instant improvements are seen. The client usually finds they have an increased freedom of breathing, less breathlessness and, more objectively, a noticeable increase in the breath-holding time after expiration (i.e., the control pause), showing there has been a change in the ventilation threshold to carbon dioxide. (Courtney, 2000, p. 21)

ENERGY THERAPIES FOR ASTHMA AND ALLERGIES

Therapeutic touch (TT), healing touch, or Reiki can offer comfort. TT has been shown to relieve anxiety and provide relaxation in several studies with various conditions (Kramer, 1990; Hughes et al, 1996; Ireland, 1998). TT may be helpful in conjunction with conventional therapy in asthma as well. Table 3-7 lists a few manipulative and body-based methods and energy therapies for asthma and allergy.

Table 3-7 Manipulative and Body-Based Methods and Energy Therapies for Respiratory Concerns

Intervention	Management	Treatment Regimen	Cautions, Precautions, Interactions	References
Chiropractic	Asthma—significant reduction in symptom severity and bronchial hyperreactivity from baseline. Significant results in both the sham and treatment group.	Chiropractic manipulation	Effect may be a function of time or type of sham treatment. Conventional asthma therapy must always be available also.	Freeman, Lawlis, 2001; Nielsen et al, 1995
Chiropractic	OM—decrease in otitis symptoms	Chiropractic treatment from one chiropractor	Retrospective, nonrandomized study of 46 children (< age 5)	Loo, 1999; Froehle, 1996
Musculoskeletal therapy in combination with Eucapnic Breathing Retraining	Asthma	Musculoskeletal massage to work muscles of breathing	Time and cost; need a skilled practitioner.	Courtney, 2000; anecdotal

Massage	Asthma, cystic fibrosis improvement. General well being, increase circulation.	20-min massage HS by trained parent. Swedish massage for relaxation, deep-tissue, or neuromuscular for areas.	Small well-done studies with good results	Field, 2000
Negative ions	Allergy and asthma	Negative ion generator	Unproven	Iker, 2000
Osteopathy	Asthma and other respiratory conditions	Osteopathic manipulation	Does not replace conventional therapy.	Chaitow et al, 2002
Reflexology	Asthma and allergy	Reflexology points for sinuses: plantar surfaces of toes and webbing between fingers. Stimulate with thumb and index finger or eraser of pencil.	Minimal study.	Iker, 2000
Therapeutic touch	Decreases anxiety in a variety of conditions.	15- to 20-min treatment	Several studies. Ask permission.	Krieger, 1993

hs, *At bedtime*; OM, *otitis media.*

REFERENCES

Adkinson NF Jr: Immunotherapy for allergic rhinitis [editorial], *N Engl J Med* 314(341):522, 1999.

Ai AL et al: Private prayer and optimism in middle-aged and older patients awaiting cardiac surgery, *Gerontologist* 42(11):70, 2002.

Al-Nakib W et al: Prophylaxis and treatment of rhinovirus colds with zinc gluconate lozenges, *J Antimicrob Chemother* 20:893, 1987.

Baker J C et al: Reduced dietary intakes of magnesium, selenium and vitamins A, C and E in patients with brittle asthma, *Thorax* 50(supp 2):A75, 1995.

Balon J et al: A comparison of active and simulated chiropractic manipulation as adjunctive treatment for childhood asthma, *N Engl J Med* 339:1013, 1998.

Battan FK, Dart RC: Emergencies, injuries, and poisoning. In Hay W et al, eds: *Current pediatric diagnosis and treatment,* ed 15, New York, 2001, McGraw-Hill.

Bensky D, Gamble A: *Chinese herbal medicine materia medica.* Seattle, 1986, Eastland Press.

Berman S et al: Ear, nose, throat. In Hay WW et al, eds: *Current pediatric diagnosis and treatment,* ed 15, New York, 2001, McGraw-Hill.

Biernacki W, Peake M: Acupuncture in treatment of stable asthma, *Res Med* 92:9, 1998.

Blumenthal M: *Herbal Medicine: Expanded Commission E monographs.* Newton, Mass, 2000, Integrative Medicine Communication.

Boericke W: *New manual of homeopathic materia medica and repertory,* New Delhi, 2000, B. Jain.

Bowler S, Green A, Mitchell C: Buteyko breathing techniques in asthma: a blinded randomized controlled trial, *Med J Aust* 169:575, 1998.

Brunton S, Saphir R: Dust mites and asthma, *Hosp Pract* 34(10):67, 1999.

Bucca C et al: Effect of vitamin C on histamine bronchial responsiveness of patients with allergic rhinitis, *Ann Allergy* 65:311, 1990.

Buckle J: Aromatherapy. In Snyder M, Lindquist R: *Complementary/alternative therapies in nursing,* ed 4, New York, 2002, Springer.

Buckle J: The role of aromatherapy in nursing care. In Colbath J, Prawlucki P, eds: *Nurs Clin North Am* 36(1):57, 2001.

Byrd RP, Krishnaswamy G, Roy TM: Difficult-to-manage asthma, *PGM* 108(6):37, 2000.

Castleman M: *Blended medicine: the best choices in healing,* Emmaus, Pa, 2000, Rodale.

Chaitow L, Bradley D, Gilbert C: *Multidisciplinary approaches to breathing pattern disorders,* St Louis, 2002, Churchill Livingstone.

Chen A, Chen J: Treatment of asthma with herbs and acupuncture, *Lotus Update* (self-published), 1999.

Christensen P et al: Acupuncture for bronchial asthma, *Allergy* 39:379, 1984.

Codina R, Lockey R: Combating allergens at home: what you need to know about preventing asthma, *Consultant* (February):279, 2000.

Coen BL et al: Effects of biofeedback-assisted relaxation on asthma severity and immune function, *Pediatr Asthma Allergy Immunol* 10:71, 1996.

Cohen H, Neuman I, Nahum H: Blocking effect of vitamin C in exercise-induced asthma, *Arch Pediatr Adolesc Med* 151:367, 1997.

Cools M et al: Long-term effects of specific immunotherapy, administered during childhood, in asthmatic patients allergic to either house-dust mite or to both house-dust mite and grass pollen, *Allergy* 55:69, 2000.

Corren J, Storms WW, eds: *21st century management of upper respiratory allergic diseases*, [Highlights from a conference: National Institutes of Health, 1997], Califon, NJ, 1998, Cardiner-Caldwell Synermed.

Courtney R: Breathe easy: Eucapnic Breath Retraining: a powerful tool for the somatic therapist, *Massage & Bodywork* 15(4):12, 2000.

Courtney R: Butey K breathing for health, www.breathingCO2.com, accessed Jan 6, 2003.

Crook W: *The yeast connection*, New York, 1986, Vintage.

Cummings S, Ullman D: *Everybody's guide to homeopathic medicine*, New York, 1997, Tarcher Putnam.

Day A: The journal as a guide for the healing journey, *Nurs Clin North Am* 36(1):131, 2001.

Deadman P: Asthma, *J Chin Med* 10:5, 1982.

DerMarderosian A: *The review of natural products*, St Louis, 2001, Facts and Comparisons.

Deter HC, Albert G: Group therapy for asthma patients: a concept for the psychosomatic treatment of patients in a medical clinic—a controlled study, *Psychother Psychosom* 40:95, 1983.

Douglas R et al: Failure of effervescent zinc acetate lozenges to alter the course of upper respiratory infection in Australian adults, *Antimicrob Agents Chemother* 31:1263, 1987.

Dunn, KS, Horgas AL: The prevalence of prayer as a spiritual self-care modality in elders, *J Holist Nurs* 18(4):337, 2000.

Durham SR et al: Long-term efficacy of grass-pollen immunotherapy, *N Engl J Med* 341:468, 1999.

Eby G, Davis D, Halcomb W: Reduction in duration of common cold by zinc gluconate lozenges in a double-blind study, *Antimicrob Agents Chemother* 25:20, 1984.

Ernst E, ed: *The desktop guide to complementary and alternative medicine: an evidence-based approach*, St Louis, 2001, Mosby.

Ewer T, Stewart D: Improvement in bronchial hyper-responsiveness in patients with moderate asthma after treatment with a hypnotic technique: ARC trial, *BMJ* 293:1129, 1986.

Farr B et al: Two randomized controlled trials of zinc gluconate lozenges therapy for experimentally induced rhinovirus colds, *Antimicrob Agents Chemother* 31:1183, 1987.

Fetrow C, Avila J: *Complementary and alternative medicines*, Springhouse, Penn, 1999, Springhouse.

Field T: *Touch therapy*, Philadelphia, 2000, Churchill Livingstone.

Flannelly LT, Inouye J: Relationships of religion, health status, and socioeconomic status to the quality of life of individuals who are HIV positive, *Issues Ment Health Nurs* 22(3):253, 2001.

Fleisher M: Sneezes and wheezes: homeopathy for hay fever and allergies, *Homeopathy Today* April/May:10, 2002.

Fluge T et al: Long-term effects of breathing exercises and yoga in patients with bronchial asthma, *Pneumologie* 48:484, 1994.

Fradet B et al: *The natural way of healing asthma and allergies*, New York, 1995, Dell.

Frawley D: *Ayurvedic healing: a comprehensive guide*, ed 2, Twin Lakes, Wisc, 2000, Lotus Press.

Frawley D, Lad V: *The yoga of herbs*, Twin Lakes, Wisc, 1998, Lotus Press.

Freedberg PD et al: effect of progressive muscle relaxation on the objective symptoms and subjective responses associated with asthma, *Heart and Lung* 16:24, 1987.

Freeman L, Lawlis G: *Complementary and alternative medicine*, St Louis, 2001, Mosby.

Friese K, Kruse S, Moeller H: Acute otitis media in children, comparison between conventional and homeopathic therapy, *HNO* (German) 44(8):462, 1996.

Froehle RM: Ear infection: a retrospective study examining improvement from chiropractic care and analyzing for influencing factors, *J Manipulative Physiol Ther* 19(3):169, 1996.

Fuller K, Casparian JM: Vitamin D: Balancing cutaneous and systemic considerations, *South Med J* 94(1):58, 2001.

Fung KP, Chow O, So SY: Attenuation of exercise-induced asthma by acupuncture, *Lancet* 2:1419, 1986.

Gamble A: Alternative medical approaches to the treatment of asthma, *Alt and Comp Ther* 1(2):61, 1995.

Gift AG, Moore T, Soeken K: Relaxation to reduce dyspnea and anxiety in COPD patients, *Nurs Res* 41:242, 1992.

Gilbert D, Moellering R, Sande M: *The Sanford guide to antimicrobial therapy*, Hyde Park, VT, 2002, Antimicrobial Therapy.

Godfrey J, Godfrey N, Novick S: Zinc for treating the common cold: review of all clinical trials since 1984, *Alt Ther* 2(6):63, 1996.

Gupta S: Tylophora indica in bronchial asthma: a double blind study, *Ind J Med Res* 69:981, 1979.

Hackman R, Stern J, Gershwin ME: Complementary/alternative therapies in general medicine: asthma and allergies. In Spencer J, Jacobs J, eds: *Complementary/alternative medicine: an evidence-based approach*, St Louis, 1999, Mosby.

Hay L: *Heal your body*, Carlsbad, Calif, 2000, Hay House.

Heap M, Aravind K: *Hartland's medical and dental hypnosis*, Edinburgh, 2002, Churchill Livingstone.

Hemila H: Vitamin C and infectious disease. In Packer L, Fuchs J, eds: *Vitamin in health and disease*, New York, 1997, Marcel Dekker.

Henry M et al: Improvement of respiratory function in chronic asthmatic patients with autogenic therapy, *J Psychosom Res* 17:265, 1993.

Hirt M, Nobel S, Barron E: Zinc nasal gel for the treatment of common cold symptoms: a double-blind, placebo-controlled trial, *Ear Nose Throat J* 79:778, 2000.

Hodge L et al: Consumption of oily fish and childhood asthma risk, *MJA* 164:137, 1996.

Huebscher R: *Honey and lemon cough syrup: An old home remedy*, 2002, unpublished recipe.

Hughes PP, Meize-Grochowski R, Harris CN: Therapeutic touch with adolescent psychiatric patients, *J Holist Nurs* 14(1):6, 1996.

Huntley A, Ernst E: Herbal medicines for asthma: a systematic review, *Thorax* 55:925, 2000.

Ireland M: Therapeutic touch with HIV-infected children: a pilot study, *J Assoc Nurs AIDS Care* 9(4):68, 1998.

Ivker R: *Sinus survival*, New York, 2000, Tarcher Putnam.

Ivker R, Nelson T: *Asthma survival*, New York, 2001, Tarcher Putnam.

Janssen GWHM: The application of Maharishi Ayur-Veda in the treatment of 10 chronic diseases: a pilot study, *Ned Tijdschr Genieskd* 5:586, 1989.

Jobst K et al: Controlled trial of acupuncture for disabling breathlessness, *Lancet* 2:1416, 1986.

Johnston C, Solomon E, Corte C: Vitamin C status of a campus population: college students get a C minus, *J Am College Health* 46:209, 1998.

Jones A: *Yoga: A step-by-step guide*, Boston, 1998, Element Books.

Keegan L: The environment as healing tool. Colbath J, Prawlucki P, eds: *Nurs Clin North Am* 36(1):73, 2001.

Keen CL, Gershwin ME: Zinc deficiency and immune function, *Annu Rev Nutr* 10:413, 1990.

Kleijnen J, ter Riet G, Knipschild P: Acupuncture and asthma: a review of controlled trials, *Thorax* 46:799, 1991.

Kornfield J: *The inner art of meditation*, Boulder, Colo, 1996, Sounds True.

Kotses H et al: Long-term effects of biofeedback-induced facial relaxation on measures of asthma severity in children, *Biofeedback Self Regul* 16:1, 1991.

Kramer NA: Comparison of therapeutic touch and casual touch in stress reduction of hospitalized children, *Pediatr Nurs* 16:483, 1990.

Krieger D: *Accepting your power to heal*, Santa Fe, NM, 1993, Bear & Co.

Kuhn M: *Complementary therapies for health care providers*, Philadelphia, 1999, Lippincott.

Lad V: *The complete book of Ayurvedic home remedies*, New York, 1998, Three Rivers Press.

Lal A, Kumar L, Malhotra S: Knowledge of asthma among parents of asthmatic children, *Indian Pediatr* 32:649, 1995.

LaValle J et al: *Natural therapeutics pocket guide*, Hudson, Ohio, 2000, LexiComp.

Lichstein K: *Clinical relaxation strategies*, New York, 1988, Wiley Interscience.

Loo M: Complementary/alternative therapies in select populations: children. In Spencer J, Jacobs J, eds: *Complementary/alternative medicine: an evidence-based approach*, St Louis, 1999, Mosby.

Maciocia G: *The practice of Chinese medicine*, New York, 1994, Churchill Livingstone.

Maher-Loughman G, McDonald N, Mason A et al: Controlled trial of hypnosis in the symptomatic treatment of asthma, *BMSH*:371, 1962.

Malo JL, Cartier A, Dolovich J: Occupational asthma due to zinc, *Eur Respir J* 6:447, 1993.

Mark J: Asthma. In Rakel D, editor: *Integrative medicine*, Philadelphia, 2003, WB Saunders.

McBride S et al: The therapeutic use of music for dyspnea and anxiety in patients with COPD who live at home, *J Holist Nurs* 17(3):229, 1999.

McDowell B: Vitamin A and beta carotene, *Alt and Comp Ther* 1(2):67, 1995.

Meisenhelder JB, Chandler EN: Prayer and health outcomes in church members, *Alt Ther Health Med* 6:56, 2000.

Miles Laboratory. Information sheet on bee sting protection, 1986.

Mittman P: Randomized, double-blind study of freeze-dried *Urtica dioica* in the treatment of allergic rhinitis, *Planta Med* 56(1):44, 1990.

Moneret-Vautrin DA, Kanny G, Thevenin F: Asthma caused by food allergy, *Rev Med Intern* 17:551, 1996.

Monteleone CA, Sherman AR: Nutrition and asthma, *Arch Intern Med* 157:23, 1997.

Morrison JB: Chronic asthma and improvement with relaxation induced by hypnotherapy, *Royal Soc Med* 81:701, 1988.

Mossad S et al: Zinc gluconate lozenges for treating the common cold: a randomized, double-blind, placebo-controlled study, *Ann Intern Med* 125(2):81, 1996.

Murray M: Food allergies, *Natural Med J* 1(7):18, 1998.

Murray MT, Pizzorno JE: Asthma. In Pizzorno J, Murray M, eds: *Textbook of natural medicine*, ed 2, vol 2, Edinburgh, 1999, Churchill Livingstone.

Nagarathna R, Nagendra HR: Yoga for bronchial asthma: a controlled study, *BMJ* 291:1077, 1985.

Nagendra HR, Nagarathna R: An integrated approach of yoga therapy for bronchial asthma: a 3-54 month prospective study, *J Asthma* 23(3):123, 1986.

Naparstek B: *A meditation to help relieve asthma*, [audio cassette recording], Cleveland, Ohio, 1992, Health Journeys/Image Paths.

Naparstek B: Staying well with guided imagery, New York, 1994, Warner Books.

National Academies Press (NAP): Dietary reference intakes: applications in dietary assessment, 2001, *www.NAP.edu/catalog/9956.html*. Accessed Jan 6, 2003.

National Institutes of Health. National Heart, Lung, and Blood Institute [NIH-NHLBI]: *Guidelines for the diagnosis and management of asthma*, Expert Panel Report 2, Bethesda, MD, 1997, NIH Publication #97-4051.

National Institutes of Health: *Acupuncture, NIH consensus statement* 15(5):1, Washington, DC, 1997, US Government Printing Office, *http://odp.od.nih.gov/-consensus/cons/107/107_statement.htm*.

National Jewish Medical and Research Center: *Medfacts. Nasal Wash Treatment*, 2000, Patient Information Sheet.

Neuman I, Nahum H, Ben-Amotz A: Reduction of exercise-induced asthma oxidative stress by lycopene, a natural antioxidant, *Allergy* 55:1184, 2000.

Nielson NH et al: Chronic asthma and chiropractic spinal manipulation: a randomized clinical trial, *Clin Exp Allergy* 25:80, 1995.

O'Connor J, Bensky D: *Acupuncture: a comprehensive text*, Seattle, 1981, Eastland Press.

Pelton R et al: *Drug-induced nutrient depletion handbook*, Hudson, Ohio, 2001, Lexi-Comp.

Pharmacist's Letter/Prescriber's Letter [PL/PL]: *Natural medicine's comprehensive database (NMCD)*, Stockton, Calif, 2002, NMCD.

Pharmacist's Letter/Prescriber's Letter: *Natural medicines in clinical management: colds and flu 2000* (4), Stockton, Calif, 2000, PL/PL.

Pharmacist's Letter/Prescriber's Letter: *The updated therapeutic uses of herbs*, Stockton, Calif, 3/15/2000, NMCD.

Pizzorno J, Murray M, Joiner-Bey H: *The clinician's handbook of natural medicine*, Edinburgh, 2002, Churchill Livingstone.

Rakel D: *Integrative medicine*, Philadelphia, 2003, WB Saunders.

Reilly D et al: Is evidence for homeopathy reproducible? *Lancet* 344:1601, 1994.

Renfroe K: Effect of progressive muscle relaxation on dyspnea and state anxiety in patients with chronic obstructive pulmonary disease, *Heart and Lung* 17:408, 1988.

Research Committee of the British Tuberculosis Association: Hypnosis for asthma—a controlled trial, *BMJ* 4(263):71, 1968.

Reuther I: Yangsheng as a complementary therapy in the management of asthma: a single-case appraisal, *J Alt Comp Med* 4(2):173, 1998.

Rockwell S: Rotation diet: a diagnostic and therapeutic tool. In Pizzorno J, Murray M, eds: *Textbook of natural medicine*, ed 2, vol 2, Edinburgh, 1999, Churchill Livingstone.

Rogers D: Mind-body interventions. In Micozzi M, ed: *Fundamentals of complementary and alternative medicine*, Edinburgh, 2001, Churchill Livingstone.

Schwartz J, Weiss ST: Dietary factors and their relation to respiratory symptoms: the second national health and nutrition examination survey, *Am J Epidemiol* 132:67, 1990.

Scott J: *Natural medicine for children*, New York, 1990, Avon Books.

Sharma H, Clark C: *Contemporary ayurveda*, Philadelphia, 2000, Churchill Livingstone.

Sharma H, et al: Modern insights into ancient medicine, *JAMA* 265(20):2633, 1991.

Shuler PA et al: The effects of spiritual/religious practices on psychological well-being among inner city homeless women, *Nurs Pract Forum* 5:106, 1994.

Shutte M, personal communication–class lecture, 3/01.

Simon D: *The wisdom of healing*, New York, 1997, Harmony Books.

Singh V, et al: Effect of yoga breathing exercises (pranayama) on airway reactivity in subjects with asthma, *Lancet* 335:1381, 1990.

Skinner S: *An introduction to homeopathic medicine in primary care*, Gaithersburg, MD, 2001, Aspen.

Slovis B, Brigham K: Obstructive lung disease. In Andreoli T et al, ed: *Cecil essentials of medicine*, ed 5, Philadelphia, 2001, Saunders.

Smyth J et al: Effects of writing about stressful experiences on symptom reduction in patients with asthma or rheumatoid arthritis, *JAMA* 281:14, 1999.

Snyder M: Progressive muscle relaxation. In Snyder M, Lindquist R, eds: *Complementary/alternative therapies in nursing*, New York, 1998, Springhouse.

Spector SL: Common triggers of asthma, *Postgrad Med* 90:50, 1991.

Speiss et al: Auswirkung von Informations-und Entspannungsgruppen auf die Lungenfunktion und psychophysische Befindlichkeit bei Asthmapatienten, *Prax Klin Pneumol* 42:641, 1988.

Spencer J, Jacobs J: Complementary/alternative medicine: An evidence-based approach, 1999.

Tashkin D et al: A controlled trial of real and simulated acupuncture in the management of chronic asthma, *J Allergy Clin Immunol* 76(6):855, 1985.

Taylor M et al: Randomized controlled trial of homeopathy versus placebo in perennial allergic rhinitis with overview of four trial series, *BMJ* 321:471, 2000.

Temes R: *Medical hypnosis: an introduction and clinical guide*, Edinburgh, 1999, Churchill Livingstone.

Thich Nhat Hanh: *The blooming of a lotus: guided meditation exercises for healing and transformation*, Boston, 1997, Beacon. (Also others from 1976.)

Tirtha S: *The Ayurvedic encyclopedia: natural secrets to healing, prevention and longevity*, ed 2, Bayville, NY, 1998, Ayurveda Holistic Center Press.

Vedanthan PK et al: Clinical study of yoga techniques in university students with asthma: a controlled study, *Allergy Asthma Proc* 19:3, 1998.

WARN (Wisconsin Antibiotic Resistance Network): *Clinical practice fact sheets for respiratory illness—2000*. Recommendations of a task force sponsored by the Wisconsin Division of Public Health, State Medical Society of Wisconsin and Marshfield Medical Research Foundation. Funding provided by USCDCP, 2000. *www.wismed.org*

Weil A: *Balanced living* at the Ask Dr. Weil website: *www.drweil.com/app/cda/drw_cda.php*, accessed Jan 6, 2003.

Wilson Q et al: Transcendental meditation and asthma, *Respiration* 32:74, 1975.

Yu D, Lee S: Effect of acupuncture on bronchial asthma, *Clin Sci Mol Sci* 51:503, 1976.

Zakay-Rones Z et al: Inhibition of several strains of influenza virus in vitro and reduction of symptoms by an elderberry extract *(Sambucus nigra)* during an outbreak of influenza B Panama, *J Alt Comp Med* 1(4):361, 1995.

GASTROINTESTINAL CONCERNS

Roxana Huebscher ▪ Helen Miller ▪ Louise Rauckhorst

NAC THERAPIES FOR COMMON GASTROINTESTINAL CONCERNS

Common gastrointestinal (GI) concerns include signs and symptoms such as constipation, diarrhea, and nausea, as well as diagnoses such as gastroesophageal reflux disease (GERD), peptic ulcer disease (PUD), irritable bowel syndrome (IBS), inflammatory bowel disease (IBD), gallbladder and liver concerns, and hemorrhoids. Preventing colon cancer is another major GI concern because colorectal cancer is the second leading cause of death resulting from malignancy in the United States; approximately 6% of Americans will develop colon cancer (McQuaid, 2002). Appropriate workup and diagnosis is necessary before any therapies because numerous disorders can be the cause of GI symptoms. Once the diagnosis is made, however, natural-alternative-complementary (NAC) therapies may be useful in conjunction with conventional care.

CONSTIPATION, DIARRHEA, AND IRRITABLE BOWEL SYNDROME

Constipation

According to the 1991 National Health Interview Survey, constipation is a GI complaint affecting approximately 4.5 million persons in the United States (National Digestive Diseases Information Clearinghouse [NDDIC], 2001), and laxative sales run in the millions of dollars. Constipation is defined as stool frequency less than two to three times per week (Heuman et al, 1997), or infrequent, hard, small stools, or excessive straining at stool (McQuaid, 2002), or incomplete emptying of stool. Some causes of constipation include dietary indiscretion, poor bowel habits, IBS, Hirschsprung's, malignancy, hypothyroidism, diabetes, and other endocrine disorders; depression; scleroderma and lupus; cystic fibrosis, Parkinson's, multiple sclerosis, spinal cord injury, and other neurologic disorders; and stroke, uremia, and medications. After appropriate diagnosis, NAC treatments are available to both prevent and treat constipation.

Diarrhea

Diarrhea, defined as loose, watery stools occurring more than three times in one day, is a common problem usually lasting only a day or two. The average adult in the United States has about four bouts of

202

diarrhea per year (NDDIC, 2001). Diarrhea can last longer than a few days, causing dehydration, which is especially serious in the very young and in older adults (NDDIC, 2001). Causes of diarrhea include dietary indiscretion; food intolerances (e.g., lactase deficiency, food allergy); virus, bacteria, bacterial toxins; parasites; medication reactions and laxative abuse; toxic substances; intestinal diseases (e.g., IBD or celiac disease); post-GI surgery; radiation; Zollinger-Ellison syndrome and other tumors; and functional bowel disorders (e.g., IBS) (Heuman et al, 1997; NDDIC, 2001; McQuaid, 2002). Appropriate diagnosis is necessary and, in conjunction with adequate diagnostic testing and appropriate treatment for the condition, oral rehydration therapy and other NAC therapy are appropriate.

Irritable Bowel Syndrome

IBS is a common chronic functional bowel disorder affecting approximately 10% to 20% of the population and is related to 20% to 50% of referrals to gastroenterologists (Achkar, 2001; Bensoussan et al, 1998; McQuaid, 2002). Symptoms often start in the late teens to early 20s and include pain and other GI symptoms that are not explained by other pathologic or disease processes or structural or biochemical abnormalities. IBS is defined as chronic lower abdominal symptoms for a period of more than 3 months that has two of the three following features:

> (1) relieved with defecation; (2) onset associated with a change in frequency of stool; (3) onset associated with a change in form (appearance) of stool. Other symptoms supporting the diagnosis include abnormal stool frequency (more than three bowel movements per day or fewer than three per week); abnormal stool form (lumpy or hard or loose or watery); abnormal stool passage (straining, urgency, or feeling of incomplete evacuation); passage of mucus; bloating or feeling of abdominal distention. (McQuaid, 2002, p. 644)

In the United States, 75% of people diagnosed with IBS are women. Up to 68% of children over age 5 who have the complaint of recurrent abdominal pain meet the adult criteria for IBS. Men with IBS tend to have diarrhea, while women tend toward constipation. (Heitkemper, Jarrett, 2001). A diagnosis is made through the process of excluding other GI diagnoses.

ALTERNATIVE HEALTH CARE SYSTEMS FOR CONSTIPATION, DIARRHEA, AND IRRITABLE BOWEL SYNDROME

Ayurveda for Constipation and Irritable Bowel Syndrome

Ayurvedic herbs have been used successfully for the management of opioid-induced constipation in patients with cancer. In one study, the treatment group received an herbal preparation called

Misrakasneham that included *Clitoria ternatea, Curcuma longa* (turmeric), and *Vitis vinifera* (grape skin, leaf, seed), as well as castor oil. Members of this group had satisfactory bowel movements (17 of 20 patients) as did the senna extract group (11 of 16 patients) but did not differ significantly between the groups (Ernst, 2001; Ramaesh, 1998).

Triphala is best for constipation in older adults according to Frawley (1989). Licorice tea after meals, castor oil, and *ghee* (clarified, boiled unsalted butter) in warm milk are other laxatives used. Enema therapy, termed *basti*, is available consisting of medicinal oils such as sesame, calamus, or herbal decoctions in a liquid. Fasting may be recommended (Lad, 1985). The constitution of the individual (whether he or she is *vata, pitta,* or *kapha*) is considered before treatments; therapies are adjusted accordingly.

From the Ayurvedic perspective, IBS is caused by vata pushing pitta into the colon. For treatment, herbal remedies and recipes are available. For chronic cases, Ayurveda recommends introducing ½ to 1 cup of sesame oil into the rectum and retaining it for 5 minutes to lubricate the colon. This basti should be done once or twice a week as needed to control the IBS (Lad, 1998).

In addition, anecdotally, yoga postures recommended for constipation are the Vitality Breath, the Cobra, the Tree, backward bend, yoga *mudra*, knee to chest, shoulder stand, and Corpse. Some individuals may not be able to do some of these postures because of mobility or balance problems or cardiovascular disorders. For example, people with glaucoma, neck pain, obesity, disc problems, or on menses should not do the shoulder stand (Jones, 1998; Lad, 1985). Easier forms of the same *asanas* (postures) that may be helpful are recommended for beginning students of yoga.

Traditional Chinese Medicine for Constipation and Irritable Bowel Syndrome

For constipation, Traditional Chinese Medicine (TCM) acupuncture has been used, as well as Chinese herbs. Acupuncturists may use the meridian points Large Intestine 4 and 11 and sometimes points on the abdomen. Chinese laxative herbs can be gentle and effective if used properly.

In TCM, IBS is a digestive disorder with the clinical symptoms of abdominal pain, loose and more frequent bowel movements, distended abdomen, rectal mucus, incomplete emptying of rectum, constipation, or any combination (Lewis, 1992). In TCM, the two most common organs involved with this imbalance are the Liver and Spleen. Other organs that may be involved are Lung, Large Intestine (LI), and Small Intestine (SI). (See Appendix B for location of the meridians.)

An explanation of the Liver and Spleen organs in TCM will help explain the TCM view. Rather than being a solid organ with very specific functions, as in Western medicine, an organ in TCM is seen as a complex system including not only the anatomic tissue, but also consisting of a corresponding emotion, sense organ, and relationships to substances and energies of the body. An organ is a dynamic entity that has balances and checks with other organs to keep the whole person functioning well (Maciocia, 1989).

The Liver ensures the smooth flow of Qi throughout the body, to all the organs, and in the correct directions. This concept is extremely important, because any stagnation of Qi produces very uncomfortable symptoms. Because Qi flow relates to the emotional state, restrained Qi causes frustration or depression that may be accompanied by a feeling of a lump in the throat, tightness in the chest, or abdominal distension. The Liver Qi assists the Stomach and Spleen in digestion. The Stomach Qi needs to move downward to aid movement of food through the system, and the Spleen Qi needs to go up to support the work of the Stomach. If stagnation is affecting the Stomach, symptoms of nausea, vomiting, or belching may be seen. If the spleen Qi is affected, diarrhea results. In addition, as one of its main functions, the Liver also stores blood and controls the contraction and relaxation of the sinews (tendons) of the body (Maciocia, 1989).

The Spleen aids the Stomach in digestion by transforming food and drink into Qi to be distributed to the rest of the body. The Spleen transports the useable nutrients to the various organs responsible for production of Qi and blood. If the Spleen Qi is weakened or impaired, the appetite will be affected, digestion will suffer, and diarrhea with abdominal distension may result. The digestion and circulation of fluids may also stagnate, causing edema or phlegm production. The Spleen controls blood to keep it in the blood vessels and helps in production of blood. The Spleen nourishes the tissues of the body, in particular, the muscles of the limbs. Also, the Spleen is responsible for level of physical energy available. Our capacity for thinking clearly, and concentrating, is dependent on the Spleen; and conversely, too much thinking will injure the Spleen (Maciocia, 1989).

The most common imbalance involved in IBS is stagnant Liver Qi invading the Spleen. This imbalance may be combined with Spleen Qi deficiency. Symptoms of stagnant Liver Qi invading the Spleen are:
- Spastic abdominal pain, aggravated by pressure
- Constipation
- Abdominal distension
- Incomplete emptying of rectum

Symptoms of Spleen Qi deficiency are:
- Loss of appetite
- Fatigue

- Abdominal distention after eating
- Diarrhea
- Mucus per rectum (Lewis, 1992)

The treatment strategy for IBS includes therapy to relieve stagnation of Qi in Liver and intestines, harmonize Liver and Spleen, and support Spleen Qi. Table 4-1 reviews research related to acupuncture and IBS or abdominal symptoms. Table 4-2 lists the TCM management of IBS, as well as other alternative health care system treatments.

Homeopathy

Case taking (history taking) is as important in homeopathy as it is in conventional care. Homeopathic remedies for constipation include *Alumina, Bryonia alba, graphites, Lycopodium clavatum, Nux vomica, opium, Plumbum metallicum, sepia, silicea,* or *sulphur* (Skinner, 2001). However, individual accompanying signs and symptoms, as well as psychosocial areas determine which remedy will be used. Skinner (2001) states that no high-quality studies using homeopathic remedies for constipation have been conducted.

Homeopathy has been used successfully in the treatment of diarrhea. Jacobs (1994) completed a randomized double-blind placebo-controlled clinical trial of children with diarrhea. The 81 children who were given individualized homeopathic treatments (i.e., remedies that fit their symptoms specifically) had a significant decrease in duration of diarrhea.

Common homeopathic treatments for gastoenteritis include *Arsenicum album, Calcarea carbonica, Chamomilla, Mercurius vivus or Mercurius solubilis, Natrum sulpuricum, Phosphorus, Podophyllum peltatum, Pulsatilla, Sulphur,* and *Veratrum album.* Individual symptoms, in addition to the gastroenteritis, point to the correct therapy (Horvilleur, 1986; LaValle et al, 2000; Skinner, 2001).

For hemorrhoids, extracts of *Aesculus hippocastanum* (1X), *Calendula officinalis* (1X), *Hamamelis virginica* (1X), and *Paeonia officinalis* (1X) in a base of almond oil, avocado oil, and cocoa butter is a soothing homeopathic remedy. The mixture is sold under the brand name of Nelson's Hemorrhoid Creme and is applied topically to the cleansed rectal area. In addition, for a hemorrhoid clot, *Lachesis 5C* is recommended; or if anal cracking appears, take *Graphites 9C, Nitricum acidum 9C, Ratanhia 9C* (Horvilleur, 1986).

Amish Folk Medicine

Amish folk medicine recipes for diarrhea include:
1. Mix 1 tsp flour with 1 tsp nutmeg, 1 tsp white sugar, and a pinch of salt in glass. Add enough water to make easy to drink. Take every 4 hours.
2. For children, give 2 tsp vinegar every 2 hours.

Table 4-1 Acupuncture and Chinese Herbal Research Related to Gastrointestinal Concerns and Irritable Bowel Syndrome

Study	Type	Number	Measure	Outcome
Bensoussan et al, 1998	Compared three treatment groups: individualized herbal treatment; standard herbal treatment; placebo group. All groups are randomized and double blinded.	Total of 116: group 1 = 38, group 2 = 43, group 3 = 35.	BSS and global improvement assessed by patients and gastroenterologists. Patients assessed degree of IBS symptoms that interfered with life. Results were measured at beginning of treatment, after 8 wks of treatment, end of treatment (16 wks), and 14 wks posttreatment.	Patients in groups 1 and 2 had improved BSS scores compared with placebo group ($P = 0.03$) and better global improvement ($P = 0.007$). Group 1 improved about the same as did group 2 but maintained improvement 14 wks posttreatment.
Cahn et al, 1978	Two groups of patients received endoscopy; first group received real acupuncture, second group received sham acupuncture for pain control.	90 patients were in study, 45 in each group.	Attending nurse reported patients' reactions, endoscopist reported number of attempts or unsuccessful test, and patient reported posttest of pain or sickness.	All criteria indicated significantly better results for the real acupuncture group. (P values given for each variable.)

Continued

Table 4-1	Acupuncture and Chinese Herbal Research Related to Gastrointestinal Concerns and Irritable Bowel Syndrome—cont'd			
Study	**Type**	**Number**	**Measure**	**Outcome**
Chan et al, 1997	Uncontrolled study; acupuncture once wkly for 4 wks for IBS symptoms.	N = 7	Well being and symptoms were recorded.	Improvement in general well being and symptoms of bloating were decreased.
Li et al, 1992	Review of research studies on effects of acupuncture on GI function.	12 studies on gastric motility; 13 studies on EMG of stomach function; 9 studies on gastric secretion; 5 studies on analgesia for endoscopy; 21 studies on various GI conditions.	Measures were not indicated.	Acupuncture was shown beneficial for regulating GI motor activity and secretions and for analgesia with endoscopy. No clear benefit was observed in specific GI disorders possibly because of poorly controlled studies.

| Yanhua, Sumei, 2000 | Scalp acupuncture treatment for acute epigastric and abdominal pain. | 86 patients total: epigastric pain (n = 15), liver and gallbladder disorders (n = 20), gynecologic pain (n = 16), urinary stones (n = 14), intestinal pain (n = 16), other causes (n = 5). | Patients reported pain and symptom cessation or relief immediately after treatment and within 2 days of treatment. | 95.35% of patients experienced marked or effective improvement based on study rating system. |

EMG, *Electromyography*; GI, *gastrointestinal*; IBS, *irritable bowel syndrome*; BSS, *bowel symptom scale*.

Table 4-2		Alternative Health Care Systems for Constipation, Diarrhea, and Irritable Bowel Syndrome		
Intervention	*Management*	*Treatment Regimen*	*Cautions, Precautions, Interactions*	*References*
Ayurveda				
Herbs	Constipation	Licorice tea; triphala; one glass of water boiled with 1 tbsp of flaxseed at hs; Misrakasneham *Clitoria ternatea, Curcuma longa* (turmeric) and *Vitis vinifera* (grape); castor oil	Fluids increased with flaxseed. Laxatives should be used on short-term basis.	Lad, 1985; PL/PL, 2002
	IBS	½ tsp of an herb mixture made up of: 1 part shatavari, ⅛ part kama dudha, ⅛ part shanka bhasma, 2 parts arrowroot. Administer mixture with a little warm water		Lad, 1998

		bid after eating. 1 tsp of psyllium husks with ½ c yogurt 1 hr after dinner, or 1 tsp flaxseed boiled in 1 c of water and administered at bedtime	Increased fluids when taking bulk laxatives.	
Oils	Constipation	Oral: castor oil; 1 tsp of ghee in glass of warm milk	Castor oil SE: nausea, cramps, electrolyte loss, dependence.	Lad, 1985; PL/PL, 2002
	IBS	Basti (enema): ½-1 c warm sesame oil into the rectum. Retain for 5 mins to lubricate colon, 1-2 times/wk to control IBS.	Oil enemas are contraindicated in those with diabetes, obesity, indigestion, low *agni*, enlarged spleen, unconsciousness.	Lad, 1998, 1985
Yoga	Constipation	Vitality Breath, the Cobra, and the Tree, Backward Bend, yoga *mudra*, knee to chest, Shoulder Stand, and Corpse	There are different poses for each of the constitutions. Those with back or orthopedic problems or poor balance may have difficulty with some poses. Modification of postures may be needed. All yoga postures should be performed while doing deep, quiet breathing.	Jones, 1998; Lad, 1985

Continued

211

Table 4-2 Alternative Health Care Systems for Constipation, Diarrhea, and Irritable Bowel Syndrome—cont'd

Intervention	Management	Treatment Regimen	Cautions, Precautions, Interactions	References
Traditional Chinese Medicine				
Acupuncture	IBS	Treatment 1-2 times/wk for 3-4 wks. Reevaluate with each treatment. When symptoms stabilize, treatment may be every 2-3 wks for 6 mos. To correct Liver Qi: Liver 3, 13 and 14, Gallbladder 34, Urinary Bladder (UB) 18. To harmonize Spleen and Stomach: Stomach 25, 36, and 37, Ren 12, UB 20, and 21. To support Spleen: Ren 6, Spleen 6. To relieve Intestines: UB 25 and 27, Lung 7.	Acupuncture points over the chest and ribs are needled obliquely to avoid puncturing the lungs.	Lewis, 1992; Maciocia, 1992

Acupuncture or acupressure	Constipation	Large intestine 4 and 11; CV (Ren mo) 6 and St 36. Sometimes points on the abdomen.	No acupuncture is performed on abdomen during pregnancy.	Gach, 1990
Moxibustion: the burning of the mugwort herb over acupuncture points to support the Qi and open the acupuncture meridians.	IBS	Performed with acupuncture treatments. Patient may be taught to treat self at home. To support Spleen Qi: moxa on ginger at Ren 6. (Treatment also helps stop diarrhea.) Salt moxa at Ren 8.	Care must be taken not to burn skin around area.	Gaeddert, 1998; Maciocia, 1994
Auricular acupuncture: a micro-acupuncture system on the ear can treat various conditions.	IBS	Use 2-3 needles with body acupuncture treatment. Sterile press tacks may be taped on the ear for up to 1 wk. To treat Liver Qi stagnation: Liver and Shenmen points. To treat Spleen Qi deficiency: Spleen and Stomach points.	If press tacks are used, patient must be instructed on care and use and must watch for signs of infection.	Gaeddert, 1998; Lewis, 1992

Continued

213

Table 4-2 Alternative Health Care Systems for Constipation, Diarrhea, and Irritable Bowel Syndrome—cont'd

Intervention	Management	Treatment Regimen	Cautions, Precautions, Interactions	References
Traditional Chinese Medicine—cont'd				
Chinese herbs: herbs are used in a formula designed for each patient. Many herbs are considered in addition to those listed.	IBS	Herbs that may be used are: Chai Hu (*Radix Bupleuri*) and Bai Shao (*Radix Paeoniae albae*) to pacify the Liver and move Liver Qi. Zhi Gan Cao (*Radix Glycyrrhizae uralensis praeparata*) and Fu Ling (*Sclerotium Poriae cocos*) to tonify the Spleen and harmonize Liver and Spleen. Take as directed. A formula to open stagnation may be used for 1-2 mos to relieve more acute symptoms; then a more supportive formula may be used to continue the healing process.	An experienced herbalist must be consulted to prescribe herbal formulas accurately and safely. Taking an inappropriate formula may worsen symptoms.	Gaeddert, 1998; Maciocia, 1994

Homeopathy

Remedies *Alumina, Bryonia alba, Graphites, Lycopodium clavatum, Nux vomica, opium, Plumbum metallicum, sepia, silicea,* or *sulphur*	Constipation (based on case finding and other signs and symptoms)	Individualize remedy. Examples: if very hard pushing is necessary to evacuate stools—*Alumina 9C.* Constipation during menstrual periods—*Graphites 9C.* Constipation with urge to defecate but being unable to—*Nux vomica 9C.*	Trained homeopathic practitioner and complete case finding are needed.	Horvilleur, 1986; Skinner, 2001
Remedies: *Arsenicum album, Calcarea carbonica, Chamomilla, Mercurius vivus* or *Mercurius solubilis,*	Diarrhea (based on case finding)	Individualize remedy. Examples: diarrhea from infectious origin—*Arsenicum album 9C.* Diarrhea worse after meals, particularly breakfast—*Natrum sulphuricum*	Trained homeopathic practitioner needed and complete case finding. Treat dehydration and see health care practitioner with prolonged or severe diarrhea.	Horvilleur, 1986; Skinner, 2001

Continued

215

Table 4-2	Alternative Health Care Systems for Constipation, Diarrhea, and Irritable Bowel Syndrome—cont'd			
Intervention	**Management**	**Treatment Regimen**	**Cautions, Precautions, Interactions**	**References**
Homeopathy—cont'd				
Remedies: cont'd *Natrum sulpuricum, Phosphorus, Podophyllum peltatum, Pulsatilla, Sulphur,* and *Veratrum album*		9C. Diarrhea after eating fatty foods—*Pulsatilla* 9C. Diarrhea and cold sweats or diarrhea during menstrual periods—*Veratrum album* 9C.		
Remedies: *Aesculus hippocastanum, Calendula officinalis, Collinsonia canadensis, Graphites,*	Hemorrhoids (based on case finding)	Examples: hemorrhoid clot *Lachesis* 5C by mouth. Anal cracking appears, take *Graphites* 9C, by mouth. Local: *Nutricium acidum* 9C,		Horvilleur, 1986

Hamamelis virginica, Lachesis, Paeonia officinalis	*Ratanhia 9C, extracts of Aesculus hippocastanum (1X), Calendula officinalis (1X), Hamamelis virginica (1X), and Paeonia officinalis (1X) in a base of almond oil, avocado oil and cocoa butter; sold under the brand name of Nelson's Hemorrhoid Creme.*

CV, Conception Vessel, also called Ren mo; hs, *at bedtime*; IBS, *irritable bowel syndrome*; PL/PL, *Pharmacist's Letter/Prescriber's Letter*; SE, *side effects*; St, *stomach*.

3. Boil carrots, then puree. Take 1 tsp every 15 minutes.
4. Cook rice until soft. For infants, give rice water with a bit of sugar and milk. For older children, eat the whole rice.
5. Mix ½ cup fresh orange juice, 1 tbsp sugar, ⅙ tsp salt, 1⅓ cup water. Give child ½ oz of the mixture every 2 hours (Quillin, 1996, p. 103).

MIND-BODY-SPIRIT INTERVENTIONS FOR CONSTIPATION, DIARRHEA, AND IRRITABLE BOWEL SYNDROME

Mind-body-spirit interventions may be useful for symptoms of constipation and IBS, and possibly chronic diarrhea. Numerous strategies can be used for a complex process such as IBS. A safe home environment is a priority. Assertiveness, biofeedback, improving bowel habits, journaling, cognitive therapy, prayer and meditation, counseling, relaxation strategies, and other stress management may help. Hypnotherapy and psychotherapy have also shown some effectiveness for IBS (Watkins, 1997; Whorwell et al, 1987; Guthrie et al, 1991).

Biofeedback for Constipation and Irritable Bowel Syndrome

Biofeedback has had positive effects in several pediatric and adult constipation studies. Ernst (2001) reviewed four pediatric randomized clinical trials (Loening, 1990; Loening-Bauke 1995; Van der Plas et al, 1996; Cox et al, 1998) in which conventional treatment was compared with biofeedback in children with constipation, encopresis, or both. "The biofeedback compared 2 to 6 weeks of training or seminars. Two studies found short-term benefit in defecation dynamics (Van der Plas et al, 1996; Loening-Baucke, 1995) and rates of soiling (Cox et al, 1998), but none found significant improvement in soiling, stool frequency, or laxative use at one year or more" (Rubin, 2002, p. 267). Also, in a recent study, biofeedback for some was found effective in outlet obstruction constipation (McKee et al, 1999; Pettit, 1999).

Ernst (2001) reports an uncontrolled study of 40 IBS patients who used computer-aided thermal biofeedback training (Leahy et al, 1998). "Patients achieved progressively deeper levels of relaxation after four 30-minute sessions. The results suggested a reduction of global and bowel symptom scores" (Ernst, 2001, p. 298-299).

Bowel Habits

Bowel habits refer to rethinking and retraining for toileting, including the recommendation that persons heed the urge to go to the bathroom at the time of the urge. This idea means that, when necessary, persons must learn to toilet outside the comfort of their own home rather than holding stool. Another part of retraining is to eat on a regular basis and then to sit down on the toilet approximately 15 to 30 minutes after eating, especially following the morning meal. When starting this routine, patients need to take in extra fluids and fiber to make the process easier. These individuals may need to try "power pudding" to wean themselves off laxatives. Caring for hemorrhoids or fissures is also part of bowel habit planning as is keeping the rectal area clean. These conditions often produce pain and discomfort and are reasons why people put off having a bowel movement; thus the stool may become harder, and the constipation cycle continues. However, with time and focus on natural strategies, new bowel habits will develop.

Psychologic Factors

Stress increases colonic motility in both normal subjects and those with IBS (Narducci et al, 1985) and "mental-emotional problems (e.g., anxiety, fatigue, hostile feelings, depression, sleep disturbances) are reported by almost all patients with IBS" (Murray, Pizzorno, 1999a, p. 1361; Svedlund et al, 1985), although the IBS symptom severity may vary with these factors. In a study comparing 25 women with IBS to 25 women with IBD:

> Patients with IBS had higher levels of depressive symptoms than did patients with IBD. They also reported significantly higher levels of the other study variables—emotional abuse, self-blame, and self-silencing. These three variables were strongly interrelated. Depression did not correlate with any of the other study variables in either group, indicating that emotional abuse, self-blame, and self-silencing can appear independently of depression. A greater percentage of patients in the IBS group had experienced sexual and physical abuse than had those in the IBD group. Emotional abuse was found to be strongly associated with IBS even when the researchers controlled for physical and sexual abuse. (Ali, 2000 in Heitkemper, Jarrett, 2001, p. 31)

Cognitive Therapy

Cognitive therapy may be helpful for many GI symptoms, especially when stress is involved. Wells-Federman and colleagues (2001) in a general discussion on what cognitive therapy is describe the process:

> Cognitive therapy is the conceptual model for a short-term intervention to modify negative irrational thinking. It teaches people to recognize that negative thinking often causes emotional distress. In the context of cognitive therapy, cognitive restructuring is a technique or series of strategies that helps people evaluate their thoughts, challenge them, and replace them with more rational responses. These responses reduce the negative consequences of stress and enhance health. Cognitive restructuring does not gloss over or deny misfortune,

suffering, or negative feelings. There are many things in peoples' lives for which it is appropriate to feel sad, anxious, angry, or depressed. Rather, cognitive restructuring is a technique that can help people become "unstuck" from these powerful moods so that they can experience a broader spectrum of feelings. (p. 97)

The goals of cognitive therapy according to Wells-Federman and colleagues (2001) are for patients to develop awareness by recognizing upsetting situations; to recognize automatic thoughts and the connection between the thoughts and their emotions; to identify errors in thinking, distortions, and self-defeating beliefs; and to choose more appropriate empowering thoughts while challenging the negative thoughts. As a simple example, when something unpleasant happens, many people say something such as, "This is always the way it is." With cognitive restructuring, people challenge negative irrational thoughts by asking, "Is this true?" Many times, the answer is "no." Individuals can then reframe and be more optimistic and realistic. It is important for the person to differentiate negative irrational from negative rational thoughts because there are times and circumstances when it is appropriate to be sad, angry, or fearful (Wells-Federman et al, 2001).

Hypnosis

In a study of 33 patients with refractory IBS, 20 improved after being treated with four 40-minute hypnotherapy sessions over a period of 7 weeks (sessions at 0, 1, 3, and 7 weeks). Patients were also instructed in autohypnosis and encouraged to use it for at least two 10-minute sessions each day. Eleven lost almost all of their symptoms (Harvey et al, 1989). "Short-term improvement was maintained for 3 months without further formal treatment. Hypnotherapy in groups of up to 8 patients was as effective as individual therapy" (p. 424). The individual and group hypnotherapy session included the following:

Induction of hypnosis by eye fixation, general relaxation was encouraged; the patient was then asked to place a hand on the abdomen and to feel a sensation of warmth and relaxation. Finally, patients were asked to imagine a riverside scene and to relate the slow flow of a calm river to the smooth rhythmic action of their own gastrointestinal tract. (Harvey et al, 1989)

In a study with 30 patients, Whorwell and colleagues (1984) compared hypnotherapy with psychotherapy and placebo. Both groups had seven ½-hour sessions of decreasing frequency over a 3-month period, and the hypnosis group was given an autohypnosis tape for daily use. Both groups showed significant improvement, but the hypnotherapy group showed dramatic improvement with the difference between the two groups being highly significant. Improvement was seen in abdominal pain, distension, general well being, and bowel habit. The control group showed improvement in the first three areas but not in bowel habit. Whorwell claims an 80% success rate and targets suggestions on gut activity rather than on relaxation and ego strengthening alone.

Relaxation, Journaling, Bibliotherapy, Creative-Expressive Arts

Studies combining relaxation and cognitive therapy have shown positive results for treatment of IBS (Neff, Blanchard, 1987; Blanchard, Schwarz, 1988 in Novey, 2000). In addition, journaling or bibliotherapy, such as poetry writing or art therapy, may be helpful. "Poetry and poetry therapy enable individuals to express what they may be unable to say in other ways" (p. 107) and is an ideally suited therapy for survivors of violence, abuse, or incest (Rojcewicz, 2000). Similarly, reading that helps the patient "get away" may be relaxing and stress relieving. Creating artwork may also be an outlet for that which a person cannot express.

Exercise, Dance, Movement Therapy

Fraenkel (2000) gives an overview of the various conditions that dance may help and, although IBS and constipation are not included *per se*, people with histories of physical and sexual abuse, eating disorders, and those with serious illness are considered excellent candidates. Dance can decrease depression, reduce anxiety, change self-concept or body image, improve relatedness and social interaction, and heighten levels of attention and cognitive processes.

Increasing exercise helps tone muscles and may therefore help bowels to move, especially exercise that works the abdominal muscles, such as rowing, walking, sit-ups, or swimming (Fontaine, 2000). A minimum of 20 to 30 minutes of exercise each day is a good recommendation. When exercising, maintaining fluid intake is important. Table 4-3 lists mind-body-spirit interventions for constipation, diarrhea, and IBS.

BIOLOGIC-BASED THERAPIES FOR CONSTIPATION, DIARRHEA, AND IRRITABLE BOWEL SYNDROME

Fluids, Food, and Fiber for Constipation

Water is important in the treatment of constipation. An old home remedy for constipation is squeezing the juice of one half of a lemon into a glass of warm water and drinking this mixture after awakening. Increasing the daily amount of fluids to eight 8-ounce glasses per day, in the form of waters and pure juices (not sweetened fruit drinks) can aid with softer stools. Ernst (2001) reports on a

Table 4-3 Mind-Body-Spirit Interventions for Constipation, Diarrhea, and Irritable Bowel Syndrome

Intervention	Management	Treatment Regimen	Cautions, Precautions, Interactions	References
Affirmation	Constipation, IBS; fear of letting go, stuck, refusing to release old ideas, insecurity	Repeat several times a day. For colon: "I easily release that which I no longer need. The past is over and I am free" (Hay, p. 25). For constipation: "As I release the past, the new and fresh and vital enter. I allow life to flow through me" (p. 26). For IBS: "It is safe for me to live. Life will always provide for me. All is well" (p. 64).	Choose the appropriate affirmation or have individual write one. Must be positive, present tense, personal.	Hay, 2000
	Diarrhea; fear, rejection, "running off"	"My intake, assimilation, and elimination are in perfect order. I am at peace with life" (p. 28)	May work well for chronic diarrhea.	Hay, 2000
Behavioral, psychotherapy,	IBS and health problems caused or	Individual sessions may help find past traumas	Person must have appropriate therapist.	Farthing, Gomborone,

222

cognitive therapy	exacerbated by stress, including nausea	or self-defeating behaviors. Brief dynamic psychotherapy may help up to two thirds of patients who do not respond to standard therapy. An example of cognitive therapy-restructuring process: (1) Stop, take a breath, release tension, realize a stressful thing has occurred. (2) Reflect, recognize automatic thoughts. Are they rational, irrational, self-defeating? (3) Choose a healthful response. Challenge unrealistic beliefs and thoughts. Several sessions are necessary.	Health care provider needs to provide choices.	1997; Wells-Federman et al, 2001 (p. 98)
Biofeedback	Constipation, IBS Encopresis; fecal incontinence, fecal retention	Several sessions are necessary. Benefits are	Need trained practitioner. Warn client that unexpected sensations, images, experiences,	Ernst, 2001; Freeman, Lawlis, 2001; Leahy, 1998; Rubin,

Continued

223

Table 4-3 Mind-Body-Spirit Interventions for Constipation, Diarrhea, and Irritable Bowel Syndrome—cont'd

Intervention	Management	Treatment Regimen	Cautions, Precautions, Interactions	References
Biofeedback, cont'd		short-term but not long-term in some	feelings, and thoughts may occur during biofeedback.	2002; Steefel, 1995
Bowel habits	Constipation, IBS; help establish habit pattern	Sit on toilet for a few mins, 20 mins after eating.		
Dance, exercise, movement therapy	Constipation and IBS through toning muscles, help promote general well being; decrease depression and anxiety; change self-concept and body image; improve social interaction	Personal preference is followed; include abdominal exercises. Exercise most days of the week.	No studies are available, but victims of abuse and people with eating disorders are considered good candidates.	Fraenkel, 2000
Education on IBS process	Constipation	Dietary changes are needed. Decrease constipating foods. Increase water and fluids.	Warnings: fiber without extra fluids can be very uncomfortable. Need to increase fluids.	

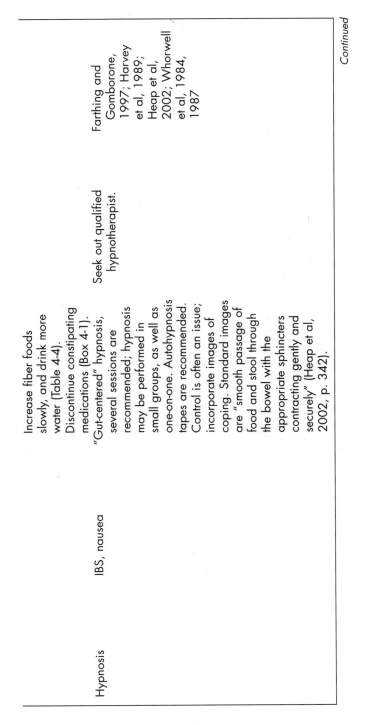

| Hypnosis | IBS, nausea | Increase fiber foods slowly, and drink more water (Table 4-4). Discontinue constipating medications (Box 4-1). "Gut-centered" hypnosis, several sessions are recommended; hypnosis may be performed in small groups, as well as one-on-one. Autohypnosis tapes are recommended. Control is often an issue; incorporate images of coping. Standard images are "smooth passage of food and stool through the bowel with the appropriate sphincters contracting gently and securely" (Heap et al, 2002, p. 342). | Seek out qualified hypnotherapist. | Farthing and Gomborone, 1997; Harvey et al, 1989; Heap et al, 2002; Whorwell et al, 1984, 1987 |

Continued

Intervention	Management	Treatment Regimen	Cautions, Precautions, Interactions	References
Imagery	IBS, nausea, assist weight gain in patients with cancer, weight loss management.	Techniques: audiotapes or guided imagery. Diagnostic imagery—short relaxation, conducive setting, patient creates an image picture expressive of the disease, then patient draws three imagery components that flow naturally (and they do not need to be anatomic or realistic): the disease, the treatment, the defenses; these symbols are examined and evaluated. End-state imagery—specific purpose is to produce a change in the body.	Not all patients will want imagery; can be very emotional experience, and provider should be knowledgeable because of possible effects. No driving or operating machinery is recommended while practicing imagery.	Fontaine, 2000; Freeman, Lawlis, 2001; Naparstek text (1994) and tapes: *Chemotherapy,* 1991; *General Wellness,* 1991; *Healing Trauma,* 1999; *Radiation Therapy,* 1999; *Stress I and II,* 1995; *Weight Loss,* 1997

Journaling	IBS; may be good for survivors of abuse or violence.	Express what cannot be said in another way.		Rojcewicz, 2000
Music	IBS, nausea; reduces vomiting and anxiety after chemotherapy	Personal preference	RCT of 33 chemotherapy patients; music used with standard therapy.	Ernst, 2001; Ezzone et al, 1998; Frank, 1985
Prayer and meditation	May help decrease anxiety, IBS, IBD symptoms.	Personal preference		
Relaxation and autogenics	GERD, IBS, nausea	Deep slow breathing, progressive muscle relaxation, autogenics, hobbies		Ernst, 2001; Farthing, Gomborne, 1997; Freeman, Lawlis, 2001

GERD, *Gastroesophageal reflux disease;* IBD, *inflammatory bowel disease;* IBS, *irritable bowel syndrome;* RCT, *randomized controlled trial.*

German-controlled clinical trial involving mineral water. The investigators studied:

> The acute effects of mineral water containing sulfate (2754 mg/L) on bowel movements and stool consistency (Gutenbrunner, Gundermann, 1998). Thirty-four healthy volunteers received either 500 ml mineral water or tap water (29 mg/L sulfate). Significant beneficial effects are reported for the time to bowel movement and stool consistency in favor of mineral water compared with tap water. (Ernst, 2001, p. 251)

Constipating foods may vary with the individual, however, cheese, processed food, ice cream, highly concentrated sugar foods, and meat have little fiber; limiting them may help relieve constipation (NDDIC, 2001). Also medications can be constipating. Box 4-1 lists medications that can cause or increase constipation. If possible, discontinue constipating medications.

The American Dietetic Association recommends 20 to 35 grams of fiber per day. Stemming from a diet of highly processed and sweetened foods, Americans tend to eat only about 5 to 20 grams a day (NDDIC, 2001). Ten to twelve grams is often all that is needed to aid in constipation relief for some (McQuaid, 2002), although more fiber may be needed for heart health and cancer prevention. Fiber is increased slowly because some patients do not tolerate a rapid increase and may suffer from abdominal discomfort, gas, and bloating (NDDIC, 2001). Importantly, when adding fiber to the diet,

---

Box 4-1

Examples of Medications that Cause Constipation

Antacids with aluminum or calcium
    Anticholinergics
    Tricyclic antidepressants
    Antihistamines
Antiepileptics
Antihypertensives and cardiovascular medications
    Calcium-channel blockers
    Clonidine
    Diuretics
Calcium supplements
Codeine, opiates, narcotics
Iron supplements
Nonsteroidal antiinflammatory drugs (NSAIDS)
Psychotropics
Sedatives
Sucralfate

increases in fluid intake are essential because the bulk of the stool will be increased by the fiber, and water is necessary for the movement through the colon.

Several "power puddings" may help alleviate constipation. Power pudding is a name given to foods with laxative potential, and the recipes tend to have the consistency of pudding. Behm (1985), with use of her special recipe, showed a decrease in the use of magnesia for constipation. A test group of 19 people who had difficulty with constipation took more than seven doses of magnesia per month. The 14 in the control group were moderate users of magnesia, taking less than five doses per month. Behm studied a number of doses of magnesia and cost per resident for a 1-year period. She divided the study into a routine timeframe and a treatment phase. November to April was the period of checking routine laxative use; then from May to October, the 19 in the treatment group received the special recipe. Doses of magnesia in the test group dropped from 7.35 per resident to 1.06, whereas the control group increased from 4.21 to 4.88 doses. Two power pudding recipes are described in Box 4-2 and Box 4-3.

Other aids include fiber. Fiber can be either soluble or insoluble. Insoluble fiber has little water and passes almost unchanged through the colon (although insoluble fiber does pick up water in the intestine). The insoluble fiber increases stool bulk and thus transit rate; helps relieve constipation; and may help prevent appendicitis, colon

---

Box 4-2

Behm's (1985) Special Recipe for Constipation

2 c applesauce
2 c unprocessed bran
1 c of 100% prune juice
Serve 1 ounce per day

Box 4-3

Charon's Power Pudding Recipe

1½ c pitted prunes
1 c applesauce
½ c bran (such as an All-Bran cereal)
1 c prune juice
½ c per day with lots of water
½ c = 1 fruit exchange

(Charon Pierson, 2001)

cancer, and diverticulosis but has little effect on intestinal bacterial growth. Insoluble fiber is in the form of cellulose, some hemicellulose, and lignin (Gutierrez, 1994).

Soluble fiber has the properties of helping normalize blood sugar and cholesterol. Soluble fiber nourishes GI tract bacteria, thus it helps increase bacterial growth and end products; produces gas and volatile fatty acids; helps synthesize vitamins; and can bind toxins and prevent absorption. (Soluble fiber can also interfere with needed nutrient absorption.) Soluble fiber is in the form of pectin, gum, mucilages, and some hemicellulose (Gutierrez, 1994).

Most fruits, vegetables, cereals, and legumes have both soluble and insoluble fiber but in varying amounts. Blonde psyllium husk, a bulk laxative that provides soluble fiber, forms a mucilaginous mass when mixed with water and is a good source of soluble fiber, having 1.7 g of fiber per dose. Additionally, it is useful for constipation, IBS, and as a secondary medication in some diarrhea (Blumenthal et al, 2000). Table 4-4 describes the approximate grams of fiber in specific servings of food.

Currently, controversy exists over fruits, vegetables, and fiber as helping in the prevention of colon cancer. Fiber does not appear to prevent the recurrence of colorectal adenomas, precursors to colon cancer, thus whether it prevents colon cancer is questionable (PL/PL, 2000; Alberts et al, 1998; Schatzkin et al, 2000; Fuchs et al, 1999). The question remains, does fiber prevent the original occurrence of polyps but not the recurrence? A recent prospective study of fruit and vegetable consumption showed no protective effect against colon cancer (Michels et al, 2000). However, because fiber, fruits, and vegetables have many nutrients needed for other concerns, and because fiber foods are a good substitute for processed and concentrated-sugar foods, encouraging fruits, vegetables, and fiber use is still warranted.

In addition, for constipation, LaValle and colleagues (2000) recommend vitamin C and *Lactobacillus acidophilus* and *Bifidobacterium bifidum*. These bacteria may help to restore normal flora to the intestine. LaValle and colleagues (2000) and The Commission E (Blumenthal et al, 2000) recommend the internal use of flaxseed for chronic constipation and for "colons damaged by abuse of laxatives, irritable colon, diverticulitis, and as mucilage for gastritis and enteritis" (Blumenthal et al, 2000, p. 136). In addition, flax is high in omega-3 fatty acids, a needed essential fatty acid, because Americans tend to eat more omega-6 fatty acids; and flax can help balance the two by providing omega 3s.

Rehydration and Oral Intake for Diarrhea

Fluids are the mainstay in the treatment of diarrhea. In conventional practice, patients are told to buy commercial rehydration solutions. However, these products are costly and, depending on circumstances,

Table 4-4	Food Fiber Content (all values are approximate)	
Increase fluid intake when increasing fiber.		
Food	**Serving Size**	**Total Fiber (in grams)**
Cereal		
Fiber One	½ c	11.9
All-Bran	⅓ c	8.6
Raison Bran	¾ c	5.3
Oatmeal	½ c uncooked	4
Whole wheat Total	1 c	2.6
Cheerios	1¼ c	2.5
Grapenuts	½ c	5
Shredded Wheat and Bran	⅔ c	2.5
Wheaties	⅔ c	2.3
Corn grits	3 tbsp uncooked quick	1.5
Other grains		
Wheat bran	½ c	12.3
Bulgur (ala) (toasted cracked wheat)	⅓ c dry	11
Barley	¼ c uncooked	5
Wheat germ	3 tbsp	3.9
Pumpernickel	1 slice	2.7
Rye flour	2½ tbsp	2.6
Whole wheat flour	2½ tbsp	2.1
Popcorn popped	3 cups	2
Whole wheat snack crackers	4	2
Cracked wheat bread	1 slice	1.9
Oat flour	2½ tbsp	1.8
Melba wheat toast	5 slices	1.8
Whole wheat bread	1 slice	1.5
Corn tortilla	1	1.4
Egg noodles cooked	½ c	1.4
Spaghetti	½ c cooked	0.9 (2.7 if whole wheat)
Macaroni	½ c cooked	0.7 (2.1 if whole wheat)
Flour tortilla	1	0.7
Rice	⅓ c cooked	0.5
Cornmeal	2½ tbsp	0.4

Continued

Table 4-4	Food Fiber Content (all values are approximate)—cont'd	
Food	**Serving Size**	**Total Fiber (in grams)**
Fruit		
Canned prunes	1 c	13.8
Blackberries, boysenberries	1 c	7.2
Avocado	½	4.8
Canned pears	½ c	3.7
Dried prunes	6	3.4
Fresh raspberries	1 c	3.3
Fresh pear	½ large or 1 small with skin	2.9
Orange	1 small	2.9
Mango	½ small	2.9
Fresh strawberries	1¼ c	2.8
Fresh apple with skin	1 small	2.8
Fresh red plum	2 medium	2.4
Banana	1 small	2.2
Canned applesauce	½ c unsweetened	2
Dried apricots	7 halves	2
Fresh apricot with skin	2	1.8
Cherries	1 c	1.8
Fresh grapefruit	½ medium	1.6
Fresh pineapple	¾ c	1.4
Cantaloupe	1 c cubed	1.1
Dates	2 ½ medium	0.9
Honeydew	1 c cubed	0.9
Watermelon	1¼ c cubed	0.6
Raisins	2 tbsp	0.4
Grapes with skin	15 small	0.4 (red) to 0.6 (white)
Vegetables		
Turnip	½ c cooked	4.8
Frozen peas	½ c cooked	4.3
Frozen okra	½ c cooked	4.1
Brussels sprouts	½ c cooked	3.8
Acorn squash	½ c baked	2.9
Sweet potato flesh	⅓ c cooked	2.7
Red cabbage	½ c cooked	2.6
Broccoli	½ c cooked	2.4

Continued

Table 4-4	Food Fiber Content (all values are approximate)—cont'd	

Food	Serving Size	Total Fiber (in grams)
Vegetables—cont'd		
Sliced carrots	½ c cooked	2
Whole kernel corn	⅓ c canned	2
Onion	½ c chopped cooked	2
Green beans	½ c canned	2
Spinach	½ c cooked	2
Potato	½ c baked with skin	2
Asparagus	½ c cooked	1.8
Peeled beets	½ c cooked	1.8
Celery	1 c chopped	1.7
Green pepper	1 c chopped	1.7
Fresh cabbage	1 c	1.5
Tomato	½ c canned	1.3
	⅓ c sauce	1.1
	1 medium fresh	1
Zucchini	½ c sliced cooked	1.2
Cauliflower	½ c cooked	1
V-8 juice	½ c	0.7
Iceberg lettuce	1 c	0.5
Fresh cucumber	1 c	0.5
Legumes, Nuts		
Almonds	½ c roasted	7.9
Red kidney beans	½ c cooked	6.9 (dark red) to 7.9 (light red)
Butter beans	½ c cooked	6.9
Navy beans, great northerns	½ c dried cooked	6.5, 7
Pinto beans, refried beans	½ c cooked	6
	½ c dried cooked	
Black beans	½ c cooked	6
Lentils	½ c dried cooked	5.2
Broad beans	½ c cooked no pods	5.1
Black-eyed peas	½ c canned	5
Lima beans	½ c	4.3
Mung beans	½ c	3.3
Peanuts	¼ c roasted	3.1
Peanut Butter	2 tbsp crunchy	2

may not be available. The World Health Organization (WHO) oral rehydration solution (ORS) is inexpensive (under $1.00) and, "despite its higher sodium content (90 mmol/L) than solutions commercially prepared in the United States (45 mmol/L), the WHO solution will correct electrolyte imbalances including hyponatremia and hypernatremia" (Ladinsky et al, 2000, p. 700). Recent studies have used a lower osmolality WHO ORS (using 74 mmol/L of sodium) and found equal safety and efficacy (Ladinsky et al, 2000).

The WHO ORS is approved by the American Academy of Pediatrics and is dispensed in a packet to be mixed with water. In a study to verify whether parents would be more satisfied with commercial or WHO ORS, parents were actually more satisfied with the WHO packet that they themselves mixed (Ladinsky et al, 2000) than they were with the commercial solution. Unfortunately, WHO ORS may not be available at many pharmacies. The WHO solution is a good alternative to commercial rehydration solutions. However, since it may be hard to find, since commercial solutions are expensive, and since inexpensive homemade rehydration solution recipes are difficult to locate, recipes from several sources are included here.

Two things are important to remember with oral rehydration. The water used to mix these solutions must be potable-clean-pure, and the recipes need to be followed accurately to obtain the right mixture of electrolytes. Boxes 4-4 through 4-7 describe several oral rehydration therapies. Remember that one household teaspoon equals 4 to 6 grams of salt or sugar.

Other rehydration solutions may also be helpful. There is less stool loss in patients given rice ORS compared with those given glucose ORS; the percentage reduction in several studies ranged from 3% to 53% (www.who.int, 1990). This effect was greater in patients with cholera than it was in those with noncholera diarrhea. Cholera

---

Box 4-4

Recipe 1—"Home Mix" Rehydration Drink

8 level tsp sugar (raw sugar or molasses can be used instead of sugar)
½ level tsp salt
1 liter of clean water
Add: ½ cup of fruit juice or coconut water or mashed ripe banana, if available. This ingredient provides potassium, which may help the child accept more food and drink.

From: Werner D: *Where there is no doctor*, Palo Alto, Calif, 1996, Hesperian Foundation.

is not a problem in the United States, however because a decreased rate of stool loss and decreased output also occurred, some individuals might prefer to use whatever it takes to lessen the diarrhea. The formula was 50 grams of cooked rice powder instead of the 20 grams of glucose of the WHO ORS recipe; the other ingredients can be

---

Box 4-5

Recipe 2—Cereal Rehydration

8 heaping tsp (or two handfuls) of powdered cereal. Powdered rice is best; or use finely ground maize, wheat flour, sorghum, or cooked and mashed potatoes.
½ tsp salt
I liter clean water
Boil for 5 to 7 minutes to form a liquid gruel.
Cool.
Add: ½ cup of fruit juice or coconut water or mashed ripe banana, if available. This ingredient provides potassium, which may help the child accept more food and drink.
Taste the drink each time before you use it to be sure it is not spoiled. Cereal drinks can spoil in a few hours in hot weather.

From: Werner D: Where there is no doctor, *Palo Alto Calif, 1996, Hesperian Foundation.*

Box 4-6

WHO Rehydration Solution and the Practical Interpretation

NaCl 3.5 grams—½ to ¾ tsp salt (table salt) (1 tsp salt=6 grams of salt)
KCl 1.5 grams—2 bananas (average banana supplies 600 mg of potassium)
$NaHCO_3$ 2.5 grams—½ tsp baking soda
Glucose 20 grams—4 to 5 tsp table sugar (1 tsp sugar=4 grams)
Water 1 liter—1 quart water
mEq/L offered by this recipe are as follows:
This solution equals 90 mmol/L of sodium, 20 of potassium, 80 of chloride, 30 of bicarbonate, and 111 of glucose. The new reduced osmolality WHO ORS has 74 mmol/L rather than 90 mmol/L of sodium.

Rehydration solution from World Health Organization, Oral and Intravenous Rehydration Solutions, annex 2, www.who.int (accessed August 1, 2001).

Box 4-7

Traveler's Recipe for Rehydration

To 1 L of potable water (bottled, boiled, or purified) add:
½ tsp table salt
½ tsp salt substitute (provides potassium chloride)
½ tsp baking soda (provides bicarbonate)
2-3 tbsp sugar or 2 tbsp honey or light corn syrup

From Paynter W: Travel medicine, Clin Rev 10(1):55, 2000.

added before or after cooking the rice (www.who.int, 1990; de Bruyn, 2001). Other solutions include water in which cereal has been cooked, salted rice water, unsweetened fruit juice, and vegetable or chicken soup, salted or unsalted. WHO recommends plain water in addition to the salted fluids.

During adult and pediatric diarrhea, after approximately 4 hours of rehydration, eating food should continue and is considered appropriate therapy; WHO recommends that food not be withheld (www.who.int/chd/publications, 1990). Foods include salted vegetable or chicken soup, cereals, and well-cooked vegetables and foods from the usual diet. Low-fat and bland foods seem to work well. The BRAT diet (bananas, rice, applesauce, tea-toast) is a bland diet, as are cooked potatoes and pastas. Apple, because of its pectin content, is a valuable food for both constipation and diarrhea. Apple has up to 17% pectin and pectic acids. Pectin absorbs water from the GI tract, thus aiding in making a formed stool (DerMarderosian, 2001). Parents are usually advised to keep their babies on breast milk or formula; however, short-term use of a lactose-free diet is associated with a shorter period of diarrhea for some individuals (Sondheimer, 2001 in Hay 2001). Patients may need to stop lactose products for a short time if they notice intolerance, but they should continue to hydrate with other fluids. The German Commission E recommends flaxseed as mucilage (gruel) for the short-term treatment of gastroenteritis and enteritis (Blumenthal et al, 2000).

Acidophilus is used at times to restore GI flora. The value of acidophilus remains unclear, but it has been shown to inhibit bacterial and fungal growth in the vagina. *In vitro* acidophilus has been shown to inhibit *Campylobacter pylori* (DerMarderosian, 2001).

Diet and Nutritional Supplements for Irritable Bowel Syndrome and Food Intolerances

With food intolerances and allergies, some of the testing may be part of the treatment. That is, while testing through food elimination to discover possible causes of the symptoms, the patient may also become better by discontinuing an allergen. Other methods can be used to test for food allergies, and several of these ways are discussed here because they often are not part of conventional health care plans for IBS and other GI symptoms.

> Food represents the largest antigenic challenge confronting the human immune system. The surface area of the GI tract is greater than the area of a tennis court, making it the largest, most active immune-reacting surface in the body. (Barrie, 1998, p. 8)

About two thirds of patients with IBS have at least one food intolerance, and some patients have several (Jones et al, 1982; Murray, Pizzorno, 1999a). In addition to food intolerances (such as to lactose), food allergies also occur. Approximately one half of patients with IBS responded to an elimination diet and were able to identify triggers (Farthing, Gomborone, 1997; Nanda, 1989). Food irritant elimination consists of eliminating a food for a number of days to see if symptoms change. Then, foods are reintroduced into the diet, one at a time. "When the relationship between ingestion of certain foods and resulting symptoms is unclear, the use of food challenge methods is warranted" (Barrie, 1999, p. 149).

IgE-mediated antibody responses cause the most severe immediate allergy symptoms, but IgG and its complex mediators may also be involved in more than 80% of food allergy reactions. These reactions are usually delayed, with people showing symptoms hours to days later. "In experimental models, IgG antibodies have been shown to increase intestinal permeability...By increasing intestinal permeability, elevated levels of IgG could result in increased exposure to antigens" (Barrie, 1998, p. 9).

Testing for food allergies or intolerances can be done in several ways. These include laboratory methods and also experiential clinical challenge tests. Laboratory tests include the radioallergosorbent test (RAST), a test that picks up IgE but not hidden allergies such as IgG. The RAST has low sensitivity. The radioallergosorbent procedure (RASP) is similar to the RAST but is more sensitive and specific and is thought to pick up some IgG. Both of these tests are expensive. There is also the enzyme linked immunosorbent assay (ELISA), a serum test requiring a reactant; the ELISA can measure IgE, IgG, IgG4 (a subclass of IgG associated with high antigens, particularly food antigens), and IgA. Being able to get a combination of IgG4 and IgE is thought to be a better correlate to food allergy than is skin testing alone. The ELISA has good sensitivity but limited research (Barrie, 1998).

Skin testing and provocation tests are also available. Skin testing consists of the skin prick, checks for IgE, has poor sensitivity, but is good for picking up inhalant allergens. Provocation-neutralization and serial-dilution tests involve diagnosing a sensitivity through provoking a response to a test dose. This process is done with intradermal serial dilutions—observing substances that provoke symptoms and "second, to discover which dilutions of those substances are appropriate for treatment" (Barrie, 1998, p. 10). Provocation can also occur using sublingual drops, especially good for children. The provocation method is appropriate (but controversial) for a wide range of food allergens, as well as for chemicals, pollens, dusts, and molds. Other laboratory tests include using a galvanometer at acupuncture points that measures the skin's electrical activity and kinesiologic testing that uses muscle testing after ingesting a small portion of suspected allergen (Barrie, 1998).

The other way to discover food allergies is through experiential challenges. One of these ways is through an elimination diet followed by reintroduction of food. A second way is through fasting followed by food challenges. People with known food allergies are not appropriate for this type of testing, especially if they have immediate or severe reactions, or both. These individuals, obviously, should avoid such substances.

In addition to being useful with IBS, elimination diets may be useful to patients with IBD and, as stated in the previous chapter, to those with allergies and asthma. The elimination diets also may be helpful with atopy and hyperactivity.

Because severe food allergy can cause anaphylaxis, people who know they have a true food allergy need to eliminate these foods entirely. Even a very small amount of an allergy-producing food (e.g., $\frac{1}{44,000}$ of a peanut) can produce a reaction in highly allergic patients (National Institute of Allergy and Infections Diseases [NIAID], 2001). Box 4-8 lists instructions for an elimination diet for food intolerance or if allergy is suggested.

Another test to consider for intestinal symptoms is the digestive stool analysis. This nonconventional test checks digestion through substances such as triglycerides, chymotrypsin, iso-butyrate, and meat and vegetable fibers; absorption through long- and short-chain fatty acids, cholesterol, total fecal fat; colonic environment through bacterial and mycology cultures; and immunology through fecal secretory IgA. Patients with low IgA may have high titers of antibodies against food antigens (Barrie, 1998).

In a study by Bland and colleagues (1995), a food-supplemented detoxification program helped in the management of chronic health problems. Prestudy, the subjects were free of serious disease but suffered from "chronic health complaints such as fatigue, myalgia, arthralgia, chronic gastrointestinal problems, headaches, sleep disturbances, and cognitive impairment of at least one year's duration" (p. 64). A total of 84 patients were in the treatment group and 22 in the control group; assignment was by self-selection. Both groups followed the same food-elimination diet, and those in the intervention group also received a food supplement. The elimination diet consisted of drinking at least 2 quarts of water daily and avoiding all alcohol, caffeine, and decaf-

Box 4-8

Elimination Diet for Irritable Bowel Syndrome

- Keep a symptom calendar for several weeks to pinpoint foods or activities that manifest symptoms. Enough diary time is needed to obtain reactions to a variety of foods.
- Eliminate all known allergens.
- Eliminate all general common allergens from diet for 7 days minimum, up to a month. General common allergens are dairy, wheat, corn, soy, peanuts, shellfish, eggs, chocolate. Also eliminate caffeine, concentrated sweets, alcohol, and nicotine. Other grains may need to be eliminated (oats, etc.).
- Start by eliminating dairy and grain if unable to do all common allergens.
- Eliminate monosodium glutamate (MSG), food additives, sulfites, dyes, sorbitol, aspartame, and any known distressing foods.
- Read labels, and remember that foods can be labeled in different ways (milk in a product may be labeled as whey, casein, lactoglobulin. MSG may be in foods labeled hydrolyzed protein, textured protein, sodium or calcium caseinate, yeast extract, seasoning).
- Add back one food at a time to see if symptoms recur. Wait 4 to 6 days before adding another to determine if symptoms reoccur.
- If you have definite known allergies, wear a medical alert bracelet, and carry a syringe with epinephrine.

From Barrie S: Food allergy testing. In Pizzorno J, Murray M, editors: Textbook of natural medicine, *Edinburgh, 1999, Churchill Livingstone.* *Rockwell S: Rotation diet: A diagnostic & therapeutic tool. In Pizzorno J, Murray M, editors:* Textbook of natural medicine, *Edinburgh, 1999, Churchill Livingstone.*

feinated coffee. In addition subjects eliminated: dairy; meats such as beef, pork, veal (chicken, turkey, lamb, cold-water fish were allowed); and gluten, including wheat, spelt, kamut, oats, rye, barley, amaranth, or malt (rice, corn, buckwheat, quinoa, gluten-free flour, potato, tapioca, and arrowroot were allowed). The treatment subjects' food supplement consisted of fiber, vitamins, and minerals and gave them extra calories (brand name *UltraClear Sustain*). After 10 weeks, the 84 subjects in the treatment group had a 52% reduction in symptoms as measured by the Metabolic Screening Questionnaire (MSQ), and the control group had a 22% reduction in symptoms. Bland and colleagues (1995) concluded that the supplement may help the "chronically unwell" and that symptoms may be a result of:

the adverse metabolic impact of toxin accumulation from both exogenous and endogenous sources, and that the symptoms are amenable to improvement through the application of a properly designed metabolic detoxification program. (p. 62)

MacIntosh and Ball (2000) completed a similar small study with 25 disease-free participants but who were symptomatic according to the MSQ. The participants followed a hypoallergenic diet consisting of a 7-day detoxification plan with a similar food supplement from the prior study. The Day 1 to 3 diet included any fruits except citrus, any vegetables except tomatoes or potatoes, Basmati white rice and legumes, peas, lentils, green beans, nuts and seeds (except peanuts), flavorings to include butter, olive oil, high-quality sunflower or flaxseed oil (cold use), and herbs and spices (except salt). Participants were not to consume dairy, wheat, concentrated sweets, caffeine, alcohol, eggs, oats, or suspected allergens-intolerances. Optional foods starting Day 4 were turkey, fish (no shellfish), and grains such as buckwheat, millet, amaranth, quinoa, and brown rice. Results showed a 47% reduction in symptoms. The authors conclude that this type of program may be appropriate for individuals without specific toxin exposure or disease diagnosis.

Ernst (2001) reports a study of 380 patients with IBS in which one group received a high-fiber diet and a supplement containing yeast, vitamin B, nicotinamide, folic acid, and herbal extracts of chamomile, angelica, valerian, and peppermint. The second group received only a high-fiber diet. Over 6 weeks, the frequency, intensity, and duration of the symptoms were reduced in the supplemented group when compared with the diet-only group (Grattagliano et al, 1998).

In addition, when adding fiber to the diet, patients with IBS need to increase fiber slowly because some patients have increased symptoms with too much fiber. IBS patients also can add lactobacillus to help restore normal GI flora and eliminate candida.

Multiple variables are involved in food digestion, absorption, and the colonic environment. Elimination-detoxification diets, rotation diets, and supplement therapies may be worth a trial for people with IBS, as well as other GI disorders.

Herbals for Constipation, Diarrhea, and Irritable Bowel Syndrome

Herbals for constipation   Herbals for constipation include psyllium, milk thistle, aloe, buckthorn, cascara sagrada, and senna (Blumenthal et al, 2000; LaValle et al, 2000). Milk thistle has mild laxative effects. Buckthorn, cascara, and senna are stimulant laxatives and have abuse potential, just as does any commercial laxative, and are for short-term use only. They can cause severe cramping and diarrhea.

Aloe latex is a "drastic cathartic" and is to be used only with caution (DerMarderosian, 2001). Dependence on laxatives can be a real problem, especially for older adults. Thus, with few exceptions, laxative herbs, whether prescribed or other over-the-counter, are to be taken with care and for a few days only.

Psyllium is a bulk-forming laxative. Psyllium seed is black or blonde and there is also psyllium husk. For constipation, as well as hemorrhoids, anal fissures, and IBS, all types are approved by German Commission E and WHO (Blumenthal, 2000). Psyllium seed also helps lower blood cholesterol.

Herbals for diarrhea   Herbs for infectious diarrhea include goldenseal (*Hydrastis canadensis*), which has been shown in a few trials to be effective for the treatment of *Escherichia coli* (*E. coli*), *Shigella*, *Salmonella*, *Klebsiella, and Cholera* (PL/PL CE, 2000, Part 2). *In vitro*, berberine, the major alkaloid in goldenseal:

> kills or inhibits many common bacteria including: *Staphylococcus*, *Streptococcus*, *Chlamydia*, *E. coli*, *Pseudomonas*, *Neisseria*, and many others. *In vitro* studies have also shown that berberine inhibits the growth of protozoa such as *Giardia* and *Trichomonas*. A clinical study in pediatric patients with giardiasis reported that berberine was as effective as metronidazole. (PL/PL [CE, part 2], 2000, p. 21)

Goldenseal is a potentially toxic drug; it is absolutely contraindicated in pregnancy. Also, tolerance is thought to develop after only a few weeks of use (Fetrow, Avila, 1999).

Other herbs for diarrhea include barberry, bilberry (huckleberry), chamomile, nutmeg (a spice), oak bark, and witch hazel. Numerous other herbs are listed by the German Commission E (Blumenthal, 2000) and the Facts and Comparison's *Review of Natural Products* (DerMarderosian, 2001).

Herbals for irritable bowel syndrome   For IBS, Buckle (1997) mentions that the essential oil peppermint has antispasmodic effects. (Note that although most essential oils are *not* for internal use, peppermint is taken internally for IBS.) In a study of endoscopy spasm, peppermint was found to relieve colonic spasm within 30 seconds (Buckle, 1997; Leicester, Hunt, 1982). Murray and Pizzorno (1999b) also recommend the use of peppermint oil for IBS and intestinal colic. Enteric-coated peppermint oil is recommended because the oil in the stomach may cause heartburn, and the enteric coating allows the peppermint oil to pass to the small and large intestine before dissolving. Once in the intestine, peppermint relaxes intestinal muscle and may relieve spasm. In addition, peppermint volatile oil may be effective against *Candida albicans* and thus useful in IBS, because an overgrowth of candida may be one of the aggravating factors.

Peppermint is also recommended for "spastic discomfort of the upper GI tract and bile ducts" (Blumenthal, 2000, p. 301). Table 4-5 outlines some biologic-based therapies for constipation, diarrhea, IBS, and a few other GI concerns.

MANIPULATIVE AND BODY-BASED METHODS AND ENERGY THERAPIES FOR CONSTIPATION, DIARRHEA, AND IRRITABLE BOWEL SYNDROME

Massage

Ernst (2001) reports four studies of massage used for constipation, all clinical trials. A total of 101 people were in the four trials. Two of the trials showed improvement in stool frequency and stool consistency, but this result was not found in the one randomized trial. Abdominal massage technique is routinely taught in massage training. Therapists are taught to follow the path of the colon (DeDomenico, Wood, 1997), and Fritz (1995) describes a pattern in "the direction of flow for emptying of the large intestine and colon" (p. 237). A gentle technique and proper amount of time are important with use of massage for constipation. Massage also may be soothing for people with IBS, using abdominal massage similar to that for constipation, in a gentle effleurage clockwise motion. However, if patients have a background of abuse, massage may bring up strong emotions for which the therapist needs to be prepared or massage may not be appropriate.

Aromatherapy Massage

Anecdotally for constipation, Fontaine (2000) recommends massaging the abdomen in a clockwise direction with orange, black pepper, ginger, or marjoram mixed in a carrier oil. Pure almond oil is a common carrier oil. Always check for allergies before using oils. Be sure to wash hands thoroughly following massage with pepper. For hemorrhoids, Fontaine recommends geranium, chamomile, or lavender essential oil mixed with a carrier oil and massaged into the rectal area by the patient. Be certain that no prior allergies are present. Anecdotally for diarrhea, Fontaine (2000) recommends a gentle abdominal massage with aromatherapy oils such as coriander, chamomile, neroli, lavender, or peppermint in a carrier oil.

Reflexology

Reflexology theory claims that points on the feet (as well as ears and hands) correspond to the organs and areas in the body; reflexology is thousands of years old but has little research. Anecdotally, for constipation and rectal problems, Byers (1991), a well-known reflexologist, describes a technique and foot reflex points to work. Areas on the feet to be stimulated include the points for liver, gall bladder, diaphragm, adrenals, lower spine, sigmoid, and ileocecal areas (see

Table 4-5 Biologic-Based Therapies for Constipation, Diarrhea, Irritable Bowel Syndrome, and Other Gastrointestinal Concerns

A complete prescribing source should be consulted before using biologic therapies. Vitamin and mineral dosing is often higher than is the standard recommended upper limit. At times of illness or deficiency, persons may need more of such supplements. Any herb can cause allergy. Herbs are generally contraindicated in women who are pregnant or lactating and with children unless research data or a long history of safe use is established.

Intervention	Management	Treatment Regimen	Cautions, Precautions, Interactions	References
Fiber, bulk-forming laxatives	Constipation; some persons with IBS. Decrease the risk of diverticulosis and possibly colon cancer.	20-35 g/day. (See Table 4-4 for fiber content of foods.) Even a lesser amount may help. Power pudding, Charon's recipe (see Box 4-3 and 4-4). Bran Methylcellulose—Citrucel; Calcium polycarbophil—FiberCon; Psyllium—Metamucil	Increase levels slowly. Take with plenty of fluids.	NDDIC, 2001
Increase fluids, water	Constipation, diarrhea, IBS	6-8 glasses/day		
Glutamine (an amino acid)	IBD, diarrhea, decreases intestinal permeability and	Dose varies depending on use.	If sensitive to MSG, patient may be sensitive to glutamine. Glutamine	Murray, Pizzorno, 1999a,c Barrie, 1998; PL/PL, 2002

Continued

Table 4-5 Biologic-Based Therapies for Constipation, Diarrhea, Irritable Bowel Syndrome, and Other Gastrointestinal Concerns—cont'd

Intervention	Management	Treatment Regimen	Cautions, Precautions, Interactions	References
Glutamine, cont'd	enhances intestinal absorption of nutrients and help patients with HIV gain weight.		may worsen hepatic encephalopathy.	
Evening primrose oil (GLA)	IBS "possibly effective" when taken for IBS exacerbated by PMS; IBD.	Large dose variations. Oil is obtained from plant seed.	SE: nausea, headache. Drug interactions may occur (anticoagulant, anesthesia, phenothiazines)	LaValle, 2000; PL/PL, 2002
Olive oil	Binds bile acids; possibly effective for prevention of colon cancer.	No specific dose established; use as substitute for other cooking oils. For gallbladder problems, olive oil is given following several wks of consumption of unfiltered apple juice. Called "Gallbladder	May cause biliary colic and is contraindicated with stones per PL/PL; however, olive oil is part of an old treatment for gallbladder problems. Has hypoglycemic effects; might allow for decreased antihypertensive drug doses	PL/PL, 2001

Vitamins, Nutrients

Folic acid (folate is necessary for DNA synthesis and repair)	Possibly decreases colon cancer risk with long-term use.	400 µg/day. Increase dietary intake or use supplement. Eat fortified foods and cereals. Difficult to get enough folic acid from food.	NAP, 2002; PL/PL, 2001
		Adult UL: 1000 mcg/day. Be sure pernicious anemia is ruled out because folate masks symptoms.	
Vitamin C (from food) for decreasing cancer risk; supplements for help with constipation	Possibly decreases colon cancer risk; aids in constipation relief; IBS; IBD (may help prevent fistula formation), possibly helps PUD.	With 200 mg/day from food, risk of colon cancer decreases.	NAP, 2002; PL/PL, 2001; LaValle et al, 2000; Murray, Pizzorno, 1999a; Zhang, 1997
		Adult UL: 2000 mg/day. Doses >1000 mg/day may lend to kidney stone formation. Interact with acetaminophen, aluminum-containing antacids, ASA, heparin, iron, warfarin. Some take dose until bowel tolerance is reached.	
Lutein (a carotenoid and antioxidant)	Possibly decreases colon cancer	Dietary sources: kale (44 mg/cup); spinach	PL/PL, 2002
		Administration with beta-carotene may	

Continued

245

Table 4-5 Biologic-Based Therapies for Constipation, Diarrhea, Irritable Bowel Syndrome, and Other Gastrointestinal Concerns—cont'd

Intervention	Management	Treatment Regimen	Cautions, Precautions, Interactions	References
Lutein, cont'd	risk with dietary intake.	(26 mg/cup); kiwi, grapes, orange juice, squash, broccoli (3 mg/cup), corn, zucchini. No specific dose established, however, 7-12 mg/day have lowest risk of macular degeneration and cataracts.	reduce bioavailability of lutein and increase bioavailability of beta-carotene.	
Quercetin (bioflavonoid)	Inflammatory bowel disease; food allergies	Onions, red wine, green tea, apples, berries, brassica vegetables. 250-500 mg tid.		Barrie, 1998; Murray, Pizzorno, 1999; PL/PL, 2002
Minerals				
Calcium	Possibly decreases risk of colon cancer.	Increase dietary intake. Increase intake of milk and dairy products. Ingestion of vitamin-D	UL: 2500 mg/day. Need proper mineral ratios. Excess can cause hypercalcemia, milk	NAP, 2002; PL/PL, 2001, 2002

	Uses	Dosage	Cautions/Notes	References
	foods increases calcium absorption.		alkali syndrome, renal insufficiency. Interactions with drugs. Use cautiously with people who have high-serum phosphate levels. Separate calcium supplementation from dairy products and other high-phosphorus foods by 2 hours (can reduce calcium absorption). Separate magnesium and calcium administration also.	
Selenium	Antioxidant, possibly decreases risk of colon cancer.	200 µg/day	Adult UL: 400 µg/day. Can increase the cytotoxic effects of cisplatin. Toxicity can occur.	NAP, 2001; PL/PL, 2001
Zinc	Diarrhea; Crohn's disease (zinc deficiency is complication of Crohn's disease).	10-40 mg/day; elemental zinc is given for acute diarrhea in malnourished or zinc-deficient children.	Adult UL: 40 mg/day. May not respond to oral or IV supplementation; may be defect in transport. Need to have adequate zinc/copper ratio.	Murray, Pizzorno, 1999; PL/PL, 2002

Continued

Table 4-5 Biologic-Based Therapies for Constipation, Diarrhea, Irritable Bowel Syndrome, and Other Gastrointestinal Concerns—cont'd

Intervention	Management	Treatment Regimen	Cautions, Precautions, Interactions	References
Herbs				
Cascara sagrada bark (*Rhamnus purshiana*)	Constipation; anal fissures, hemorrhoids, after rectoanal surgery. Is a stimulant laxative.	Various forms. Infusion: steep 1-2 g in 150 ml boiling water for 10-15 mins.	SE: cramps. Electrolyte imbalance. Abuse potential. Short-term use only. Try diet measures and bulk-formers first.	Blumenthal, 2001; PL/PL, 2002
Cat's claw (*Uncaria tomentosa*)	IBS, diverticulitis, colitis, hemorrhoids, parasites, leaky bowel.	Root and bark used. Freeze-dried extract. Dose varies with type of preparation.	SE: headache, dizziness, vomiting. May lower blood pressure; do not use with antihypertensives. No clinical trials.	Fetrow, Avila, 1999; PL/PL, 2002
German chamomile (*Chamomilla recutita*)	Diarrhea—faster resolution; GI spasm and inflammatory diseases.	Can make tea; will help with hydration as well. 3 g of whole flower heads in 150 ml water tid to qid.	Allergy. Should not be used if person is allergic to ragweed, asters, chrysanthemums. Be sure to use German chamomile.	DerMarderosian, 2001; Blumenthal et al, 2000

Chlorella pyrenoidosa (green freshwater algae)	Ulcerative colitis symptom relief as scored on the disease activity index (DAI); decreased stool frequency, less inflammation on sigmoidoscopy, physician assessment significant improvement; quality of life improvement.	In this study subjects had 2 months of taking: took solid tablets and a liquid (Chlorella has amino acids, vitamin and minerals). As a general dietary supplement, 3 gms daily of chlorella tablets or 30 ml daily of liquid extract (PL/PL, 2002)	Small study (N = 8). Had to take 50 Chlorella tablets and 100 ml Chlorella extract a day for this study.	Merchant, Andre, 2001; PL/PL, 2002
Garlic (Allium sativum)	Decrease colon cancer risk; aid selenium absorption.	1 to 7 cloves wkly, fresh or cooked	Odor, GI upset.	PL/PL 2001
Goldenseal (Hydrastis canadensis)	Diarrhea: berberine (one of the main chemical alkaloids) shown to shorten the	Various doses. Plant is an endangered species.	SE and adverse effects: bradycardia, CNS depression, GI symptoms, seizures, paralysis,	Fetrow, Avila, 1999; PL/PL, 2000, 2002

Continued

249

Table 4-5 Biologic-Based Therapies for Constipation, Diarrhea, Irritable Bowel Syndrome, and Other Gastrointestinal Concerns—cont'd

Intervention	Management	Treatment Regimen	Cautions, Precautions, Interactions	References
Goldenseal, cont'd	duration of acute Vibrio cholera, some species of Giardia, Salmonella, Shiegella, and some Enterobacteriaceae		paresthesia. Likely unsafe when used orally in high doses or long-term. Interferes with laboratory tests.	
Grapefruit seed extract (Citrus paradisi)	IBS, intestinal parasites	No typical dose.	Use preservative-free extract. Numerous possible drug interactions. Alters drugs metabolized by cytochrome P450 enzyme system.	LaValle, 1999; PL/PL, 2002
Peppermint oil and peppermint leaf (Mentha x piperita)	IBS (with diarrhea-predominant symptoms), enteritis; flatulence; possibly dissolve gallstones	Oil: 0.2 ml bid to tid between meals. Leaf: 3-6 g/day of cut leaf for infusions and extracts.	Contraindicated in obstruction of bile ducts, gallbladder inflammation, severe liver damage. Peppermint oil should not be used on the face.	Blumenthal, 2001; Murray, Pizzorno, 1999; Pittler, Ernst, 1998; PL/PL, 2002

Psyllium (both black and blonde seed and husk are for constipation)	Chronic constipation, IBS, anal fissures, hemorrhoids, secondary treatment in diarrhea (blonde husk and blonde seed).	Dose forms vary. 10 to 30 g/day of whole or ground black seeds. 7 to 8 oz of water is needed with the dose. Start slowly. Try bulk laxatives and fiber 1 mo before judging results.	SE: allergy. Contraindicated in stenosis of the GI tract or suspect obstruction or difficulties in regulating diabetes. May decrease insulin needs. Must take fluids with this herb. Blonde psyllium husk is good source of soluble fiber.	Blumenthal, 2001
Senna pod (fruit) and senna leaf (*Senna alexandrina*)	Constipation; a stimulant laxative.	Taken as tea or swallowed in powder form. Senna is in OTC Correctol, ExLax, Senokot, Smooth Move.	SE: cramps. Electrolyte imbalance. Abuse potential. Short-term use only. Try diet measures and bulk-formers first.	Blumenthal, 2001
Witch hazel	Hemorrhoids— itching, discomfort, and burning.	Local application. 5-10 g of leaf and bark per 250 ml water. Also suppositories up to six/day.	Contact dermatitis	PL/PL, 2002

Continued

Table 4-5	Biologic-Based Therapies for Constipation, Diarrhea, Irritable Bowel Syndrome, and Other Gastrointestinal Concerns—cont'd			
Intervention	**Management**	**Treatment Regimen**	**Cautions, Precautions, Interactions**	**References**
Other				
Lactobacillus	Normalize bowel flora; rotavirus in children, antibiotic-associated diarrhea, traveler's diarrhea.	1-10 billion viable organisms daily in 3 to 4 divided doses	SE: flatulence that subsides with use; possibility of infection.	PL/PL, 2002

ASA, Acetylsalicylic acid; bid, twice a day; CNS, central nervous system; DNA, deoxyribonucleic acid; GI, gastrointestinal; GLA, gamma linolenic acid; HIV, human immunodeficiency virus; IBD, inflammatory bowel disease; IBS, irritable bowel syndrome; IV, intravenous; MSG, monosodium glutamate; NAP, National Academies Press; NDDIC, National Digestive Diseases Information Clearing House; OTC, over-the-counter; PL/PL, Pharmacist's Letter/Prescriber's Letter; PMS, premenstrual syndrome; PO, by mouth; PUD, peptic ulcer disease; qid, four times a day; SE, side effects; tid, three times a day; UL, upper limits—the maximum level of daily nutrient that is likely to pose no risk of adverse effects. Includes intake from food, water, and supplements.

Appendix E). Ernst (2001) reports on 130 postoperative women who were randomized to either reflexology or leg-foot massage or talking; treatments were 15 minutes for 5 days. Results reported no significant differences in stool frequency after the treatment or after 4 days of follow-up. Ernst does not report any other details (the study is not in English) (Kesselring et al, 1998). More details would be helpful regarding the kind of leg and foot massage that was done and if a difference existed from baseline for both massage and reflexology groups combined. Regarding organ points on the foot, Byers writes that reflexology is not the same as massage; however, the foot is being manipulated during massage, and this manipulation may have been as helpful as was the reflexology. Byers writes:

> When we think of colon problems or constipation, it is necessary that we do not just think of working the intestinal tract. Here is where our *helper areas* are important. Our key helper areas for constipation would be the liver because it produces and manufactures the bile, also the diaphragm—solar plexus because emotions have a great effect on our digestive system. But we must also think of working the adrenal glands, because the adrenals help us with muscle tone, which in turn helps with the peristaltic action in the intestinal tract. Another area to think about is the lower back reflex for the nerves that supply the colon (Byers, 1991, p. 154).

Therapeutic touch, healing touch, Reiki, or Qi gong may reduce anxiety or relieve symptoms for IBS or constipation. These therapies have had little published GI research; however, health care practitioners practicing energy work experientially know the comfort such therapies bring. Table 4-6 lists manipulative and body-based methods and energy therapies for constipation, diarrhea, and IBS.

DYSPEPSIA, NAUSEA, GASTROESOPHAGEAL REFLUX DISEASE, AND PEPTIC ULCER DISEASE

Dyspepsia

Dyspepsia is a general term usually referring to upper abdominal or epigastric symptoms such as belching, indigestion, discomfort, fullness, "heartburn," nausea, or GERD symptoms. Dyspepsia is very common, occurring in about 25% of the population and accounting for about 3% of general office visits (McQuaid, 2002).

Nausea

Nausea is an intensely uncomfortable abdominal feeling of queasiness that may or may not lead to vomiting. Nausea is a common feeling in the first half of pregnancy; as a side-effect of chemotherapy and radiation therapy; postoperatively; with GI irritants, bulimia, and food poisoning; in hepatobiliary or pancreatic disorders; from various infections; with headaches, inner-ear disturbance (including

Table 4-6 Manipulative and Body-Based Methods and Energy Therapies for Constipation, Diarrhea, and IBS

Intervention	Management	Treatment Regimen	Cautions, Precautions, Interactions	References
Massage	Constipation, enhanced digestion and elimination	Abdominal rubbing in direction of colon (up right side, across abdomen, and down left), gentle strokes.	Skilled practitioner needed. Ernst found four clinical trials that say "abdominal massage is a promising treatment."	Ernst, 2001; Fritz, 1995
Aromatherapy massage	Diarrhea	Aromatherapy oils such as coriander, chamomile, neroli, lavender, or peppermint in a carrier oil such as almond oil. 15- to 20-min session or as tolerated	Allergy. Be sure to use only a few drops of pure essential oils and to dilute them.	Fontaine, 2000
Healing touch, Reiki, Therapeutic Touch	Nausea, irritable bowel		Need skilled practitioner. Request permission	Fontaine, 2000

motion sickness), and intracranial pressure; and as a side effect of substances, including medications. Nausea may also be present with cardiac and kidney disorders, as well as with diabetes, uremia, and adrenocortical crisis (McQuaid, 2001).

Gastroesophageal Reflux Disease

GERD refers to a weakness in the lower esophageal sphincter (LES) that allows gastric contents to reflux back into the esophagus and potentially damage the mucosa (Heuman et al, 1997). GERD has a number of natural therapies that can help decrease symptoms (Castell et al, 1998).

Peptic Ulcer Disease

A peptic ulcer is a break in the duodenal or gastric mucosa "that arises when the normal mucosal defensive factors are impaired or are overwhelmed by aggressive luminal factors such as acid and pepsin" (McQuaid, 2002, p. 618). In the majority of non-NSAID PUD, *Helicobacter pylori*, is the cause; thus antibiotics are first-line therapy. Chronic NSAID use, stress, smoking, and Zollinger-Ellison syndrome are also causes or aggravators of PUD.

ALTERNATIVE HEALTH CARE SYSTEMS FOR DYSPEPSIA, NAUSEA, GASTROESOPHAGEAL REFLUX DISEASE, AND PEPTIC ULCER DISEASE

Ayurveda for Gastroesophageal Reflux Disease

Because the stomach is the site of the first stage of digestion, Ayurveda views most digestive disorders as beginning in the stomach or being first noted there. Because the stomach is a kapha organ, the stomach reflects the general state of kapha in the body. If the mind-body physiology is in balance, a sense of contentment, nourishment, and happiness is present; however, the stomach is a sensitive organ that is easily upset by either the wrong diet or emotional disturbances or worry (Frawley, 2000).

The heartburn and sour taste in the mouth associated with GERD usually indicates excessive pitta in the small intestine. The cause is viewed as mainly being dietary: too much spicy or sour foods or alcohol. Excessive amounts of sweet foods can also cause hyperacidity via fermentation and consequent acid production.

Treatment of hyperacidity (GERD) includes an antipitta diet emphasizing antacid foods such as milk or ghee and whole grains. Sour foods such as pickles, yogurt, wine, and vinegar should be avoided, as well as bananas (which have a sour aftertaste). Herbs with demulcent and bitter properties are helpful in ameliorating this condition and include aloe gel, shatavari, and amalaki. If digestion is weak, a formula such as Trikatu can help to improve the digestive fire.

Ayurveda for Peptic Ulcer Disease

Ulcers related to hyperacidity most frequently reflect a pitta condition wherein excess acid causes inflammation of the gastric mucosa and results in the experience of a hot, burning sensation that may be accompanied by sharp pain. Vata-types may also develop stomach ulcers because of their nervous sensitivity and worry that cause untimely secretion of acid. Vata ulcers involve more pain and less burning sensation, and other vata-type symptoms will be present, such as bloating, constipation, and insomnia. If a kapha deficiency is also present, the protective mucous layer in the stomach that normally prevents direct contact of the acid secretions with the mucosa may be lessened.

Treatment of pitta-type ulcers includes small frequent meals with a bland diet with whole grains and other easy-to-digest foods. Initially, a few days of a milk fast (3 to 4 glasses of warm milk per day) may be helpful. Alcohol, smoking, bananas, eggplant, and spicy, sour, and fermented foods should be eliminated. In regard to herbal treatment, the same demulcent and bitter herbs helpful in treating GERD are recommended to regulate stomach acidity and protect the mucous membrane. Herbal teas (for example, jatamamsi and brahmi tea before bedtime) may help relieve stress and reduce acid secretions. Yoga postures that are beneficial include Leg Lift, Camel, Cobra, Bow, Bridge, and Spinal Twist. Breathing exercises such as Cooling Breath (breathing through curled tongue) and Moon Breath (breathing through left nostril only) for 5 to 10 minutes may be helpful.

For vata-type ulcers, application of heat to the stomach will bring relief (whereas, pitta-type ulcer discomfort will not be relieved by heat). The key to management of vata-type ulcers is regularizing eating habits and diminishing stress and worry. Excessive dry, light, spicy, cold, and raw foods should be avoided, and the individual should eat sufficient food at regular intervals to regularize acid secretion. A bland diet with mild spices is recommended.

Kapha-type individuals seldom develop PUD because they seldom worry, and because they have a good supply of mucous to protect the gastric mucosa. Kapha ulcers may be associated with overeating sweet or oily foods, or experiencing the emotions of grief, greed, or attachment, or both. In contrast with pitta- or vata-type ulcers, individuals with kapha-type ulcers experience increased phlegm, nausea, lack of appetite, and a sense of dull pain and heaviness in the epigastric area. For treatment, a light antikapha diet is recommended along with spices that stimulate digestion, such as cayenne, dry ginger, black pepper, cloves, or herbal formulas (e.g., Trikatu). The demulcent herbs used to treat pitta- or vata-type ulcers should be avoided because they may aggravate the condition (Frawley, 2000; Lad, 1998).

Finally, Tirtha (1998) acknowledges the current Western view that peptic ulcers are caused by bacteria and thus recommends the use of different antibacterial herbs for each type of ulcer in addition to the previously listed antiinflammatory measures: pitta-type—goldenseal, aloe, sandalwood, jasmine, and turmeric; vata-type—garlic, sandalwood, jasmine, turmeric; kapha-type—garlic, goldenseal, sandalwood, and turmeric.

Traditional Chinese Medicine

Acupuncture for nausea, vomiting, and gastroesophageal reflux disease   A National Institutes of Health (NIH) consensus panel has recognized acupuncture as effective for nausea of pregnancy, adult postoperative nausea, and chemotherapy nausea and vomiting, as well as for postoperative dental pain (NIH Consensus Development Panel on Acupuncture, 1997, 1998). Dundee and colleagues (1986) studied acupuncture immediately after a gynecologic preoperative opiate injection that had a significant effect on postoperative nausea and vomiting; they also studied the use of eltroacupuncture for patients with cancer with resultant reduced cisplatin-induced nausea and vomiting (Dundee, 1987, 1989). Acupuncture points for GERD include Liver 14 on the rib cage, the stomach channel on the chest above the nipple, and Ren 17 (Conception Vessel) on the chest between the breasts. Ren 12 with Stomach 36 regulates GI motility (Li et al, 1992).

Acupressure for nausea   Acupressure-point wristbands work well for nausea. Acupressure has positive study evidence for the conditions of nausea of pregnancy, postoperative, and for motion sickness (Dundee et al, 1988; Hyde, 1989; Harmon et al, 1999; Alkaissi et al, 1999). Pericardium 6 (P 6), the Neiguan point, is usually used for the acupressure band or needles. This point is on the forearm between the two tendons and is 3-finger widths from the wrist crease (Stern et al, 2001). The best type of wristband is adjustable, and patients are told to apply rotating pressure on the band button if they have any symptoms. Stern and colleagues (2001) studied P 6 with this type acupressure band and reported that:

> subjects reported significantly fewer symptoms of motion sickness on days when wearing the Acuband on the wrist or the arm than they did on control days (when they worn no Acuband). Subjects also showed less abnormal gastric activity on the days when wearing an Acuband than they did on control days. (p. 91)

The difference between the acupressure band used in the Stern study and the band used in two studies in which acupressure did not work was that the unsuccessful studies (Bruce et al, 1990; Warwick et al, 1991) used nonadjustable bands, and patients were not told to push on the bands when they had symptoms.

Homeopathy for Nausea and Peptic Ulcer Disease

Some of the more common homeopathic remedies for nausea are *Ipecacuanha, Nux vomica, Pulsatilla, Tabacum, Phosphorus* (LaValle et al, 2000; Skinner, 2001). Case finding (taking a history) to match symptoms and other patient characteristics to the nausea are needed so that a proper remedy is chosen. In addition, several remedies are available for PUD, including *Bismuthum oxydatum, Hydrastis Canadensis,* and *Nux vomica* (LaValle, 1999). Table 4-7 lists alternative health care systems methods for dyspepsia, nausea, GERD, and PUD.

MIND-BODY-SPIRIT INTERVENTIONS FOR DYSPEPSIA, NAUSEA, GASTROESOPHAGEAL REFLUX DISEASE, AND PEPTIC ULCER DISEASE

Biofeedback, hypnosis, relaxation, and music therapy have been studied for nausea and vomiting. In reviews of studies with these modalities, Ernst (2001) reports that all methods have a positive effect except biofeedback, although there were "earlier promising case studies" (p. 317). Some of these studies included children. "Hypnosis, used in children as young as 4 years old, led to a decrease in severity and duration of nausea" and "nausea resulting from chemotherapy can be ameliorated by the use of hypnosis," including self-hypnosis (Primack, 1999, p. 156). Fontaine (2000) recommends imagery as a modality with nausea. Naparstek has numerous tapes and compact discs (CDs) that may be helpful with GI problems. Music and imagery help reduce vomiting and anxiety in postchemotherapy patients (Ezzone et al, 1998; Frank, 1985). Box 4-9 gives lifestyle modifications that can help GERD. Visualization-imagery, autogenics, meditation, prayer, and relaxation also may help manage symptoms, especially if stress is a component. These modalities are helpful for any GI complaints that are aggravated by stress (Freeman, Lawlis, 2001; Weil, 2001).

In the 1980s, hypnosis reduced the relapse rate of duodenal ulcers (Colgan et al, 1988). Thirty patients, endoscopically diagnosed as having ulcers and then diagnosed endoscopically as healed, were divided into a medical treatment group and a group combining medical treatment and hypnosis. The treatment group learned and practiced hypnosis. After 1 year, a relapse rate of 53% resulted for hypnosis patients and 100% for the controls. This finding was at a time when the routine recurrence rate for ulcers was approximately 85% because providers were not treating *Helicobacter pylori* (Freeman, Lawlis, 2001). Hypnosis possibly decreased gastric secretion. In addition, the relaxation and stress-reduction techniques used with hypnosis may have helped because they may:

> ...strengthen immune function, most specifically T-cell function.
> Bacteria in the body are controlled by T cells. Therefore a strength-
> ening of immune function, leading to the natural destruction of

Table 4-7 Alternative Health Care Systems for Dyspepsia, Nausea, Gastroesophageal, and Peptic Ulcer Disease

Intervention	Management	Treatment Regimen	Cautions, Precautions, Interactions	References
Ayurveda				
	GERD (usually excess pitta)	Antipitta diet: antacid foods, such as milk or ghee, and whole grains. Avoid sour foods such as pickles, yogurt, wine, vinegar, and bananas. Demulcent herbs with bitter properties: aloe gel, shatavari, amalaki. If weak digestion: Trikatu (herbal formula)	Aloe gel can be contaminated with anthraquinones, which can be a drastic cathartic	Frawley, 2000; Lad, 1998
	Pitta-type ulcers.	Initially, a milk fast (three to four glasses of warm milk/day). Small, frequent meals with a bland diet with whole grains and other easy-to-digest foods. Avoid alcohol, smoking,		

Continued

Table 4-7	Alternative Health Care Systems for Dyspepsia, Nausea, Gastroesophageal, and Peptic Ulcer Disease—cont'd			
Intervention	**Management**	**Treatment Regimen**	**Cautions, Precautions, Interactions**	**References**
Ayurveda—cont'd				
		bananas, eggplant, and spicy, sour, and fermented foods. Herbs: same demulcent and bitter herbs helpful in treating GERD. Herbal teas (e.g., jatamamsi and brahmi tea before bedtime). Yoga postures: Leg Lift, Camel, Cobra, Bow, Bridge, and Spinal Twist. Breathing exercises: Cooling Breath (breathing through curled tongue) and Moon Breath (breathing through left nostril only) for 5-10 minutes/day.		
	Vata-type ulcers	Heat to the stomach. Bland diet with mild spices.		

	Sufficient food at regular eating intervals. Diminish stress and worry. Avoid excessively dry, light, spicy, cold, and raw foods.	
Kapha-type ulcers	Antikapha diet. Avoid overeating sweet or oily foods. Use spices that stimulate digestion such as cayenne, dry ginger, black pepper, cloves or herbal formulas such as Trikatu. Deal with grief, greed, attachment issues. Avoid the demulcent herbs.	
Ulcers caused by bacteria	In addition to the above treatments. Pitta-type: goldenseal, aloe, sandalwood, jasmine, and turmeric. Vata-type: garlic, sandalwood, jasmine, turmeric. Kapha-type: garlic, goldenseal, sandalwood, turmeric	Tirtha, 1998

Continued

Table 4-7 Alternative Health Care Systems for Dyspepsia, Nausea, Gastroesophageal, and Peptic Ulcer Disease—cont'd

Intervention	Management	Treatment Regimen	Cautions, Precautions, Interactions	References
Traditional Chinese Medicine				
Acupuncture	GERD	Include Liver 14 on the rib cage, the stomach channel on the chest above the nipple, and Ren 17 (Conception Vessel) on the chest between the breasts. Ren 12 with Stomach 36 regulates GI motility.	Acupuncture points over the chest and ribs are needled obliquely to avoid puncturing the lungs.	Li et al, 1992.
Acupressure	Nausea	Pericardium 6 (P 6), the Neiguan point; can also use wristbands		Dundee et al., 1988; Hyde, 1989; Harmon, 1999; Alkaissi et al, 1999

GERD, *gastroesophageal reflux disease;* GI, *gastrointestinal.*

Box 4-9

Gastroesophageal Reflux Disease—Lifestyle Modifications, and Nutritional-Herbal Treatments

Discontinue smoking
No lying down for at least 2 to 3 hours after eating
Lie on left side—moves gastric contents away from entrance of esophagus
Elevate head of bed 4 to 6 inches
Keep a food diary for 1-2 weeks to identify food offenders
Weight loss
No eating within 2 hours of bedtime
Diet modifications including:
Small meals
Low fat
Stop food offenders
Discontinue caffeine, chocolate, alcohol, carminatives (peppermint, spearmint)
Limit carbonated beverages, acidic foods
Suck hard candy or chew gum to increase saliva
Drink chamomile tea
If possible, discontinue drugs that worsen GERD (calcium-channel blockers, progesterone, anticholinergics, theophylline, nitrates, beta agonists, alpha-adrenergic antagonists)

Mind-body-spirit processes that may help symptoms
Affirmations
Visualization and imagery
Autogenics and relaxation

H. pylori, may have also been a contributing factor to the differences between groups. (Freeman, Lawlis, 2001, p. 246)

Table 4-8 lists mind-body-spirit interventions that may be useful for the treatment of upper GI problems.

BIOLOGIC-BASED THERAPIES FOR DYSPEPSIA, NAUSEA, GASTROESOPHAGEAL REFLUX DISEASE, AND PEPTIC ULCER DISEASE

Nutrients
Vitamin B6 may be helpful for the nausea of pregnancy. Two randomized clinical trials used 30 mg and 75 mg a day. Although nausea was improved, vomiting was not affected (Ernst, 2001).

Table 4-8 Mind-Body-Spirit Interventions For Dyspepsia, Nausea, Gastroesophageal, and Peptic Ulcer Disease

Intervention	Management	Treatment Regimen	Cautions, Precautions, Interactions	References
Affirmation	Heartburn (fear, clutching fear); ulcer (fear; a strong belief that you are not good enough. What is eating away at you?)	Heartburn: "I breathe freely and fully. I am safe. I trust the process of life" (p. 39). Ulcer: "I love and approve of myself. I am at peace. All is well" (p. 69)	If makes own affirmations, need to be positive, personal, present tense.	Hay, 2000
Autogenics, relaxation	Stress reduction; GERD, PUD, dyspepsia	Autogenics, progressive relaxation, relaxation tapes	No operating vehicle or machinery with tapes.	Freeman, Lawlis, 2001; Payne, 2001; Weil, 2001
Distraction (music and video)	Nausea and vomiting from cancer treatment in children	Music decreased duration but not severity of nausea. Video games decreased anticipatory and posttreatment nausea.	Personal preference for music is important.	Keller, 1995

Hypnosis	Anticipatory nausea in children, chemo nausea.	Self-hypnosis	Sustained after only 2 mos of self-hypnosis (n = 20 in study).	Genius, 1995; Jacknow et al, 1994; Primack, 1999
	PUD; decrease recurrence	Hands-on-abdomen technique with suggestions of warmth, control of gastric secretions and healing of the ulcers.	Had seven sessions.	Colgan et al, 1988; Heap, Aravind, 2002
Imagery-visualization	Nausea, stress related to symptoms	*Chemotherapy* audiotape.	No operating vehicle or machinery while listening to tapes.	Naparstek, 1991
Prayer-meditation	Decrease anxiety; PUD, dyspepsia, GERD	Personal preference		

GERD, *Gastroesophageal reflux disease;* PUD, *peptic ulcer disease.*

Several nutritional practices are available for GERD. Box 4-9 reviews these practices, some of which are more lifestyle modifications, while others deal with food products. The important thing is not to eat what makes the GERD worse and keep a food diary to help determine what those foods are. Pay attention to fats and oils that are consumed to see if any specific type may cause more symptoms than do others.

Herbs

In a recent nausea study in Thailand, 32 pregnant women were given a supplement containing 1 gram of ginger for 4 days. These participants experienced less nausea and vomiting than did 35 control-group subjects who took a placebo (Vutyavanich, 2001). No side effects to mothers or babies were experienced. Buckle (1997) recommends a sliver of ginger root in hot water for relief of nausea from pregnancy, or for postradiation and chemotherapy.

Other herbs for nausea include chamomile (LaValle et al, 2000) and peppermint oil. The German Commission E recommends artichoke leaf and cinnamon for dyspeptic problems. They also recommend inhaled or local application (diluted) of mint oil for flatulence and functional GI disorders.

Peptic Ulcer Disease—Biologic-Based Therapies

Cabbage juice is an old "home remedy" for ulcers dating back to the work of Garnett Cheney, MD in the late 1950s:

> who reported curing many ulcer patients with about one quart of raw cabbage juice [per day]. To render the juice more palatable, Dr. Cheney often added celery juice, made from both stalk and greens, pineapple juice, tomato juice or citrus juice. Chilling the "cocktail" also helps to improve the flavor. The juice...should not be taken all at once, but in numerous glasses throughout the day. (Bricklin, 1985)

Chamomile (*Matricaria recutita*), also called German or Hungarian chamomile, has antispasmodic, GI antiinflammatory, antimicrobial activities; it is used to treat PUD and spasms of the GI tract (PL/PL [CE Part 1], 2000). Roman-English chamomile (*Anthemis nobilis*), also called scotch, garden, lawn, sweet, and true or common chamomile, is a related, but not identical, herb; it is the chamomile of choice in Britain. English chamomile is contraindicated in pregnancy and reported to be an abortifacient and to affect the menstrual cycle (DerMarderosian, 2001; Fetrow, Avila, 1999; PL/PL [CE Part 1], 2000). However, the Commission E says that no restrictions are known regarding the use of German chamomile in pregnancy. The Commission recommends German chamomile for "gastrointestinal spasms and inflammatory diseases of the gastrointestinal tract" (Blumenthal et al, 2000, p. 59).

Deglycyrrhizinized licorice (DGL) is recommended for PUD; it has a mild antiinflammatory effect (Blumenthal et al, 2000; Fetrow, Avila, 1999). DGL chewable tablets are available. Chronic high doses can be toxic and cause sodium and water retention and potassium loss (Blumenthal et al, 2000). DGL interacts with several drugs, including antihypertensives, corticosteroids, digoxin, terfenadine, and quinidine. Avoid use in hypokalemic states, hypertension, heart failure, edematous states, and in persons with hepatic or renal damage. DGL is contraindicated in pregnancy and lactation (LaValle et al, 2000). Before taking this herb, seek full herbal information, or use a qualified herbalist.

Commission E recommends dandelion root with herb for disturbances of bile flow, loss of appetite, and dyspepsia, as well as for diuresis (Blumenthal et al, 2000). Dandelion root with herb consists of the entire plant, *Taraxacum officinale*, which is gathered while it is flowering. Several forms of dosing are available.

Aromatherapy

Anecdotally for nausea, Fontaine (2000) recommends compresses with ginger, lavender, or peppermint. Specific aroma probably depends on the preference of the consumer. Fontaine also recommends teas of peppermint, catnip, ginger, or chamomile for morning sickness. Be sure the chamomile is the German chamomile and not the English, because the English chamomile is contraindicated in pregnancy (DerMarderosian, 2001). Buckle (1997) recommends Cardamom (*Elettaria cardamomum*), the essential oil, a few drops for inhalation on a tissue, for the relief of nausea from radiation or chemotherapy. Table 4-9 lists biologic-based therapies for dyspepsia, nausea, GERD, and PUD.

MANIPULATIVE AND BODY-BASED METHODS AND ENERGY THERAPIES FOR DYSPEPSIA, NAUSEA, GASTROESOPHAGEAL REFLUX DISEASE, AND PEPTIC ULCER DISEASE

Massage is generally contraindicated with nausea. However, the appropriate aromatherapy by inhalation, as previously listed, may be helpful. Anecdotally for nausea, Fontaine (2000) recommends healing touch, Reiki, and therapeutic touch. These methods may be helpful to relieve anxiety associated with GERD, dyspepsia, or PUD.

BIOLOGIC-BASED THERAPIES FOR LIVER AND GALLBLADDER CONCERNS

The following is a brief overview of a few biologic-based therapies for other GI disorders. Table 4-10 discusses biologic-based therapies for liver and gall bladder concerns, and Table 4-11 reviews herb drug potential interactions that can interfere with liver metabolism.

Table 4-9 Biologic-Based Therapies for Dyspepsia, Nausea, Gastroesophageal, and Peptide Ulcer Disease

A complete prescribing source should be consulted before using biologic therapies. Vitamin and mineral dosing is often higher than is the standard recommended upper limit. At times of illness or deficiency, persons may need more of such supplements. Any herb can cause allergy. Herbs are generally contraindicated in pregnancy, lactation, and with children unless research data or a long history of safe use has been established.

Intervention	Management	Treatment Regimen	Cautions, Precautions, Interactions	References
Foods	Decrease in gastric cancer occurrence rate	Increased garlic and onion intake	Breath odor, GI symptoms	You et al, 1989; Primack, 1999
	Ulcers	Cabbage juice, 1 quart/day, taken throughout the day. Add celery, pineapple, tomato, or citrus juice to make it more flavorful.	Anecdotal	Bricklin, 1985
Vitamin B6	Nausea of pregnancy	RDA is 1.9 mg in pregnancy. Recommendation for nausea is 30-75 mg/day	Pregnancy UL: is 100 mg/day over age 18 and 80 mg/day under age 18. Toxic symptoms can occur. Sensory neuropathy has	Ernst, 2001; NAP, 2002

Vitamin C	Possibly help PUD	With 200 mg/day from food, the risk of colon cancer drops; some take vitamin C to bowel tolerance (diarrhea).	occurred. Needs to be balanced with other B vitamins. Adult UL: 2000 mg/day. Doses greater than 1000 mg/day may possibly lead to kidney stone formation. Interact with acetaminophen, aluminum containing-antacids, ASA, Heparin, iron, warfarin.	NAP, 2002; PL/PL, 2001; La Valle et al, 2001; Murray, Pizzorno, 1999a
Bismuth subcitrate (bismuth is a natural occurring mineral)	*H. pylori*	240 mg bid before meals	SE: darkening of tongue and stool. Needs to be compounded.	Murray, Pizzorno, 1999c
Hydrochloric acid	Chronic indigestion with hypochlorhydria	Start with one tablet of 10 grains (600 mg) at large meal. If no aggravation, take tablets with large meals until feel warmth in stomach	Contraindicated in ulcer, bleeding, GERD. After determining the largest dose that can take at large meals without feeling warmth, maintain that	Murray, Pizzorno, 1999c

Continued

Table 4-9 Biologic-Based Therapies for Dyspepsia, Nausea, Gastroesophageal, and Peptide Ulcer Disease—cont'd

Intervention	Management	Treatment Regimen	Cautions, Precautions, Interactions	References
Hydrochloric acid, cont'd		or reach seven tablets, whichever is first. Take tablets throughout the meal. Continue taking with meals. If feel symptoms of warmth, decrease dosing. Every 3 days, decrease dose by 1 capsule per meal. If warmth continues, decrease more rapidly.	dose with large meals and take fewer with small meals. Decrease dosing and discontinue use as stomach warmth occurs.	
Bromelain (Ananas comosus); other name: pineapple enzyme	Dyspepsia (when combined with pancreatic extract of trypsin, amylase, and lipase). Mild IBD	80-320 mg bid to tid PO for 8-10 days	Allergy. SE: GI disturbance. Increases levels of tetracycline. Might increase risk of bleeding with anticoagulants and NSAIDS. Contraindicated in bleeding (GI etc.)	Blumenthal et al, 2000; LaValle et al, 2000

Catnip tea	Indigestion, colic	1 to 2 tsp with 6 oz boiling water. Flowering tops are used	Large amounts may cause vomiting. No studies.	PL/PL, 2002
Cat's claw (*Uncaria tomentosa*)	PUD	Root and bark; freeze dried extract	SE: headache, dizziness, vomiting. May lower blood pressure; do not use with antihypertensives. No clinical trials.	Fetrow, Avila, 1999; PL/PL, 2002
German chamomile (*Chamomilla recutita*)	GERD, peptic ulcer	Can make tea.	Allergy. Should not be used if person allergic to ragweed, asters, chrysanthemums. Be sure to use German chamomile.	DerMarderosian, 2001; Blumenthal et al, 2000
Dandelion (whole plant) (*Taraxacam officinale*)	Dyspepsia, loss of appetite, disturbances in bile flow	Various dosing forms. Infusion: steep 1 tbsp cut root and herb in 150 ml water or 3 to 4 gms of powdered whole plant steeped in 150 ml of water.	GI upset caused by bitter quality. Contraindicated in obstruction of the bile duct.	Blumenthal, 2001; PL/PL, 2002
Ginger (*Zingiber officinale*)	Nausea, dyspepsia	Dose depends on formulation. 2-4 g/day of cut rhizome or dried extract.	Caution if have gallstones.	Blumenthal et al, 2000

Continued

Table 4-9 Biologic-Based Therapies for Dyspepsia, Nausea, Gastroesophageal, and Peptide Ulcer Disease—cont'd

Intervention	Management	Treatment Regimen	Cautions, Precautions, Interactions	References
Licorice, DGL (*Glycyrrhiza glabra*)	PUD, gastritis, bloating, indigestion	Chewable tablets	Chronic high doses toxic and can cause sodium and water retention, potassium loss, and hypertension. Drug interactions including antihypertensives, corticosteroids, digoxin, terfenadine, quinidine. Avoid use in hypokalemic states, hypertension, heart failure, edematous states and in persons with hepatic or renal damage. DGL is contraindicated in pregnancy and lactation. Contraindication in liver disorders. DGL studies for ulcer are inconclusive.	Blumenthal et al, 2000; LaValle et al, 1999; PL/PL, 2002

Peppermint leaf and peppermint oil	Gastritis, dyspepsia, nausea, vomiting	Various preparations	Can increase colic in persons with gallstones.	PL/PL, 2002
Aromatherapy	Nausea	Compresses with ginger, lavender, or peppermint.	Personal preference important. Essential oils must be diluted and must not be applied directly to the skin.	Fontaine, 2000
	Nausea from radiation or chemotherapy	Cardamom, a few drops on a tissue for inhalation.		Buckle, 1997
	Abdominal cramps, colic, dyspepsia	Lavender (Lavandula angustifolia) 1 to 5 gtts diluted in a carrier oil (such as sweet almond oil) and rubbed on affected area		Buckle, 2001

ASA, Acetylsalicylic acid; bid, twice a day; DGL, deglycyrrhizinized licorice; GERD, gastroesophageal reflux disease; GI, gastrointestinal; gtts, drops; IBD, inflammatory bowel disease; NAP, National Academies Press; NSAIDs, nonsteroidal antiinflammatory drugs; PL/PL, Pharmacist's Letter/Prescriber's Letter; PO, by mouth; PUD, peptic ulcer disease; RDA, Recommended Daily Allowance; SE, side effects; tid, three times a day; UL, upper limits—the maximum level of daily nutrient that is likely to pose no risk of adverse effects. Includes intake from food, water, and supplements.

Table 4-10 Biologic-Based Therapies for Liver and Gallbladder Concerns

A complete prescribing source should be consulted before using biologic therapies. Any herb can cause allergy. Herbs are generally contraindicated in women who are pregnant or lactating and with children unless research data or a long history of safe use has been established.

Intervention	Management	Treatment Regimen	Cautions, Precautions, Interactions	References
Unfiltered apple juice	Gallbladder symptom relief	Several glasses apple juice per day for a few wks followed by one time dose of an ounce of olive oil	Note that unfiltered apple juice is used pasteurized juice should be used.	Anecdotal
Dandelion (whole plant)	Disturbances in bile flow, gallstones	Various dosing forms; infusion: steep 1 tbsp cut root and herb (or 3-4 gms of powdered whole plant) in 150 ml water	GI upset caused by bitter quality. Contraindicated in obstruction of the bile duct. Can exhibit hypoglycemic effects. Theoretical drug interactions.	Blumenthal, 2001; PL/PL, 2002
Goldenseal (Hydrastis canadensis)	Liver disorders	Various doses. Plant is an endangered species.	SE and adverse effects: bradycardia, CNS depression, GI symptoms, seizures,	Fetrow, Avila, 1999; PL/PL, 2000, 2002

Herb	Indications	Dosage	Cautions/Side effects	References
Milk thistle (*Silybum marianum*)	Hepatoprotective; cirrhosis, death cap mushroom poisoning, hepatitis, alcoholic liver disease, occupational toxic chemical exposure, for the improvement of liver function tests	Formulations standardized to 70% to 80% silymarin. IV for amanita phalloides mushroom poisoning. IV silibinin not available in United States.	paralysis, paresthesia. Likely unsafe when used orally in high doses or long-term. Unsafe in pregnancy and children. Short-term use only. Interferes with laboratory tests	Blumenthal et al, 2000; Castleman, 1995; Evidence Report/Tech Assessment #21, 2000; PL/PL, 2002
Peppermint oil	Nonulcer dyspepsia; possibly gallstones	0.2-0.4 ml diluted in liquid tid; (average daily amount is 6 to 12 gtts)	Allergic reactions and cross reactions with ragweed, marigold, daisy, mum. SE: mild laxative effect. Problems in study designs. Interacts with antacids and H2 antagonists. Not to be used with achlorhydria.	Murray, Pizzorno, 1999b; PL/PL, 2002

CNS, *Central nervous system;* GI, *gastrointestinal;* gtts, *drops;* IV, *intravenous;* PL/PL, *Pharmacist's Letter/Prescriber's Letter;* SE, *side effects;* tid, *three times a day.*

Table 4-11 Liver Metabolism*

Drug Category	Herbs that May Alter Liver Enzymes	Herbs that May Cause Hepatotoxicity from Pyrrolizidine Alkaloids
ACE inhibitors	American mandrake (*Podophyllum peltatum*); Balmony (*Chelone glabra*); Barberry (*Berberis vulgaris*); Blue flag (*Iris versicolor*); Button Bush (*Cephalanthus spp*); Fringetree (*Chionanthus virginicus*); Goldenseal (*Hydrastis canadensis*); Greater Celandine (*Chelidonium majus*); Leptandra (*Veronicastrum virginicum*); Oregon grape (*Berberis aquifolium*); Sagebrush (*Artemisia tridentata*); Virginia Snakeroot, Serpentaria (*Aristolochia serpentaria*); Wahoo, Burning Bush (*Euonymus atropurpureus*)	Coltsfoot (*Tussilago farfara*); Comfrey (*Symphytum officinale*); Hound's Tongue (*Cynoglossum officinalis*); Life Root, Squaw Weed (*Senecio aureus*)
Antiasthmatics		
Anticoagulants		
Anticonvulsants		
Antidepressants (tricyclic)		
Glucocorticoids		
Oral contraceptives		

*The liver metabolizes many pharmaceutical drugs, and any alteration of this metabolism can cause either an increase or decrease in the drug's pharmacologic effects. Some herbs also tend to increase liver metabolism by stimulating the liver directly or indirectly. Patients taking the following pharmaceuticals along with the listed herbs should be advised to use caution with herbs that may potentially alter liver function.
ACE, angiotensin-coverting enzyme.
From LaValle J et al: Herb/drug potential interactions: liver metabolism. In Natural therapeutics pocket guide, Hudson, Ohio, 2000, LextComp.

Foods

Unfiltered apple juice is an old home remedy for gallstone symptoms. Natural unfiltered (pasteurized) apple juice daily for a few weeks followed by one dose of an ounce of olive oil is the therapy.

In addition, coffee may decrease the incidence of gallstones. In the Harvard Health Professionals Follow-Up Study (Leitzmann et al, 1999), the relative risk was significantly lower for men who drank two or more cups of coffee per day. Decaffeinated coffee was not associated with a decreased risk.

Herbs

Milk thistle's (*Silybum marianum*) value has been demonstrated "in more than 100 rigorous scientific experiments. Unfortunately, the vast majority of these studies has been European, mostly German, and few mainstream American physicians read German botanical medicine journals" (Castleman, 1995, p. 18). Milk thistle is used for alcoholic cirrhosis, death cap mushroom poisoning, hepatitis, occupational toxic chemical exposure, for the improvement of liver function tests, and for psoriasis (Castleman, 1995; PL/PL, 2000). Studies used formulations standardized to 70% silymarin, 200 to 400 mg/daily.

Silibinin, part of the silymarin complex, improves survival when used intravenously as supportive treatment for liver damage caused by death cap (*Amanita phalloides*). The commonly used dose is 20 to 50 mg/kg of body weight over 24 hours, divided into four infusions, each administered over a 2-hour period. This regimen is started within 48 hours of mushroom ingestion. However, intravenous silibinin is not available in the United States (PL/PL, 2000).

Goldenseal's (*Hydrastis canadensis*) active alkaloid, berberine, may stimulate the secretion of bile and bilirubin. In a study of chronic cholecystitis, "berberine treatment resulted in a disappearance of clinical symptoms, a decrease in bilirubin level, and an increase in bile volume of the gallbladder" (PL/PL [CE Part 2], 2000, p. 22). Goldenseal also helped decrease cholera. Goldenseal is a dangerous drug in high doses and is definitely contraindicated in pregnancy. Tolerance is thought to develop after only a few weeks of use (Fetrow, Avila, 1999).

Dandelion root with herb (i.e., the entire plant) is recommended for disturbances in bile flow and for hepatobiliary disorders (Blumenthal et al, 2000). Dandelion is contraindicated in obstruction of the bile duct and should be used for gallstones under supervision only.

Menthol, the principal component of peppermint oil, has been shown to dissolve gallstones in combination with related terpenes.

This approach to gallstone removal offers an effective alternative to surgery and has been shown to be safe even when consumed for prolonged periods of time [up to 4 years]. Terpenes, like menthol, help to dissolve gallstones by reducing bile cholesterol levels while increasing bile acid and lecithin levels in the gall bladder. (Murray, Pizzorno, 1999b, p. 829)

Enteric-coated peppermint oil may offer the same benefit.

REFERENCES

Achkar E: Common clinical manifestations of gastrointestinal disease. In Andreoli T, ed: *Cecil essentials of medicine*, Philadelphia, 2001, Saunders.

Alberts DS et al: Lack of effect of a high-fiber cereal supplement on the recurrence of colorectal adenomas. Phoenix Colon Cancer Prevention Physicians' Network, *N Engl J Med* 342:1156, 2000.

Ali A et al: Emotional abuse, self-blame, and self-silencing in women with irritable bowel syndrome, *Psychosom Med* 62(1):76, 2000.

Alkaissi A, Stalnert M, Kalman S: Effect and placebo effect of acupressure (P6) on nausea and vomiting after outpatient gynaecological surgery, *Acta Anaesthesiol Scand* 43:270, 1999.

Barrie S: Food allergy testing. In Pizzorno J, Murray M, editors: *Textbook of natural medicine*, Edinburgh, 1999, Churchill Livingstone.

Barrie S: Food allergies, *Natural Med J* 1(7):6, 1998.

Behm RM: A special recipe to banish constipation, *Geriatric Nurs* 6(4):216, 1985.

Bensoussan A et al.: Treatment of irritable bowel syndrome with Chinese herbal medicine: a randomized controlled trial, *JAMA* 280(18):1585, 1998.

Blanchard EB, Schwarz SP: Two-year follow-up of behavioral treatment of irritable bowel syndrome, *Behav Ther* 19:67, 1988.

Bland J et al: A medical food-supplemented detoxification program in the management of chronic health problems, *Altern Ther Health Med* 1(5):62, 1995.

Bricklin M: *Natural remedies for what ails you*, Emmaus, Penn, 1985, Rodale.

Buckle J: *Clinical aromatherapy in nursing*, San Diego, Calif, 1997, Singular.

Blumenthal M, Goldberg A, Brinckmann J: *Herbal medicine: expanded Commission E monographs*, Newton, Mass, 2000, Integrative Medicine Communications.

Bruce DG et al: Acupressure and motion sickness, *Aviat Space Environ Med* 60:361, 1990.

Byers D: *Better health with foot reflexology*, St Petersburg, Fla, 1991, Ingham Publishing.

Cahn A et al: Acupuncture in gastroscopy, *Lancet* 1(8057):182, 1978.

Castell D et al: GERD: management algorithms for the primary care physician and the specialist, *Pract Gastroenterol* April:18, 1998.

Castleman M: Milk thistle: nature's liver protector, *Herb Q* 66:18, 1995.

Chan J, Carr I, Mayberry JF: The role of acupuncture in the treatment of irritable bowel syndrome: a pilot study, *Hepato-Gastroenterol* 44:1328, 1997.

Colgan SM, Faragher EB, Whorwell PJ: Controlled trial of hypnotherapy in relapse prevention of duodenal ulceration, *Lancet* 1(8598):1299, 1988.

Cox DJ et al: Contribution of behaviour therapy and biofeedback to laxative therapy in the treatment of pediatric encopresis, *Ann Behav Med* 20:70, 1998.

De Bruyn G: Diarrhea. In Barton S, ed: *Clinical evidence*, London, 2001, BMJ.

DeDomenico G, Wood EC: *Beard's massage*, Philadelphia, 1997, Saunders.

DerMarderosian A, ed: *The review of natural products*, St Louis, 2001, Facts and Comparisons.

Dundee JW et al: Traditional Chinese acupuncture: a potential useful antiemetic? *BMJ* 293:583, 1986.

Dundee JW et al: Acupuncture to prevent cisplatin-associated vomiting [letter], *Lancet* 8541:1083, 1987.

Dundee JW et al: P6 acupressure reduces morning sickness, *J R Soc Med* 81:456, 1988.

Dundee JW et al: Acupuncture prophylaxis of cancer chemotherapy-induced sickness, *J R Soc Med* 82:268, 1989.

Ernst E: *The desktop guide to complementary and alternative medicine*, St Louis, 2001, Mosby.

Evidence Report/Technology Assessment #21: *Milk thistle: effects on liver disease and cirrhosis and clinical adverse effects*, AHRQ publication #01-E025, 2000. *www.ahrq. gov/clinic/evrptfiles.htm.*

Ezzone S et al: Music as an adjunct to antiemetic therapy, *Oncol Nurs Forum* 25:1551, 1998.

Farthing M, Gomborone J: Abdominal symptoms and the mind. In Watkins A, ed: *Mind-body medicine*, Edinburgh, 1997, Churchill Livingstone.

Fetrow C, Avila J: *Professional's handbook of complementary and alternative medicine*, Springhouse, Penn, 1999, Springhouse.

Fontaine K: *Healing practices*, Upper Saddle River, NJ, 2000, Prentice Hall.

Fraenkel D: Dance/movement therapy. In Novey D, ed: *Clinician's complete guide to complementary and alternative medicine*, St Louis, 2000, Mosby.

Frank JM: The effects of music and guided visual imagery on chemotherapy induced nausea and vomiting, *Oncol Nurs Forum* 12:47, 1985.

Frawley D: *Ayurvedic healing: a comprehensive guide*, ed 2, Twin Lakes, Wisc, 2000, Lotus Press.

Frawley D: *Ayurvedic healing: a comprehensive guide*, Salt Lake City, Utah, 1989, Passage.

Freeman L, Lawlis GF: *Mosby's complementary and alternative medicine*, St Louis, 2001, Mosby.

Fritz S: *Mosby's fundamentals of therapeutic massage*, St Louis, 1995, Mosby.

Fuchs CS et al: Dietary fiber and the risk of colorectal cancer and adenoma in women, *N Engl J Med* 340:169, 1999.

Gach MR: *Acupressure's potent point*, New York, 1990, Bantam Books.

Gaeddert A: *Healing digestive disorders: natural treatments for gastrointestinal conditions*, Berkeley, Calif, 1998, North Atlantic Books.

Genuis M: The use of hypnosis in helping cancer patients control anxiety, pain, and emesis: a review of recent empirical studies, *Am J Clin Hypn* 37(4):316, 1995.

Grattagliano A et al: Studie clilncio randomizzato sull'efficacia di un integratore biologico nei pazienti affetti da sindrome dell'intestino irritabile, *Minerva Gastroenterol Dietol* 44:51, 1998.

Gutenbrunner C, Gundermann G: Kontrollierte Studie uber die abfuhrende Wirkung eines Heilwassers, *Z Allg Med* 74:648, 1998.

Guthrie E et al: A controlled trial of psychological treatment for the irritable bowel syndrome, *Gastroenterol* 100:450, 1991.

Gutierrez Y: *Nutrition in health maintenance and health promotion*, San Francisco, 1994, University of California at San Francisco.

Harmon D et al: Acupressure and the prevention of nausea and vomiting after laparoscopy, *Br J Anaesth* 82:387, 1999.

Harvey R et al: Individual and group hypnotherapy in treatment of refractory irritable bowel syndrome, *Lancet* 1(8635):424, 1989.

Hay L: *Heal your body*, Carlsbad, Calif, 2000, Hay House.

Heap M, Aravind K: *Hartland's medical and dental hypnosis*, Edinburgh, 2002, Churchill Livingstone.

Heitkemper M, Jarrett M: Irritable bowel syndrome, *AJN* 101(1):26, 2001.

Heuman DM, Mills AS, McGuire HH: *Gastroenterology*, Philadelphia, 1997, Saunders.

Horvilleur A: *The family guide to homeopathy*, Arlington, Va, 1986, Health and Homeopathy Publishing.

Hyde E: Acupressure therapy for morning sickness, *J R Soc Med* 81:456, 1989.

Jacknow D et al: Hypnosis in the prevention of chemotherapy-related nausea and vomiting in children: a prospective study, *J Dev Behav Pediatr* 15:258, 1994.

Jacobs J et al: Treatment of acute childhood diarrhea with homeopathic medicine: A randomized clinical trial in Nicaragua, *Pediatrics* 93(5):719, 1994.

Jones A: *Yoga: a step-by-step guide*, Boston, 1998, Element.

Jones V et al: Food intolerance: a major factor in the pathogenesis of irritable bowel syndrome, *Lancet* 2:1115, 1982.

Keller V: Management of nausea and vomiting in children, *J Ped Nurs* 10(5):280, 1995.

Kesselring A, Spichiger E, Muller M: Fussreflexzonenmassage, *Pflege* 11:213, 1998.

Lad V: *The complete book of Ayurvedic home remedies*, New York, 1998, Three Rivers Press.

Lad V: *Ayurveda: The science of self-healing*. Wilmot, Wisc, 1985, Lotus Press.

Ladinsky M et al: The World Health Organization oral rehydration solution in US pediatric practice, *Arch Pediatr Adolesc Med* 154:700, 2000.

LaValle J et al: Herb/drug potential interactions: liver metabolism. In *Natural therapeutics pocket guide*, Hudson, Ohio, 2000, LexiComp.

Leahy A et al: Computerised biofeedback games: a new method for teaching stress management and its use in irritable bowel syndrome, *J Roy Soc Phys Lond* 32:552, 1998.

Leicester RJ, Hunt RH: Peppermint oil to reduce colonic spasm during endoscopy, *Lancet* 2:989, 1982.

Leitzmann JF et al: A prospective study of coffee consumption and the risk of symptomatic gallstone disease in men, *JAMA* 281:2106, 1999.

Lewis P: Irritable bowel syndrome: emotional factors and acupuncture treatment, *J Chin Med* 40:9, 1992.

Li Y et al: The effect of acupuncture on gastrointestinal function and disorders, *Am J Gastroenterol* 87(10):1372, 1992.

Loening BV: Modulation of abnormal defecation dynamics by biofeedback treatment in chronically constipated children with encopresis, *J Pediatr* 116:214, 1990.

Loening-Baucke V: Biofeedback treatment for chronic constipation and encopresis in childhood: long term outcome, *Pediatr* 96:105, 1995.

MacIntosh A, Ball K: The effects of a short program of detoxification in disease-free individuals, *Altern Ther Health Med* 6(4):70, 2000.

Maciocia G: *The foundations of Chinese medicine*, New York, 1989, Churchill Livingstone.

Maciocia G: *The practice of Chinese medicine*, New York, 1994, Churchill Livingstone.

McKee RF et al: Identification of patients likely to benefit from biofeedback for outlet obstruction constipation, *Br J Surg* 86:355, 1999.

McQuaid K: Alimentary tract. In Tierney L, McPhee, S, Papadakis M, editors: *Current medical diagnosis and treatment*, New York, 2002, McGraw Hill.

Merchant R, Andre C: A review of recent clinical trials of the nutritional supplement *Chlorella pyrenoidosa* in the treatment of fibromyalgia, hypertension, and ulcerative colitis, *Altern Ther Health Med* 7(3):79, 2001.

Michels KB et al: Prospective study of fruit and vegetable consumption and incidence of colon and rectal cancers, *J Am Cancer Inst* 92:1740, 2000.

Murray M, Pizzorno J: Irritable bowel syndrome. In Pizzorno J, Murray M, editors: *Textbook of natural medicine*, ed 2, vol 2, Edinburgh, 1999a, Churchill Livingstone.

Murray M, Pizzorno J: Mentha piperita. In Pizzorno J, Murray M, editors: *Textbook of natural medicine*, ed 2, vol 1, Edinburgh 1999b, Churchill Livingstone.

Murray M, Pizzorno J: Maldigestion. In Pizzorno J, Murray M, editors: *Textbook of natural medicine*, ed 2, vol 2, Edinburgh, 1999c, Churchill Livingstone.

Nanda R et al: Food intolerance and the irritable bowel syndrome, *Gut* 30:1099, 1989.

Naparstek B: *Chemotherapy* [audiotape], Akron, Ohio, 1991, Health Journeys. *www.healthjourneys.com*

Narducci F et al: Increased colonic motility during exposure to a stressful situation, *Dig Dis Sci* 30:40, 1985.

National Academies Press (NAP): Vitamins, minerals, 2002, *www.nap.edu*, accessed Jan, 2003.

National Digestive Diseases Information Clearing House [NDDIC]: Diarrhea. Constipation. Irritable Bowel Syndrome. Crohn's Disease. National Institute of Diabetes and Digestive and Kidney Diseases, 2001. *http://www.niddk.nih.gov/health/digest/pubs.htm*.

Neff DF, Blanchard EB: A multicomponent treatment for irritable bowel syndrome, *Behav Ther* 18:70, 1987.

NIH Concensus Development Panel on Acupuncture: NIH Panel Issues consensus statement on acupuncture, *NIH News Release*, Nov 5, 1997.

NIH Concensus Development Panel on Acupuncture: Acupuncture, *JAMA* 280(17):1518, 1998.

Novey D: *Clinician's complete reference to complementary and alternative medicine*, St Louis, 2000, Mosby.

Paynter W: Travel medicine, *Clin Rev* 10(1):55, 2000.

Pettit J: Biofeedback, *Clin Rev* 9(10):113, 1999.

Pharmacist's Letter/Prescriber's Letter [PL/PL]: *Natural medicines comprehensive database*, Stockton, Calif, 2002, Therapeutic Research Faculty.

Pharmacist's Letter/Prescriber's Letter: *Natural medicines in clinical management: colon cancer prevention 2001*, vol 2, Stockton, Calif, 2001, Therapeutic Research Faculty.

Pharmacist's Letter/Prescriber's Letter: *Natural medicines in clinical management: colds and flu 2000*, vol 4, Stockton, Calif, 2002, Therapeutic Research Faculty.

Pharmacist's Letter/Prescriber's Letter CE: *The updated therapeutic uses of herbs*, part 1 and 2, Continuing Education Booklet, Stockton, Calif, 2000, Therapeutic Research Faculty.

Pittler M, Ernst E: Peppermint oil for IBS: A critical review and meta analysis, *Am J Gastroenterol* 93(7):765, 1998.

Pizzorno J, Murray M: editors: *Textbook of natural medicine*, ed 2, vol 2, Edinburgh, 1999, Churchill Livingstone.

Primack A: Complementary/alternative therapies in the prevention and treatment of cancer. In Spencer J, Jacobs J, editors: *Complementary/alternative medicine*, St Louis, 1999, Mosby.

Quillin P: *Amish folk medicine*, Sarasota, Fla, 1996, Book World Services.

Ramaesh P et al: Managing morphine-induced constipation: a controlled comparison of an Ayurvedic formulation and senna, *J Pain Symptom Manage* 16:240, 1998.

Rockwell S: Rotation diet: A diagnostic & therapeutic tool. In Pizzorno J, Murray M, editors: *Textbook of natural medicine*, ed 2, vol 2, 1999, Churchill Livingstone.

Rojcewicz S: Poetry therapy. In Novey D, ed: *Clinician's complete reference to complementary and alternative medicine*, St Louis, 2000, Mosby.

Rubin G: Constipation. In Barton S, ed: *Clinical evidence*, issue 6, London, 2002, BMJ Publishing.

Schatzkin A et al: Lack of effect of a low-fat diet on the recurrence of colorectal adenomas. Polyp Prevention Trial Study Group, *N Eng J Med* 342:1149, 2000.

Skinner S : *An introduction to homeopathic medicine in primary care*, Gaithersburg, Md, 2001, Aspen.

Sondheimer J: Gastrointestinal tract. In Hay W et al, editors: *Current pediatric diagnosis and treatment*, New York, 2001, McGraw Hill.

Steefel L: Establishing a biofeedback program in your clinical practice, *Alt Comp Ther* 1(2):103, 1995.

Stern R et al: Acupressure relieves the symptoms of motion sickness and reduces abnormal gastric activity, *Alt Ther Health Med* 7(4):91, 2001.

Svedlund J et al: Upper gastrointestinal and mental symptoms in the irritable bowel syndrome, *Scand J Gastroenterol* 20:595, 1985.

Tirtha S: *The Ayurvedic encyclopedia: natural secrets to healing, prevention and longevity*, ed 2, Bayville, NY, 1998, Ayurveda Holistic Center Press.

Van der Plas R, Benninga M, Büller H et al: Biofeedback training in treatment of childhood constipation: A randomized controlled study, *Lancet* 348:776, 1996.

Vutyavanich T, Kraisarin T, Ruangsri R: Ginger for nausea and vomiting in pregnancy: Randomized, double-masked, placebo-controlled trial, *Obstet-Gynecol* 97:577, 2001.

Warwick-Evans LA, Masters IJ, Redston SB: A double-blind controlled evaluation of acupressure in the treatment of motion sickness, *Aviat Space Environ Med* 62:776, 1991.

Weil A: The Andrew Weil website, *www.askdrweil.com: Steering clear of GERD*, 1999, accessed Jan, 2003.

www.niaid.nih.gov/factsheets.ffod.htm: Food allergy and intolerances, 2001, accessed July 26, 2002.

www.who.int/chd/publications/cdd: Oral and intravenous rehydration solutions, 1990, accessed August 1, 2001.

www.who.int/chd/publications/newslet/update: Rice-based oral rehydration salts. Division of Child Health Development Update #7, 1990, accessed August 1, 2001.

Watkins A, ed: *Mind body medicine*, Philadelphia, 1997, Churchill Livingstone.

Wells-Federman C, Stuart-Shor E, Webster A: Cognitive therapy. In Colbath J, Prawlucki P, editors: *Nurs Clin North Am: Holist Nurs Care* 36(1):93, 2001.

Werner D: *Where there is no doctor: a village health care handbook*, Palo Alto, Calif, 1996, Hesperian Foundation. (Note: this text comes in approximately 30 different languages.)

Whorwell P, Prior A, Faragher E: Controlled trial of hypnotherapy in the treatment of severe refractory irritable-bowel syndrome, *Lancet* 2(8414):1232, 1984.

Whorwell PJ, Prior A, Colgan SM: Hypnotherapy in severe irritable bowel syndrome, *Gut* 28:423, 1987.

Yanhua S, Sumei Y: The treatment of 86 cases of epigastric and abdominal pain by scalp acupuncture, *J Chin Med* 62:27, 2000.

You W et al: Allium vegetables and reduced risk of stomach cancer, *J Natl Cancer Inst* 81:162, 1989.

Zhang M: Vitamin C inhibits the growth of a bacterial risk factor for gastric carcinoma: *H. pylori, Cancer* 80(10): 897, 1997.

DERMATOLOGIC CONCERNS

Roxana Huebscher

NAC THERAPIES FOR DERMATOLOGIC CONCERNS

Numerous factors play a role in skin disorders. Because the skin, especially the skin on the face, is the first thing that others see, people who have skin conditions are often self-conscious and sensitive about their image. These individuals may avoid public and social activities, and thus skin disorders are not only physically difficult, but also mentally, emotionally, and spiritually challenging. For example, in a survey of the psychosocial effects of psoriasis, 86% of respondents said they hated the public's ignorance, 72% avoided swimming, 64% avoided buying short-sleeved clothing, 57% believed people stared at them, 55% thought that nonsufferers regarded psoriasis as contagious and untouchable, 50% believed their sexual relationships were affected, and 40% avoided playing sports (Ramsay, O'Reagan, 1988). Therefore the treatment of skin disorders includes not only the dressings, herbal preparations, and medications, but also, more importantly, the compassion, caring, and help with psychosocial aspects. Health care providers (HCPs) need appropriate referrals and resources at hand, and they need knowledge of the many natural-alternative-complementary (NAC) therapies available.

NAC therapies covered in this chapter include treatments for common conditions such as acne, eczema, fungal infections, herpes, pruritus, poison ivy, psoriasis, rosacea, and warts, as well as wounds, abrasions, and sunburn. The coverage is not exhaustive yet gives a flavor of the numerous NAC therapies that are available.

ALTERNATIVE HEALTH CARE SYSTEMS FOR DERMATOLOGIC CONCERNS

Ayurveda

Several herbs have been used for skin conditions. These herbs include ashwagandha, coriander, and guggul. Lad (1985) mentions coriander juice as having antipitta properties. Used for rash, hives, and dermatitis, coriander can be applied to the skin as a pulp to relieve burning. Lad also mentions turmeric with a pinch of salt as a paste to be applied to abrasions, bruises, or traumatic swelling. In addition, black pepper "mixed with ghee relieves pitta disorders such as dermatitis and hives" (Lad, 1985, p. 140).

Traditional Chinese Medicine

Anecdotally, acupressure points have been reported for self-care treatment of skin disorders. Acupressure, a treatment form in traditional oriental medicine, is similar to acupuncture except pressure is applied to the meridian points instead of inserting needles. Appendix B gives the meridians and points mentioned in the table. Chinese herbs also may be helpful for atopic eczema. Spencer and Jacobs (1999) reviewed the evidence from several studies on both adults and children. Although people usually get individualized herbal formulas with Traditional Chinese Medicine (TCM), six studies have used the same 10-herbal formula and found good results. In one study, 23 of the 37 children treated showed improvement (Sheehan, Ahterton, 1992, 1994). All the children originally had extensive nonexudative atopic eczema.

Homeopathy

According to case finding, the recommended homeopathic remedy is based on the symptoms and other life factors that accompany the skin signs. For example, *Hepar sulphuris calcareum* is for acne on the face and forehead that is painful to touch, and *sulphuris* is for the acne of "intellectually active patients with strong self-esteem who are sensitive to heat, kick the covers off at night and may have a history of other skin problems; they may be untidy" (Skinner, 2001, p. 159). Other homeopathic remedies for acne, eczema, psoriasis, and rosacea are listed with biologic information.

Home Remedies

Old home remedies abound for skin conditions, such as applying the inside skin of a banana peel to a wart. For warts, Amish folk remedies include applying juice from milkweed or dandelion, or rubbing with raw potato peelings or garlic, or topically applying a castor oil-soaked bandage (Quillan,1996). *Amish Folk Medicine* suggests vinegar as an underarm deodorant after bathing, as a hair rinse, or applied to insect stings. For itching, the authors advocate a poultice of cornstarch, application of witch hazel, or 3 cups of cooked oatmeal in a cheesecloth bag soaked in warm water for 15 minutes and then rubbed over the itchy area (Quillan, 1996). Table 5-1 lists a few alternative health care system therapies for skin concerns.

Table 5-1	Alternative Health Care Systems for Dermatologic Concerns			
Intervention	Management	Treatment Regimen	Cautions, Precautions, Interactions	References
Ayurveda Herbs				
Ashwagandha (*Withania somnifera*)	Carbuncles, scabies, ulcers, swelling	Topical: bruised leaves and ground root are applied topically.	May alter level of benzodiazepines and decrease tolerance to opiates when taken internally. May protect against cyclophosphamide-induced leukopenia. Contraindicated in pregnancy.	Mishra et al, 2001; LaValle et al, 2000; DerMarderosian, 2001; PL/PL, 2002
Black pepper	Dermatitis and hives	Topical: Black pepper is mixed with ghee and applied.	Wash hands thoroughly. Avoid eyes.	Lad, 1985
Coriander (*Coriandrum sativum*)	Rash, hives, dermatitis, burning	Topical: make pulp with juice and apply.	Allergic reactions; photosensitivity (Is in carrot family)	Lad, 1985; PL/PL, 2002
Guggul (*Commiphora mukul*), the same	Nodulocystic acne	A dose of gugulipid equivalent to 25 mg guggulsterone/day.	GI effects are reported when taken internally; has thyroid-stimulating	Mishra et al, 2001; LaValle et al, 2000;

286

genus as myrrh; also called gugulipid			properties. Interacts with propranolol, diltiazem, thyroid drugs.	DerMarderosian, 2001; PL/PL, 2002
Turmeric (*Curcuma longa*)	Abrasions, bruises, swelling, ringworm	Topical: Turmeric is applied with a pinch of salt as a paste.		Lad, 1985; PL/PL, 2002

Traditional Chinese Medicine (TCM)

Chinese herbs	Eczema, pediatric patients	Specific formulation of 10 herbs: *Ledebouriella seseloides, Potentilla chinensis, Clematis armandii, Rehmannia glutinosa, Paeonia lactiflora, Lophatherum gracile, Dictamnus dasycarpus, Tribulus terrestris, Glycyrrhiza uralensis, Schizonepeta tenuifolia*; other herbs	In follow-up after 1 yr, 23 of 37 children showed improvement; 4 dropped out because of the unpalatability of herbs and 10 because of lack of response. Brand name Zemaphyte.	Sheehan, Ahterton, 1992, 1994 in Spencer, Jacobs, 1999; Hackman, 1999
Acupuncture	Acne	Specific individual meridian points are selected; ear acupuncture also can be used.		Liu, 1993; Xu, 1989

Continued

Intervention	Management	Treatment Regimen	Cautions, Precautions, Interactions	References
TCM—cont'd				
Acupressure	Skin disorders that are caused or worsened by stress, tension, or fatigue, acne, eczema; self-care by patient using pressure to points. Can be used by patient or by an acupressure practitioner.	Participant sits forward in chair; UB 23 and UB 47 are briskly rubbed with backs of patient or practitioner's hands. For 1 min, St 36 is briskly rubbed with heel of one of patient's leg to below outside of knee on opposite leg. Back of neck is grasped with one hand, and UB 10 is pressed. For 1 min, gentle firm pressure is applied on St 2 and St 3 on cheeks. For 1 min, light pressure is applied to TW (SJ or San Jiao) 17 and SI 17 under earlobes; and participant	Anecdotal. See Appendix B for meridians and points. Practice breathing exercise and regular exercise, and proper diet also. Practitioner or patient may apply the acupressure.	Gach, 1990

		breathes deeply. For 2 min, palms are brought together; middle and index fingers lightly touch GV (Du Mo) 24.5. (the Third Eye point). Concentrate and breathe deeply.		Gach, 1990
Traditional oriental breathing exercises	Eczema	Participant stands with arms at sides; inhales as arms are raised over head; exhales as arms are lowered. Repeat 10-20 times.	Anecdotal; avoid hyperventilation; perform slowly.	
Homeopathy	See Table 5-5 through 5-8 for remedies for many skin conditions.	Varies with symptoms, signs.	Symptom-specific for remedies. Educated practitioner is needed.	Boericke, 1999, 2000; Cummings, Ullman, 1997; Skinner, 2001
Amish home remedies	Warts	Topical: Juice from milkweed or dandelion is applied, or raw potato peelings or garlic are		Quillan, 1996

Continued

Table 5-1 Alternative Health Care Systems for Dermatologic Concerns—cont'd

Intervention	Management	Treatment Regimen	Cautions, Precautions, Interactions	References
Amish home remedies, cont'd				
	Itching	rubbed onto wart; or a castor oil-soaked bandage is topically applied. Poultice of cornstarch or witch hazel is applied, or 3 c of cooked oatmeal in a cheesecloth bag is soaked in warm water for 15 min and then rubbed over itchy area.		
	Underarm deodorant	Topical: Vinegar is applied after bathing.		
	Hair rinse	Vinegar is applied.		
	Insect stings	Topical: Vinegar is applied on sting.		

GI, Gastrointestinal; St, stomach; tid, three times a day; TW, triple warmer (also called San Jiao); UB, urinary bladder; SI, small intestine; GV, governing vessel (also called Du Mo).

MIND-BODY-SPIRIT INTERVENTIONS FOR DERMATOLOGIC CONCERNS

Support Groups

Support groups may help people with skin conditions gain confidence and improve self-image. Burr and Gradwell (1996) report on their facility's skin disorders support group and provide an evaluation from the group that had met for 1 year. The group began with initial meetings of 5 to 10 people and, at the end of the year, had 30 to 35 members. Fourteen people completed an opinion survey, and various emotions emerged within the group:

> All respondents felt that the presence of nurses at the meetings provided an essential link between the individuals and the hospital. All respondents felt that doctors should be able to attend, but by invitation only. Seventy-five percent of respondents reported that their confidence had increased and they felt less isolated as a result of attending the support group. One woman felt depressed at the meetings as she had time to confront issues about her condition which she usually put to the back of her mind. One man felt that the sessions were the only times he was able to relax. Ninety-five percent of respondents felt that it was beneficial to share feelings, although one woman felt that the presence of a professional [counselor] was needed. (Burr, Gradwell, 1996, p. 1181)

Autogenics

Ernst (2001) reports on a controlled trial (Ehlers et al, 1995) for atopic eczema showing autogenics superior to an education program and as effective as cognitive behavioral therapy. Section II outlines an autogenic procedure. This type of relaxation may be comforting and stress reducing for those who have skin conditions aggravated by stress.

Hypnosis

Hypnosis has been used in skin conditions with some success. Freeman and Lawlis (2001) report on several studies using hypnosis as wart treatment. The authors state that there tends to be less recurrence with hypnosis than with conventional treatment. Ferreira and Duncan (2002) report a case study of a young man who had numerous therapies for warts; he was finally referred for biofeedback-assisted hypnotherapy and experienced complete remission of 22 warts in less than 12 weeks.

Freeman and Lawlis (2001) also discuss a dramatic case of hypnosis effect on ichthyosis. In addition, they advocate the use of hypnosis with burn pain:

> Even though hypnosis is the most frequently cited nonpharmacologic intervention for burn pain in adults, nearly all published reports of

hypnosis for burn pain are anecdotal with few clinically controlled trials. Case studies often fail to document pain measurement, drug dosages, or treatment failures. Even when the poor quality and low number of studies are considered, the number of favorable outcomes and reports of dramatic benefits would suggest that some burn victims benefit from hypnosis interventions. (Freeman, Lawlis, 2001, p. 244)

In a study of 61 burn patients, who averaged 13.5% of their body burned, hypnosis versus sham hypnosis was employed (Patterson, Ptacek, 1997). Only those treatment patients having the highest baseline level of pain had a difference when compared with those with highest baseline level of pain in the control group. Freeman and Lawlis (2001) speculate that the sham group may have induced a state of self-hypnosis and that having a control group employed may have verified this opinion.

Hypnosis may be useful in patients with chronic skin conditions. Ernst (2001) reports that reasonable evidence from clinical trials exists for the use of hypnosis in a variety of health conditions, including dermatologic conditions, citing a recent review reporting empirical findings on the use of hypnosis in medicine (Pinnell, Covino, 2000).

Other mind-body-spirit interventions include affirmation, imagery, meditation, prayer, relaxation therapy, and biofeedback. Table 5-2 describes a few mind-body-spirit interventions for dermatologic concerns.

BIOLOGIC-BASED THERAPIES FOR DERMATOLOGIC CONCERNS

The reader is instructed to consult one of the many herbal references for complete information on biologics and herbs because the tables are quite abbreviated. A few examples are discussed.

Dietary Modifications

Murray and Pizzorno (1999b) advocate a sound nutritional program for psoriasis and eczema, citing a few studies that documented food being related to psoriasis:

> The evaluation of 316 psoriasis patients with 366 controls, both groups being in the age range 16-65 years, found that psoriasis was positively associated with body mass index and inversely related to intake of carrots, tomatoes, fresh fruits, and the index of beta-carotene intake (Naldi, 1996). Research at a Swedish hospital studying the effects of fasting and vegetarian regimens on chronic inflammatory disease found that such diets helped psoriatic patients (Lithell, 1983). The improvement was probably due to decreased levels of gut-derived toxins and polyamines. Patients have also benefited from gluten-fee and elimination diets. (Murray, Pizzorno, 1999b, p. 1515; Bazex, 1976; Douglass, 1980)

Table 5-2	Mind-Body-Spirit Interventions for Dermatologic Concerns			
Intervention	**Management**	**Treatment Regimen**	**Cautions, Precautions, Interactions**	**References**
Affirmations	Psoriasis, itching, eczema, acne	Psoriasis: "I am alive to the joys of living. I deserve and accept the very best in life. I love and approve of myself" (p. 58). Itching: "I am at peace just where I am. I accept my good, knowing all my needs and desires will be fulfilled" (p. 45). Eczema: "Harmony and peace, love and joy surround me and indwell me. I am safe and secure" (p. 30). Acne: "I am a Divine expression of life. I love and accept myself where I am right now" (p. 10).	Positive, personal, present tense statements	Hay, 2000

Continued

Intervention	Management	Treatment Regimen	Cautions, Precautions, Interactions	References
Hypnosis or biofeedback-assisted hypnosis	Atopic dermatitis Warts	Various numbers of sessions	Experienced hypnotherapist who is knowledgeable of anatomy, physiology of condition for appropriate suggestions.	Stewart, Thomas, 1995 Freeman, Lawlis, 2000; Ferreira, Duncan, 2002
	Burns	Hypnosis: preceding burn treatment	Qualified practitioner is recommended. In study, highest pain level benefited when compared with highest pain level in control group. Others showed no difference between sham hypnosis and hypnosis. Sham was relaxation, however.	Patterson, Ptacek, 1997
	Congenital ichthyosis	Practiced over a period of weeks. Hypnosis in sessions that asked a 16-year-old to clear arms,	Case study recorded; photographs were included.	Mason, 1952

Therapy	Indications	Application	Comments	References
Imagery	Any skin disorder, burns	then legs, then trunk. Dramatic improvement was shown. Variable results, depending on condition. Example: *General Wellness* (1991 audiotape) or individual guided imagery.	Experienced practitioner, who is knowledgeable of the anatomy, physiology of condition, for appropriate suggestions, is recommended. Experienced practitioner with an awareness of the complexity of the burn unit is necessary.	Achterberg, 1985; Naparstek, 1991
Meditation-prayer	Enhances well being and insight; improves self-image and optimism, relieves stress; is a positive form of coping.	Patient wishes are followed. Meditation tapes are available. Use intercessory or personal prayer, as desired.		Bush, 1999; King, 1994; Dunn, Horgas, 1994; Flannelly, Inouye, 2001; Meisenhelder, Chandler, 2000; Shuler et al, 1994
Relaxation-autogenics	Anxiety; atopic eczema	Quiet place is recommended; deep	Therapy takes practice and time.	Ehlers et al, 1995; Ernst, 2001;

Continued

Table 5-2	Mind-Body-Spirit Interventions for Dermatologic Concerns—cont'd			
Intervention	**Management**	**Treatment Regimen**	**Cautions, Precautions, Interactions**	**References**
Relaxation-autogenics, cont'd		breathing is performed; participant relaxes from head to toe. Tapes are available. (See Section II for autogenic information.)		Freeman, Lawlis, 2001.
Biofeedback	Anxiety	Various forms are available—temperature, skin, muscle. Biofeedback can be combined with hypnosis.	An experienced practitioner is recommended to teach technique.	
Stress management; psychologic interventions	Psoriasis	Showed improvement of psoriasis symptoms.	May be costly.	Zachariae et al, 1996
Support groups	Skin disorders (e.g., psoriasis, eczema, rosacea)	Nurse-facilitator role: Organize, delegate group responsibilities; minimize group leader domination (leader may be professional, paraprofessional, or a layperson); Supply	Referral resources need easy access, including crisis support. Some support groups can become negative or reinforce negativity; strategies need to be both realistic yet	Burr, Gradwell, 1996; Kinney et al; 1992

		affirming so that negative behavior and actions are not reinforced.
		information; encourage expression of experiential knowledge and feelings from participants; emphasize individual group member's personal responsibility, control, and active coping; offer resource referrals; plan strategies; develop problem-solving techniques; evaluate the group process and progress.
Resources	Allergic skin disorders; asthma	National Jewish Medical and Research Center, 800-222-LUNG, www.nationaljewish.org
	Psoriasis	National Psoriasis Foundation, 800-723-9166. www.psoriasis.org
	Rosacea	National Rosacea Society, 888-No-Blush (662-5874)
	Eczema	National Eczema Association, 800-818-7546, www.eczema assn.org

Chapter 4 (Gastrointestinal Concerns) discusses allergy and elimination diets and gives information on use.

Zinc

Zinc is a necessary oral nutrient mineral and also has been used for years topically to treat skin conditions. It is necessary for the functioning of more than 300 enzymes and is highly concentrated in the skin, as well as the liver, pancreas, kidneys, bone, muscles, and other tissues (LaValle et al, 2000). Zinc is used for treatment of numerous skin conditions, including acne, aphthous ulcers, oral herpes, diaper rash, eczema, wound healing, and psoriasis. Zinc needs to be in balance with copper.

Tea Tree Oil

Tea tree oil *(Melalueuca alternifolia)* has antibacterial, antiviral, and antifungal conditions and has been used topically for numerous conditions, including acne, tinea pedis, onychomycosis, boils, carbuncles, corns, calluses, impetigo, herpes, psoriasis, ringworm, wound infections, burns, cuts, scrapes, insect bites, lice, and vaginitis. Tea tree oil is also useful for smelly feet (Sierpina, 2001; LaValle et al, 2000; Murray, Pizzorno, 1999b).

An Australian study found significant improvement in acne with either 5% gel of tea tree oil or 5% benzoyl peroxide lotion (Bassett et al, 1990 in Murray, Pizzorno, 1999a, 1999b). The substances were given randomly to 124 patients and were applied two times daily topically.

> After 3 months, both treatments produced a significant improvement in the mean number of both non-inflamed and inflamed lesions, although with non-inflamed lesions benzoyl peroxide was found to be more effective. An important finding was that there were fewer reports of side effects (dryness, [pruritus], stinging, burning, and skin redness) with tea tree oil (44% vs. 79%). (Murray, Pizzorno, 1999b, p. 819)

Sarsaparilla

In a study of sarsaparilla used for psoriasis, 62% improved and 18% cleared the disease (Thurman, 1942). Sarsaparilla binds endotoxins; high endotoxin levels in the circulation are associated with conditions such as liver disease, psoriasis, and fevers, as well as inflammatory processes, and all seem to improve with sarsaparilla (DerMarderosian, 2001; Murray, Pizzorno, 1999a).

> Endotoxins are cell wall constituents of bacteria that are absorbed from the gut. Normally, the liver plays a vital role by filtering these, and other, gut-derived compounds before they reach the general

circulation. If the amount of endotoxin absorbed is excessive or if the liver is not functioning adequately, the liver can become overwhelmed and endotoxins will spill into the blood. If endotoxins are allowed to circulate, activation of the alternate complement system occurs. This system plays a critical role in aggravating inflammatory processes, and activation of complement is responsible for much of the inflammation and cell damage that occurs in many diseases including gout, arthritis, and psoriasis. Historically, these conditions have been treated with sarsaparilla. (Murray, Pizzorno, 1999a, p. 940)

Anecdotal Herbal Use

Jewelweed (*Impatiens L*), or touch-me-not, is a traditional herbal for prevention of poison ivy and for topical irritation caused by poison ivy. Jewelweed is a tender succulent plant.

Plantain is a topical agent for skin problems such as insect bites, poison ivy, dermatitis, ulcers, herpes, boils, and infections. Plantain also has been used as an antiinflammatory. Plantain is a perennial weed with worldwide distribution.

Soapwort is used to make "natural" soaps and shampoos. The plant is commonly seen along roadsides (DerMarderosian, 2001).

Potentially Dangerous Herbs

Coltsfoot (*Tussilago farfara*) is rich in zinc and can be applied topically to relieve skin conditions (Dominick, 1996). However, coltsfoot has possible adverse effects, including elevating blood pressure (pressor effects); the U.S. Food and Drug Administration has classified this herb as of "undefined safety," and Canada has banned its use (DerMarderosian, 2001; Fetrow, Avila, 1999). Similarly, comfrey, also called knitbone, is no longer recommended as a therapy either topically or orally. Comfrey has been shown to be hepatotoxic and is potentially fatal (DerMarderosian, 2001). Comfrey had been used for many years as topical treatment for bruises, burns, and sprains.

Tables 5-3 and 5-4 describe some of the biologic-based therapies used for the treatment of skin conditions, including dietary practices, vitamins, minerals, and herbs. In addition, Tables 5-5 through 5-8 give an overview of natural products to consider for acne, eczema, psoriasis, and rosacea, including homeopathic remedies.

MANIPULATIVE AND BODY-BASED METHODS FOR DERMATOLOGIC CONCERNS

People with skin conditions may be deprived of physical or skin contact and touch, and thus massage to areas not affected by the malady may be helpful. Hand and foot massage is easy and soothing.

Table 5-3 Biologic-Based Therapies for Dermatologic Concerns

A complete prescribing source should be consulted before using biologic therapies. Nutrient doses may be above the recommended daily allowance or tolerable upper limit. In illness or deficiency, such doses may be acceptable; however, long-term use is not suggested.

Intervention	Management	Treatment Regimen	Cautions, Precautions, Interactions	References
Nutrients				
Dietary modifications	Psoriasis, eczema	Keep a diet-symptom diary. Avoid known dietary allergens and irritants for specific condition. Elimination and rotation diets (eliminate certain foods for up to a month to see if symptoms improve. Add only one food at a time back into diet). (See Chapter 4.)	Takes time, patience. Need to read labels.	Murray, Pizzorno, 1999b; Naldi et al, 1996; Lithell et al, 1983; Bazex, 1976; Douglass, 1980
Fish oils, omega-3 fatty acids. EPA and DHA are omega-3 fatty acids found in	Psoriasis, acne, eczema, rosacea	Suggest dietary sources: mackerel, herring, tuna, halibut, salmon, sardines. IV dosing may be more effective than oral	High doses can cause GI upset, loose stools. May alter glucose regulation. Effects of drugs with hypoglycemic activity	Fontaine, 2000; LaValle et al, 2000; PL/PL, 2002

fish oil.		supplementation for psoriasis. Oral doses range from 1 to 4 g/day	may be potentiated. Contraindicated in active bleeding. Can inhibit platelet aggregation. Use caution with anticoagulants. Discontinue 14 days before surgery.	
Flaxseed oil and flaxseed. (Rich source of the omega-3 fatty acid called ALA). Precursor for EPA and DHA. Flaxseed also has omega-6 fatty acids.	Acne, psoriasis, abscesses; deficiency symptoms of omega 3 include skin and hair problems; thus LaValle recommends high omega-3 for acne.	Oral: 1 to 2 tbsp/day of oil or eat ground flaxseeds for acne. Topical: Can make poultice (30-50 g flaxseed flour made into semisolid paste and applied to skin). Traditionally mixed with mustard seed powder when used as poultice, or can make compress with 30-50 g flour and warm water.	Refrigerate oil. Flaxseeds must be taken with plenty of water. Flaxseeds contraindicated in ileus; extreme caution is recommended or flaxseed should not be used in those with dysphagia. Can cause esophageal blockage. May increase bleeding time.	Blumenthal et al, 2000; LaValle et al, 2000; PL/PL, 2002
LA and BB	Eczema, rosacea	LA: 5-10 billion CFU/day BB: 5-10 billion CFU/day	Refrigerate LA and BB. Antibiotics eliminate LA. Refrigerate. Use of antibiotics can cause a	LaValle et al, 2000

Continued

Table 5-3   Biologic-Based Therapies for Dermatologic Concerns—cont'd

Intervention	Management	Treatment Regimen	Cautions, Precautions, Interactions	References
Nutrients—cont'd				
LA and BB, cont'd			greater need for bifidobacteria.	
Betaine hydrochloride (contains hydrochloric acid)	Rosacea	Works as digestive aid; 325-650 mg qd after a protein meal.	Do not use with those with ulcers; high doses cause GI irritation.	LaValle et al, 2000; PL/PL, 2002.
Vitamin A	Acne, eczema, psoriasis, rosacea	Adult RDA: men, 900 μg/day, women 700 μg/day. Pregnancy 750-770 mg/day. Adult UL = 3 mg or 3000 μg.	Fat-soluble vitamin, so toxicity can occur; pregnant women should not take more than 2800-3000 μg/day (UL) 1 μg of vitamin A = 3.33 units of vitamin A.	LaValle et al, 2000; NAP, 2002
Vitamin B complex	Rosacea	B Complex-25 to 50 mg/day	Provides support for a variety of biologic activity and ensures adequate amount of vitamin B.	LaValle et al, 2000
Vitamin B3 niacinamide	Acne	RDA: men, 16 mg/day, women 14 mg/day.	Doses over 2.5 g/day can cause liver damage	LaValle et al, 2000; NAP,

	Acne: 4% niacinamide topical gel. Adult UL = 35 mg niacin. Involved with vitamin B; may be best to take in combination.	and glucose intolerance. Toxicity symptoms: HA, nausea, flushing, tingling, sweating. Estrogen-containing medications, antibiotics, isoniazid cause depletion of niacin.	2002; Shalita, 1995
Vitamin C	Eczema, gingivitis, psoriasis, sunburn, wound healing	RDA: men, 90 mg/day, women, 75 mg/day. Adult UL = 2000 mg. Diarrhea is common side effect.	Doses greater than 1000 mg/day may contribute to kidney stones. Large intake in diabetics can cause falsely elevated blood glucose readings. Vitamin C can cause increased absorption of iron and decreased absorption of copper. Vitamin C regenerates vitamin E back to active antioxidant status. Oral contraceptives, indomethacin, tetracyclines, aspirin &	LaValle et al, 2000; NAP 2002

Continued

Table 5-3	Biologic-Based Therapies for Dermatologic Concerns—cont'd			
Intervention	Management	Treatment Regimen	Cautions, Precautions, Interactions	References
Nutrients—cont'd				
Vitamin C, cont'd			other salicylates can cause depletion of vitamin C	
Vitamin D (also known as calciferol)	Psoriasis	AI: 5-15 μg/day (1 μg calciferol. = 40 IU of vitamin D.) Adult UL = 50 μg.	Fat soluble, potentially toxic. Cholestyramine, anticonvulsants, corticosteroids, isoniazid, rifampin, H2 receptor antagonists, mineral oil can cause depletion of vitamin D. Vitamin D can cause increase in absorption of calcium and phosphorus. Vitamin A antagonizes some of activity of vitamin D.	LaValle et al, 2000; Fontaine, 2000; Morimoto, 1990; NAP, 2002
Vitamin E (as d′ alpha tocopherol)	Acne, dry skin and hair, eczema,	Adult RDA = 15 mg/day. Adult UL: 1000 mg/day.	Fat soluble. Can prolong prothrombin time and	LaValle et al, 2000; NAP,

Nutrient	Uses	Dosage	Comments	Reference
	psoriasis, sunburn, wound healing		cause impairment in hemostasis; stop 1 wk before surgery. Cholestyramine, colestipol, orlistat, and mineral oil interfere with absorption of vitamin E. Iron can bind and inactivate vitamin E. Large doses of vitamin E can interfere with absorption of vitamin A. Vitamin C regenerates vitamin E back to its active antioxidant state.	
Copper (needed in conjunction with zinc)	Acne	RDA: 900 µg/day. UL = 10,000 µg/day (10 mg).	Contraindicated in Wilson's disease. Need proper zinc/copper ratio (< 15:1). Zinc and iron can inhibit absorption of copper (and excess copper can cause depletion of zinc). Large doses of vitamin C can lead to depletion of copper.	LaValle et al, 2000; NAP, 2002

Continued

305

Table 5-3 Biologic-Based Therapies for Dermatologic Concerns—cont'd

Intervention	Management	Treatment Regimen	Cautions, Precautions, Interactions	References
Nutrients—cont'd				
Selenium	Acne	RDA: 55 μg/day. UL = 400 μg	Toxicity can occur with large doses including loss of hair and nails, skin lesions, digestive dysfunction, nervous system abnormalities.	LaValle et al, 2000; NAP, 2002
Zinc	Acne, aphthous ulcers, oral herpes, diaper rash, eczema, wound healing, psoriasis, and other skin conditions	PO: RDA: men, 11 mg/day, women, 8 mg/day. Adult UL: 40 mg. Condition-specific doses will vary (e.g., for acne: 25 mg/day only until clear). Topical: zinc oxide, glycine cream. This formulation allows better absorption than other zinc preparations.	Zinc can be toxic in excess. Need proper zinc/copper ratio because zinc can inhibit copper absorption. Ratio of zinc to copper fed to humans of 2:1, 5:1, and 15:1 had limited effects on copper absorption, thus best to stay in that range. Elevated copper, calcium, iron can cause a depletion of zinc. Also, vegetarians and	PL/PL, 2002; Godfrey et al, 2001; LaValle et al, 2000; NAP, 2002

Other Preparations

		people with diarrhea may need more zinc.	
Baking soda (sodium bicarbonate)	Soothing the itch of poison ivy, contact dermatitis, or minor skin irritation	Make paste with water and apply directly on unbroken irritated skin.	Also can use in bath. Caution: Causes slippery tub.	Anecdotal.
Oatmeal	Sooths irritated skin; decreases itching.	Mix in bath water. Can buy commercial products.	Caution: causes a very slippery tub; is messy.	Anecdotal reports
Tar	Atopic eczema, psoriasis. May reduce need for more potent corticosteroid use.	Topical, inexpensive, works on some persons and not others; is an old remedy.	Stains, smells. Can cause skin dryness or irritation. Do not use on "red hot" (extremely severe or acute) disease.	Boguniewicz, Leung, 2001
Duct tape	Warts (Verruca vulgaris)	Topical duct tape occlusion over wart for maximum of 2 months was more effective than cryotherapy. Duct tape cut close to the size of wart and kept in place 6 days. After 6 days, tape removed, area soaked in water and then wart debrided		Focht et al, 2002.

Continued

Table 5-3 Biologic-Based Therapies for Dermatologic Concerns—cont'd

Intervention	Management	Treatment Regimen	Cautions, Precautions, Interactions	References
Other Preparations—cont'd				
Duct tape, cont'd		with emery board or pumice stone. Tape left off overnight and reapplied the next day. Self-care.	Duct tape can cause allergy.	

AI, Adequate intake; ALA, alpha-linolenic acid; BB, Bifidobacterium bifidum; CFU, colony-forming units; DHA, Docosahexaenoic acid; EPA, eico-sapentaenoic acid; GI, gastrointestinal; HA, headache; hx, history; IU, international units; IV, intravenous; LA, Lactobacillus acidophilus; NAP, National Academies Press; PL/PL, Pharmacist's Letter/Prescriber's Letter; PO, by mouth; RDA, recommended daily allowance; Sx, symptoms; UL, upper limits—the maximum level of daily nutrient that is likely to pose no risk of adverse effects. Includes intake from food, water, and supplements.

Dietary Recommended Intake (DRI) values expand on the RDAs and contain four categories of recommendations (i.e., RDA, AI, UL, EAR [estimated average requirement]). The latest data should be consulted.

Both the AI and the RDA are goals for intakes but are defined differently.

RDA is the intake at which risk of inadequacy is very small (2% to 3%); RDA is expected to meet the nutrient needs of 97% to 98% of the individuals in a life stage and gender group.

AI is the observed average or experimentally set intake by a defined population or subgroup that appears to sustain a defined nutritional status, such as growth rate, normal circulating nutrient values, or other functional indicators of health. AI is used if sufficient scientific evidence is not available to derive an EAR. AI IS NOT RDA.

EAR is the intake that meets the estimated nutrient needs of one half of the individuals in a group.

(References from the Food & Nutrition Board National Academy of Sciences Institute of Medicine, www.nap.edu.)

Table 5-4 Biologic-Based Therapies for Dermatologic Concerns—Herbs

A complete prescribing source should be consulted before using biologic therapies. Herbs may cause allergic reactions and interactions. Herbs are generally contraindicated or not recommended for women who are pregnant or lactating and for children unless research data or a long history of safe use has been established.

Intervention	Management	Treatment Regimen	Cautions, Precautions, Interactions	References
Aloe vera gel (Aloe africana, arborescens, perryi, spicata)	Sunburn, minor burns, wounds, frostbite, chronic leg ulcers, acne, seborrhea, psoriasis	Topical gel (from 98% to 100% strength). Use 3 to 5 times a day.	Skin burning. Adverse reaction if contaminated with anthraquinones and taken orally (strong cathartic).	DerMarderosian, 2001; Fontaine, 2000; Murray, Pizzorno 1999a; PL/PL, 2002; Sierpina, 2001
Arnica flower (Arnica Montana or chamissonis)	Acne, boils, bruises, rashes, sprains, wounds	Topical use only. Do not apply to open skin. Arnica is anti-inflammatory, analgesic.	Prolonged use may cause allergies. FDA has classified drug as unsafe; is poisonous. However, German Commission E has approved use of arnica flower.	Blumenthal et al, 2000; DerMarderosian, 2001; Fetrow, Avila, 1999; Fontaine, 2000; PL/PL, 2002
Calendula (Calendula officinalis)	Inflammation of oral and pharyngeal mucosa; poorly	Gargle with tea made of 1 to 2 g of dried flowers in 150 ml boiling water	Allergy. Is in ragweed, marigold, mum, daisy family. No known	Blumenthal et al, 2000; PL/PL, 2002

Continued

309

Table 5-4 Biologic-Based Therapies for Dermatologic Concerns—Herbs—cont'd

Intervention	Management	Treatment Regimen	Cautions, Precautions, Interactions	References
Calendula, cont'd	healing wounds (e.g., leg ulcers, bruises, boils, rashes)	for 5-10 min. Pour tea over cloth and apply as poultice. Infusions and tinctures; topical ointment for wounds; contains 2 to 5 g of herb in 100 g ointment.	contraindications or interactions.	
Chasteberry (*Vitex agnus*)	Acne	Dosing depends on formulation.	May affect hormone levels; not to be used if patient has cancer or fibroids.	LaValle et al, 2000; PL/PL, 2002
Coleus (*Coleus forskolin*)	Eczema, psoriasis	No dose given for skin problems. Inhibits histamine release from mast cells.	May cause hypotension and alter platelet aggregation. Numerous theoretical interactions. Discontinue 14 days before surgical procedures.	LaValle et al, 2000; PL/PL, 2002
German chamomile flower	Eczema, skin cracks, bruises, frostbite,	Tea for mouth rinse or gargle: 3 g of dried	Allergy. Highly concentrated tea can	Blumenthal et al, 2000;

Herb	Indications	Preparation/Dosage	Precautions	References
(Matricaria, recutita)	insect bites, irritations and infections of mouth and gums, hemorrhoids. Mucositis induced by radiation or chemotherapy	flower heads in 150 ml of boiling water for 5-10 min. Strain. External: bath additive 50 g per 2.5 gal. Poultice: semisolid paste or plaster. 3%-10% ointments and gels.	cause vomiting. Some drug interactions. Topical: may be as good or better than hydrocortisone cream. Avoid topical use near eyes.	Ernst, 2001; PL/PL, 2002
Echinacea (Echinacea purpurea)	Inflammatory skin conditions, poorly healing wounds, chronic ulcerations	External preparation: semisolid with at least 15% pressed juice; also ointments of at least 15% pressed juice in base of petrolatum jelly or anhydrous lanolin and vegetable oil.	Do not take longer than 8 wks. Oral has several drug interactions. Not recommended for HIV+, TB, MS or immuno-compromised individuals.	Blumenthal et al 2000; PL/PL, 2002; WHO, 1999
Evening primrose (Oenothera biennis)	Eczema, psoriasis, rosacea	Standardized to contain 8%-9% gamma-linolenic acid and at least 72% linoleic acid per dose. Oral use.	Contraindicated in those with active bleeding, seizure disorders, schizophrenia, or those receiving antipsychotic or antiseizure medications. Discontinue 2 wks before dental surgery. Potential interaction	LaValle et al, 2000

Continued

Table 5-4 Biologic-Based Therapies for Dermatologic Concerns—Herbs—cont'd

Intervention	Management	Treatment Regimen	Cautions, Precautions, Interactions	References
Evening primrose, cont'd			with NSAIDS, anticoagulants.	
Flaxseed (Linum usitatissimum)	Abscesses, ulcers	Topical: Semisolid paste with 30-50 g flaxseed flour for moist heat application	No contraindications for external use.	Blumenthal et al, 2000
Gotu kola (Centella asiatica)	Psoriasis; postsurgical and trauma wounds, fistulas, gynecologic perineal lesions, burns, ulcerations; varicosities and venous insufficiency; prevention of keloid and scars; shingles; hemorrhoids. May stabilize connective tissue growth in scleroderma	Topical: 0.2%-0.4% bid to tid to wound areas; tinctures and creams; oral for venous insufficiency	May cause burning, contact dermatitis. May be abortifacient. May be sedating orally.	LaValle, et al, 2000; PL/PL, 2002; Murray, Pizzorno, 1999c

312

Grapefruit seed extract (Citrus paradisi)	Mild skin irritations, eczema, rosacea	Antifungal, antibacterial, antiparasitic preparation. Topical and internal as oral drops and oral rinse.	Numerous theoretical drug interactions, especially if extract acts similar to grapefruit juice.	LaValle et al, 2000; PL/PL, 2002
Lemon balm (Melissa officinalis)	Herpes labialis (cold sores)	Topically apply cream or ointment containing 1% of a 70:1 lyophilized aqueous extract 2-4/day at first symptoms; or apply a saturated cotton ball of the tea made with 2-3 g of cut leaf in 150 ml boiling water boiled for 5-10 min.	May cause contact dermatitis.	LaValle et al, 2000; PL/PL, 2002
Mayapple (podophyllum)	Warts, condyloma, plantar warts	Topical: resin (potent poison)	Systemic toxicity even with topical applications except for fruit. Entire mayapple is toxic.	DerMarderosian, 2001; Fetrow, Avila, 1999
Milk thistle (Silybum marianum)	Eczema, rosacea, psoriasis	Oral: Liver protectant. Concentrated extract recommended 70%-80% silymarin per dose.	Mild laxative; Commission E approves use as liver protectant and for digestive disorders.	Blumenthal et al, 2000; LaValle et al, 2000; PL/PL, 2002
Myrrh (Commiphora molmol)	Mild inflammation of oral and	Topical: Mouthwashes, rinses, and paints.	Dermatitis	Blumenthal et al, 2000;

Continued

Table 5-4 Biologic-Based Therapies for Dermatologic Concerns—Herbs—cont'd

Intervention	Management	Treatment Regimen	Cautions, Precautions, Interactions	References
Myrrh, cont'd	pharyngeal mucosa (gingivitis, ulcers, stomatitis); minor skin inflammation	Tincture, resin applied in various dilutions.		DerMarderosian, 2001; PL/PL, 2002
Oak bark (Quercus robur, petraea, alba)	Inflammatory skin diseases; contact dermatitis, eczema, hemorrhoids, nail fissures, small burns, gargle for pharyngitis-tonsillitis, laryngitis, bleeding gums	Topical: bath (5 g/1 L water). Bathe only affected area. Tinctures: compresses, gargles—boil 20 g drug per 1 L water for 10-15 min; use strained.	Hepatotoxicity with internal use. Avoid use over extensive areas of open skin.	Blumenthal et al 2000; Fetrow, Avila, 1999
Oat straw (Avena sativa)	Inflammatory and dry, itching skin conditions	Topical baths; 100 g cut herb to one full bath qd to bid	Contact dermatitis	Blumenthal et al, 2000; DerMarderosian, 2001; Fetrow, Avila, 1999
Olive leaf (Olea europaea)	Herpes, acne, eczema		Insufficient evidence for use other than	LaValle et al, 2000;

314

	Antiviral, antibacterial, antifungal. Oral: Tea.		lowering blood pressure (PL/PL). Possible hypoglycemic effects. Do not use with individuals with gallstones.	PL/PL, 2002
Plantain (*Plantago lanceolata and major*)	Burns, wounds, poison ivy, inflammatory reactions of skin	Topical: cold macerate for rinse, gargle, or cataplasm. Soak 1.4 g cut herb in 150 ml cold water for 1-2 hrs, stirring often. Apply to affected area.	Dermatitis, is quite allergenic.	Blumenthal et al, 2000; DerMarderosian, 2001; Fetrow, Avila, 1999
Sarsaparilla (*Smilax* varieties)	Psoriasis, eczema, pruritus, rashes, wound care, leprosy	Oral: dried root: 1-4 g or by decoction tid. Liquid extract and solid extract also.	Unsafe when used in excessive amounts (including kidney impairment). Occupational asthma reported once from sarsaparilla root dust.	DerMarderosian, 2001; Fetrow, Avila, 1999; Murray, Pizzorno, 1999a; Thurman, 1942; PL/PL, 2002
Tea tree oil (*Melaleuca alternifolia*)	Antibacterial, antiviral and antifungal. Topically for acne, tinea pedis,	Topical concentrations from 0.4%-100%. Acne: 5%-15% solution (possibly more effective with inflamed lesions) for	Contact dermatitis. Keep in amber-colored bottle because light can affect potency. Use a dropper and separate bottle for	Bassett et al, 1990; Carson et al 1995,1998; Fetrow, Avila 1999; LaValle

Continued

Intervention	Management	Treatment Regimen	Cautions, Precautions, Interactions	References
Tea tree oil, cont'd	onychomycosis, boils, carbuncles, corns, calluses, impetigo, herpes, psoriasis, ringworm, wound infections, burns, cuts, scrapes, insect bites, lice, vaginitis. Also for smelly feet.	3 mos. Tinea pedis: 8% to 10% tea tree oil, cream or 40% solution. Onychomycosis: 100% tea tree oil for 6 mos.	application to avoid contamination. Do not ingest.	et al 2000; Sierpina, 2001; Murray, Pizzorno, 1999a, 1999b; Tong et al 1992; PL/PL, 2002
Walnut leaf (*Juglans regia*)	Excessive perspiration of the hands and feet; scalp itching, dandruff, herpes, eczema, slow healing wounds, sunburn; mild superficial inflammation of skin	Topical: compresses and partial baths; 2-3 g cut leaf per 100 ml cold water; simmer 15 min after boiling.	Avoid occlusive dressings and application to large areas.	Blumenthal et al, 2000

Herb	Uses	Dosage/Preparation	Comments/Precautions	References
Witch hazel (*Hamamelis virginiana*)	Anal and vaginal itching, hemorrhoids, varicose veins, swelling, inflammation of gums or mouth, bruises, sprains, eczema	Topical: hemorrhoid pads, compresses, ointment, gel; as gargle; salve, tincture. For compresses and irrigations, simmer 5 to 10 g leaf and bark per 250 ml water. For poultice, use witch hazel water undiluted or diluted 1:3 with water. Also are semisolid preparations and suppositories.	Contact dermatitis, excess internal use not recommended—tannins can cause hepatic damage	Blumenthal et al, 2000; DerMarderosian, 2001; Fetrow, Avila, 1999; PL/PL, 2002
Yarrow (*Achillea millefolium*)	Slow-healing wounds (stops wound bleeding); eczema	Sitz bath: 100 g of yarrow (above ground parts) per 5 gal warm or hot water. Wrap upper body in towels. Soak 10-20 min.	Contact dermatitis is common with use; uterine stimulant.	Blumenthal et al, 2000; DerMarderosian, 2001; Fetrow, Avila, 1999; PL/PL, 2002

bid, Twice a day; FDA, U.S. Food and Drug Administration; HIV, human immunodeficiency virus; MS, multiple sclerosis; NSAIDs, nonsteroidal antiinflammatory drugs; PL/PL, Pharmacist's Letter/Prescriber's Letter; qd, daily; TB, tuberculosis; tid, three times a day.

Table 5-5	Acne Vulgaris	
Category	**Natural Products to Consider**	**Documentation**
Herb	Chasteberry, vitex	HD
	Tea tree (topical)	HD
	Olive leaf	PA
Vitamin, mineral, trace element, nutraceutical	Vitamin A, condition-specific dose: 5000-10,000 IU/day	HD
	Zinc, condition-specific dose: 25 mg/day until clear WITH copper, condition-specific dose: 2 mg/day until clear	HT
	Vitamin B3 (niacinamide), condition-specific dose: 4% topical (if available)	HT
Homeopathic remedy	Homeopathic combination formulas are available for many conditions. Following list includes some of the most common single homeopathic remedies for acne vulgaris.	
	Baptista tinctoria	PD
	Hepar sulphuris calcareum	PD
	Kall bromatum	PD
	Pulsatilla	PD
	Sulphur	PD
Additional supplements	Fish oils, condition-specific dose: 750 mg 2-3 times/day OR Flaxseed oil, condition-specific dose: 1 tbsp/day	HD
	Selenium, condition-specific dose: 200 µg/day.	HD

Continued

Table 5-5	Acne Vulgaris—cont'd	
Category	**Natural Products to Consider**	**Documentation**
	WITH Vitamin E, condition-specific dose 200-400 IU/day	

HD, *Human data*—*case reports and anecdotal evidence reported in the literature but not as scientifically sound as human trials;* HE, *historic evidence*—*traditional uses of particular natural product for some conditions have been reported, as well as other reports of clinical experience;* HT, *human trials*—*published data, structured studies (e.g., double-blind, placebo-controlled, and randomized clinical trials) that support a relationship between natural product and specific condition of use;* IU, *international units;* PA, *pharmacologic activity*—*potential benefit may be observed for specific condition based on proposed pharmacologic activity of natural product;* PD, *proving data*—*information exists to support value of using specific homeopathic remedy for particular condition.*
From LaValle J et al: Natural therapeutics pocket guide, Hudson, Ohio, 2000, LexiComp.

After the feet or hands are washed, the patient can rest in a comfortable position while a massage therapist, a reflexologist, a trained family member, or a trained health care provider gives the massage. Some people do not like having their hands or feet rubbed, so, if feasible, a head and scalp massage also can be provided as an alternative.

The essential oil lavender can be diluted in a carrier oil and used for numerous skin conditions including burns, acne, mild eczema, insect bites, psoriasis, and ringworm (Buckle, 2001). The oil has shown *in vitro* activity against some bacteria. Buckle, a nurse and internationally known aromatherapist, recommends two to five drops of lavender in 5 ml of aloe vera gel to produce a 2% to 5% solution. Essential oils must be pure.

Field (2000) studied parental massage that was done in a proscribed manner for children with atopic dermatitis. Parents applied any prescribed topical medications with the massage. The control group continued with standard medical care but did not receive massage. The study surveyed 20 children with atopic dermatitis who were stratified to group randomly by the severity of their atopy. The massage group showed significant focal improvement in redness, lichenification, excoriation, and pruritus by the last day of treatment. The central group had improvement in scaling only. Dermatologists who were blinded as to the children's group assignment performed the

Table 5-6	Eczema	
Category	*Natural Products to Consider*	*Documentation*
Herb	Milk thistle	PA, HE
	Evening primrose	PA
	Grapefruit seed extract	PA
	Olive leaf	PA
	Artichoke	PA
Vitamin, mineral, trace element, nutraceutical	*Lactobacillus acidophilus* and *Bifidobacterium bifidum*, condition-specific dosage: 10-15 billion CFU twice daily (dairy free) for 2 weeks, then 1-2 billion CFU twice daily	HD
	Fish oils, condition-specific dose: 750 mg 2-3 times/day	HT
	Vitamin A, condition-specific dose: 10,000-35,000 IU/day	PA
	Vitamin C, condition-specific dose: 250-1000 mg/day	HT
Homeopathic remedy	Homeopathic combination formulas are available for many conditions. Following list includes some of the most common single homeopathic remedies for eczema.	
	Calcarea carbonica	PD
	Cantharis	PD
	Croton tiglium	PD
	Graphites	PD
	Mezereum	PD
	Sulphur	PD
Additional supplements	Selenium, condition-specific dose: 200 μg/day	HD
	Vitamin E, condition-specific dose: 200-400 IU/day	PA

Continued

Table 5-6	Eczema—cont'd	
Category	**Natural Products to Consider**	**Documentation**
	Zinc, condition-specific dose: 15-35 mg/day	HD

CFU, *Colony-forming units;* HD, *human data—case reports and anecdotal evidence reported in the literature but not as scientifically sound as human trials;* HE, *historic evidence—traditional uses of a particular natural product for some conditions have been reported, as well as other reports of clinical experience;* HT, *human trials—published data, structured studies (e.g., double-blind, placebo-controlled, randomized clinical trials) that support a relationship between the natural product and a specific condition of use;* IU, *international units;* PA, pharmacologic activity—potential benefit may be observed for specific condition based on the proposed pharmacologic activity of natural product;* PD, *proving data—information exists to support value of using specific homeopathic remedy for particular condition.*
From LaValle J et al: *Natural therapeutics pocket guide,* Hudson, Ohio, 2000, LexiComp.

dermatologic assessment. In addition, parents' anxiety decreased in the massage group, and the parents' evaluation of the child's coping showed improvement. The child's activity level and affect also improved.

Pressure sores are another area of concern. Many homebound or bedridden individuals get skin breakdown. Massage for these individuals is mandatory:

> Patients who lie quietly in bed due to paralysis or weakness should receive a good massage to areas where pressure is apt to cause decubitus ulcers. Combined with frequent changes of position and proper resting positions, massage can help prevent the formation of decubitus ulcers. Deep strokes that bring blood to the area should be applied each time the patient is moved...Effleurage and [pétrissage] may be applied with depth. Stroking *toward* the pressure areas will encourage capillary dilation. Friction can also be applied around the pressure area. (Tappan, 1988, p. 112)

ENERGY THERAPIES FOR DERMATOLOGIC CONCERNS
Wound Healing
Finch (1997) reported that noncontact therapeutic touch (NCTT) hastened wound healing in two studies (Wirth, 1990; Wirth et al, 1993) and did not have an effect in three other studies (Wirth et al

Table 5-7 Psoriasis

Category	Natural Products to Consider	Documentation
Herb	Coleus	PA
	Milk thistle	PA, HE
	Gotu kola	HD
	Evening primrose	PA
Vitamin, mineral, trace element, nutraceutical	Zinc, condition-specific dose: 50 mg plus 2 mg of copper daily (note this is a high zinc to copper ratio)	HT
	Fish oils, condition-specific dose: 750 mg 2-3 times/day	HT
	Flaxseed oil, condition-specific dose: 1 tbsp/day	PA
Homeopathic remedy	Homeopathic combination formulas are available for many conditions. Following list includes some of the most common single homeopathic remedies for psoriasis.	
	Arsenicum album	PD
	Graphites	PD
	Sulphur	PD
Additional supplements	Vitamin A, condition-specific dose: 10,000 IU/day	PA
	Vitamin C, condition-specific dose: 1000 mg/day	PA
	Vitamin E, condition-specific dose: 800 IU/day	PA

HD, Human data—case reports and anecdotal evidence reported in the literature but not as scientifically sound as human trials; HE, historic evidence—traditional uses of a particular natural product for some conditions have been reported, as well as other reports of clinical experience; HT, human trials—published data, structured studies (e.g., double-blind, placebo-controlled, randomized clinical trials) that support a relationship between natural product and specific condition of use; IU, international units; PA, pharmacologic activity—potential benefit may be observed for specific condition based on proposed pharmacologic activity of the natural product; PD, proving data—information exists to support value of using specific homeopathic remedy for particular condition.

From LaValle J et al: Natural therapeutics pocket guide, Hudson, Ohio, 2000, LexiComp.

Table 5-8	Rosacea	
Category	**Natural Products to Consider**	**Documentation**
Herb	Cat's claw	PA
	Chasteberry, vitex	PA
	Milk thistle	PA
	Grapefruit seed extract	PA
	Evening primrose	PA
Vitamin, mineral, trace element, nutraceutical	*Lactobacillus acidophilus* and *Bifidobacterium bifidum*, condition-specific dose: 10-15 billion CFU twice daily for 2 wks, then 1-2 billion CFU twice daily (dairy free)	PA
	Betaine hydrochloride, condition-specific dose: 325-650 mg with meals three times/day as needed	PA
	Vitamin A, condition-specific dose: 10,000 IU/day	PA
	Fish oils, condition-specific dose: 1000 mg twice daily	PA
Homeopathic remedy	Homeopathic combination formulas are available for many conditions. Following list includes some of the most common single homeopathic remedies for rosacea.	
	Atropa belladonna	PD
	Lachesis mutus	PD
	Sanguinaria canadensis	PD
	Sepia	PD
	Thuja occidentalis	PD
Additional supplements	Vitamin B complex-25, condition-specific dose: 25-50 mg twice daily	PA

CFU, *Colony-forming units;* HD: *Human data—case reports and anecdotal evidence reported in the literature but not as scientifically sound as human trials;* HE, *historic evidence—traditional uses of a particular natural product for some conditions have been reported, as well as other reports of clinical experience;* HT, *human trials—published data, structured studies (e.g., double-blind, placebo-controlled, randomized clinical trials) that support relationship between*

natural product and specific condition of use; PA, pharmacologic activity—
potential benefit may be observed for specific condition based on proposed
pharmacologic activity of natural product; PD: proving data—information
exists to support value of using specific homeopathic remedy for particular
condition.
From LaValle J et al: Natural therapeutics pocket guide, *Hudson, Ohio,*
2000, LexiComp.

1994; Wirth, Barrett, 1994; Wirth et al, 1996). However, the latter three studies contained confounding variables: in one study, the healing was done by trainee healers; in the second study, all participants were aware of the reasons for the study and were familiar with previous wound-healing experiments; and in the third study, the healer was in "ill health" having "influenza-like symptoms." "These persisted throughout the experiment and 81% of the treatment group exhibited similar symptoms despite there having been no physical contact between the practitioner and the subjects" (Finch, 1997, pp. 502-503). Thus drawing conclusions from the studies is difficult.

The use of microcurrent electrical therapy (MET) to promote wound healing and to promote lymphatic drainage has support in the research literature (Barron, Jacobson, 1986; Carey, Wainapel, 1985; Lulndeberg et al, 1992; Mercola, Kirsch, 1995). After several days of MET, contaminated wounds tend to become sterile and heal faster. MET was shown to be a catalyst in wound healing by increasing the generation of adenosine triphosphate (ATP), as well as enhancing amino acid transport and protein synthesis (Cheng et al, 1982).

Burns

Turner and colleagues (1998) report a study comparing therapeutic touch (TT) with sham TT on 99 severely burned patients. A significant decrease in pain, anxiety, and CD8+ lymphocytes for the TT group was reported. No decreased analgesic was used.

When people have skin conditions, they face physical, mental, emotional, and spiritual challenges because of the visibility of many disorders. NAC therapies can help relieve some of the discomfort and suffering. When the HCP has knowledge of all types of therapy, more options may be provided. Table 5-9 gives an overview of manipulative and body-based methods and energy therapies for dermatologic concerns.

Table 5-9 Manipulative and Body-Based Methods and Energy Therapies for Dermatologic Concerns

Intervention	Management	Treatment Regimen	Cautions, Precautions, Interactions	References
Massage	To provide general relaxation and touch for person with skin disorders	Massage over skin that does *not* exhibit rash or abnormal area (i.e., foot or hand massage if a person has acne or rosacea). Person with skin condition may be sensory deprived.	No massage over areas of skin disorder, acne, eczema, psoriasis, or rosacea. See Section II for more discussion of massage techniques.	Beck, 1994
	Atopic dermatitis; improves focal area, redness, lichenification, excoriation, pruritus. Decreases anxiety in parents and children	Daily 20-min massage. (Parents in the research study were trained and followed a written description and videotape.) Performed with emollient with medication.	Pediatric population massage by parents. Both treatment and control children's groups continued with routine care, and medications.	Field, 2000
	Treatment for pressure sore areas	Massage with effleurage, pétrissage to areas of pressure.	Avoid massage over open areas.	Tappan, 1988
Hand and foot reflexology	Appropriate form of massage when	Use lotion for hand and foot massage	Wash patients feet and hands before massage	

Continued

Table 5-9 Manipulative and Body-Based Methods and Energy Therapies for Dermatologic Concerns—cont'd

Intervention	Management	Treatment Regimen	Cautions, Precautions, Interactions	References
Hand and foot reflexology, cont'd	not able to touch a skin abnormality		or reflexology. Some people do not like their hands or feet massaged. Do not massage if open lesions or fungal infection exists. Use gloves if needed.	
Hand and foot massage	Good for those who cannot or do not want other areas of body touched	Use cream or lotion on hands and feet. Nonscented, nonallergenic preparation.	Wash feet and hands before massage. Same instruction as above.	
Aromatherapy massage	Burns, acne, mild eczema, insect bites, psoriasis, ringworm; pruritis in patients undergoing hemodialysis	2-5 drops of lavender in 5 ml of aloe vera gel to produce a 2% to 5% solution. Significant decrease in pruritis with 7-min massage on upper arm and palm (arm	Use may cause allergy. Oil must be pure essential oil. Pure oils are quite expensive.	Buckle, 2001; Ro, 2002

Heliotherapy (sunshine)	Psoriasis	without fistula). Lavender and tea tree oil were used. Sweet almond and jojoba were the carrier oils. Diluted to 5%. 4 wks of supervised heliotherapy versus no intervention showed significant improvement and decreased use of treatment in year after heliotherapy.	Avoid overexposure to sunshine. Risk of skin cancer.	Snellman et al, 1993; Cooper, 1999 (discusses UVB and PUVA therapies and risks)
TT	Decreases pain and anxiety in burn patient.	Recommended time for TT is 15-20 min. daily; experienced practitioner is recommended.	Obtain participant's permission. Time for treatment in this study was 5-20 min.	Turner et al, 1998
TT	Accelerates wound healing	5 min. daily treatments; experienced practitioner is recommended	Obtain permission. Trained practitioner is recommended; TT practitioners in study had 5 or more years experience.	Wirth, 1990, 1993, 1994, 1996

Continued

Table 5-9   Manipulative and Body-Based Methods and Energy Therapies for Dermatologic Concerns—cont'd

Intervention	Management	Treatment Regimen	Cautions, Precautions, Interactions	References
MET	Promotes wound healing	Treatment varies with individual.	Used with caution. Do not use for patient with pacemaker (resuscitation may be required).	Barron et al, 1986; Carey et al, 1985; Cheng et al, 1982; Lulndeberg et al, 1992; Mercola, Kirsch, 1995

MET, *microcurrent electrical therapy*; TT, *therapeutic touch*.

REFERENCES

Achterberg J: *Imagery in healing: Shamanism and modern medicine*, Boston, 1985, New Science Library.

Barron J, Jacobson W: Treatment of decubitus ulcers: a new approach, *Minn Med* 68:103, 1986.

Bassett IB et al: A comparative study of tea-tree oil versus benzoyl peroxide in the treatment of acne, *Med J Aust* 153:455, 1990.

Bazex A: Diet without gluten and psoriasis, *Ann Derm Symp* 103:648, 1976.

Beck M: *Milady's theory and practice of therapeutic massage*, ed 2, Albany, New York, 1994, Milady/Delmar.

Blumenthal M, Goldberg A, Brinckmann J: *Herbal medicine: expanded Commission E monographs*, Newton, Mass, 2000, Integrative Medicine Communications.

Boericke W: *New manual of homoeopathic materia medica and repertory*, ed 2, New Delhi, 2000, Jain.

Boericke W: *Pocket manual of homoeopathic materia medica and repertory*, New Delhi, 1999, Jain.

Boguniewicz M, Leung D: Allergic disorders. In Hay W et al, eds: *Current pediatric diagnosis and treatment*, New York, 2001, McGraw-Hill.

Buckle J: The role of aromatherapy in nursing care. In Colbath J, Prawlucki P, editors: *Nurs Clin North Am* 36(1):57, 2001.

Burr S, Gradwell C: The psychosocial effects of skin diseases: need for support groups, *Br J Nurs* 5(19):1177, 1996.

Bush E et al: Religious coping with chronic pain, *Appl Psychophysiol Biofeedback* 24(4):249, 1999.

Carey P, Wainapel S: Electrotherapy for acceleration of wound healing: low intensity direct current, *Arch Physical Med Rehab* 66:443, 1985.

Carson CF et al: Susceptibility of methicillin-resistant *Staphyloxxus aureus* to the essential oil *Melaleuca alternifolia*, *J Antimicrob Chemother* 35:421, 1995.

Carson CF, Riley TV, Cookson BD: Efficacy and safety of tea tree oil as a topical antimicrobial agent, *J Hosp Infect* 40(3):175, 1998.

Cheng N et al: The effects of electric currents on ATP generation, protein synthesis and membrane transport in rat skin, *Clin Orthoped* 171:264, 1982.

Cooper K et al: Psoriasis: New clues to causation, new ways to treat, *Patient Care* May 18, 1999, p. 154.

Cummings S, Ullman D: *Everybody's guide to homeopathic medicines*, New York, 1997, Tarcher/Putnam.

DerMarderosian A: *The review of natural products*, St Louis, 2001, Facts and Comparisons.

Dominick AW: Coltsfoot, *Herbal Q* 69:37, 1996.

Douglass JM: Psoriasis and diet, *Calif Med* 133:450, 1980.

Dunn K, Horgas A: The prevalence of prayer as a spiritual self-care modality in elders, *J Holist Nurs* 18(4):337, 2000.

Ehlers A, Stangier U, Gieler U: Treatment of atopic dermatitis: a comparison of psychological and dermatological approaches to relapse prevention, *J Consult Clin Psychol* 63:624, 1995.

Ernst E: *The desktop guide to complementary and alternative medicine*, St Louis, 2001, Mosby.

Ferreira J, Duncan B: Biofeedback-assisted hypnotherapy for warts in an adult with developmental disabilities, *Alt Ther Health Med* 8(3):142, 2002.

Fetrow C, Avila J: *Complementary and alternative medicines*, Springhouse, Penn, 1999, Springhouse.

Field T: *Touch therapy*, Philadelphia, 2000, Saunders.

Finch B: Therapeutic touch and wound healing, *J Wound Care* 6(10):501, 1997.

Flannelly L, Inouye J: Relationships of religion, health status, and socioeconomic status to the quality of life of individuals who are HIV positive, *Issues Ment Health Nurs* 22(3):253, 2001.

Focht D, Spicer C, Fairchok M: The efficacy of duct tape vs cryotherapy in the treatment of verruca vulgaris (the common wart), *Arch Pediatr Adolesc Med* 156:971, 2002.

Fontaine K: *Healing practices: alternative therapies for nursing*, Upper Saddle River, NJ, 2000, Prentice Hall.

Freeman LW, Lawlis GF: *Mosby's complementary and alternative medicine*, St Louis, 2001, Mosby.

Gach M: *Acupressure's potent points*, New York, 1990, Bantam.

Godfrey H et al: A randomized clinical trial on the treatment of oral herpes with topical zinc oxide/glycine, *Alt Ther Health Med* 7(3):49, 2001.

Hackman R, Stern J, Gershwin M: Complementary/alternative therapies in general medicine: asthma and allergies. In Spencer J, Jacobs J, editors: *Complementary/alternative medicine: an evidence-based approach*, St Louis, 1999, Mosby.

Hay L: *Heal your body*, Carlsbad, Calif, 2000, Hay House.

King D et al: Beliefs and attitudes of hospital inpatients about faith, healing and prayer, *J Fam Pract* 39:349, 1994.

Kinney C, Mannetter R, Carpenter M: Support groups. In Bulechek G, McCloskey J, eds: *Nursing interventions*, ed 2, Philadelphia, 1992, Saunders.

Lad V: *Ayurveda: the science of self-healing*, Wilmot, Wisc, 1985, Lotus.

LaValle J et al: *Natural therapeutics pocket guide*, Hudson, Ohio, 2000, LexiComp.

Lithell H et al: A fasting and vegetarian diet treatment trial on chronic inflammatory disorders, *Acta Derm Vener* (Stockholm) 63:397, 1983.

Liu J: Treatment of adolescent acne with acupuncture, *J Tradit Chin Med* 13(3):187, 1993.

Lulndeberg T, Eriksson S, Malm M: Electrical nerve stimulation improves healing of diabetic ulcers, *Ann Plastic Surg* 29(4):328, 1992.

Mason AA: A case of congenital ichthyosiform erythrodermia of Brocq treated by hypnosis, *BMJ* 23:422, 1952.

Meisenhelder J, Chandler E: Prayer and health outcomes in church members, *Alt Ther Health Med* 6:56, 2000.

Mercola J, Kirsch D: The basis for microcurrent electrical therapy (MET) in conventional medical practice, *J Adv Med* 8(2):107, 1995.

Mishra L, Singh B, Dagenais S: Healthcare and disease management in Ayurveda, *Alt Ther Health Med* 7(2):44, 2001.

Morimoto S et al: Inverse relation between severity of psoriasis and serum 1,25-dihydroxy-vitamin D level, *J Dermatol Sci* 1(4):277, 1990.

Murray M, Pizzorno J: Aloe vera and *Melaleuca alternifolia* (tea tree). In Pizzorno J, Murray M, eds: *Textbook of natural medicine*, vol 1, Edinburgh, 1999a, Churchill Livingstone.

Murray M, Pizzorno J: Acne and psoriasis. In Pizzorno J, Murray M, editors: *Textbook of natural medicine*, vol 1, Edinburgh, 1999b, Churchill Livingstone.

Murray M, Pizzorno J: Centella asiatica (gotu kala). In Pizzorno J, Murray M, editors: *Textbook of natural medicine*, vol 1, Edinburgh, 1999c, Churchill Livingstone.

Naldi L et al: Dietary factors and the risk of psoriasis: results of an Italian case-controlled study, *Br J Dermatol* 134:101, 1996.

Naparstek B: *General wellness* [audiotape], Akron, Ohio, 1991, Image Paths.

National Academies Press (NAP) element references. Vitamin references, www.nap.edu, 2002. Accessed Jan., 2003.

Patterson D, Ptacek J: Baseline pain as a moderator of hypnotic analgesia for burn injury treatment, J Consult Clin Psychol 65(1): 60, 1997.

Pharmacist's Letter/Prescriber's Letter [PL/PL]: Natural medicines comprehensive database, Stockton, Calif, 2002, Therapeutic Research Faculty.

Pinnell CM, Covino NA: Empirical findings on the use of hypnosis in medicine: a critical review, Int J Clin Exp Hypn 48:170, 2000.

Quillan P: Amish folk medicine, Canton, Ohio, 1996, Leader.

Ramsay B, O'Reagan M: A survey of the social and psychological effects of psoriasis, Br J Dermatol 118:195, 1988.

Ro Y et al: The effects of aromatherapy on pruritis in patients undergoing hemodialysis, Dermatol Nurs 14(4):231, 2002.

Shalita AR et al: Topical nicotinamide compared with clindamycin gel in the treatment of inflammatory acne vulgaris, Int J Dermatol 34(6):434, 1995.

Sheehan MP, Ahterton DJ: One-year follow-up of children treated with Chinese medicinal herbs for atopic eczema, Br J Dermatol 130:488, 1994.

Sheehan MP, Ahterton DJ: A controlled trial of traditional Chinese medicinal plants in widespread nonexudative atopic eczema, Br J Dermatol 126:179, 1992.

Shuler P et al: The effects of spiritual/religious practices on psychological well-being among inner city homeless women, NP Forum 5:106, 1994.

Sierpina V: Top twenty herbs for primary care. In Micozzi M, editor: Fundamentals of complementary and alternative medicine, Edinburgh, 2001, Churchill Livingstone.

Skinner S: An introduction to homeopathic medicine in primary care, Gaithersburg, Md, 2001, Aspen.

Snellman E et al: Supervised four-week heliotherapy alleviates the long-term course of psoriasis, Acta Derm Venereol 73:388, 1993.

Spencer J, Jacobs J: Complementary/alternative medicine, St Louis, 1999, Mosby.

Stewart A, Thomas S: Hypnotherapy as a treatment for atopic dermatitis in children and adults, Br J Dermatol 132(5):778, 1995.

Tappan F: Healing massage techniques, ed 2, Norwalk, Conn, 1988, Appleton and Lange.

Thurman FM: The treatment of psoriasis with sarsaparilla compound, N Engl J Med 227:128, 1942.

Tong MM, Altman PM, Barnetson RS: Tea tree oil in the treatment of tinea pedis, Australas J Dermatol 33:145, 1992.

Turner J et al: The effect of therapeutic touch on pain and anxiety in burn patients, J Adv Nurs 28(1):10, 1998.

Wirth D: The effect of noncontact therapeutic touch (TT) on the healing rate of full thickness dermal wounds, Subtle Energies 1(1):1, 1990.

Wirth D, Barrett M, Eidelman W: Non-contact TT and wound epitheliazation: An extension of previous research, Compl Ther Med 2:187, 1994(a).

Wirth D, Barrett: Complementary healing therapies, Int J Psychosomatics 41:1, 1994(b).

Wirth D et al: Non-contact TT intervention and full thickness wounds: A replication, Compl Ther Med 4:237, 1996.

Wirth D et al: Full thickness dermal wounds treated with noncontact TT: A replication and extension, Comp Ther Med 1:127, 1993.

Xu Y: Treatment of acne with ear acupuncture—a clinical observation of 80 cases, J Trad Chin Med 9(4):238, 1989.

Zachariae R et al: Effects of psychologic intervention on psoriasis: a preliminary report, J Am Acad Dermatol 34:1008, 1996.

CHAPTER 6

CARDIOVASCULAR CONCERNS

Pamela Shuler ▪ Roxana Huebscher ▪ Helen Miller ▪ Louise Rauckhorst

NAC THERAPIES FOR HEART HEALTH

The first section of this chapter deals with natural-alternative-complementary (NAC) modalities for heart health, meaning promotion and preventive measures for hearts that are healthy, measures to heal sick hearts and select some NAC treatments for heart failure and coronary disease. Clinicians need to focus on preventing heart disease in patients and to work with those who have been diagnosed with coronary heart disease (CHD) in an effort to reestablish a healthy heart. The goal of therapy is either to prevent development of CHD or to reverse the process of atherosclerosis. The second section of the chapter deals with NAC therapies for hypertension and stroke. Many of the cardiovascular NAC therapies have little research base.

Most Americans are at risk for cardiovascular disease; over 60 million Americans have some form of cardiovascular disease; almost 13 million have CHD, and close to 50 million are hypertensive. Over 10 million Americans are diabetic, and over 100 million have elevated cholesterol levels. Furthermore, close to 50 million adult Americans smoke cigarettes, over 25% do not participate in physical activity on a regular basis, and over 100 million are overweight or obese (American Heart Association [AHA], 2002; National Heart, Lung and Blood Institute [NHLBI], 2001). Thus all appropriate therapies, NAC and conventional, should be used to keep hearts healthy and work with cardiovascular concerns.

Coronary Heart Disease

CHD refers to atherosclerosis of the epicardial coronary arteries (Fauci et al, 1998). Certain lifestyle risk factors such as cigarette smoking, physical inactivity, and obesity can contribute to the untoward effects of CHD (AHA, 2001). CHD is the single leading cause of death in the United States and is present in many individuals who are unaware that they even have a heart problem, because atherosclerosis, the underlying cause of CHD, may not present itself in the form of angina pectoris. The first sign of a heart problem may be a cardiac arrest (sudden death) or a myocardial infarction (MI). Patients may be more likely to have chest pain if they have coexiting health problems, including hypertension, elevated cholesterol levels, and diabetes mellitus, because these conditions can intensify the progression of CHD (AHA, 2001; Ornish, 1990a,b). However, some individuals have "silent" MIs. In addition, patients with metabolic syndrome have an increased risk for the development of, or progression of, CHD (NHLBI, 2001). Metabolic syndrome refers to "a constellation of major risk factors, life-habit risk factors and emerging risk factors related to CHD. Factors characteristic of the metabolic syndrome are abdominal obesity, atherogenic dyslipidemia (elevated triglyceride, small LDL [low-density lipoprotein] particles, and low HDL [high-density lipoprotein] cholesterol), elevated blood pressure, insulin resistance (with or without glucose intolerance) and prothrombotic and proinflammatory states," (NHLBI, 2001 pp. 5-6). Therefore the NHLBI report (2001) stresses the importance of assessing all patients with this syndrome for CHD and establishing a treatment plan that not only targets reduction of LDL cholesterol levels, but also targets reduction of the identified "metabolic syndrome" factors.

Heart Failure

Heart failure is a condition that results from a myocardial function abnormality. This condition "results in the inability of the heart to deliver enough oxygenated blood to meet the metabolic needs of the body. When the right and left ventricles fail as pumps, pulmonary and systemic venous hypertension ensues, resulting in the syndrome of CHF" (Fletcher, Thomas, 2001, p. 249). Congestive heart failure (CHF) may be from systolic or diastolic dysfunction and presents with symptoms that may include dyspnea, orthopnea, edema, fatigue, and decreased exercise tolerance. Diastolic dysfunction refers to an impaired diastolic filling of the left ventricle and loss of muscle elasticity. Systolic dysfunction is:

> characterized by an ejection fraction of less than 40%, is defined as a depression in the contractile force of the myocardium and often results in a thin and dilated heart muscle that is incapable of maintaining an adequate cardiac output. (Fletcher, Thomas, 2001, p. 250)

ALTERNATIVE HEALTH CARE SYSTEMS FOR HEART HEALTH

Ayurveda and Traditional Chinese Medicine have numerous therapies to deal with cardiovascular concerns. Massage, yoga, tai chi, qi gong, and acupuncture are a few possible therapies. Acupuncture may help promote weight loss (Li, 1999); yoga and tai chi can improve overall fitness and improve balance (DiCarlo et al, 1995); meditation can help decrease stress, and massage can promote relaxation and increase circulation (Mishra et al, 2001). Table 6-1 lists a few alternative health care system modalities for heart health.

Table 6-1 Alternative Health Care Systems for Heart Health

Intervention	Management	Treatment Regimen	Cautions, Precautions, Interactions	References
Ayurveda				
Ayurvedic massage	MI, ischemic heart disease, functional heart disease, cold hands and feet caused by bad circulation, varicose veins	Trained practitioner is recommended	Do not use with fever, indigestion, or with patients undergoing *panchkarma* (cleansing processes)	Mishra et al, 2001
TM	Relieves stress	Daily practice recommended	Can decrease health care costs in general in those who meditate	Sharma, 2000; Telles, 1995
Yoga	Reduces stress; loosens chronically tense muscles; improves relaxation, promotes general fitness	Varies with individuals; daily practice is encouraged	Need instructor to ensure correct movements; avoid learning from videotapes; often combined with meditation and prayer and with breathing, relaxation techniques	DiCarlo et al, 1995; Ornish 1990a; Sharma 2000

Traditional Chinese Medicine

Acupuncture	May help increase weight loss, may help lower cholesterol and BP levels	Result varies with individual	Must select practitioner familiar with treatment of obesity; most effective in lowering BP and cholesterol levels when combined with diet therapy	Li , 1999
Qi gong	Builds muscle strength, improves balance, relieves stress, improves depression	Sancier study showed that after 1 yr of Qi gong, older patients in "heart energy deficient" group had increased cardiac output and decreased peripheral resistance	Daily practice is recommended; need instructor to ensure correct movements	Horstman, 1999; Luskin, 1998; Sancier, 1996
Tai chi	May result in positive cardiovascular changes and respiratory benefit; builds muscle strength, improves balance, relieves stress, improves mood	Daily practice recommended; promotes relaxed breathing and mental attention; low-impact exercise is encouraged	Need instructor to ensure correct movements	Brown et al, 1989; Jin, 1992; Lai J et al, 1993; Luskin, 1998; Wolf, et al, 1996; Wolfson et al, 1996; Zhuo, 1984

BP, *Blood pressure*; MI, *myocardial infarction*; TM, *transcendental meditation*.

MIND-BODY-SPIRIT INTERVENTIONS FOR HEART HEALTH

Ornish and colleagues (1990a, 1990b, 1991, 1993) demonstrated that lifestyle changes can reverse the progression of atherosclerotic plaques in the coronary arteries. In their study, the researchers used a low-fat vegetarian diet, smoking cessation, stress-management training, and moderate exercise:

> The intervention began with a week-long residential retreat at a hotel to teach the lifestyle intervention to the experimental-group patients. Patients then attended regular group support meetings (4 [hours] twice a week)...The stress management techniques included stretching exercises, breathing techniques, meditation, progressive relaxation, and imagery. (Ornish et al, 1990b, p. 130)

Results showed a reversal of coronary artery stenosis with these many strategies. The conclusion was that "comprehensive lifestyle changes may be able to bring about regression of even severe coronary atherosclerosis after only 1 year, without use of lipid-lowering drugs" (Ornish et al, 1990b, p. 129).

Stress relief measures were abundant in the study, including the social support and time given to the patients. Social support may be especially important (Gliksman et al, 1995; Williams et al, 1992). Other personal stress measures that can be used for heart health, and that do not require a health care provider, include yoga (Ornish, 1990a,b), personal prayer (Shuler et al, 1994), hobbies, creative and expressive arts, listening to music, journaling, pet therapy, and numerous relaxation techniques (Jacobs et al, 1986). Guided imagery (Naparstek, 1997; Wynd, 1992) can help with smoking cessation. See Chapter 2 and Chapter 12 for more mind-body-spirit information. Chapter 2 gives points on assertiveness, affirmations, thought stopping, and attitude and personality characteristics of healthy individuals.

Regular exercise can aid weight loss and help in heart failure (AHA, 2001; NHLBI, 2001; Ornish, 1990a,b; Puffer, 2001). A study of patients with heart failure, using a low-intensity program with light-step aerobics and the exercise bicycle three times a week (starting with 20 minutes and working up to 50 minutes by the end of a 12-week program) was successful in increasing peak flow, exercise tolerance, and workload (Sturm et al, 1999). The patients all had cardiomyopathy with ejection fractions of approximately 18%. No adverse outcomes were reported. Casual walking or low-intensity pool exercises are also choices for initial exercise routines (Fletcher, Thomas, 2001).

Another example for heart failure therapy is biofeedback and relaxation. In one study, 40 patients from a cardiac step-down unit who had advanced heart failure were assigned to one skin-temperature biofeedback intervention or to routine care. In addition to biofeedback, the intervention group had imagery of hand warmth and modified progressive muscle relaxation. The control group had the same measurements taken but no intervention. The intervention group was able to raise their skin temperature in finger and foot, increase cardiac output, and decrease systemic vascular resistance and respiratory rate. No changes in oxygen consumption or catecholamine levels were seen, and no changes in the control group occurred (Moser et al, 1997). Table 6-2 presents a selection of mind-body-spirit therapies for heart health.

BIOLOGIC-BASED THERAPIES FOR HEART HEALTH

Diet modifications and the use of nutritional supplements such as carnitine, lecithin, psyllium, magnesium, vitamin B complex, and zinc may promote weight loss (Abdel-Aziz et al, 1984; AHA, 2001; Balch, Balch et al, 2000; Eades, Eades, 1996; Feskens, Kromhout, 1993; Lininger et al, 1999; McDougall et al, 1995; NHLBI, 2001; Northrup, 1998; Onofrj et al, 1995; Ornish, 1998). Diet, vitamins, and minerals play an important role in heart health. For example, magnesium deficiency can cause metabolic changes that may contribute to heart attacks and strokes (Altura, Altura, 1995; Caspi et al, 1995; Ravn et al, 1996). Some evidence suggests that low body stores of magnesium increase the risk of abnormal heart rhythms (Institute of Medicine, 1999), which may increase the risk of complications associated with a heart attack. Population surveys have associated higher blood levels of magnesium with lower risk of CHD (Ford, 1999; Liao et al, 1998; Gartside, Glueck, 1995). Further studies are needed to understand the complex relationships among dietary magnesium intake, indicators of magnesium status, and heart disease (ods@nih.gov, 2001).

Similarly, herbs have been used for cardiovascular problems. For example, hawthorn, also called hawthorn berry or maybush, has been used for angina, heart failure, tachycardia, hypertension, arteriosclerosis, and Buerger's disease (Fetrow, Avila, 1999; La Valle et al, 2000; Pharmacist's Letter/Prescriber's Letter [PL/PL], 2001, 2002). Hawthorn:

> may be therapeutically useful in the treatment of New York Heart Association (NYHA) functional class II (mild to moderate) heart failure. Patients with NYHA functional class II heart failure receiving a daily dose of 600 mg of hawthorn extract showed significant clinical improvement over an 8-week period. (Schmidt et al, 1994) Hawthorn, either alone or with coenzyme Q-120, was found to be beneficial and favors comparably to captopril in patients with heart failure (Tauchert et al, 1994; Fetrow, Avila, 1999, p. 325).

Table 6-2 Mind-Body-Spirit Interventions for Heart Health

Intervention	Management	Treatment Regimen	Cautions, Precautions, Interactions	References
ACE factors	People who are tuned in to their mind-body signals of discomfort, pain, fatigue, distress, sadness, anger, and pleasure psychologically cope better and have a better immune profile and healthier cardiovascular system	Inform people; teach ACE concepts; enhance with biofeedback, guided imagery, meditation; refer for counseling as needed	People who need to develop ACE factors are repressors; communication that this (repressing) is not a sickness but a talent; helps maintain emotional stability; this repressing coping mechanism may not be needed; can learn new ways of coping; can be compared with a heavy coat in the summertime; participant can take repressing off until needed	Dreher, 1995; Schwartz, 1983; (See Chapter 2 for more information.)
Affirmations	Heart problems	"Joy. Joy. Joy. I lovingly allow joy to flow through my mind and body and experience" (p. 39)		Hay, 2000

Treatment	Effects	Comments	Notes	References
Biofeedback	Increases cardiac output, decreases systemic vascular resistance, decreases response rate, increases finger and foot skin temperature in those with advanced heart failure (ejection fraction mean 21% to 22%)	Biofeedback and relaxation combination; subjects in study were hospitalized and had one session of treatment	N = 40; need biofeedback practitioner	Dracup et al, 1993; Good, 1998; Moser et al, 1997
Exercise	Improves exercise tolerance and lowers extremity Sx with peripheral vascular disease.	Limited walking, 3-4 times/wk and progress to daily exercise		Powers et al, 1999
	Improves HF in those with cardiomyopathy (initial ejection fractions were approximately 18%). Increases VO_2,	Low-intensity exercise program for those with CHF under supervision; patient preference is recommended	Need supervision, start slowly; activity depends on functional class of disease; N = 29 in Sturm study.	Fletcher, Thomas, 2001; Sturm et al, 1999

Continued

Table 6-2 Mind-Body-Spirit Interventions for Heart Health—cont'd

Intervention	Management	Treatment Regimen	Cautions, Precautions, Interactions	References
Exercise, cont'd	exercise tolerance and workload Reduces BP, promotes weight loss, improves cardiovascular functioning, reduces risk for CAD	30 min 2 times/wk initially, increase to 45 min 5 times/week Long-term goal: 30 min daily	Sustained physical activity important for cardiovascular conditioning and weight management; start exercising slowly, gradually increase intensity; important to develop positive attitude about physical activity and incorporate it into lifestyle	AHA, 2001; Lininger et al, 1999; NHLBI, 2001; Ornish, 1990a,b; Puffer, 2001
Forgiveness	Decreases anger (poor anger management may be predictor of heart disease); trait anger decreases,	Brief forgiveness training recommended; referral is necessary	HCP needs referral sources	Luskin, 1998

participant becomes more willing to forgive, increases hope and self-efficacy toward emotional management

Modality	Benefits	Notes	Precautions	References
Guided imagery and visualization (with or without music)	Helps improve mood, relieve depression and fatigue, decrease cortisol levels; promote abstinence from cigarettes in ex-smokers, may help with smoking cessation; promotes healing; strengthens immune system	Therapy varies with individual; audiotapes and CDs are recommended or individual tapes can be made; audiotapes: *A Meditation to Help You Stop Smoking* (1997); *Healthy Heart and Cholesterol* (1999); *Stress I and II* (1995); *Weight Loss* (1997)	No driving or operating machinery while listening to tapes; often combined with meditation, prayer, relaxation techniques, or yoga for maximal benefit	McKinney et al, 1997; Naparstek, 1994 and audiotapes; Ornish, 1990a,b; Samuels et al, 1988; Wynd, 1992
Hypnosis	Helps reduce obesity and stress; assists smoking cessation, decreases heart rate and BP; controls vasodilation,	Several sessions may be needed; most effective as part of multidimensional approach	Need experienced practitioner familiar with physiology of concern	Luskin, 1998

Continued

Table 6-2 Mind-Body-Spirit Interventions for Heart Health—cont'd

Intervention	Management	Treatment Regimen	Cautions, Precautions, Interactions	References
Hypnosis, cont'd	peripheral blood flow, cardiac arrhythmias; reduces pain and anxiety during surgery			
Meditation	Helps lower BP, decrease premature heartbeats, reduce cholesterol levels, control anger	Therapy varies with individual	Often combined with prayer, relaxation techniques, visualization or yoga for maximal benefit	Benson, 1977; Ornish 1990a,b
Music	Reduces heart rate after MI, postoperative; decreases BP after MI; diminishes myocardial oxygen demand; can "entrain" the heart rate to rhythm	Patient preference is recommended	Prepare individual and environment; unpleasant memories may be associated with some music, so participant's input important	Bason, 1972; Haas, 1986; Luskin, 1998; White, 2001
Pet therapy	Increases survival after MI, buffers	Ownership or visitation	Pet responsibility; allergy can be a concern	Huebscher, 2000;

Continued

	physiologic responses, helps relieve stress, promotes family cohesion			Jennings, 1997
Personal and intercessory prayer; spirituality	Reduces pain; promotes emotional, physical, and spiritual healing; reduces stress, depressive symptoms, alcohol and drug use, perceived worries; controls anger	Therapy varies with individual	HCPs are not expected to serve the role of spiritual advisor to participants; however, HCPs can encourage participants to explore potential benefits that prayer may have on their physical and mental well being	Ai, 2002; Bush, 1999; Byrd 1988; Dunn, 2000; King, 1994; Luskin, 1998; Meisenhelder, 2000; Ornish, 1990a,b; Shuler et al, 1994; Wirth et al, 1994
Relaxation techniques	Help strengthen immune response; reduce stress; improve flexibility; reduce blood pressure; control anger; enhance well being	Therapy varies with individual	Some relaxation techniques use various yoga techniques; often combined with meditation, prayer, visualization, or yoga for maximal benefit	Jacobs et al, 1986; Kiecolt-Glaser et al, 1984; Ornish, 1990a,b

Table 6-2 Mind-Body-Spirit Interventions for Heart Health—cont'd

Intervention	Management	Treatment Regimen	Cautions, Precautions, Interactions	References
Religious practices, church attendance	Participant may be less likely to smoke; has positive effect on morbidity and mortality; increased social support	Personal preference is recommended		Luskin, 1998
Smoking cessation	Reduces cardiovascular risk	Various NAC therapies; hand hobby; finger foods, behavioral strategies; self-massage, guided imagery; audiotapes: *A Meditation to Help You Stop Smoking* (1997); herbs and vitamins in cardiac tables	Book resource: *No If's, And's or Butts, the Smoker's Guide to Quitting* (Krumholz, Phillips, 1993, Avery Publishing; individuals exposed to second-hand smoke may regularly need herbs and supplements	Balch et al, 2000; Ornish, 1990a,b; Naparstek, 1997; Spiegel, 1993; Wynd, 1992
Social support	Influences cardiovascular risk factors, improves quality of life	Social support is assessed; refer as needed. "Hook" people up with possible positive social networks and resources	Amassing a database is time-consuming many family and cultural factors are involved	Friedman, 1995; Gliksman, 1995; Luskin, 1998, Ornish,

			1990a,b; Uchino, 1996; Williams, 1992
Weight reduction	Helps lower cholesterol and triglyceride levels; lowers BP and risk for CAD	Diet, exercise, and behavior modification are "gold standard" of treatment	Selection of diet is individual and partially depends on ID; a nutritionally sound diet that is low in saturated fat and high in carbohydrates that have a low glycemic index and contains large amounts of fiber (e.g., beans, most vegetables, fruits) is recommended; If ID is present, a diet low in fat and carbohydrates and high in protein is appropriate	AHA, 2001; Aronne, 2001; Northrup, 1998

ACE, *Attend, connect, and express;* AHA, American Heart Association; BP, *blood pressure;* CAD, *coronary artery disease;* CDs, *compact discs;* CHF, *coronary heart failure;* HCP, *health care practitioner;* HF, *heart failure;* ID, *insulin dependence;* NAC, *natural-alternative-complementary;* NHLBI, *National Heart, Lung and Blood Institute;* Sx, *symptoms;* VO₂, *volume of O₂.*

With respect to smoking cessation, the supplements coenzyme Q10, grape seed extract, vitamin B complex, vitamin E, vitamin C, vitamin A, and zinc may provide support for some patients who are striving to overcome addiction to cigarettes (Anderson, 2001, Balch, Balch, 2000; Frei, 1991; Levine et al, 1996; Lininger et al, 1999; Rimm et al, 1993; Stampfer et al, 1993; Stephens et al, 1996; Weber et al, 1994).

Serum cholesterol and triglyceride levels may be reduced by nutritional supplements, including carnitine (Abdel-Aziz et al, 1984), chromium (Riales, Albrink, 1981; Wang et al, 1989), evening primrose oil (Reichert, 1995), and lecithin (Lininger et al, 1999). Several foods have cholesterol-lowering properties. Among these foods are flaxseed, which is high in the essential fatty acid alpha-linolenic acid. Lignins, a form of fiber, are also good for lowering cholesterol. Garlic (Neil et al, 1996; Silagy, Neil, 1994; LaValle et al 2000; Lau, 2001; Sierpina 2001; Stevinson et al, 2000; Yeh, 2001), walnuts (Zambon et al, 2000), artichoke (Kirchhoff et al, 1994; LaValle et al, 2000) and fish oil (PL/PL 2002) may also lower cholesterol.

Help with lowering blood sugar may be possible following NAC supplements, biotin (Coggeshall et al, 1985), coenzyme Q10 (Gaby, 1996; Shigeta et al, 1966), chromium (Riales, Albrink, 1981), and magnesium (Lininger et al, 1999).

Table 6-3 lists some biologic-based therapies for heart health. Table 6-4 lists cardioactive herbs of which providers need to be aware; especially if patients are using them with cardioactive conventional medications (LaValle et al, 2000). Table 6-5 lists anticoagulant herbs with bioactive constituents (LaValle et al, 2000). The practitioner must obtain a thorough knowledge of conventional therapies being used by the patient if heart problems have been diagnosed to ensure safe introduction of NAC regimens.

MANIPULATIVE AND BODY-BASED METHODS AND ENERGY THERAPIES FOR HEART HEALTH

Self-massage of the hand or ear can help with smoking cessation, and general massage can provide stress reduction and improve circulation (DePaoli, 1995; Hernandez-Reif et al, 1999). Similarly, Therapeutic Touch, healing touch, or Reiki may provide general relaxation and relief from anxiety (Krieger, 1993; Mentgen, 2001). (Table 6-6.)

NAC THERAPIES FOR HYPERTENSION AND STROKE PREVENTION AND TREATMENT

Hypertension

The Joint National Committee on Prevention, Detection, Evaluation, and Treatment of High Blood Pressure (JNC VI, 1997) defines hypertension as systolic blood pressure of 140 mm Hg or greater,

Table 6-3 Biologic-Based Therapies for Heart Health

A complete prescribing source should be consulted before using biologic therapies. Nutrient doses may be above the recommended daily allowance or tolerable upper limit. In illness or deficiency, such doses may be acceptable; however, long-term use may not be appropriate.

Intervention	Management	Treatment Regimen	Cautions, Precautions, Interactions	References
Dietary				
Diet modification	May lower cholesterol levels; lowers BP and triglycerides	Eliminate transfatty acids (hydrogenated fat); reduce saturated fat, cholesterol, and total fat intake; reduce simple sugars; reduce alcohol intake; increase plant foods, soluble fiber, and fish consumption	Must adhere to strict elimination or reduction of products in diet to fully benefit; may want to eliminate one food type at a time	AHA, 2001; Feskens et al, 1993; NHLBI, 2001; Ornish, 1990a,b
	Reduces ischemic vascular disease	Increase fruits and vegetables		Barton, 2001
High-protein diet	For those with hyperinsulinemia and insulin resistance; may promote weight loss, reduce	Establish daily adherence to diet; increase fluids	Should check patient's serum insulin level in a fasting state; if reading is > 10 mU/ml (milli-units/milliliter),	Eades et al, 1996; Northrup, 1998

Continued

Table 6-3 Biologic-Based Therapies for Heart Health—cont'd

Intervention	Management	Treatment Regimen	Cautions, Precautions, Interactions	References
High-protein diet, cont'd	serum cholesterol, triglycerides, blood sugar, and BP		hyperinsulinemia *is* present; diet is most effective when combined with exercise program	McDougall et al, 1995; Ornish, 1990a,b
Low-fat, complex carbohydrate diet (vegan optional)	For patients *without* hyperinsulinemia and insulin resistance, may lower serum cholesterol and BP	Establish daily adherence to diet	Check patient's serum insulin level in a fasting state; if reading is < 10 mU/ml, hyperinsulinemia is *not* present; most effective when combined with exercise	
Mediterranean diet	Improves vascular and cardiovascular health	High number of fruit, vegetables, unprocessed foods, monounsaturated fats (olive oil); meat is viewed as a condiment		Powers et al, 1999; Katsouyanni et al, 1991
Vegan diet	May prevent heart disease or may benefit heart health	Vegan diet is total vegetarian with no dairy products	Ensure adequate nutrient, vitamin, mineral intake	Ornish, 1990a,b

Flavonoids (polyphenolic antioxidants that occur in fruits (e.g., apples) vegetables, onion, tea, red wine; quercetin is a flavonoid	Average flavonoid intake is inversely related to CHD mortality (Hertog); flavonoid and quercetin intake were highly correlated in the study, with quercetin representing 39%-100% of total flavonoid intake	Increase consumption of foods highest in flavonoid: onion, kale, French bean, broccoli, endive, celery, cranberry, as well as lettuce, tomato, red pepper, broad bean, strawberry, apple, grape, red wine, tea tomato juice	Barton, 2001; Hertog et al, 1995
Flaxseed (alpha linolenic acid) and other omega-3 essential fatty acids	Helps lower LDL	Seeds or oil; oil must be refrigerated	Haggerty, 1999; Cunnane et al, 1995; Birenbaum et al, 1993; PL/PL, 1999
		Is a bulk laxative. Seeds should be ground and must be taken with adequate fluid intake.	
Oat bran and other soluble fiber	Reduces LDL and triglyceride levels	Begin slowly; drink plenty of fluids when increasing fiber	PL/PL, 1999
		Can cause obstruction; because oat bran has gluten, can cause a reaction in those with gluten allergy	

Continued

Table 6-3 Biologic-Based Therapies for Heart Health—cont'd

Intervention	Management	Treatment Regimen	Cautions, Precautions, Interactions	References
Psyllium	Lowers cholesterol, LDL, and triglyceride levels; can aid in weight loss	1-2 tsp powdered seeds in large glass of water or juice daily	Contraindicated in poorly controlled diabetes and swallowing difficulties; must be taken with adequate fluid intake because of risk of esophagus blockage	Blumenthal et al, 1998; Lininger et al, 1999; PL/PL, 1999
Fish oil (rich source of omega 3 fatty acids)	May lower triglycerides and ↑HDL and reduce risk of postmenopausal myocardial infarction.	Anchovies, herring, mackerel, salmon, sardines 1-4 g/day of supplement	GI upset, loose stools, nausea, bad breath. Can inhibit platelet aggregation. Greater than 3g/day may affect immune function. May ↑LDL	Stark, 2000 ; PL/PL, 2002
Soy protein	Lowers total cholesterol and LDL levels; may raise HDL level	25-40 g soy protein/day Use food sources	Must include the isoflavones for best effect	Anderson, 1995; Baum, 1998; Crouse, 1999; Kurowska, 1997

Decrease sugars	May increase risk of heart disease with excess	Decrease sucrose, fructose, lactose	Has been a debate over the relationship between heart risk and sugars	Grant, 1998
Vitamins				
Vitamin B complex (including folic acid, B6, B12)	May lower risk of CAD, peripheral occlusive disease; stroke. Reduces high homocysteine levels that are related to heart and peripheral arterial occlusive disease; deficiency in B vitamins may contribute to binge eating in women	B complex 50 mg daily; folic acid at least 400 µg daily	The B vitamins work together in the body and should always be taken together; a deficiency in one often indicates a deficiency in another; do not take more than 100 mg of B6 daily, because neuropathies can occur	Balch et al, 2000; Northrup, 1998; Robinson et al, 1998; Selhub et al, 1993; Stamfer et al, 1992
Nicotinic acid	Decreases cholesterol, LDL, and triglyceride levels	1.5-3.0 g daily; take 325 mg ASA or 200 mg ibuprofen 30 min before to avoid flushing; this is also a conventional treatment. Begin treatment	GI distress; take with food; hepatotoxicity—check liver function; may increase uric acid; avoid in those with gout; more likely to	PL/PL, 1999, 2002

Continued

Table 6-3 Biologic-Based Therapies for Heart Health—cont'd

Intervention	Management	Treatment Regimen	Cautions, Precautions, Interactions	References
Nicotinic acid, cont'd		slowly and titrate up. Niacin RDA is 14-16 mg/day. Adult UL 35 mg/day.	flush if also using nicotine patch	
Vitamin C	Has antioxidant effect; may reduce risk of mortality from cardiovascular disease	Adult RDA 75-90 mg/day; smokers need an additional 35 mg/day; dietary sources best; for slowing progression of atherosclerosis slow release 250 mg in combination with 136 IU of vitamin E has been given. Others may supplement approximately 500-1000 mg daily. Adult UL 2000 mg/day	Can cause diarrhea; can increase absorption of iron—use with caution for patients with hemochromatosis or hemosiderosis; avoid using more than 200 mg daily if patient has history of kidney stones	Frei, 1991; Levine et al, 1996; PL/PL, 2002
Vitamin E (15 mg of vitamin E from food = 22 IU of RRR-alpha)	Dietary intake may possibly decrease risk of heart disease and cardiovascular	Food sources: wheat germ, almonds, safflower oil, corn and soybean oil, turnip greens, mango,	Use of vitamin E supplementation for preventing heart diseases controversial;	Barton, 2001; PL/PL, 1999, 2002; Rimm et al, 1993;

tocopherol (natural) or 33 IU of synthetic vitamin E	events; use as supplement is controversial	peanuts; adult RDA 15 mg/day; supplement recommendation varies: 200-800 IU daily; use the RRR-alpha tocopherol ("natural"), which may have better biologic activity. Adult UL: 1000 mg/day.	FDA will not allow labeling claims for prevention of heart disease; vitamin E interferes with production of clotting factors dependent on vitamin K; can interact with warfarin and increase bleeding; has drug interactions	Stampfer et al, 1993; Stephens et al, 1996; PL/PL, 2002
Minerals Calcium	May help lower cholesterol levels and BP	Adult AI: 1200 mg daily; used in combination with low-fat diet, 400 mg tid of calcium carbonate reduced LDL and increased HDL. Adult UL 2500 mg/day.	Use 800 mg of CCM if patient has history of calcium oxalate kidney stones; CCM is best absorbed; however, calcium carbonate can be used (if no history of kidney stones exists) if desire to swallow fewer pills; avoid using bone meal, dolomite, or	Bell et al, 1992; Burros, 1997; Miller et al, 1988; Osborne et al, 1996; Pak, 1987; PL/PL, 2002; Sheikh et al, 1987

Continued

Table 6-3 Biologic-Based Therapies for Heart Health—cont'd

Intervention	Management	Treatment Regimen	Cautions, Precautions, Interactions	References
Calcium, cont'd			oyster shell, because high levels of lead may be present	
Chromium	Stabilizes metabolism of glucose; may lower cholesterol levels; improves insulin resistance; may increase HDL level in those taking beta-blocker medication; chromium deficiency may contribute to binge eating in women	200-600 µg daily; adult AI: 20-35 µg/day Adult UL not determined.	Vitamin C can increase absorption of chromium; daily dose of chromium higher than 300 µg is not recommended for extended periods, because the risk of toxicity is unclear; oral trivalent form generally well tolerated	Northrup, 1998; Offenbacher, 1994; PL/PL, 2002; Riales et al, 1981; Wang et al, 1989
Magnesium	Improves insulin resistance; may help lower BP; may help decrease cholesterol and LDL	Adult RDA: 310-420 mg/day depending on age; adult UL 350 mg/day; (magnesium UL represents	Separate calcium and magnesium dosing times; diuretics and digoxin are thought to decrease magnesium	Kawano et al, 1998; Lininger et al, 1999; PL/PL, 2000,

	levels. Magnesium deficiency may contribute to binge eating in women	supplementation only and not food and water); 20-130 mg/day elemental magnesium for deficient patients. 200-1000mg/day has been used to decrease BP and serum lipids	levels so check for deficiency if patients on these medications; drug interactions are possible	2001, 2002; Northrup, 1998
Potassium	Helps regulate BP	99 mg daily	Supplementation is not always needed if hypertensive medications are potassium sparing; potential drug interactions	Cappuccio et al, 1991
Selenium	Risk of ischemic heart disease increases with low blood selenium concentrations; Possible cardiac antiarrhythmic agent antioxidant effects	RDA: 55 μg/day. Adult UL 400 μg/day.	Safety and toxicity factors exist; can be toxic with increase of only 4-5 times of what is normally ingested	Badmaev et al, 1996; Barton, 2001; Lehr, 1994; selenium in www.cc.nih.gov, 2003

Continued

Table 6-3 Biologic-Based Therapies for Heart Health—cont'd

Intervention	Management	Treatment Regimen	Cautions, Precautions, Interactions	References
Zinc	Zinc is associated with insulin action; has antioxidant effects; zinc deficiency may contribute to binge eating in women	RDA: 8-11 mg/day. Adult UL 40 mg/day.	Zinc can inhibit copper absorption; can also lead to depletion of iron, calcium, and magnesium, therefore a multimineral supplement should also be taken; potential drug interactions exist	Anderson, 2001; Lininger et al, 1999; Northrup, 1998; PL/PL, 2002
Decrease iron intake	May decrease risk of vascular disease	RDA: 8-18 mg/day. Adult UL 45 mg/day		Kiechl et al, 1997
Other Substances				
CQ10 or ubiquinone, a vitamin-like co-factor found mostly in mitochondria; high levels present in heart	Possibly effective as a treatment for angina, hypertension; reduces toxicity associated with doxorubicin chemotherapy;	90-150 mg/day or 100 mg/day PO divided into 2-3 doses; angina—50 mg tid; hypertension—225 mg/day; cardiotoxicity associated with doxorubicin—50 mg/day	GI upset may occur; CQ 10 levels can increase with biliary-hepatic insufficiency; may have additive effect with hypertensive medications; can reduce anticoagulant	DerMarderosian, 2001 Digiesi et al, 1992; Fetrow, Avila, 1999; Folkers et al, 1982; Fujioka et al, 1983;

and liver; widely used in Japan	likely effective for insomnia related to CHF; decreases dyspnea and other Sx of CHF; provides antioxidant effect for heart and lungs; aids metabolic reactions; modulates immunity and BP; may lower blood sugar level in those with diabetes		effects of warfarin; may take several months to show beneficial effects; take with meals to increase absorption; WARNING: patients taking CQ10 with CHF should not discontinue use abruptly, must be weaned off. See potential drug interactions	Gaby, 1996; Kamikawa et al, 1985; LaValle et al, 2000; Morisco et al, 1993; Mortensen et al, 1985; PL/PL, 2000, 2001; Shigeta et al, 1966; Sinatra, 1997; Weber et al, 1994
Chinese red yeast rice	Lowers lipids similar to commercial statins	Heber study used 2.4 g/day for 12 wks (1200 mg bid per PL/PL). Best if taken with CQ10.	Participants should also follow a 30% fat, < 10% saturated fat and < 300 mg cholesterol diet	Heber et al, 1999; Morelli, Zoorob, 2000; PL/PL, 2002
L-carnitine (Carnitine is synthesized in liver, kidneys, and	May improve exercise tolerance in those with chronic stable	HF and chronic stable angina—1 g bid; after MI—2-6 g/day;	The body produces carnitine, if adequate amounts of iron, niacin,	Abdel-Aziz et al, 1984; Balch et al,

Continued

Table 6-3 Biologic-Based Therapies for Heart Health—cont'd

Intervention	Management	Treatment Regimen	Cautions, Precautions, Interactions	References
L-carnitine, cont'd brain from lysine and methionine)	angina; improves symptoms with HF; aids in fat metabolism and weight loss; helps lower triglyceride and cholesterol levels; may reduce pain associated with peripheral neuropathy; diabetics are at risk for carnitine deficiency	peripheral vascular disease—2 g bid	vitamin B6, vitamin C, and methionine are present. Vegetarians are more likely to be deficient in carnitine because it is not present in vegetable protein; L-carnitine is the best supplement form of carnitine; do not use DL-carnitine because it may cause toxicity	2000; LaValle, 2000; Lininger et al, 1999; PL/PL, 2000, 2002; Onofrj et al, 1995
Lecithin	Is a phospholipid. May help lower cholesterol; aids in weight loss	1.2-2.4 g/day typical dose; 20-30 g/day used in study	Initial use may cause abdominal bloating or diarrhea	Balch et al, 2000; DerMarder-osian, 2001; Lininger et al, 1999; PL/PL, 2002

Inositol nicotinate (composed of six niacin molecules linked to an inositol molecule; inositol is essential component of cell membrane phospholipids)	Is used for intermittent claudication, Raynaud's disease, hyperlipidemia	1500-4000 mg/day in divided 2-4 doses for peripheral vascular disease and increased lipids	Several weeks of treatment may be necessary before seeing results; may increase liver enzymes; has numerous interactions with diseases or conditions, including diabetes, cardiac arrhythmias; contraindicated in peptic ulcer disease and liver-gallbladder disease	O'Hara et al, 1988; Eliopoulos, 1999; PL/PL, 2000, 2002

Herbs

Evening primrose oil (*Oenothera biennis*)	Possibly lowers cholesterol levels; reduces effects of peripheral neuropathy	3-4 g/day	Inadequate vitamin C, magnesium, zinc, and B vitamins can interfere with therapeutic effect; therefore it should be taken with a multivitamin; avoid during pregnancy	Horrobin et al, 1983; PL/PL, 2002

Continued

Table 6-3 Biologic-Based Therapies for Heart Health—cont'd

Intervention	Management	Treatment Regimen	Cautions, Precautions, Interactions	References
Fenugreek (Trigonella foenum-graecum)	Lowers cholesterol levels in rats and dogs possibly because of fiber, saponin, and nicotinic acid	Seeds: 1-2 g seeds PO tid; tea: steep 500-mg seed in 150 ml cold water for 3 hrs and strain; maximum dose is 6 g seed/day	Bleeding, bruising, hypoglycemia can occur with large doses. Possible enhanced effect of anticoagulants and antidiabetic agents; other drug interactions exist; contraindicated in pregnancy	Fetrow, Avila, 1999; PL/PL, 2002
Garlic (Allium sativum)	Lowers LDL and triglyceride levels; prevents excessive platelet adhesion	Chew one whole garlic clove daily or take 300-450 mg bid daily. Most studies have used standardized garlic powder extract containing 1.3% alliin content.	Most effective when combined with a diet low in saturated fats and cholesterol; active ingredient in garlic is allicin; if using garlic supplements, allicin content should be standardized	PL/PL, 2002; Law, 2001; Kiesewetter, 1991
Ginkgo (Ginkgo biloba)	Provides antioxidant activity in the	60-120 mg bid	May affect seizure activity	Blumenthal et al, 1998;

Agent	Action/Uses	Dosage	Comments	References
	cardiovascular system; prevents excessive platelet adhesion; increases walking distance with intermittent claudication		Headache or indigestion can occur with initial use. Numerous drug interactions. Platelet aggregation affected.	Clostre, 1988; Ferrandini et al, 1993; Pittler, Ernst, 2000; PL/PL 2002
Grape seed extract (Vitis vinifera); has procyanidins	Provides antioxidant effects; strengthens capillaries; promotes venous strength and integrity; improves symptoms of chronic venous insufficiency; enhances effects of vitamin C	50-100 mg bid or tid for 3 wks followed by maintenance of 40-80 mg/day; for venous insufficiency, 150-300 mg/day	Research has been done in France and results are published in French	Bergqvist et al, 1981; Dartenuc et al, 1980; Delacroix, 1981; Lininger et al, 1999; PL/PL, 2002; Rehn et al, 1996
Gugulipid (extract of gum guggal)	Reduces serum lipids in up to 70% of patients	Gugulipid 100-500 mg/day	May affect bioavailability of cardiovascular drugs (e.g., propranolol, diltiazem). Can interfere with thyroid function and therapy.	PL/PL, 1999, 2002

Continued

Table 6-3 Biologic-Based Therapies for Heart Health—cont'd

Intervention	Management	Treatment Regimen	Cautions, Precautions, Interactions	References
Hawthorn (Crataegus laevigata)	Is likely effective in increasing cardiac output and exercise tolerance; decreases Sx in mild HF by increasing heart contraction and coronary blood flow and by causing vasodilation; protects blood vessels from damage; improves exercise tolerance for those with angina.	Oral: hawthorn leaf with flower extract, 160-900 mg/day in divided doses bid to tid; or herbal berry extract, berry preparations, or tincture	Hawthorn may take 1-2 mo for maximal effect and should be considered a long-term therapy; SE: nausea, GI complaints, fatigue, sweating, rash on hands, palpitations, headache, dizziness, sleeplessness, agitation, circulatory disturbances. Drug interactions: with antiarrhythmics, cardiac glycosides, (digoxin), CNS depressants, and other cardiovascular drugs.	Brown, 1996; Fetrow, Avila, 1999; Hanack et al, 1983; LaValle et al, 2000; Lianda, 1984; Mavers et al, 1974; PL/PL, 2002; Schmidt, 1994; Tauchert, 1994; PL/PL, 2001; Weikl et al, 1993

ACE, Angiotensin-converting enzyme; AHA, American Heart Association; AI, adequate intake; ASA, acetylsalicylic acid; bid, twice a day; BP, blood pressure; CAD, coronary artery disease; CCM, calcium citrate-malate; CHD, coronary heart disease; CHF, coronary heart failure; CNS, central nervous system; FDA, U.S. Food and Drug Administration; GI, gastrointestinal; HDL, high-density lipoprotein; IU, international units; LDL, low-density lipoprotein; NHLBI, National Heart, Lung and Blood Institute; PL/PL, Pharmacist's Letter/Prescriber's Letter; PO, by mouth; CQ10, coenzyme Q10; RDA, recommended daily allowance; RRR, natural vitamin E; SE, side effects; Sx, symptoms; tid, three times a day; UL, upper limits—the maximum level of daily nutrient that is likely to pose no risk of adverse effects. Includes intake from food, water, and supplements.

Dietary recommended intake (DRI) values expands on the RDAs and contains four categories of recommendations (i.e., RDA, AI, UL, EAR [estimated average requirement]). Latest data should be checked.

Both the AI and the RDA are goals for intakes, but are defined differently.

RDA is the intake at which risk of inadequacy is small (2% to 3%); RDA is expected to meet the nutrient needs of 97% to 98% of the individuals in a life stage and gender group.

AI is the observed average or experimentally set intake by a defined population or subgroup that appears to sustain a defined nutritional status (e.g., growth rate, normal circulating nutrient values, other functional indicators of health). AI is used if sufficient scientific evidence is not available to derive an EAR. AI IS NOT RDA.

EAR is the intake that meets the estimated nutrient needs of one half of the individuals in a group.

(References from the Food and Nutrition Board National Academy of Sciences Institute of Medicine, www.nap.edu.)

Table 6-4 Cardioactive Herbs

A qualified health care provider should use these herbs with caution, especially in cardiac patients and those taking cardioactive medications.

The most commonly used herbs are in **bold print.**

Cardioactive Herbs and Plant Part	Bioactive Constituent(s) with Potential Adverse Effect
Broom (Cytisus scoparius) tops	Alkaloid content has cardio-depressant activity
Kola (Cola spp) nut	Caffeine content
Coltsfoot (Tussilago farfara) leaf	Calcium channel-blocking ability; SHOULD NOT BE TAKEN INTERNALLY due to pyrrolizidine alkaloids
Devil's Claw (Harpagophytum procumbens) tubers	May have chronotropic and inotropic effects; cardiotonic
Dogbane (Apocynum cannabinum) root	Contains cardiac glycosides
Figwort (Scrophularia nodosa) whole plant	Contains cardiac glycosides
Foxglove (Digitalis purpurea) whole plant	Contains cardiac glycosides
Fumitory (Fumaria officinalis) whole plant	Contains cardiotonic alkaloids
Ginger (Zingiber officinalis) root	Cardioactive constituents; avoid large and prolonged doses
Ginseng, panax (Panax ginseng) root	Cardiotonic activity
Goldenseal (Hydrastis canadensis) rhizome	Cardioactive alkaloid (berberbine)

Hawthorn (*Crataegus oxyacantha*) leaf, flower, berry	Cardiotonic activity
Immortal (*Asclepias asperula*) root	Contains cardiac glycosides
Lily-of-the-valley (*Convallaria majalis*) whole plant	Contains cardiac glycosides
Lime, linden (*Tilia spp*) flower	Cardiotoxic in large doses
Mistletoe (*Viscum spp*) leaf	Contains viscotoxin (may have a negative inotropic effect)
Motherwort (Leonurus cardiaca) whole plant	Contains cardiac glycosides
Night-blooming cereus (**Cactus grandiflorus**) fruit	Cardiotonic amines and tyramine; not for use with monoamine oxidase inhibitors
Pleurisy (*Asclepias tuberosa*) root	Contains cardiac glycosides
Prickly ash (*Zanthoxylum spp*) bark	May interfere with sodium, potassium, adenosinetriphosphatase (ATPase)
Quassia, Jamaican (*Picrasma excelsa*) stem wood	Quinine-like properties; larger doses may interfere with cardiac medications

From Herb/drug potential interactions. In LaValle J et al, eds: Natural therapeutics pocket guide, Hudson, Ohio, 2000, Lexi-Comp.

Table 6-5 Anticoagulant Herbs

Anticoagulant herbs are contraindicated in individuals with active bleeding (e.g., peptic ulcer, intracranial bleeding). Caution should be taken in individuals with a history of bleeding, hemostatic disorders, or drug-related hemostatic problems. Caution should also be taken with individuals taking anticoagulant medication, including warfarin, aspirin, aspirin-containing products, nonsteroidal antiinflammatory drugs, antiplatelet agents (e.g., ticlopidine, clopidogrel, dipyridamole) or herbs with antiplatelet activity (e.g., garlic, ginkgo, ginseng), and vitamin E. Use should be discontinued before dental or surgical procedures (generally at least 14 days before). The following list includes some of the most commonly recognized anticoagulant botanical constituents. It should be noted that there might be unidentified constituents in these botanicals that may have anticoagulant activity. The most commonly used herbs are in **bold print**.

Anticoagulant Herbs	*Bioactive Constituents*
Alfalfa *(Medicago sativa)*	Coumarin constituents
Angelica *(Angelica archangelica)*	Coumarin constituents
Anise *(Pimpinella anisum)*	Coumarin constituents
Arnica, leopard's bane *(Arnica Montana)* NOT FOR INTERNAL USE	Hispidulin
Asafetida *(Ferula asafetida)*	Coumarin constituents
Bilberry *(Vaccinium myrtillus)*	Proanthocyanidins
Birch *(Betula barosma)*	Salicylate constituents
Bladderwrack *(Fucus vesiculosis)*	Unknown constituents
Bromelain *(Ananas comosus)*	Bromelain enzyme
Cat's claw *(Uncaria tomentosa)*	Proanthocyanidins
Celery *(Apium graveolens)*	Coumarin constituents
Coleus *(Coleus forskohlil)*	Forskolin
Cordyceps *(Cordyceps sinensis)*	Adenosine
Dong quai *(Angelica sinensis)*	Furocumarins
Evening primrose *(Oenothera biennis)*	Gamma-linolenic acid
Fenugreek *(Trigonella foenum-graecum)*	Coumarin constituents
Feverfew *(Tanacetum parthenium)*	Parthenolides
Garlic *(Allium sativum)*	Ajoene, Allicin, alliin
Ginger *(Zingiber officinalis)*	Kaempferol, coumarin constituents
Ginkgo *(Ginkgo biloba)*	Catechin, ginkgolides, kaempferol
Ginseng, American *(Panax quinquifolium)*	Ginsenosides
Ginseng, panax *(Panax ginseng)*	Ginsenosides

Table 6-5	Anticoagulant Herbs—cont'd
Anticoagulant Herbs	*Bioactive Constituents*
Ginseng, Siberian *(Eleutherococcus senticosus)*	Eleutherosides
Grape seed *(Vitis vinifera)*	Proanthocyanidins
Green tea *(Camellia sinensis)*	Catechins
Guggul *(Commiphora mukul)*	Guggulsterones
Horse chestnut *(Aesculus hippocastanum)*	Coumarin constituents
Horseradish *(Radicula armoracia)*	Kaempferol
Prickly ash *(Zanthoxylum spp)*	Coumarin constituents
Quassia *(Picrasma excelsa)*	Coumarin constituents
Red clover *(Trifolium pratense)*	Coumarin constituents
Reishi *(Ganoderma lucidum)*	Adenosine
Turmeric *(Curcuma longa)*	Curcuminoids
Sweet clover *(Melilotus spp)*	Coumarin constituents
White willow *(Salix alba)*	Salicylate constituents

From LaValle J et al, eds: Natural therapeutics pocket guide, *Hudson, Ohio, 2000, Lexi-Comp.*

diastolic blood pressure of 90 mm Hg or greater, or taking antihypertensive medication. The purpose of treating hypertension is to decrease the risk of cardiovascular morbidity and mortality, including stroke. Many individuals do not have symptoms with hypertension, and taking medication may be a particular challenge because the side effects of medication may make patients feel worse than when not on medications.

In addition to treatment, the need for preventative measures is great as well. Many lifestyle modifications lend themselves to both prevention of cardiovascular disease and maintenance of a lower or normal blood pressure. Among these modifications are exercise, weight loss, smoking cessation, stress management, and numerous dietary and dietary supplement modifications.

Stroke

Stroke is a cerebral infarct (thrombotic or embolic) or hemorrhage characterized by sudden onset of a neurologic deficit and neurologic signs originating in the involved brain region. Stroke is the third leading cause of death in the United States, even though the incidence in the last few decades has decreased. The patient often has a history of atherosclerosis, hypertension, diabetes, or valvular heart disease. A transient ischemic attack (TIA) is a sudden onset of

Table 6-6 Manipulative and Body-Based Methods and Energy Therapies For Heart Health

Intervention	Management	Treatment Regimen	Cautions, Precautions, Interactions	References
SM (hand or ear)	Adjunct therapy for smoking cessation; reduces anxiety; improves moods; reduces nicotine withdrawal symptoms; helps reduce number of cigarettes smoked	At least three times daily	Patients must be taught to perform self-massage on hand or ear	Hernandez-Reif et al, 1999
Massage	General relaxation	Gentle rhythmic strokes; concentrates on the hands, feet, neck, head, face	Qualified massage therapist is needed	DePaoli, 1995
Healing touch, Therapeutic Touch, Reiki	Decreases stress; relieves anxiety; promotes relaxation and comfort	Preferably several sessions	Obtain permission; qualified practitioner is needed	Heidt, 1981; Krieger, 1993; Mentgen, 2001; Olson, Sneed, 1995

SM, *Self-massage.*

neurologic deficit that resolves completely within 24 hours, whereas a stroke persists beyond this time period. Whether a stroke is an infarction or hemorrhage is often clinically difficult to determine. A computerized tomography (CT) scan can determine hemorrhage, but a magnetic resonance imaging (MRI) scan may be needed to determine other causes (Aminoff, 2001).

ALTERNATIVE HEALTH CARE SYSTEMS FOR HYPERTENSION AND STROKE

Ayurveda

According to Tirtha (1998), imbalance in any of the three primary doshas (vata, pitta, or kapha) can result in hypertension. Excess vata is associated with constriction of blood vessels that can cause sudden changes in blood pressure, when associated with temporary mental stress or worry; or persistent hypertension, when there is a chronic vata excess. Excess pitta is associated with hormonal imbalance that leads to more forceful pumping of blood, flushed face, headache, sensitivity to light, anger, and irritability. In contrast, excess kapha is associated with obstruction of the blood channels caused by thickening of blood vessel walls and increased blood viscosity, resulting in constant high blood pressure. Kapha-type hypertension is usually accompanied by obesity, fatigue, edema, and high cholesterol levels.

In regard to treatment of hypertension, Tirtha (1998) cautions that long-term use of antihypertensive herbs or medicines without attending to the balancing of the underlying cause will eventually lead to the development of side effects. Lad (1998) adds that Ayurvedic treatments (especially herbal therapy) should be used only as an adjunct to conventional care and that they should be used only with the knowledge and approval of the individual's personal health care provider (HCP). The use of these treatments, however, may enable prescription antihypertensive medications to be discontinued or to be effective at reduced dosages.

Traditional Chinese Medicine for Hypertension

For hypertension, acupuncturists can use auricular points. Translated from Chinese, the author Liqun (1995) states that the clinical effect of auriculotherapy in the treatment of vascular hypertension is beneficial. The short-term effects are similar to hypotensive medication and the long-term results are better than medication (interpretation/review of the Liqun Chinese article). Correct points, correct location, and proper method are important with this therapy. Points are divided into three groups. Group one consists of fast-acting points that lower blood pressure, Group two settles the nervous and endocrine system, and blood vessels. Group three regulates the Heart and Liver and calms the mind, while regulating involvement of nutrients and fluids (Liqun, 1995). Box 6-1 describes the ear points for stimulation and Appendix B shows an ear with point areas.

The procedure is to needle 7 of the 14 points every other day on alternating ears for several weeks. For chronic cases, ear pellets may also be used; these are magnetite balls or seeds of *Semen vaccariae*, which are taped onto the ear points so that the patient may produce pressure by stimulation of the pellets; the pressure should produce sufficient stimulation. Patients press these pellets three to four times per day for 1 minute; pellets should be renewed every 3 to 5 days. Treatment is for not less than 2 months. Bloodletting of 5 to 10 drops, after massage of the ear, may also be done for serious or acute cases, as well as electro-acupuncture (Liqun, 1995).

Box 6-1

Auricular Points for Hypertension

Group 1
Retroauricular groove
Ear apex

Group 2
Subcortex
Sympathetic nervous system
Endocrine
Brainstem
Shen Men
Occiput

Group 3
Heart
Liver
Kidney
Spleen
Triple warmer (San Jiao point)
In addition, therapy may be done on the forehead point for headache and dizziness, and external ear and points for palpitations.

From English translation of Liqun Z: How to promote the therapeutic effect of auriculotherapy in the treatment of vascular hypertension, J Trad Chin Med 50:37, September, 1995.

The blood pressure lowers during the first 1 to 2 weeks, with best results after 8 to 10 weeks. Liqun suggests reducing hypotensive medication gradually "by one half after one week and withdrawn after 2 weeks; in severe cases medication should be reduced after signs of lowering of blood pressure" (Liqun, 1995, p. 37).

Traditional Chinese Medicine for Stroke

In Chinese medicine, stroke, or the condition of bleeding in the brain, is called "wind-stroke." Four pathologic factors are involved with the development of wind-stroke: internal wind, phlegm, fire, and Blood stasis (Maciocia, 1994). Wind-stroke is described as a crisis involving an upward attack of wind complicated by phlegm and fire, causing Qi and blood to lose control. This event causes severe imbalance of yin and yang, leading to change of consciousness and function.

Internal wind is a condition in Chinese medicine that is characterized by rapid onset, quick changes in signs and symptoms, and migratory symptoms. Wind may cause tremors, convulsions, stiffness, or paralysis. Internal wind is always related to an imbalance of the Liver, with heat or excess energy rising suddenly to the head. Usually a lower body deficiency of Blood occurs, allowing the upper body energy to lose control (Maciocia, 1989).

Phlegm originates from an inability of the Spleen to process and transport the fluids of the body. Phlegm may also result from the effect of heat on body fluids, causing it to thicken and stagnate. Phlegm can affect the Lungs, Heart, Kidney, and Stomach. The nature of phlegm is heavy and can cause stagnation in the organs, acupuncture channels, or under the skin (Maciocia, 1989).

Fire is an extreme form of heat. Heat causes symptoms such as red tongue, thirst, rapid pulse, and fever. Fire not only moves upward and is more drying than heat, but it can also cause bleeding. The nature of fire is to rise to the head, injure the blood, deplete the Qi of the body, and possibly affect the mind by causing delirium or unconsciousness (Maciocia, 1989).

Blood stasis is slowing of the circulation of the Blood. Blood stasis can be the result of poor circulation of Qi, drying of Blood from heat, or from the influence of cold on the body (Maciocia, 1989).

Some combination of at least three of these four factors must be present to facilitate onset of wind-stroke, along with deficiency of Qi, Blood, or yin. There are two types of wind-stroke:

1. Severe type—attacks the internal organs and the acupuncture channels. This type is characterized by coma, paralysis, aphasia, and numbness.
2. Mild type—attacks only the acupuncture channels. This type results in unilateral paralysis, numbness, and slurred speech. No coma or loss of consciousness results (Maciocia, 1994).

The main organs involved in wind-stroke are the Heart, Liver, Spleen, and Kidney. Long-term pathology of these organs provides the background for the development of the factors previously mentioned and creates the acute situation of wind-stoke.

Wind-Stroke Treatment

Treatment is focused on dispelling wind, removing obstructions from the channels, and regulating circulation of Qi and Blood in the channels. This action will relieve spasms, alleviate numbness, and restore strength and activity to paralyzed limbs (Maciocia, 1994).

Acupuncture

During the acute phase of severe wind-stroke, acupuncture is not the treatment of choice; however, acupuncture may be combined with Western medical treatments to encourage resolution of coma. Acupuncture should be instituted within 7 to 10 days, or as soon as the acute hemorrhage has stopped. If treatment is begun within 20 to 40 days, the chance of significant improvement of the sequelae of stroke will be better; with the mild type of stoke, acupuncture should be started within 2 to 3 days (Canruo, 1986). Table 6-7 describes acupuncture treatment for specific symptoms. Table 6-8 reviews research related to acupuncture and stroke. See Appendix B for the meridian locations.

Scalp Acupuncture

Problems involving the central nervous system and brain can be treated using acupuncture on the zones of the head corresponding to the motor and sensory areas. Hemiplegia is treated using the contralateral side of the scalp in the areas specific to the upper or lower limb or both. An advantage to scalp acupuncture is that the patient is able to exercise the affected limbs at the same time the treatment is given to maximize effectiveness of treatment (O'Connor, Bensky, 1981).

Moxibustion

Moxibustion is a method of burning the mugwort herb on the acupuncture needles or above the skin at the acupuncture points. The heat is warming to the Qi and Blood, improving the circulation and flow of the channels. Moxibustion is especially useful if patients are very deficient of energy or their condition has become chronic. Caution must be used to avoid burning the skin, especially if numbness is present (O'Connor, Bensky, 1981).

Chinese Herbal Therapy

The HCP needs to consult an experienced herbalist who can accurately and safely prescribe herbal formulas. The focus with the use

Table 6-7   Acupuncture Treatment for Specific Stroke Symptoms

Hemiplegia: Electric current may be added to the needles to strengthen stimulation of the points.	Yang channels: Points on the affected side are used.	Yin channels: Points are needled on the unaffected side to balance the activity of the yang channels.
Two or three points are selected on each limb with treatment 2-3 times/wk.	Arms: Large Intestine 4,10,11,15, and 16; Triple Warmer 3, 5, and 14; Small Intestine 3	Arms: heart or pericardium channel.
	Legs: Gallbladder 29, 30, 31, 34, and 39; Stomach 32, 36, 41; Urinary Bladder 40, 57.	Legs: spleen, liver, or kidney channel.
Aphasia: To open the tongue, ease the throat and promote speech.		Ren 23, Heart 5, Kidney 6
Stiffness and contracture of muscles can occur in late stages of wind-stroke.	Points are selected as above for hemiplegia but are more specific for the area of the joints involved.	Yin points are added more liberally to nourish the muscles and sinews.

Table 6-8 Research Related to Acupuncture and Stroke Treatment

Study	Intervention	Number of Subjects	Measure	Outcome
Chen, Fang, 1990	Acupuncture treatment within 3 wks after cerebral insult vs more than 3 wks	108 participants with hemiplegia caused by stroke	Retrospective review; controlled trials and clinical findings	Early treatment more successful
Johansson et al, 1993	PT and OT vs PT and OT plus acupuncture	78 patients: 40 in PT and OT group; 38 in acupuncture group	Motor function, balance, and ADL (Barthel's Index) assessed before treatment and at 1, 3, and 12 mos after stroke; Nottingham Health Profile for quality of life assessed at 3, 6, and 12 mos after stroke	Acupuncture group recovered faster and to greater extent than did PT or OT control group ($p < 0.02$) at 1 and 3 mos for mobility, walking, and balance; acupuncture group regained ADL sooner and to greater extent; effect remained at 12 mos

| Naeser et al, 1994 | Acupuncture treating hand paresis in chronic and acute patients after stroke. Compared outcomes in relation to CT scan lesion sites | 13 total: 8 patients at least 6 mos after stroke (chronic), 3 patients 2 mo after stroke (acute), 2 chronic untreated patients | Six hand-motor evaluations assessed: pretreatment, after the 20th treatment, after the 40th treatment, and at 2 and 4 mos after treatment | 11 treated patients reported good response (improvement on 4 of 6 hand tests); all patients had CT scan lesions involving ½ or < ½ of motor pathway areas |
| Naeser et al, 1992 | Real vs. sham acupuncture in acute stroke patients. Examined results in relationship to CT scan lesion sites. | 16 patients: 10 received real acupuncture, 6 received sham acupuncture; no other control group | Boston Motor Inventory test for active range of motion administered before treatment and within 5 days of completing treatment | More patients had good response after real acupuncture than sham acupuncture if CT lesion was in one half or less than one half of the motor pathway areas ($p < 0.013$); no patients had good response in sham group |

ADL, *Activities of daily living*; CT, *computed tomography*; PT, *physiotherapy*; OT, *occupational therapy*.

Table 6-9	Some Chinese Herbs for Wind-Stroke	
Chinese Name	**Latin Name**	**Function**
Tian Ma	*Rhizoma Gastrodiae elatae*	Subdues Liver wind
Mu Li	*Concha ostreae* (Oyster shell)	Sedates the Liver and calms anxiety
Dang Gui	*Radix Angelicae sinensis*	Circulates and harmonizes Blood
Shi Gao	*Gypsum*	Clears fire
Bai Zhu	*Rhizoma Atractylodis macrocephalae*	Clears phlegm

of herbal formulas is to open the channels and disperse the pathologies as previously listed (wind, phlegm, fire, and Blood stasis). Diagnosis of the individual patient is of the *utmost* importance to keep their condition stable and enhance resolution of their symptoms. In addition, herbs would be included to improve the patient's energy and address specific symptoms such as dizziness, headache or other pain, muscle stiffness, or any combination (Fruehauf, 1994; Maciocia, 1994). Table 6-9 provides an overview of some Chinese herbs that may be used for wind-stroke. Table 6-10 lists NAC hypertension and stroke therapies from an alternative health care system perspective.

MIND-BODY-SPIRIT INTERVENTIONS FOR HYPERTENSION AND STROKE

Stroke Units

A routine part of care for a person who has had a stroke can be a specialized stroke unit. These units are sometimes part of conventional care, but not always.

> One systematic review of randomized control trials (RCTs) has found that people with stroke who are managed in specialist stroke rehabilitation units are more likely to be alive and living at home a year after the stroke than those managed in general medical wards, and that stroke unit care reduces time spent in hospital. Observational studies have found that these results are reproducible in routine clinical settings. (Gubitz, Sandercock, 2001, p. 128)

Exercise and Movement

Exercise is recommended by JNC VI (1997) as a routine natural therapy for hypertension:

Table 6-10	Alternative Health Care Systems for Hypertension and Stroke			
Intervention	Management	Treatment Regimen	Cautions, Precautions, Interactions	References
Ayurveda				
Diet	Helps reduce hypertension Promotes mild diuresis, vasodilation; reduces cholesterol	Follow appropriate dosha-balancing diet Drink 1 c mango juice; 30 min later, drink ½ cup warm milk with pinch cardamom and nutmeg; add 1 tsp ghee unless cholesterol is high. Mix ½ - 1 c orange juice (2 parts) and coconut water (1 part) and drink bid or tid. Mix watermelon with pinch of coriander and cardamom; Cucumber raita (yogurt-based condiment); Mix mung dal soup with	Avoid salty, fatty, fried, and hot, spicy foods See Ayurvedic practitioner for dosing and timing	Lad, 1998 Lad, 1998

Continued

377

Table 6-10	Alternative Health Care Systems for Hypertension and Stroke—cont'd			
Intervention	**Management**	**Treatment Regimen**	**Cautions, Precautions, Interactions**	**References**
Ayurveda—cont'd				
	Helps reduce hypertension	cilantro, cumin, and pinch of turmeric; Add 1 tsp honey and 5-10 gtts cider vinegar to 1 c hot water and drink in early morning Drink magnetic water; place 1 cup water (in glass container) next to north pole magnet for 2 hrs; drink 1 cup bid		
Rasayanas (herbals)	Helps reduce hypertension	*Coleus forskohlii* 1% forskolin or 18% forskolin. 50 mg qd to bid standardized to contain 18% forskolin per dose	May alter platelet aggregation; may interact with NSAIDs, antihistamines, decongestants, anticoagulants, antihypertensives; discontinue before surgery.	Mishra et al, 2001; LaValle, 2000

Helps reduce all types hypertension	Arjuna (heart tonic with mild diuretic action); punarnava, passionflower (1 part each) and hawthorn berry (2 parts); steep ½ tsp in 1 cup hot water 5-10 min and drink after lunch and dinner	See Ayurvedic practitioner for dosing and timing. See Ayurvedic practitioner for dosing and timing.	Tirtha, 1998 Lad, 1998
	Jatmamsi, Musta (2 parts each) and Tagar (1 part); prepare and ingest after lunch and dinner	Avoid licorice. See Ayurvedic practitioner for dosing and timing.	Pelletier, 2000
Helps reduce vata-type hypertension	Brain tonics such as Brahmi (gotu kola), garlic, Ashwagandha	Follow prescribing precautions for each herbs. See Ayurvedic practitioner for dosing and timing.	Tirtha, 1998

Continued

Intervention	Management	Treatment Regimen	Cautions, Precautions, Interactions	References
Rasayanas (herbals), cont'd	Helps reduce pitta-type hypertension	Aloe vera gel and harmonizing herbs (Shatavari, Musta, Triphala, Brahmi)		
	Helps reduce kapha-type hypertension	Guggul trikata		
Oils *(Shirodhara)*	Helps reduce hypertension	Externally apply warm oil: continuous stream of warm oil is poured on forehead for 45+ min, daily application for 7-14 days is ideal, otherwise, weekly or monthly sessions are recommended	See Ayurvedic practitioner for dosing and timing.	Tirtha, 1998
Meditation	Helps reduce hypertension	Mantra meditation, or focus on breath to achieve restful alertness; Practice 30 min bid (ideally in		Cooper et al, 1978; Lad, 1998

| Yoga asanas (postures) Pranayama (breathing exercises) | Helps reduce hypertension; also reduces anxiety, depression; lowers BP; medication use decreased in Sundar study; BP returned to restudy levels in those who left yoga practice group | morning and early evening) Serpent and Savasana poses, yoga mudra, Moon Salutation Forward Bend, Moon Sequence, alternate nostril breathing, meditation | Practice consistently 30+ min/day; maintain savasana (Corpse pose) 10 to 15 min; trained instructor is recommended; start slowly; perform postures that are comfortable; some postures may not be possible with certain musculoskeletal concerns. Although yoga can improve balance, some postures require a certain amount of balance to begin and may not be appropriate for someone at risk for falls | Tirtha, 1998; Lad, 1998 Jones, 1998; Mishra et al, 2001; Patel, 1973, 1975; Sundar et al, 1984; Telles, 1993 |

Continued

Table 6-10	Alternative Health Care Systems for Hypertension and Stroke—cont'd			
Intervention	Management	Treatment Regimen	Cautions, Precautions, Interactions	References
Traditional Chinese Medicine				
Acupuncture and herbs	Stroke treatment	See Tables 6-7, 6-8, and 6-9 for specific acupuncture treatment, research, and Chinese herbs	Trained practitioner is needed	Canruo, 1986; Maciocia, 1994
Qi gong	Helps reduce hypertension and risk for stroke; decreased BP and stroke rate in the Qi gong group; may be able to decrease medications	Practice 30 min bid	Trained practitioner is needed	Farrell et al, 1999; Luskin, 1998; McGee, Chow, 1994; Sancier, 1996
Tai chi	Helps lower BP in those who are sedentary	Comparable decrease in BP is realized whether performing Tai chi or moderate intensity of	Balance and safety is important; proper instruction is necessary	Farrell et al, 1999; Young et al, 1998

Traditional Oriental Medicine

		aerobic exercise for 12 wks in older adults	
Shiatsu	Helps reduce hypertension	Ohashi suggestions: Large Intestine 11, Stomach 9 and 36, Kidney 1, Bladder 15 and 22, Gallbladder 21; pull middle and little fingers; Ampuku is important if constipation accompanies high BP (Ampuku is a form of shiatsu that deals with the *Hara*—between rib cage and pelvic bone); give neck shiatsu	Anecdotal: no shiatsu is recommended if systolic BP is over 200 Hg mm; must have trained practitioner with knowledge of pathophysiology; some points in neck are near carotid arteries and may not be appropriate	Ohashi, 1993; Namikoshi, 1995

Homeopathy

	Treatment of Broca's aphasia	Individualized therapy; remedy varies depending on accompanying symptoms; *Bothrops*	No statistical analysis was performed on data; skilled practitioner is needed	Reported in Chapman et al, 1999

Continued

Table 6-10 Alternative Health Care Systems for Hypertension and Stroke—cont'd

Intervention	Management	Treatment Regimen	Cautions, Precautions, Interactions	References
Homeopathy—cont'd		*lanceolatus* (remedy from venom of snake) was used in > 50% of cases in study; 22 of 24 in treatment group improved vs. 3 of 12 in placebo group		

bid, *Twice a day;* BP, *blood pressure;* gtts, *drops;* NSAIDs, *nonsteroidal antiinflammatory drugs;* qd, *every day;* tid, *three times a day.*

Regular aerobic physical activity—adequate to achieve at least a moderate level of physical fitness—can enhance weight loss and functional health status and reduce the risk for cardiovascular disease and all-cause mortality. (JNC VI, 1997, p. 2422)

Thirty to forty five minutes of brisk walking on most days of the week can lower blood pressure. Sedentary people have a 20% to 50% increased risk of developing hypertension. Thus movement and exercise is important for hypertension prevention, for good cardiovascular health in general, and for maintaining mobility for the person who has had a stroke; exercise and movement are imperative for the stroke patient (Westcott, 1967).

Home Blood Pressure Monitoring

Home blood pressure monitoring is a better indicator of target organ damage than is office monitoring because home blood pressure monitoring gives a better indication of the blood pressure throughout the day (Verdecchia, 1994; Mann, 2000). HCPs can develop a plan for teaching the technique and can explore purchase options for a blood pressure cuff and stethoscope.

Repressed Emotions, Defensiveness, Anger, and Anxiety

After working 2 decades specializing in hypertension, Samuel Mann, MD, postulates that hypertensives more often than normotensive individuals display two patterns of *not feeling* emotions. The two patterns Mann describes are:

1. a defensive pattern of coping with stress in which, on a day-to-day basis, unwanted emotions are automatically and unknowingly kept from awareness, and
2. the keeping from awareness of painful emotions related to severe emotional trauma, particularly that occurred during childhood. The first pattern has been the subject of investigation...the second, remarkably, has not (Mann, 2000, p. 41).

Studies of defensiveness indicate that:

hypertensive individuals report less emotional distress and are more defensive, than normotensive individuals (Jorgensen et al, 1996; Sommers-Flanagan, Greenberg, 1989). Studies in which defensiveness is assessed by questionnaires such as the Marlowe-Crowne Scale of Social Desirability (Crowne, Marlowe, 1960) have found a consistent relationship between defensiveness and hypertension. (Jorgensen et al, 1996; Mann, James, 1998; Sommers-Flanagan, Greenberg, 1989) In a recent study, a high score, indicative of defensiveness, was associated with more than a threefold risk of having hypertension. (Mann, James, 1998, p. 41)

Thomas (1997) showed in her study on anger that women who suppressed anger at home had higher blood pressure, both systolic and diastolic, than did women who expressed their anger; and the Framingham study showed that in middle-aged men, anxiety levels were predictive of later incidence of hypertension (Markovitz et al, 1993).

Because of defensiveness, anger, and repressed emotions in some patients, mind body spirit–types of therapy are appropriate. Mann discusses the various therapies that have been shown to help lower blood pressure, including biofeedback, meditation, group psychotherapy, and church attendance. Yet, no solid validated research exists, possibly because of the elusiveness and various personal characteristics that cannot be taken into account. Part of the inconsistency of research results with mind-body-spirit therapies is that trying to quantify emotions and personal traits is difficult. Although patterns may exist, such traits are markedly individual. Thus determining repressed feelings may be impossible; how is a concept that is kept from conscious awareness tapped into? The practitioner must work with the individual patient, take an adequate history to make such discoveries, and then provide appropriate referrals.

Furthermore, people who volunteer for psychologic hypertension studies may be different than those with hypertension who refuse to be in a study. Mind-body-spirit therapies for hypertension need to be individualized and chosen with mutual interaction by both patient and HCP; and when mind-body-spirit therapies are not an option, "appreciation of when a mind/ body origin is operative can still help treatment, by helping identify the medication best suited for the individual patient" (Mann, 2000, p. 43).

Stress-Management Techniques

Numerous stress-management strategies and NAC therapies can be used to work with people who have elevated blood pressure, have had a stroke, or who have problems with repressed emotions, defensiveness, anger, or anxiety related to hypertension. Biofeedback (Yucha et al, 2001), breathing exercises with interactive music (Grossman et al, 2001; Schein et al, 2001), relaxation techniques, imagery, hypnosis, meditation, music, and autogenics may help lower blood pressure. For hypertension, Benson (1974, 1975, 1977) reported on the beneficial effects of the relaxation response and meditation. In a review of autogenic studies for hypertension, four out of five studies had positive results (Ernst, 2001; Kanji et al, 1999). Prayer, meditation creative and expressive arts such as writing, painting, or sculpting may also be useful for expressing feelings that cannot be spoken or as an outlet for anger or anxiety. In addition, positive social support, support groups, movement therapies, and psychotherapy may also be helpful. Table 6-11

Table 6-11 Mind-Body-Spirit Interventions for Hypertension and Stroke

Intervention	Management	Treatment Regimen	Cautions, Precautions, Interactions	References
Affirmations	Help reduce high blood pressure	"I joyously release the past. I am at peace." (p. 19)	Positive, present tense, personal statements	Hay, 2000
	Treatment of stroke	"Life is change, and I adapt easily to the new. I accept life—past, present and future." (p. 66)		
Aromatherapy	Help decrease blood pressure (Hungarian research)	Pure essential oil: *Rose otto* (means that it is a steam distillate of the aromatic plant and 100% pure); lavender has calming effects	Allergy. Use *Rose otto* and not rose *absolute* that is extracted with petrochemicals. Personal preference for scents	Buckle, 2001
Anger management	Helps treat stroke: Also help manage blood pressure (BP) since suppressed anger leads to increased BP	Attend anger management classes; therapy will teach participant to learn how to express feelings constructively.	See Chapter 2 for stress management techniques; provider needs to amass resources and referrals	Angerer et al, 2000; Thomas, 1997

Continued

387

Table 6-11 Mind-Body-Spirit Interventions for Hypertension and Stroke—cont'd

Intervention	Management	Treatment Regimen	Cautions, Precautions, Interactions	References
Anger management, cont'd	Assertiveness (rather than aggression) is practiced			
AT	Help lower blood pressure and increase relaxation	Typically needs 8-10 sessions to learn technique	Positive findings on studies; Ernst cautions "no assessment of quality of studies"	Ernst, 2001; Kanji et al, 1999
Biofeedback and self-management training	Treat stroke; help lower blood pressure; increase relaxation; manage anger, anxiety, and depression; help achieve personal control; change appraisals of threat; improve problem-solving techniques	Varies with individual. Biofeedback training uses breathing techniques and temperature or skin conductance, or EMG most effective when combined with cognitive therapy and relaxation training	Time intensive; needs skilled practitioner	Diamond, 1999; Nakagawa-Kogan, 1994; Good,1998; Yucha et al, 2001
Breathing exercises with interactive	May help reduce blood pressure;	Practice 10 min daily	Patients must be trained to perform music-	Grossman et al, 2001; Ornish, 1990b;

music, breathing techniques	provides relaxation		guided breathing exercises	Schein et al, 2001
Creative and expressive arts	May help lower blood pressure and help with stroke rehabilitation physically, mentally, emotionally, and spiritually	Adhere to patient preference: painting, drawing, sculpting, writing, crafts, etc.		
Exercise-movement	Help lower blood pressure, relieve depression, help with weight loss	Perform regular exercise 30-45 min most days of the week (brisk walking) and aerobic exercise 3-4 times/wk	May need cardiac workup before performing aerobic exercise. Safety: If BP is extremely high, no exercise is recommended at that time.	JNC VI, 1997; Westcott, 1967
	Treat signs and symptoms of stroke	Practice various exercises; work with physical therapist or occupational therapist		
Guided imagery and relaxation	Provide general relaxation; help decrease BP	Listen to personal audiotape; or listen to Miller audiotape: Healing Journey and	Driving or operating equipment is not recommended when using imagery-	Benson et al, 1974; Miller, 1980, 1985; Naparstek, 1994, 1999; Ornish, 1990b

Continued

Table 6-11	Mind-Body-Spirit Interventions for Hypertension and Stroke—cont'd			
Intervention	**Management**	**Treatment Regimen**	**Cautions, Precautions, Interactions**	**References**
Guided imagery and relaxation, cont'd		*Down with High Blood Pressure;* Naparstek audiotape: *Healthy Heart and Cholesterol*	relaxation tapes	
Hypnosis	After stroke for hemiplegic limbs (case studies with patients who had therapy within 1 yr after stroke); help with speech and with anxiety, anger management	Several sessions may be required; more effective if therapy is part of multidimensional approach to result in behavior change	Need trained therapist	Diamond, 1999; Holroyd et al, 1989; Luskin et al, 1998; Manganiello, 1986
IPT	Help lower blood pressure, help decrease anxiety	Combined biofeedback and traditional supportive therapy; focuses on titrating and developing patient control over BP reactivity during human dialog	Case study report.	Craig et al, 2001

	Work on defensiveness, unconscious emotional concerns, past traumas	Patient has to be willing to work in these areas. Provider awareness of patient characteristics may help choice of meds.	Mann, 2000
Cognitive-behavioral therapy	May help lower BP, or decrease dose of BP medications; decreases cardiovascular risk; may help with anxiety level, anger management, defensiveness	Education, skill training, motivation training are recommended	Need trained practitioner	Emmelkamp et al, 1993; Luskin et al, 1998; Shapiro et al, 1997
Meditation and prayer	Provide general relaxation; enhance well being; help decrease BP; possibly reduce risk of stroke; give insight, hope,	Practice intercessory or personal prayer as desired; TM or relaxation-meditation is recommended; videotape—Kornfield, 1996; Naparstek		Ai, 2002; Alexander, 1989; Benson, 1975, 1977; Bush, 1999; Byrd, 1988; Dunn, 2000; Hafner, 1982; King, 1994; Meisenhelder, 2000;

Continued

Table 6-11 Mind-Body-Spirit Interventions for Hypertension and Stroke—cont'd

Intervention	Management	Treatment Regimen	Cautions, Precautions, Interactions	References
Meditation and prayer, cont'd	strength; method of anger management; reduce stress; improve quality of life; improve optimism; provide positive form of coping	audiotapes, *Stress I and II* (1995), *Healthy Heart and Cholesterol* (1999), *Healing Trauma* (1999)		Naparstek, 1994, 1995; Ornish, 1990b; Schneider et al, 1992, 1995 in Spencer, Jacobs, 1999; Shuler et al, 1994; Wenneberg, 1997
Music	Encourages verbal and nonverbal communication following stroke. May help reduce anxiety.	Varies with individual	Patient preference is important	Diamond et al, 1999; Guzzetta, 1989; Luskin, 1998
Pet therapy	Help lower BP	In study, petting a dog decreased BP; companion or pet visitation is recommended; pets are trainable as pet assistants	Patient may have pet allergies; safety is a concern; pet needs affection and care	Huebscher, 2000; Jennings, 1997

Smoking cessation	Numerous benefits, including decreasing risk of cardiovascular disease	Many mind-body-spirit interventions; stress management techniques; imagery, hypnosis	See Heart Health section in Table 6-2	Naparstek, 1997
Stress reduction	Help reduce anxiety	See various stress-reduction strategies in Chapter 2	Choose method that is appropriate for individual	Ornish, 1990b; Schneider et al, 1995
Stroke units	Stroke treatment	Produces better outcomes	Availability may be a problem	Gubitz et al, 2001
Social support	Reduce risk for angina pectoris; also used as treatment for people who have had stroke	Love and support from spouse even in the presence of high-risk factors decreases risk; helps patients with stroke to cope	Some patients have limited social support resources. HCP needs to compile SOC support information	Angerer et al 2000; Medalie; Goldbourt, 1976
Weight reduction	Reduction in BP in those with hypertension who are obese	Modest weight reduction (3%-9% of weight) achievable in motivated adults; may get modest reductions of BP in obese individuals with hypertension	Difficult to maintain weight loss; also, necessary to work with behavioral aspects	Murphy et al, 2001

AT, *Autogenic training*; BP, *blood pressure*; EMG, *electromyography*; IPT, *interpersonal psychophysiological therapy*; TM, *transcendental meditation.*

describes some of the mind-body-spirit interventions that are available for hypertension and stroke. Refer also to the heart health tables.

BIOLOGIC-BASED THERAPIES FOR HYPERTENSION AND STROKE

Dietary Measures, Minerals, and Vitamins

Natural dietary measures for hypertension control include attaining ideal weight, decreasing sodium, and increasing potassium:

> The Hypertension Prevention Trial Research Group [HPTRG] (1990) studied 841 healthy men and women with diastolic blood pressure of 78 to 89 mm Hg, showing benefit from dietary measures. They utilized four different dietary programs and a control group. The dietary programs were: reduced calories, reduced sodium, reduced sodium and calories, or increased potassium. All four dietary counseling treatment groups had lower mean blood pressures than the control group. The largest net reduction in blood pressure occurred in the calorie group: diastolic pressure was 2.8 mm Hg and 1.8 mm Hg and systolic pressure, 5.1 mm Hg and 2.4 mm Hg at 6 months and 3 years, respectively. All four dietary counseling treatment groups experienced fewer hypertensive events; significantly fewer occurred in the sodium groups. (HPTRG, 1990, p. 153)

In addition, the Dietary Approaches to Stop Hypertension (DASH) study suggests that high blood pressure can be significantly lowered by a diet high in magnesium, potassium, and calcium, and low in sodium and fat (Sacks et al, 1995, 1999; Svetkey et al, 1999; Reusser, McCarron, 1994).

Evidence suggests that magnesium plays an important role in regulating blood pressure (Institute of Medicine, 1999; Kawano et al, 1998). Diets that provide plenty of fruits and vegetables, which are good sources of potassium and magnesium, are consistently associated with lower blood pressure (Appel, 1999; Simopoulos, 1999; Appel et al, 1997). In another study, the effect of various nutritional factors on incidence of high blood pressure was examined in over 30,000 U.S. male health professionals. After 4 years of follow-up, results indicated that greater magnesium intake was associated with a lower risk of hypertension (Ascherio et al, 1992). Thus maintaining an adequate magnesium intake is a positive lifestyle modification for preventing and managing high blood pressure (NHLBI, 1997; Schwartz, Sheps, 1999; Kaplan, 1998; Office of Dietary Supplements [ods@nih.gov], 2001). In addition, dietary surveys suggest that a higher magnesium intake is associated with a lower risk of stroke (Ascherio et al, 1998).

Increasing calcium in the diet may also be helpful, although the reduction in blood pressure is thought to be modest (Osborne et al, 1996: PL/PL, 2002).

Fish oils and flaxseed contain omega-3 fatty acids that can help lower blood pressure. Most people are deficient in omega-3s and ingest an excess of omega-6s, making an incorrect ratio. Both fish oil and flaxseed add omega-3s; importantly flaxseed contains three times more omega-3 than it does omega-6 and thus can help balance the ratio (LaValle, 2000).

Low intake of vitamin C may be related to stroke. Study results from Japanese research documented an inverse relationship between serum vitamin C concentration and 20-year incidence of stroke (Yokoyama et al, 2000). The vitamin C intake was in the form of fruits and vegetables. Reduction of stroke was most pronounced (58% lower) in people who ate vitamin C–rich foods 6 to 7 days a week. In addition, vitamin C may be helpful in treating high blood pressure. With a dose of 500 mg a day for 1 month, hypertensives had a reduction of 9%, whereas the placebo group had only a 2.7% reduction (Duffy et al, 1999). (Note: blood pressure also went down with placebo, an interesting finding.)

Vitamin D also may have a role in blood pressure regulation:

> Increased blood pressure has been shown to be associated with low 25-hydroxyvitamin D levels. (Krause et al 1998; Scragg, 1995; O'Connell, Simpson, 1991) Another study found a relationship between latitude and blood pressure: rates of hypertension increase further from the equator (Rostrand, 1997). A clinical report showed that patients with mild hypertension who were exposed to total body UVB [ultraviolet B] radiation therapy increased their 25-hydroxyvitamin D levels and reduced their blood pressure. (Krause et al, 1998; Fuller, Casparian, 2001, p. 60; www.sma.org/smj/index)

The new 1998 dietary reference intake (DRI) for vitamin D is 5 μg (200 international units [IU]) as cholecalciferol per day from infant to age 50; 10 μg per day (400 IU) from age 50 to 70; and 15 μg per day (600 IU) over age 70. The increased recommendation for the older adult is because the older adult produces less vitamin D. Exposure to sunlight is essential for vitamin D production:

> Endogenous vitamin D production begins with ultraviolet B (UVB) radiation interacting with skin, therefore avoidance of UVB radiation can potentially result in vitamin D deficiency...When skin is exposed to sufficient UVB (290 to 320 nm), the hormonal cascade for the endogenous production of vitamin D is activated. (Fuller, Casparian, 2001, pp. 58-59)

Other nutritional supplements that may help lower blood pressure include coenzyme Q10, also called ubiquinone (Digiesi et al, 1992), a "class of lipid-soluble benzoquinones that are involved in mitochondrial electron transport. They are found in the majority of aerobic organisms, from bacteria to mammals" (DerMarderosian, 2001,

p. 605) and are naturally occurring compounds involved in adenosine triphosphate (ATP) generation. Ubiquinone, an antioxidant and membrane stabilizer, may help lower blood pressure, as well as being effective in CHF (LaValle, 1999; PL/PL, 2002).

Herbals

LaValle (2000) suggests garlic, hawthorn, and coleus as natural products to consider for hypertension. In addition, historic-folkloric herbs to lower blood pressure include barberry (*Mahonia vulgaris*), lemongrass (*Cymbopogon citratus*), Morinda (*Morinda citrifolia*), yellow root (*Xanthorhiza simplicissima*), and yucca (*Yucca*). Other herbs have known hypotensive physiologic effects, some with degrees of clinical evidence. These herbs include: cat's claw (*Uncaria tomentosa*), celery juice (*Apium graveolens*), evening primrose oil (*Oenothera biennis*), jiaogulan (*Gynostemma pentaphyllum*), black seed or black cumin (*Nigella sativa*), olive leaf and oil (*Olea europaea*), periwinkle (*Catharanthus roseus*), reishi mushroom (*Ganoderma lucidum*), stevia (*Stevia rebaudiana*), and *veratrum* species (DerMarderosian, 2001).

Table 6-12 lists common biologic-based therapies for hypertension. Table 6-13 lists herbs that have potential hypotensive effects. Table 6-14 lists herbs that raise blood pressure and should not be used in people with hypertension or who have a tendency toward elevated blood pressure. In addition, note that eleuthera root, also called Siberian ginseng, is contraindicated in hypertension (DerMarderosian, 2001).

MANIPULATIVE AND BODY-BASED METHODS AND ENERGY THERAPIES FOR HYPERTENSION AND STROKE

Table 6-15 lists body-based methods and energy therapies that may be helpful for treatment of hypertension or stroke. General Swedish massage, reflexology, Feldenkrais or the "M" Technique are listed as possible comforting methods of care. Massage may stimulate nerves and increase circulation, as well as reduce spasticity in hemiplegia (Diamond et al, 1999). The "M" Technique, a special, very gentle massage technique developed by Buckle (2000), a nurse and aromatherapist, may be especially helpful for the critically ill.

Therapeutic touch (TT) may allay anxiety or decrease pain in any condition. Healing touch, TT, and Reiki therapy may be appropriate for people with hypertension, poststroke patients, or for anxiety and stress management (Heidt, 1981; Olson, Sneed, 1995). In addition, transcutaneous electrical stimulation may also help lower blood pressure (Jacobsson et al, 2000). Electromagnetic therapies have been used for stroke-related hemiplegia:

A number of electromagnetic therapies that might be considered alternative in many medical fields are used conventionally in rehabil-

Table 6-12 Biologic-Based Therapies for Hypertension and Stroke

Intervention	Management	Treatment Regimen	Cautions, Precautions, Interactions	References
DASH diet	Decreases BP in stage 1 (140-159/90-99); 70% of patients decreased BP after an 8-wk diet; decreases risk of stroke	Include fruits, vegetables, whole grains, fish, poultry, nuts, low-fat dairy products; foods low in cholesterol, saturated and total fat, red meats, refined sugars; increase foods high in fiber, K, Ca, Mg, and foods moderately high in protein; DASH servings: 7-8 servings of grains and grain products per day; 4-5 servings of vegetables per day; 4-5 servings of fruit per day; 2-3 servings of low-fat or nonfat dairy per day; no more than 1-2 servings	Servings are based on 2000 calories/day; adjust as needed	Conlin et al, 2000; Sacks, 1997; Joshipura et al, 1999

Contin

Table 6-12   Biologic-Based Therapies for Hypertension and Stroke—cont'd

Intervention	Management	Treatment Regimen	Cautions, Precautions, Interactions	References
DASH diet, cont'd		of meat, poultry, fish per day; 4-5 servings of nuts, seeds, legumes per week		
Vegetarian diet	Vegetarians have lower BP than do nonvegetarians; fruits and vegetables protect against risk of stroke	Increase plant foods in diet; lacto-ova diet includes dairy and eggs; vegan diet has no dairy products	Need to ensure intake of all needed nutrients	Gillman et al, 1995; Murray, 1997; Rouse, 1983; McDougall 1995
Soy	Can lower BP by 5 mm Hg diastolic; helps lower lipids.	Include soy-containing foods; approximately 25 g/day		PL/PL, 1999
Whole grain foods	Helps prevent ischemic stroke in women, especially among nonsmokers	Increase whole grain consumption	May need to do slowly because increased fiber can cause GI upset	Liu et al, 2000
Fish oil—good source of omega-3	Helps lower BP, decreases risk of MI in postmenopausal	Food sources: anchovies, herring, mackerel, salmon, sardines, tuna; or supplement 750 mg	Bad breath, fishy taste; may alter glucose regulation contraindicated in	LaValle, 2000; Morris et al, 1993; Murphy et al, 2001; PL/PL, 2002; Stark, 2000

women		bid to tid or up to 4g/day	those with bleeding disorders; can interact with NSAIDs, warfarin, antiplatelet agents; discontinue use 14 days before surgery	Keli et al, 1996; Murphy et al, 2001
Flavonoids	Helps decrease risk of stroke	Increase consumption of foods highest in flavonoid: onion, kale, French bean, broccoli, endive, celery, cranberry, lettuce, tomato, red pepper, broad bean, strawberry, apple, grape, red wine, tea tomato juice		
Flaxseed oil—good source of omega-3	May help lower BP.	1 tbsp/day	Must be refrigerated; immature seed pods are poisonous	LaValle, 2000
Vitamins				
B vitamins	Help lower homocysteine levels and stroke risk;	Stroke recovery: 100 mg B6; 200 μg B12; 800 μg folic	Normal homocysteine is approximately 8-14 μmol/L but aim	Perlmutter, 2000

Continued

Table 6-12 Biologic-Based Therapies for Hypertension and Stroke—cont'd

Intervention	Management	Treatment Regimen	Cautions, Precautions, Interactions	References
B vitamins, cont'd	good for stroke recovery	acid; 100 mg B3	for a level below 10	
Vitamin C	Lowered BP; 9% compared with placebo 2.7%	500 mg/day; UL 2000mg/day	Vitamin C causes diarrhea when bowel tolerance is reached	Bulpitt, 1990; Duffy et al 1999; Ness, 1996; Yokoyama et al, 2000 ; PL/PL, 2002
	Helps prevent stroke; In study serum vitamin C was inversely related to subsequent incidence of both cerebral infarction and hemorrhagic stroke	Increase fruits and vegetables that are high in vitamin C in diet; eat 6 to 7 days/ week; check serum vitamin C levels for those who are hypertensive	Cohorts in this study received all vitamin C from foods; vitamin C content will vary depending on freshness of food	Yokoyama et al, 2000; Joshipura et al, 1999
Vitamin D (also known as calciferol) (1 µg of calciferol = 40 IU vitamin D)	BP regulation: increased BP shown to be associated with low 25-hydroxy-vitamin D levels.	200 IU/day (up to age 50); 400 IU/day up to age 70; 600 IU/day over age 70; UL = 2000 IU (50 µg/ day); some recommend	Sunscreen affects absorption by preventing skin from making vitamin D; 15-20 min/day of sunlight exposure	Curry, Hogstel, 2002; Fuller, Casparian, 2001; NAP, 2002

		without sunscreen required for acquiring preVit D. Caution: avoid excess sunlight exposure	
	up to 800 IU for those over age 70; sunshine on a regular basis without sunscreen will obtain preVit D because UV rays from the sun trigger vitamin D synthesis.		
Minerals			
Calcium	May help reduce systolic BP; may help prevent stroke. Data from Nurses Health Study showed reduced risk of ischemic stroke in highest quintile of Ca	Nondairy dietary Ca (400-600 mg of Ca supplements) had a somewhat lower risk of stroke, *but* milk, yogurt, hard cheese, and ice cream reduced risk more so. AI is 1000-1300 mg/day. Adult UL 2500 mg/day.	Drugs that cause Ca depletion: loop diuretics, K-sparing diuretics, anticonvulsants, barbiturates, phenytoin, corticosteroids, isoniazid, neomycin, H2-receptor antagonists, digoxin, magnesium and aluminum antacids, tetracycline
			Iso et al, 1999; JNC VI, 1997; LaValle, 2000; Murphy et al, 2001

Continued

Biologic-Based Therapies for Hypertension and Stroke—cont'd

Intervention	Management	Treatment Regimen	Cautions, Precautions, Interactions	Reference
Calcium, cont'd	intake; increased risk in lowest quintile			
Magnesium	May help lower BP	RDA: 310-420 mg/day. Adult UL 350 mg/day	May cause diarrhea; caution any use recommended with renal impairment or heart block. Drugs can cause depletion of Mg (e.g., oral contraceptives, estrogens, loop diuretics, thiazides, digoxin, tetracycline)	Iso et al, 1999; LaValle, 1999
Potassium	May protect against developing hypertension; improves BP control; inadequate intake may increase BP	No established DRI; usual daily intake is 40-80 mEq/day; JNC recommends obtaining K from fresh fruits and vegetables. Safe and adequate intake is 1.8-5.6 g/day.	Drugs can deplete K (e.g., loop diuretics, thiazides, corticosteroids, calcium-channel blockers, penicillin); ACE inhibitors may increase K. Caution	Iso et al, 1999; JNC VI, 1997; LaValle, 2000; Murphy et al, 2001; Patki et al, 1990; Pelton, 2001; PL/PL, 2002

Decrease sodium	Helps lower elevated BP	Average banana, about 600 mg; 3-4 oz raw spinach, 775 mg; 2 oz peanuts, 575 mg. 1 g = 13.4 mEq	Reduce processed food; read labels; learn sodium-salt contents; JNC recommends 6 g of NaCl or 2.4 g Na per day	regarding overdosing	JNC VI, 1997
Other Substances					
Acetyl-L-carnitine (helps shuttle fuel to mitochondria; assists in removal of by-products); is converted to L-carnitine	Stroke treatment	1500 mg/daily	May need to take 1-6 mos before improvement is seen; may cause GI upset		PL/PL, 2000; Perlmutter, 2000
Ubiquinone (coenzyme Q10); fat-soluble,	May help decrease BP, aids in stroke recovery	60 mg bid	May decrease response to warfarin; drugs that cause depletion		DerMarderosian, 2001; Langsjoen, 1994; LaValle et al, 2000;

Continued

Table 6-12 Biologic-Based Therapies for Hypertension and Stroke—cont'd

Intervention	Management	Treatment Regimen	Cautions, Precautions, Interactions	References
vitamin-like co-factor and compound			of coenzyme Q10: hydralazine, thiazides, HMG-CoA reductase inhibitors, sulfonylureas, beta-blockers, tricyclics, chlorpromazine, clonidine, methyldopa, diazoxide., biguanides, haloperidol	PL/PL, 2002
Herbs				
Celery (Apium graveolens)	May help lower BP; is a mild diuretic	Celery juice or four ribs of celery/day	Allergy, dermatitis; no studies are available	DerMarderosian, 2001; Murray, 1997; PL/PL, 2002
Garlic (Allium sativum)	Modest decrease in BP	200 to 400 mg (200-600 tid) of standard-ized extract or 4 g fresh garlic qd (one fresh clove is 2-5 g)	SE: odor; not known for sure which is the main pharmacologic constituent of garlic or if more than one	Estrada, Young, 1993; Fetrow, Avila, McMahon, Vargas, 1993; PL/PL, 2002; Silagy, Neil, 1994;

		needed. Aging garlic to reduce odor will significantly decrease alliin content, the precursor to allicin. Odorless garlic may not be as active. Garlic may interact with anticoagulants and antiplatelets and increase risk of bleeding	Rahman, 2001; Kiesewetter et al, 1991
Ginkgo (Ginkgo biloba)	Increases blood flow; improves attention, reaction time, and short-term memory; also improves intermittent claudication. May improve motor function (experimental model)	40-80 mg tid, standardized	Two small studies reviewed by Ernst; one was as a treatment after subarachnoid hemorrhage (although ginkgo has been associated with bleeding and inhibits platelet aggregation). Interactions with NSAIDs, anticoagulants and other drugs	Diamond, 1999; Ernst, 2001; LaValle, 2000; PL/PL, 2002

Continued

Table 6-12	Biologic-Based Therapies for Hypertension and Stroke—cont'd			
Intervention	Management	Treatment Regimen	Cautions, Precautions, Interactions	References
Hawthorn (Crataegus laevigata)	May help treat hypertension and other cardiovascular conditions (CHF, arrhythmias, Buerger's disease)	Standardized to 2% vexitin, 20% procyanidins, or both	Toxic in high doses; may interact with antiarrhythmic and antihypertensive medications, ACE inhibitors, cardiac glycosides (digoxin). Should be used only under an HCP's supervision	DerMarderosian, 2001; LaValle, 2000; PL/PL, 2002
Olive leaf (Oleae folium)	May help lower BP	1 cup tea tid to qid; steep 2 tsp dried leaf in 150 ml boiling water for 30 min; strain	May increase hypotension; may enhance effects of other antihypertensive medications; may cause hypoglycemic effects; use with caution with diabetics.	DerMarderosian, 2001; PL/PL, 2002

ACE, angiotensin converting enzyme; AI, adequate intake; bid, twice a day; BP, blood pressure; Ca, calcium; CHF, congestive heart failure; DASH, Dietary Approaches to Stop Hypertension; DRI, dietary recommended intake; GI, gastrointestinal; HCP, health care practitioner; HG, mercury; HMG-CoA, hydroxymethylglutaryl-coenzyme A (the "statins"); IU, international units; K, potassium; Mg, magnesium; MI, myocardial infarction; Na, sodium; NaCl, sodium chloride; NSAIDs, nonsteroidal antiinflammatory drugs; PL/PL, Pharmacist's Letter/Prescriber's Letter; qd, daily; qid, four times a day; RDA, recommended daily allowance; SE, side effects; tid, three times a day; UL, upper limits—the maximum level of daily nutrient that is likely to pose no risk of adverse effects. Includes intake from food, water, and supplements.

Dietary Recommended Intake (DRI) values expand on the RDAs and contain four categories of recommendations (i.e., RDA, RDA, AI, UL, EAR [estimated average requirement]). Check for the latest data.

Both the AI and the RDA are goals for intakes, but are defined differently.

RDA is the intake at which risk of inadequacy is very small (2% to 3%); RDA is expected to meet the nutrient needs of 97% to 98% of the individuals in a life stage and gender group.

AI is the observed average or experimentally set intake by a defined population or subgroup that appears to sustain a defined nutritional status, such as growth rate, normal circulating nutrient values, or other functional indicators of health. AI is used if sufficient scientific evidence is not available to derive EAR. AI IS NOT RDA.

EAR is the intake that meets the estimated nutrient needs of one half of the individuals in a group.

UL is the tolerable upper intake levels; the maximum level of daily nutrient intake that is likely to pose no risk of adverse effects.

References from the Food and Nutrition Board National Academy of Sciences Institute of Medicine, www.nap.edu.

Table 6-13	Hypotensive Herbs

These herbs have been reported to lower blood pressure. Caution should be taken when used with hypotensive individuals. Caution should also be taken with individuals who are taking antihypertensive medications; these herbs may lower blood pressure even further. The most commonly used herbs are in **bold print.**

Aconite, monkshood *(Aconitum columbianum)*
Arnica, leopard's bane *(Arnica Montana)*
Baneberry *(Actaea spp)*
Black cohosh *(Cimicifuga racemosa)*
Bryony *(Bryonia alba)*
California poppy *(Eschscholzia californica)*
Choke cherry, wild cherry *(Prunus serotina)*
Coleus *(Coleus forskohlii)*
Goldenseal *(Hydrastis Canadensis)* (in high doses)
Green or false hellebore *(Veratrum alba)*
Hawthorn *(Crataegus oxyacantha)*
Immortal *(Asclepias asperula)*
Indian tobacco *(Lobelia inflata)*
Jaborandi *(Pilocarpus jaborandi)*
Mistletoe, European *(Viscum album)*
Night blooming cereus *(Cactus grandiflorus)*
Pasque flower *(Anemone pulsatilla)*
Periwinkle *(Vinca major)*
Pleurisy root *(Asclepias tuberosa)*
Quinine *(Cinchona spp)*
Shepherd's purse *(Capsella bursa-pastoris)*

Herb/drug potential interactions. In LaValle J et al, eds: Natural therapeutics pocket guide, *Hudson, Ohio, 2000, Lexi-Comp.*

itation...Functional neuromuscular stimulation is a form of electrical stimulation in which muscles are activated sequentially to allow performance of motor tasks. (Diamond et al, 1999, p. 182)

And hyperbaric oxygen (HBO) therapy has been advocated for stroke (Diamond et al, 1999; Perlmutter, 2000). Some studies show improvement in mobility with HBO use. (Neubauer, End, 1980) There are some safety issues involved with HBO. Pressures need to be kept "at 1.5 to 2 atmospheres (atm), limiting exposure time, and following more rigorous procedures during compression and decompression." (Diamond et al, 1999, p. 190)

Table 6-14   Hypertensive Herbs

These herbs have been reported to increase blood pressure and should not be used in individuals who are hypertensive or susceptible to hypertension.

This table contains a classification of specific herbs whose constituents or actions (proven or reputed) may potentially interact with conventional pharmaceutical drugs. The botanical classifications are based on the known chemical constituents of each herb, the pharmacologic properties, and the side effects of each classification according to scientific principles and accepted theory. The potential interactions listed are based on the chemical constituent properties of the herbs, and most of the interactions are theorized. Many plants have constituents that may balance any potential adverse effect. Throughout this table, the most commonly used herbs are in **bold print**.

Hypertensive Herb	Biologic Effects
Bayberry *(Myrica cerifera)*	Myristicin mineralo-corticoid effects
Blue cohosh *(Caulophyllum thalictroides)*	Nicotinic action is caused by methyl-cytisine; alkaloidal effect
Broom *(Sarothamnus scoparius)*	Alkaloidal effect
Cayenne *(Capsicum annum)*	Increased catecholamine secretion
Coltsfoot *(Tussilago farfara)*	Pressor activity; NOT FOR INTERNAL USE
Ephedra *(Ephedra sinica)*	Sympathomimetic; elevated heart rate
Ginger *(Zingiber officinalis)*	Increased catecholamine secretion
Ginseng, American *(Panax quinquilfolium)*	Ginsenosides (Rg-1) may increase blood pressure in high doses or long-term use
Kola *(Cola spp)*	Vasoconstriction due to caffeine content
Licorice *(Glycyrrhiza glabra)*	Mineralocorticoid effect
Mate *(Ilex paraguariensis)*	Vasoconstriction due to caffeine content

From LaValle J et al, eds: Natural therapeutics pocket guide, Hudson, Ohio, 2000, Lexi-Comp.

Table 6-15 Manipulative and Body-Based Methods and Energy Therapies for Hypertension and Stroke

Intervention	Management	Treatment Regimen	Cautions, Precautions, Interactions	References
Massage	Stroke; massage before exercise can help reduce spasticity or stimulate nerves and increase circulation, provide comfort, assist venous return, reduce stress, restore a sense of calm	Administer gentle massage; need to massage at least 30 min	Skilled therapist knowledgeable of pathophysiology is necessary; side effects of patient medications must be known	Calenda, Weinstein, 2001; Diamond et al, 1999; Miesler, 2000; Westcott, 1967
Reflexology	Stroke	Specific points on body	A case series-positive outcomes for stroke reported	Diamond et al, 1999
Feldenkrais "M" Technique ("M" stands for manual)	Hemiplegia Acute illness—is a technique for the critically ill, fragile, or dying; a specific massage technique	Regular sessions Uses a set of repetitions of three; mild pressure that always stays the same	Anecdotal support Anecdotal support	Diamond et al, 1999 Buckle, 2000
Healing touch, TT, Reiki	Hypertension, after stroke to provide relaxation, helps	Routine sessions; TT a minimum of 15 min	Always ask permission	Anecdotal. Krieger, 1993; Mentgen, 2001

	decrease blood pressure			
HBOT	Stroke recovery; can improve gait, speech, mental function, motor activity; can reduce spasticity	Oxygen under increased atmospheric pressure (1.5-2 atmospheres); treatment lasts a few hours	Availability; some safety issues are involved; use caution; limit exposure time; expert practitioner is needed	Perlmutter, 2000
Magnetic stimulation	Animal studies suggest pulsed electromagnetic fields for treatment of stroke	Pulsed field; functional neuromuscular stimulation	Most studies are for diagnosis rather than treatment	Diamond et al, 1999
TENS	May help reduce blood pressure in patients not responding to pharmaceutical treatment	Daily	Effectiveness of treatment may not be evident until 1 mo	Jacobsson et al, 2000

HBOT, *Hyperbaric oxygen therapy;* TENS, *transcutaneous electric nerve stimulation;* TT, *therapeutic touch*

REFERENCES

Abdel-Aziz MT et al: Effects of carnitine on blood lipid pattern in diabetic patients, *Nutr Rep Int* 29:1071, 1984.

Ai Al et al: Private prayer and optimism in middle-aged and older patients awaiting cardiac surgery, *Gerontologist* 42(11):70, 2002.

Alexander CN et al: Transcendental meditation, mindfulness, and longevity: an experimental study with the elderly, *J Personality Social Psychol* 57(6):950, 1989.

Altura BM, Altura BT: Magnesium and cardiovascular biology: an important link between cardiovascular risk factors and atherogenesis, *Cell Mol Biol Res* 41:347, 1995.

American Heart Association [AHA], 2002, Cholesterol, http://www.americanheart.org. Accessed 1/15/2003.

American Heart Association [AHA], 2002, Heart facts, http://www.americanheart.org. Accessed 1/15/2003.

American Heart Association [AHA], 2003, Heart disease and stroke statistics, 2003 update, http://www.americanheart.org. Accessed 1/15/2003.

Aminoff R: Nervous system. In Tierney L, McPhee S, Papadakis M, eds: *Current medical diagnosis and treatment*, New York, 2001, McGraw Hill.

Anderson JW, Johnstone BM, Cook-Newell ME: Meta-analysis of the effects of soy protein intake on serum lipids, *N Engl J Med* 333:276, 1995.

Anderson RA et al: Potential antioxidant effects of zinc and chromium supplementation in people with type 2 diabetes mellitus, *J Am Coll Nutr* 20:212, 2001.

Angerer P et al: Impact of social support, cynical hostility and anger expression on progression of coronary atherosclerosis, *J Am Coll Cardiol* 36:1781, 2000.

Appel LJ: Nonpharmacologic therapies that reduce blood pressure: a fresh perspective. *Clin cardiol* 22:1111, 1999.

Appel LJ et al: A clinical trial of the effect of dietary patterns on blood pressure, *N Engl J Med* 336:1117, 1997.

Aronne LJ: Treating obesity: a new target for prevention of coronary heart disease, *Prog Cardiovasc Nurs* 16:98,115, 2001.

Ascherio A et al: Intake of potassium, magnesium, calcium, and fiber and risk of stroke among US men, *Circulation* 98:1198, 1998.

Ascherio A et al: A prospective study of nutritional factors and hypertension among US men, *Circulation* 86:1475, 1992.

Badmaev V, Majeed M, Passwater R: Selenium: a quest for better understanding, *Alt Ther Health Med* 2(4):59, 1996.

Balch PA, Balch JF: *Prescription for nutritional healing*, ed 3, New York, 2000, Avery.

Barton S, ed: *Clinical evidence*, ed 6, London, 2001, BMJ Publishing Group.

Bason B, Celler B: Control of the heart rate by external stimuli, *Nature* 4:279, 1972.

Baum JA et al: Long-term intake of soy protein improves blood lipid profiles and increases mononuclear cell low-density-lipoprotein receptor messenger RNA in hypercholesterolemic postmenopausal women, *Am J Clin Nutr* 68:545, 1998.

Bell L et al: Cholesterol-lowering effects of calcium carbonate in patients with mild to moderate hypercholesterolemia, *Arch Inter Med* 152:2441, 1992.

Benson H: Systemic hypertension and the relaxation response, *N Engl J Med* 296(20):1152, 1977.

Benson H: *The relaxation response*, New York, 1975, Avon.

Benson H et al: Decreased blood pressure in pharmacologically treated hypertensive patients who regularly elicited the relaxation response, *Lancet* i:289, 1974.

Bergqvist D et al: A double-blind trial of O-(s-hydroxyethyl)-rutosides in patients with chronic venous insufficiency, *Vasa* 10:253, 1981.

Birenbaum ML, Reichstein R, Watkins TR: Reducing atherogenic risk in hyperlipidemic humans with flaxseed supplementation: a preliminary report, *J Am Coll Nutrition* 12:501, 1993.

Blumenthal M et al, eds: *The complete Commission E monographs: therapeutic guide to herbal medicines,* Boston, Mass, 1998, Integrative Medicine Communications.

Brown D et al: Cardiovascular and ventilatory responses during formalized t'ai chi chuan exercises, *Res Q Exerc Sport* 60(3):246,1989.

Brown DJ: *Prescriptions for better health,* Rocklin, Calif, 1996, Prima Publishing.

Buckle J: The role of aromatherapy in nursing care. In Colbath J, Prawlucki P, eds: *Nurs Clin North Am* 36(1):57, 2001.

Buckle J: The "M" technique, *Massage and Bodywork* 15(1):52, 2000.

Bulpitt CJ: Vitamin C and blood pressure, *J Hypertension* 8:1071, 1990.

Burros M: Testing calcium supplements for lead, *New York Times* June 4:B7, 1997.

Bush E: Religious coping with chronic pain, *Appl Psychophysiol Biofeedback* 24(4):249, 1999.

Byrd R: Positive therapeutic effects of intercessory prayer in a coronary care unit population, *Alt Ther in Health & Med* 3:87, 1997.

Byrd RC: Positive therapeutic effects of intercessory prayer in a coronary care unit population, *South Med J* 81:826, 1988.

Calenda E, Weinstein S: Therapeutic massage. In Weintraub M, ed: *Alternative and complementary treatment in neurologic disorders,* New York, 2001, Churchill Livingstone.

Canruo S: The treatment of wind-stroke by acupuncture, *J Chin Med* 22:17, 1986.

Cappuccio FP, MacGregor GA: Does potassium supplementation lower blood pressure? A meta-analysis of published trials, *J Hypertens* 9:465, 1991.

Caspi J et al: Effects of magnesium on myocardial function after coronary artery bypass grafting, *Ann Thorac Surg* 59:942, 1995.

Chapman E, Wilson J: Homeopathy in rehabilitation medicine. In Schulman R, Cotter A, Harmon R, eds: *Phys Med Rehab Clin North Am* 10(3):705, 1999.

Chen Y, Fang Y: 108 cases of hemiplegia caused by stroke: the relationship between CT scan results, clinical findings and the effect of acupuncture treatment, *Acupunct Electrother Res* 15:9, 1990.

Clostre F: From the body to the cellular membranes: the different levels of pharmacological action of ginkgo biloba extract. In Funfgeld EW, ed: *Rokan (ginkgo biloba): recent results in pharmacology and clinic,* Berlin, 1988, Springer-Verlag.

Coggeshall JC et al: Biotin status and plasma glucose in diabetes, *Ann NY Acad Sci* 447:389, 1985.

Conlin PR, Chow D, Miller ER: The effect of dietary patterns on blood pressure control in hypertensive patients: results from the Dietary Approaches to Stop Hypertension (DASH) trial, *Am J Hypertens* 13:949, 2000.

Cooper M, Aygen M: Effect of meditation on blood cholesterol and blood pressure, *J Israel Med Assoc* 95:1, 1978.

Craig F et al: A novel psychophysiological therapy for the treatment of hypertension: analysis of a 16-year case study, *Alt Ther Health Med* 7(1):104, 2001.

Crouse JR III et al: A randomized trial comparing the effect of casein with that of soy protein containing varying amounts of isoflavones on plasma concentrations of lipids and lipoproteins, *Arch Int Med* 159:2070, 1999.

Crowne DP, Marlowe D: A new scale of social desirability independent of psychopathology, *J Cons Psychol* 24:349, 1960.

Cunnane SC et al: Nutritional attributes of traditional flaxseed in healthy young adults, *Am J Clin Nutri* 61:62, 1995.

Curry L, Hogstel M: Osteoporosis, *AJN* 102(1):26, 2002.

Dartenuc JY et al: Resistance capillaire en geriatrie etude d'un microangioprotecteur, *Bordeax Med* 13:903, 1980 (in French).

Delacroix P: Etude en double avengle de l'Endotelon dans l'insuffisance veineuse chronique, *Therapeutique, la Revue de Med* September 27–28:1793, 1981 (in French).

DerMarderosian A: *The review of natural products*, St Louis, 2001, Facts and Comparisons.

DePaoli C: *The healing touch of massage*, New York, 1995, Sterling.

Diamond B et al: Complementary/alternative therapies in the treatment of neurologic disorders. In Spencer J, Jacobs J, eds: *Complementary/alternative medicine: an evidence-based approach*, St Louis, 1999, Mosby.

DiCarlo L et al: Cardiovascular, metabolic, and perceptual responses to hatha yoga standing poses, *Med Exerc Nutr Health* 4:107, 1995.

Digiesi V et al: Mechanism of action of coenzyme Q10 in essential hypertension, *Curr Ther Res* 51:668, 1992.

Dracup K, Woo M, Stevenson L: Use of biofeedback in patients with advanced heart failure to reduce systemic vascular resistance, *AACN Clin Issues Crit Care* 3:40, 1993.

Dreher H: *The immune power personality*, New York, 1995, Dutton.

Duffy S et al: Treatment of hypertension with ascorbic acid, *Lancet* 354(9195):2048, 1999.

Dunn K, Horgas A: The prevalence of prayer as a spiritual self-care modality in elders, *J Holistic Nurs* 18 4:337, 2000.

Eades MR, Eades MD: *Protein power*, New York, 1996, Bantam Books.

Eliopoulos C: *Integrating conventional and alternative therapies*, St Louis, 1999, Mosby.

Emmelkamp P, Van Oppen P: Cognitive interventions in behavioral medicine, *Psychother Psychosom* 59:116, 1993.

Ernst E: *The desktop guide to complementary and alternative medicine*, St Louis, 2001, Mosby.

Estrada CA, Young MJ: Patient preferences for novel therapy: an n of 1 trial of garlic in the treatment of hypertension, *J Gen Int Med* 8:619, 1993.

Farrell SJ, Marr Ross AD, Sehgal K: Eastern movement therapies. In Schulmann R, Cotter A, Harmon R, eds: *Phys Med Rehab Clin North Am* 10(3):617, 1999.

Fauci AS et al: *Harrison's principles of internal medicine*, ed 14, New York, 1998, McGraw Hill.

Ferrandini et al, eds: *Ginkgo biloba extract as a free radical scavenger*, Paris, 1993, Elsevier.

Feskens EJ, Kromhout D: Epidemiologic studies on Eskimos and fish intake, *Ann NY Acad Sci* 14:9, 1993.

Fetrow CW, Avila JR: *Professional's handbook of complementary and alternative medicines*, Springhouse, Penn, 1999, Springhouse.

Fletcher L, Thomas D: Congestive heart failure: understanding the pathophysiology and management, *JAANP* 13(6):249, 2001.

Folkers K et al: Increase in levels of IgG in serum of patients treated with coenzyme Q10, *Res Comm Pathol Pharmacol* 38:335, 1982.

Ford ES: Serum magnesium and ischemic heart disease: findings from a national sample of US adults, *Intl J Epidem* 28:645, 1999.

Frei B: Ascorbic acid protects lipids in human plasma and low-density lipoprotein against oxidative damage, *Am J Clin Nutr* 54:1113S, 1991.

Friedman H et al: Psychosocial and behavioral predictors of longevity, *Am Psychol* 23(2):69, 1995.

Fruehauf H: Stroke and post-stroke syndrome, *J Chin Med* 44:23, 1994.

Fujioka T et al: Clinical study of cardiac arrhythmias using a 24-hour continuous electrocardiographic recorder (5th report)—antiarrhythmic action of coenzyme Q10 in diabetics, *Tohoku J Exp Med* 141:453, 1983.

Fuller K, Casparian M: Vitamin D: balancing cutaneous and systemic considerations, *South Med J* 94(1):58, 2001, www.sma.org/smj/index.htm. Accessed 1/15/03.

Gaby AR: The role of coenzyme Q10 in clinical medicine: Part II. Cardiovascular disease, hypertension, diabetes mellitus and infertility, *Alt Med Rev* 1:168, 1996.

Gartside P, Glueck C: The important role of modifiable dietary and behavioral characteristics in the causation and prevention of coronary heart disease hospitalization and mortality: the Prospective NHANES I Follow-Up Study, *J Am Coll Nutr* 14:71, 1995.

Gillman M et al: Protective effect of fruits and vegetables on development of stroke in men, *JAMA* 273:1113, 1995.

Gliksman M et al: Social support, marital status, and living arrangement correlates of cardiovascular disease risk factors in the elderly, *Soc Sci Med* 40:811, 1995.

Good M: Biofeedback. In Snyder M, Lindquist R, eds: *Complementary/alternative therapies in nursing*, ed 3, New York, 1998, Springer.

Grant W: The role of milk and sugar in heart disease, *Am J Natural Med* 5(9):19, 1998.

Grossman E et al: Breathing-control lowers blood pressure, *J Hum Hypertens* 15:263, 2001.

Gubitz G, Sandercock P: Stroke management. In Barton S, ed: *Clinical evidence*, London, 2001, BMJ Publishing.

Guzzetta C: Effects of relaxation and music therapy on patients in a coronary care unit with the presumptive diagnosis of acute myocardial infarction, *Heart Lung* 18(6):609, 1989.

Haas F, Distenfield S, Axen K: Effects of perceived musical rhythm on respiratory pattern, *J Applied Physiol* 61:1185, 1986.

Hafner RJ: Psychological treatment of essential hypertension: a controlled comparison of meditation and meditation plus biofeedback, *Biofeedback Self-Regulation* 7:305, 1982.

Haggerty WJ: Flax: ancient herb and modern medicine, *HerbalGram* 45:51, 1999.

Hanack T et al: The treatment of mild stable forms of angina pectoris using Crataegutt novo, *Therapiewoche* 33:4331, 1983 (in German).

Hay L: *Heal your body*, Carlsbad, Calif, 2000, Hay House.

Heber D et al: Cholesterol-lowering effects of a proprietary Chinese red-yeast rice dietary supplement, *Am J Clin Nutr* 69:231, 1999.

Heidt P: The effect of therapeutic touch on anxiety level of hospital patients, *Nurs Res* 30(1):32, 1981.

Hernandez-Reif M et al: Smoking cravings are reduced by self-massage, *Prev Med* 28:28, 1999.

Hertog et al: Flavonoid intake and long-term risk of coronary heart disease and cancer in the seven country study, *Arch Intern Med* 155:381, 1995.

Holroyd J, Hill A: Pushing the limits of recovery: hypnotherapy with a stroke patient, *Int J Clin Exp Hypn* 37(2):120, 1989.

Horrobin DF, Mankum S: How do polyunsaturated fatty acids lower plasma cholesterol levels? *Lipids* 18(8):558, 1983.

Horstman J: *The arthritis foundation's guide to alternative therapies*, Atlanta, 1999, Arthritis Foundation.

Huebscher R: Pets and animal-assisted therapy, *NP Forum* 11(1):1, 2000.

Hypertension Prevention Trial Research Group [HPTRG]: The hypertension prevention trial: three-year effects of dietary changes on blood pressure, *Arch Intern Med* 150:153, 1990.

Institute of Medicine. Food and Nutrition Board: *Dietary reference intakes: calcium, phosphorus, magnesium, vitamin d and fluoride*, Washington, DC, 1999, National Academy Press.

Iso H et al: Prospective study of calcium, potassium, and magnesium intake and risk of stroke in women, *Stroke* 30:1772, 1999.

Jacobs RG et al: Relaxation therapy for hypertension, *Arch Intern Med* 146:2335, 1986.

Jacobsson F et al: The effect of transcutaneous electric nerve stimulation in patients with therapy-resistant hypertension, *J Hum Hypertens* 14:795, 2000.

Jennings L: Potential benefits of pet ownership in health promotion, *J Holistic Nurs* 15(4):358, 1997.

Jin P: Efficacy of tai chi, brisk walking, meditation and reading in reducing mental and emotional stress, *J Psychosom Res* 36(4):361, 1992.

Johansson K et al: Can sensory stimulation improve the functional outcome in stroke patients? *Neurology* 43:2189, 1993.

Joint National Committee on Prevention, Detection, Evaluation, and Treatment of High Blood Pressure [JNC VI]: the Sixth Report, *Arch Intern Med* 157:2413, 1997.

Jones A: *In a nutshell yoga: a step-by-step guide*, Boston, 1998, Element.

Jorgensen RS et al: Elevated blood pressure and personality: a meta-analytic review, *Psychol Bull* 120:293, 1996.

Joshipura KJ et al: Fruit and vegetable intake in relation to risk of ischemic stroke, *JAMA* 282:1233, 1999.

Kamikawa T et al: Effects of coenzyme Q10 on exercise tolerance in chronic stable angina pectoris, *Am J Cardiol* 56:247, 1985.

Kanji N, White AR, Ernst E: Anti-hypertensive effects of autogenic training: a systemic review, *Perfusion* 12:279, 1999.

Kaplan NM: Treatment of hypertension: insights from the JNC-VI report, *Am Fam Physician* 58:1323, 1998.

Katsouyanni K et al: Diet and peripheral vascular occlusive disease: the role of poly-, mono-, and saturated fatty acids, *Am J Epidemiol* 133(1):24, 1991.

Kawano Y et al: Effects of magnesium supplementation in hypertensive patients, *Hypertension* 32:260, 1998.

Keli SO et al: Dietary flavonoids, antioxidant vitamins and incidence of stroke, *Arch Intern Med* 156:637, 1996.

Kiechl S et al: Body iron stores and the risk of carotid atherosclerosis: prospective results from the Bruneck study, *Circulation* 96(10):3300, 1997.

Kiecolt-Glaser JK et al: Psychosocial modifiers of immunocompetence in medical students, *Psychosom Med* 46:7, 1984.

Kiesewetter H et al: Effect of garlic on thrombocyte aggregation, microcirculation and other risk factors, *Int J Pharm Ther Toxicol* 29:151, 1991.

King D et al: Beliefs and attitudes of hospital inpatients about faith, healing and prayer, *J Fam Pract* 39:349, 1994.

Kirchhoff R et al: Increase in choleresis by means of artichoke extract, *Phytomedicine* 1:107, 1994.

Kornfield J: *The inner art of meditation* [videotape], Boulder, Colo, 1996, Sounds True.

Krause R et al: Ultraviolet B and blood pressure, *Lancet* 352:709, 1998.

Krieger D: *Accepting your power to heal*, Santa Fe, NM, 1993, Bear and Co.

Kurowska EM et al: Effects of substituting dietary soybean protein and oil for milk protein and fat in subjects with hypercholesterolemia, *Clin Invest Med* 20:162, 1997.

Lad V: *The complete book of Ayurvedic home remedies*, New York, 1998, Three Rivers Press.

Lai J-S et al: Two-year trends in cardiorespiratory function among older tai chi chuan practitioners and sedentary subjects, *J Am Geriatr Soc* 43:1222, 1993.

Langsjoen P et al: Treatment of essential hypertension with coenzyme Q10, *Mol Aspects Med* 15(suppl):S265, 1994.

Lau B: Recent advances on the nutritional effects associated with the use of garlic as a supplement: suppression of LDL oxidation by garlic, *J Nutr* 131:985S, 2001.

LaValle J et al: *Natural therapeutics pocket guide,* Hudson, Ohio, 2000, LexiComp.

Lehr D: A possible beneficial effect of selenium administration in antiarrhythmic therapy, *J Am Coll Nutr* 13(5):496, 1994.

Levine M et al: Vitamin C pharmacokinetics in healthy volunteers: evidence for a recommended dietary allowance, *Proc Natl Acad Sci* (USA) 93:3704, 1996.

Li J: Clinical experience in acupuncture treatment of obesity, *J Trad Chin Med* 19:48, 1999.

Lianda l et al: Studies on hawthorn and its active principle I effect on myocardial ischemia and hemodynamics in dogs, *J Trad Chin Med* 4:283, 1984.

Liao F, Folsom A, Brancati F: Is low magnesium concentration a risk factor for coronary heart disease? The Atherosclerosis Risk in Communities (ARIC) Study, *Am Heart J* 136:480, 1998.

Lininger SW et al: *The natural pharmacy,* ed 2, Roseville, Calif, 1999, Prima Publishing.

Liqun Z: How to promote the therapeutic effect of auriculotherapy in the treatment of vascular hypertension, *J Trad Chin Med* 50:37, 1995.

Liu S et al: Whole grain consumption and risk of ischemic stroke in women: a prospective study, *JAMA* 284(12):1534, 2000.

Luskin F et al: A review of mind-body therapies in the treatment of cardiovascular disease. Part 1: implications for the elderly, *Alt Ther Health Med* 4(3):46, 1998.

Maciocia G: *The practice of Chinese medicine,* New York, 1994, Churchill Livingstone.

Maciocia G: *The foundations of Chinese medicine,* New York, 1989, Churchill Livingstone.

Mann S: The mind/body link in essential hypertension: time for a new paradigm, *Alt Ther Health Med* 6(2):39, 2000.

Manganiello AJ: Hypnotherapy in the rehabilitation of a stroke victim: a case study, *Am J Clin Hypnosis* 29(1):64, 1986.

Mann SJ, James GD: Defensiveness and essential hypertension, *J Psychosom Res* 45:139, 1998.

Markovitz J et al: Psychological predictors of hypertension in the Framingham Study, *JAMA* 270(20):2439, 1993.

Mavers VW et al: Changes in local myocardial blood flow following oral administration of a Crataegus extract to non-anesthetized dogs, *Arzneim Forsch* 24:783, 1974.

McDougall J et al: Rapid reduction of serum cholesterol and blood pressure by a twelve-day, very low fat, strictly vegetarian diet, *J Am Coll Nutr* 14:491, 1995.

McGee C, Chow E: *Miracle healing from China...qigong,* Coeur d'Alene, Idaho, 1994, MediPress.

McKinney T et al: Effects of guided imagery and music (GIM) therapy on mood and cortisol in healthy adults, *Health Psychol* 16:390, 1997.

McMahon FG, Vargas R: Can garlic lower blood pressure? A pilot study, *Pharmacother* 13(4):406, 1993.

Medalie JH, Goldbourt U: Angina pectoris among 10,000 men: psychosocial and other risk factors, *Am J Med* 60:910, 1976.

Meisenhelder J, Chandler E: Prayer and health outcomes in church members, *Alt Ther Health Med* 6:56, 2000.

Mentgen J: Healing touch. In Colbath J, Prawlucki P, eds: *Nurs Clin North Am: Holistic Nurs Care* 36(1):143, 2001.

Miesler D: Stroke rehab part 2, *Massage and Bodywork,* June/July:108, 2000.

Miller E: *Down with high blood pressure,* Stanford, Calif, 1985, Source Tapes.

Miller E: *Healing journey* [audiotape], Stanford, Calif, 1980, Source Tapes.

Miller J et al: Calcium absorption from calcium carbonate and a new form of calcium (CCM) in healthy male and female adolescents, *Am J Clin Nutr* 48:1291, 1988.

Mishra L, Singh B, Dagenais S: Healthcare and disease: management in Ayurveda, *Alt Ther Health Med* 7(2):44, 2001.

Morelli V, Zoorob RJ: Alternative therapies: part II: congestive heart failure and hypercholesterolemia, *Am Fam Physician* 62:1325, 2000.

Morisco C et al: Effect of coenzyme Q10 therapy in patients with congestive heart failure. A long-term multicenter, randomized study, *Clin Invest* 71(suppl):134, 1993.

Morris MC et al: Does fish oil lower blood pressure? A meta-analysis of controlled trials, *Circulation* 88(2):523, 1993.

Mortensen SA et al: Long-term coenzyme Q10 therapy: a major advance in the management of resistant mycoardial failure, *Drug Exptl Clin Res* 11:581, 1985.

Moser et al: Voluntary control of vascular tone by using skin-temperature biofeedback-relaxation in patients with advanced heart failure, *Alt Ther Health Med* 3(1):51, 1997.

Murphy M et al: Primary prevention. In Barton S et al, eds: *Clinical evidence issue*, ed 5, London, 2001, BMJ Publishing.

Murray M: *Heart disease and high blood pressure*, Rocklin, Calif, 1997, Prima.

Naeser M et al: Acupuncture in the treatment of hand paresis in chronic and acute stroke patients—improvement observed in all cases, *Clin Rehab* 8:127, 1994.

Naeser M et al: Real versus sham acupuncture in the treatment of paralysis in acute stroke patients: a CT scan lesion site study, *J Neuro Rehab* 6:163, 1992.

Nakagawa-Kogan H: Self-management training: potential for primary care, *NP Forum* 5(2):77, 1994.

Namikoshi T: *Shiatsu: Japanese finger pressure therapy*, New York, 1995, Japan Publications.

Naparstek B: *Healthy heart and cholesterol* [audiotape], Akron, Ohio, 1999, Image Paths.

Naparstek B: *A meditation to help you stop smoking* [audiotape], Akron, Ohio, 1997, Image Paths.

Naparstek B: *Weight loss*, [audiotape], Akron, Ohio, 1997, Image Paths.

Naparstek B: *Stress I and II* [audiotape], Akron, Ohio, 1995, Image Paths.

Naparstek B: *Staying well with guided imagery*, New York, 1994, Warner.

National Heart Lung and Blood Institute [NHLBI]. Joint National Committee on Prevention, Detection, Evaluation, and Treatment of High Blood Pressure. The Sixth Report of the Joint National Committee on Prevention, Detection, Evaluation, and Treatment of High Blood Pressure, *Arch Intern Med* 157:2413, 1997.

National Heart Lung and Blood Institute [NHLBI]. The Third Report of the Expert Panel on Detection, Evaluation, and Treatment of High Blood Cholesterol in Adults (ATP III). 2001, http://www.NHLBI.org. Accessed 1/15/2003.

Neil H et al: Garlic powder in the treatment of moderate hyperlipidemia: a controlled trial and a meta-analysis, *J R Coll Phys* 30:329, 1996.

Ness AR et al: Vitamin C status and blood pressure, *J Hyperten* 14:503, 1996.

Neubauer R, End E: Hyperbaric oxygenation as an adjunct therapy in strokes due to thrombosis: a review of 122 patients, *Stroke* 11(3):297, 1980.

Northrup C: *Women's bodies, women's wisdom*, New York, 1998, Bantam Books.

O'Connor J, Bensky D: *Acupuncture a comprehensive text*, Seattle, 1981, Eastland Press.

Offenbacher EG: Promotion of chromium absorption by ascorbic acid, *Trace Elements Electrolytes* 11:178, 1994.

Office of Dietary Supplements [ODS]: Vitamins and Minerals, 2002, http://dietary-supplements.info.nih.gov. Accessed 1/15/2003.

O'Hara JO, Jolly PN, Nocol Cg: The therapeutic efficacy of isositol nicotinate in intermittent claudication: a controlled trial, *Brit J Clin Pract* 42:377, 1988.

Ohashi W: *Do-It-Yourself shiatsu: how to perform the ancient Japanese art of acupuncture without needles*, New York, 1976, 1993 update, Dutton.

Olson M, Sneed N: Anxiety and therapeutic touch, *Ment Health Nurs* 16:97, 1995.

Onofrj M et al: L-acetylcarnitine as a new therapeutic approach for peripheral neuropathies with pain, *Int J Clin Pharmacol Res* 15:9, 1995.

Ornish D: Opening your heart: Anatomically, emotionally, and spiritually, *Noetic Sci Rev*, Winter:4, 1993.

Ornish D: Can you prevent—and reverse—CAD? *Patient Care* October(15):25, 1991.

Ornish D: *Reversing heart disease*, New York, 1990a, Ballentine Books.

Ornish D et al: Can lifestyle changes reverse coronary heart disease? *Lancet* 336:129, 1990b.

Osborne CG et al: Evidence for the relationship of calcium to blood pressure, *Nutr Rev* 54:365, 1996.

Pak CY: Nephrolithiasis from calcium supplementation, *J Urol* 137:1212, 1987.

Patel C: Twelve-month follow-up of yoga and biofeedback in the management of hypertension, *Lancet* 1:62, 1975.

Patel C: Yoga and biofeedback in the management of hypertension, *Lancet* 10:1053, 1973.

Patki PS et al: Efficacy of potassium and magnesium in essential hypertension: a double-blind, placebo-controlled, crossover study, *BMJ* 301(6751):521, 1990.

Pelletier K: *The best alternative medicine: What works? What doesn't?* New York, 2000, Simon & Shuster.

Pelton R et al: *Drug-induced nutrient depletion handbook*, ed 2, Hudson, Ohio, 2001, LexiComp.

Perlmutter D: *BrainRecovery.com: powerful therapy for challenging brain disorders*, Naples, Fla, 2000, Perlmutter.

Pharmacist's Letter/Prescriber's Letter [PL/PL]: *Natural medicines comprehensive database*, Stockton, Calif, 2002, Therapeutic Research Faculty.

Pharmacist's Letter/Prescriber's Letter [PL/PL]: *Natural medicines comprehensive database*, Stockton, Calif, 2000, Therapeutic Research Faculty.

Pharmacist's Letter/Prescriber's Letter Continuing Education Booklet: *Natural medicines in clinical management: congestive heart failure* Spring(2):21, 2001.

Pharmacist's Letter/Prescriber's Letter Continuing Education Booklet: *Natural medicines in clinical management: atherosclerosis* 99(4):42, 1999.

Pittler MH, Ernst E: The efficacy of gingko biloba for treatment of intermittent claudication: a meta-analysis of randomized controlled trials, *Am J Med* 108:276, 2000.

Powers K, Vacek J, Lee S: Noninvasive approaches to peripheral vascular disease, *Postgrad Med* 106(3):52, 1999.

Puffer JC: Exercise and heart disease, *Clin Cornerstone* 3:1, 2001.

Rahman K: Recent advances on the nutritional effects associated with the use of garlic as a supplement, *J Nutr* 131:977S, 2001.

Ravn HB et al: Magnesium inhibits platelets activity—an infusion study in healthy volunteers, *Thromb Haemot* 75:939, 1996.

Rehn D et al: Investigation of the therapeutic equivalence of different galenica preparations of (s-hydroxyethyl)-rutosides following multiple dose per oral administration, *Arzneim Forsch* 46:488, 1996.

Reusser ME, McCarron DA: Micronutrient effects on blood pressure regulation, *Nutr Rev* 52:367, 1994.

Riales R, Albrink MJ: Effect of chromium chloride supplementation on glucose tolerance and serum lipids including high-density lipoprotein of adult men, *Am J Clin Nutr* 34:2670, 1981.

Rimm EB et al: Vitamin E consumption and the risk of coronary heart disease in men, *N Eng J Med* 328:1450, 1993.

Robinson K et al for the European COMAC group: Low circulating folate and vitamin B6 concentrations: risk factors for stroke, peripheral vascular disease, and coronary artery disease, *Circulation* 97:437, 1998.

Rostrand SG: Ultraviolet light may contribute to geographic and racial blood pressure differences, *Hypertens* 30:150, 1997.

Rouse IL et al: Vegetarian diet and blood pressure, *Lancet* ii:742, 1983.

Sacks FM et al: A dietary approach to prevent hypertension: a review of the Dietary Approaches to Stop Hypertension (DASH) Study, *Clin Cardiol* 22:6, 1999.

Sacks FM et al: Rationale and design of the Dietary Approaches to Stop Hypertension trial (DASH). A multicenter controlled-feeding study of dietary patterns to lower blood pressure, *Ann Epidemiol* 5:108, 1995.

Samuels M, Samuels N: *The well adult*, New York, 1988, Summit Books.

Sancier K: Medical applications of Qi gong, *Alt Ther Health Med* 2(1):40, 1996.

Schein MH et al: Treating hypertension with a devise that slows and regularizes breathing: a randomized, double-blind controlled study, *J Hum Hypertens* 15:271, 2001.

Schmidt U et al: Efficacy of the hawthorn (*Crategus*) preparation LI 132 in 78 patients with chronic congestive heart failure defined as NYHA functional class II, *Phytomedicine* 1:17, 1994.

Schneider et al: A randomized controlled trial of stress reduction for hypertension in older African-Americans, *Hypertens* 26:820, 1995.

Schneider RH, Alexander CN, Wallace RK: In search of an optimal behavioral treatment for hypertension: a review and focus on transcendental meditation. In Gentry WD, Julius S, eds: *Personality, elevated blood pressure, and essential hypertension*, Washington DC, 1992, Hemisphere.

Schwartz GE: Disregulation theory and disease: applications to the repression/cerebral disconnection/cardiovascular disorder hypothesis, *Int Rev Appl Psychol* 32:95, 1983.

Schwartz GL, Sheps SG: A review of the sixth report of the Joint National Committee on Prevention, Detection, Evaluation, and Treatment of High Blood Pressure, *Curr Opin Cardiol* 14:161, 1999.

Scragg R: Sunlight, vitamin D, and cardiovascular disease. In Crass MF II, Avioli LV, eds: *Calcium-regulating hormones and cardiovascular function*, Boca Raton, Fla, 1995, CRC Press.

Selhub J et al: Vitamin status and intake as primary determinants of homocystinemia in an elderly population, *JAMA* 270:2693, 1993.

Shapiro D et al: Reduction in drug requirements for hypertension by means of a cognitive behavioral intervention, *Am J Hypertens* 10:9, 1997.

Sharma H, Clark C : *Contemporary ayurveda*, Edinburgh, 2001, Churchill Livingstone.

Sheikh M et al: Gastrointestinal absorption of calcium from milk and calcium salts, *N Engl J Med* 317:532, 1987.

Shigeta T et al: Effect of coenzyme Q7 treatment on blood sugar and ketone bodies of diabetics, *J Vitaminol* 12:293, 1966.

Shuler PA et al: The effects of spiritual/religious practices on psychological well-being among inner city homeless women, *Nurs Pract Forum* 5:106, 1994.

Sierpina V: Top twenty herbs for primary care. In Micozzi M, ed: *Fundamentals of complementary and alternative medicine*, Edinburgh, 2001, Churchill Livingstone.

Silagy C, Neil A: A meta-analysis of the effect of garlic on blood pressure, *J Hypertens* 12:463, 1994.

Silagy C, Neil A: Garlic as a lipid lowering agent—a meta-analysis, *J R Coll Physicians Lond* 28:39, 1994.

Simopoulos AP: The nutritional aspects of hypertension, *Compr Ther* 25:95, 1999.

Sinatra S: Coenzyme Q10: a vital therapeutic nutrient for the heart with special application in congestive heart failure, *Conn Med* 61(11):707, 1997.

Sommers-Flanagan J, Greenberg RP: Psychosocial variables and hypertension: a new look at an old controversy, *J Nerv Ment Dis* 177:15, 1989.

Spencer J, Jacobs J: *Complementary/alternative medicine: an evidence-based approach*, St Louis, 1999, Mosby.

Spiegel D et al: Predictors of smoking abstinence following a single-session restructuring intervention with self-hypnosis, *Am J Psychiatr* 150(7):1090, 1993.

Stampfer MJ et al: Vitamin E consumption and the risk of coronary heart disease in women, *N Engl J Med* 328:1444, 1993.

Stampfer MJ et al: A prospective study of plasma homocystine and risk of MI in physicians, *JAMA* 268(7):877, 1992.

Stark K et al: Effect of a fish-oil concentrate on serum lipids in postmenopausal women receiving and not receiving hormone replacement therapy in a placebo-controlled, double-blind trial, *Am J Clin Nutrition* 72, 389, 2000.

Stephens NG et al: A randomized controlled trial of vitamin E in patients with coronary disease: Cambridge Heart Antioxidant Study, *Lancet* 347:781, 1996.

Stevinson C, Pittler MH, Ernst E: Garlic for treating hypercholesterolemia: a meta-analysis of randomized clinical trials, *Ann Intern Med* 133(6):420, 2000.

Sturm B et al: Should patients with severe chronic heart failure step to the beat? *Arch Phys Med Rehabil* 80:746, 1999.

Sundar et al: Role of yoga in management of essential hypertension, *Acta Cardiol* 39:203, 1984.

Svetkey LP et al: Effects of dietary patterns on blood pressure: subgroup analysis of the Dietary Approaches to Stop Hypertension (DASH) randomized clinical trial, *Arch Int Med* 159:285, 1999.

Tauchert M et al: Effectiveness of hawthorn extract LI 132 compared with the ACE inhibitor captopril: multicenter double-blind study with 132 NYHA Stage II, *Munch Med* 136(suppl):S27, 1994.

Telles S, Nagarantha R, Nagendra H: Autonomic changes during "OM" meditation, *Indian J Physiol Pharmacol* 39(4):418, 1995.

Telles S: Physiological changes in sports teachers following three months training in yoga, *Indian J Med Sci* 47(10):235, 1993.

Thomas S: Women's anger: relationship of suppression to blood pressure, *Nurs Res* 46(6):324, 1997.

Tirtha S: *The Ayurvedic encyclopedia: natural secrets to healing, prevention and longevity*, ed 2, Bayville, New York, 1998, Ayurveda Holistic Center Press.

Uchino N, Cacioppo J, Keicolt-Glaser J: The relationship between social support and physiological processes: a review with emphasis on underlying mechanisms and implications for health, *Psychol Bull* 119(3):488, 1996.

Verdecchia P et al: Ambulatory blood pressure. An independent predictor of prognosis in essential hypertension, *Hypertens* 24:793, 1994.

Wang MM et al: Serum cholesterol of adults supplemented with brewer's yeast or chromium chloride, *Nutr Res* 9:989, 1989.

Weber C et al: Antioxidative effect of dietary coenzyme Q10 in human blood plasma, *Int J Vit Nut Res* 64:311, 1994.

Weikl A et al: The influence of Crataegus on global cardiac insufficiency, *Herz Gefabe* 11:516, 1993.

Wenneberg SR et al: A controlled study of the effects of the transcendental meditation program on cardiovascular reactivity and ambulatory blood pressure, *Int J Neurosci* 89:15, 1997.

Westcott EJ: Traditional exercise regimens for the hemiplegic patient, *Am J Phys Med* 46(1):1012, 1967.

White J: Music as intervention. In Colbath J, Prawlucki P, eds: *Nurs Clin North Am* 36(1):83, 2001.

Williams R et al: Prognostic importance of social and economic resources among medically treated patients with angiographically documented coronary artery disease, *JAMA* 267:520, 1992.

Wirth D, Cram, J: The psychophysiology of nontraditional prayer, *Int J Psychsom* 41:68, 1994.

Wolf SL et al: Reducing frailty and falls in older persons: an investigation of tai chi and computerized balance training, *J Am Geriatr Soc* 44:489, 1996.

Wolfson LR et al: Balance and strength training in older adults: intervention gains and tai chi maintenance, *J Am Geriatr Soc* 44:498, 1996.

www.cc.nih.gov/ccc/supplements, *Selenium*, 2001, NIH Clinical Center. (Accessed 8/11/01.)

Wynd CA: Relaxation imagery used for stress reduction in the prevention of smoking relapse, *J Adv Nurs* 17:294, 1992.

Yeh Y, Lijuan L: Cholesterol-lowering effect of garlic extract and organosulfur compounds: human and animal studies, *J Nutr* 131:989S, 2001.

Yokoyama T et al: Serum vitamin C concentration was inversely associated with subsequent 20-year incidence of stroke in a Japanese rural community. The Shibata Study, *Stroke* 31:2287, 2000.

Young DR, Appel LJ, Jee SH: Effects of aerobic exercise and t'ai chi on blood pressure in the elderly, *Circulation* 97:828, 1998.

Yucha CB et al: The effect of biofeedback in hypertension, *Appl Nurs Res* 14:29, 2001.

Zambon D et al: Walnuts lower cholesterol levels in hypercholesterolemic individuals, *Ann Intern Med* 132:538, 2000.

Zhou D et al: Cardiorespiratory and metabolic response during tai chi chuan exercise, *Can J Sprot Sci* 9:7, 1984.

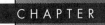
MUSCULOSKELETAL CONCERNS

Pamela Shuler ▪ Roxana Huebscher ▪ Helen Miller ▪ Louise Rauckhorst

NAC THERAPIES FOR MUSCULOSKELETAL CONCERNS

One third or more of the general population in the United States is using natural-alternative-complementary (NAC) therapies for various health problems (Eisenberg et al, 1998; Astin, 1998). Moreover, during the last 5 years, arthritis and low back pain were among the most common conditions for which people over the age of 65 used such therapies (Deyo, 1998; Eisenberg et al, 1998). To help manage the discomfort associated with these disorders, providers and patients can mutually explore the use of NAC therapies that are low risk, comforting, and cost-effective. This chapter covers some selected NAC therapies for common musculoskeletal problems.

NAC THERAPIES FOR FIBROMYALGIA

The Arthritis Foundation reports that fibromyalgia is the most common rheumatic cause of chronic diffuse pain (Freundlich, Leventhal, 1997). Fibromyalgia can be defined as a condition or syndrome presenting with a history of widespread pain for a duration of at least 3 months and pain in 11 of 18 specific tender-point sites evident on digital palpation (Burckhardt, 2001; Klippel, 1997). Pain can be either widespread or focused in multiple tender points. Tenderness in characteristic sites upon palpation with moderate pressure is usual. In addition to pain, aching, and stiffness, a sleep disorder and fatigue are usually present. Irritable bladder or bowel, paresthesia, dizziness, headaches, tempomandibular joint dysfunction, hypotension, and morning stiffness may also occur. Some people also complain of psychologic distress and cognitive dysfunction, such as forgetfulness or "fuzzy" thinking. Women are affected more often than are men; prevalence in the United States is approximately 3% to 5% of adult women and about 0.5% of adult men (Burckhardt, 2001). The cause of fibromyalgia is unknown. Patients may have no underlying disease, or they may have concomitant or underlying chronic diseases such as rheumatoid arthritis, osteoarthritis, Lyme disease, or sleep apnea (Freundlich, Leventhal, 1997). The practitioner should obtain a thorough knowledge of conventional fibromyalgia therapies that the patient currently uses to ensure safe introduction of NAC regimens.

Laboratory and radiographic abnormalities are absent. However, the chronic physical and mental affects of fibromyalgia can be disabling; patients report a lower quality of life than do patients with rheumatoid arthritis. Patients may develop reactive depression as a result of this chronic and poorly understood condition; however, fibromyalgia is not common in patients with major depressive disorder (Burckhardt, 2001).

The goal of using NAC therapies for patients with fibromyalgia is to improve sleep, reduce the number of tender points, diminish fatigue, decrease depression, relieve pain, and provide comfort.

ALTERNATIVE HEALTH CARE SYSTEMS FOR FIBROMYALGIA

Acupuncture, Qi gong, and homeopathy have had some study for fibromyalgia (Buckelew et al, 1998; Creamer et al, 1998; DeLuze, 1992; Fisher et al, 1989; Singh et al, 1998). In one homeopathy study (Fisher et al, 1989), *Rhus toxicodendron* 6C (poison ivy) was used. The type of pain appropriate for *Rhus toxicodendron* is "worse from cold and wet weather, and better from heat and continued motion" (Chapman, Wilson, 1999, p. 715). Thus case-taking is needed in more depth than simply having the appropriate amount of tender points. The group that received homeopathy reported greater reduction of number of tender points, reduced pain, and improved sleep.

Acupuncture may also help with tender points. Similarly, acupressure can be used from an acupressure provider, or the patient may use finger pressure on the points. Other therapies such as yoga or Tai chi may provide comfort and help increase mobility. Table 7-1 describes a few alternative health care systems for fibromyalgia.

MIND-BODY-SPIRIT INTERVENTIONS FOR FIBROMYALGIA

Examples of mind-body-spirit interventions that may help fibromyalgia symptoms include biofeedback, coping skills, exercise, hypnosis, meditation, music, and stress-management techniques such as relaxation and imagery. In addition, balneotherapy (therapeutic baths) may be helpful in reducing pain, and the addition of valerian to the bath may improve sleep and well being (Ernst, 2001). Patients with fibromyalgia have used these bath therapies to reduce fatigue, depression, sleep disturbances, and pain, as well as to relieve anxiety. In addition, prayer may be useful for any patient. Health care practitioners (HCPs) may wish to read Freeman and Lawlis (2001), who provide a chapter on the general topic of spiritual medicine, or Dossey (2001), who has written eloquently on prayer, healing, and what illness means.

Chapter 2 in this text also provides interventions that may help with sleep, depression, coping skills, and stress management. A combination of therapies is important with fibromyalgia because of

Table 7-1 Alternative Health Care Systems for Fibromyalgia

Intervention	Management	Treatment Regimen	Cautions, Precautions, Interactions	References
Traditional Chinese Medicine				
Acupuncture	Decreases pain and number of tender points; points are selected for general balance of system and pain control	For general balance, used on Stomach 36, Large Intestine 4; for pain control, used on local tender points, depending on individual; electroacupuncture may be used; treatment, 1-2 times/wk until condition stabilizes; may require treatment every 3-4 wks for several months	Need qualified practitioner; inform practitioner of all medications, especially anticoagulants, glucocorticoids, anticonvulsants	Deluze et al, 1992; Sprott et al, 1996, 1998; see Appendix B for meridians and points
Acupressure	May decrease pain, improve flexibility, and provide relaxation	Finger pressure on Large Intestine 4 and 11, Triple Warmer 5, Stomach 36, Gallbladder 20	Qualified practitioner needed, or patient may self-administer; no study conducted	Gach, 1990; see Appendix B for meridians and points

Continued

Table 7-1 Alternative Health Care Systems for Fibromyalgia—cont'd

Intervention	Management	Treatment Regimen	Cautions, Precautions, Interactions	References
Qi gong	Improves coping skills; increases pain threshold; relieves depression; improves function	Daily practice includes meditation, physical movement, and breathing exercises	Qualified instructor needed for teaching	Creamer et al, 1986; Singh et al, 1998
Homeopathy				
Remedies	Reduces number of tender points; helps relieve pain; improves sleep	Remedy depends on case-taking; remedy is taken for a variable period; in one study, *Rhus toxicodendron* was used in patients with fibromyalgia matched by case-taking for this remedy	Qualified practitioner needed	Chapman et al, 1999; Fisher et al, 1989

psychologic distress that the discomfort causes. Table 7-2 lists mind-body-spirit interventions for fibromyalgia.

BIOLOGIC-BASED THERAPIES FOR FIBROMYALGIA

S-adenosylmethionine (SAMe), capsaicin, and magnesium plus malic acid are the natural medicines thought to have efficacy in treating fibromyalgia (Pharmacist's Letter/Prescriber's Letter [PL/PL], 2001, 2002). The use of 5-hydroxytryptophan (5-HTP), a precursor to serotonin, is discouraged as a result of safety concerns; 5-HTP has been implicated in eosinophilia-myalgia syndrome. It also may have additive effects with antidepressants, including selective serotonin reuptake inhibitors (SSRIs), as well as with tryptophan, SAMe, and St. John's wort (La Valle, 2000; PL/PL, 2001). Two other substances to avoid are gamma-hydroxybutyric acid (GHB) and gamma-butyro-lactone (GBL); they are also considered unsafe, and GBL has been associated with numerous adverse effects and at least one death (PL/PL, 2001).

SAMe is produced from methionine and adenosine triphosphate (ATP) and is found in almost all body tissues; its synthesis is related to vitamin B12 and folate metabolism and, if these B vitamins are deficient, then SAMe concentration may be less in the central nervous system (PL/PL, 2002). Although the way in which SAMe works is unknown, theories suggest that SAMe may increase serotonin turnover and elevate dopamine and norepi-nephrine; or SAMe may alter neuron membranes so that the "neu-rotransmitters work more efficiently" (PL/PL, 2001, p. 31). SAMe seems to decrease pain, fatigue, and morning stiffness, and also alter mood.

Capsaicin, a pepper that is meant for topical use, is thought to relieve pain by depleting substance P (a neuropeptide "released in the dorsal horn by C fibers in response to nociceptive neurons [pain receptors]") (Devine, 2002, p. 1091). Magnesium is a mineral, and malic acid is an alpha-hydroxy acid. Malic acid is found in some fruits such as apples (La Valle, 2000). Both magnesium and malic acid are needed for the generation of ATP and are given in combi-nation for patients with fibromyalgia. There is no evidence that either works alone in the treatment of fibromyalgia (PL/PL, 2001, 2002).

In a double-blind, placebo-controlled study, magnesium was stud-ied in patients with chronic fatigue syndrome, a condition that shares many of the same symptoms as does fibromyalgia. Improved energy and a reduction of pain and emotional symptoms occurred in the magnesium group. However, later open studies found no deficiency in participants with chronic fatigue and no benefit from magnesium injections (Ernst, 2001). Table 7-3 provides a few bio-logic-based therapies for fibromyalgia.

Table 7-2 Mind-Body-Spirit Interventions or Fibromyalgia

Intervention	Management	Treatment Regimen	Cautions, Precautions, Interactions	References
Biofeedback	Relieves symptoms	EMG biofeedback training showed improvement of symptoms	Skilled practitioner needed	Ferraccioli et al, 1987; Freeman, Lawlis, 2001; Taylor, 1999
Coping skills training	Helps patient cope with condition, including pain, fatigue, anxiety, and depression; imparts options and hope	Regimen includes: (1) educating about condition, treatments, options, resources; (2) pacing to maximize energy for value activities; (3) monitoring current self-management to see how different activities affect process; and (4) teaching techniques such as relaxation, imagery, cognitive restructuring	Need to amass resources and referrals or obtain instructor to teach coping skills; see Chapter 2 for more information	Burckhardt, 2001
Exercise	Improves symptoms and quality of life;	Stretching at least once/day is encouraged;	Patient's deconditioned state must be taken into	Buckelew, 1998;

	provides significant changes in pain, aerobic capacity, and physical function with aerobic exercise	aerobics (walking) or combination of flexibility and strength exercises with biofeedback is recommended; begin slowly 3-10 minutes at a time, several times/day, and increase by 1-2 min/wk up to 30 min/day; water exercises in warm pool are acceptable	account; start below what patient thinks can be accomplished, because success is a strong motivator, and injury is less likely; never hold a stretch to the point of pain	Burckhardt, 1994, 2001; Ernst, 2001
Hypnosis	Relieves pain; reduces fatigue; improves sleep	Training and sessions vary, but usually takes several sessions; self-hypnosis can be learned	Hypnotherapists are not regulated; check credentials of therapist carefully	Haanen et al, 1991
Imagery	Relieves symptoms; reduces pain; provides coping skills	Use Naparstek audiotapes: *Pain* (1995); *Stress I and Stress II* (1995); *Staying Well with Guided Imagery* (1994); also use Miller tape: *Healing Journey*, (1980); see Chapter 8 for a pain and a headache script	No driving or operating machinery while listening to tapes	Miller, 1980; Naparstek, 1994 and audiotapes

Continued

Table 7-2	Mind-Body-Spirit Interventions or Fibromyalgia—cont'd			
Intervention	**Management**	**Treatment Regimen**	**Cautions, Precautions, Interactions**	**References**
Meditation	Reduces chronic pain and anxiety; relieves stress; provides positive form of coping	Goal: daily, self-performing practice after learning technique; study was for 10 wks; found moderate or great improvement in 51% of participants	Most beneficial when combined with a relaxation program or Qi gong	Kaplan et al, 1993
Music	Reduces pain and disability	Patient preference is recommended	German study conducted on patients with chronic pain, including fibromyalgia	Ernst, 2001
Prayer	Relieves stress; improves quality of life and optimism; provides positive form of coping; enhances well being	Respect individual preference; intercessory prayer or personal prayer is encouraged		Bush, 1999; Dossey, 2001; Dunn et al, 2000; Freeman, Lawlis, 2001; King et al, 1994;

Stress-management training	Relieves pain; decreases number of tender points	Daily to weekly routines with various modalities recommended; techniques include relaxation, affirmation, and assertiveness. See Chapter 2.	Stress management most effective when combined with behavior modification therapy and exercise in group settings	Meisenhelder et al, 2000; Shuler et al, 1994
Support groups	Provides social support (like-minded individuals)	Local support groups can be located through the Fibromyalgia Network, P.O. Box 31750, Tucson, AZ 85751-1750, (602) 290-5508	Chronic complaining can be a hazard in a support group; encourage positive talk	Bennett et al, 1996

EMG, *Electromyogram.*

Table 7-3 Biologic-Based Therapies for Fibromyalgia

A complete prescribing source should be consulted before using biologic therapies. Herbs may cause allergic reactions and interactions. Herbs are generally contraindicated or not recommended for women during pregnancy and lactation and for children unless research data or a long history of safe use has been established.

Intervention	Management	Treatment Regimen	Cautions, Precautions, Interactions	References
Ascorbigen and broccoli powder	May relieve pain and improve quality of life	100 mg ascorbigen and 400 mg broccoli powder daily for 1 month is recommended	Results from one preliminary study look promising, but further research (a larger, double-blind study) is needed	Bramwell, 2000
Capsaicin (cayenne or red peppers)	May relieve pain	Applied topically as cream with 0.075% capsaicin: apply cream 3-4 times/day to tender points; use diluted vinegar solution to remove cream	Avoid use on broken skin; do not use with heating pad; initially, application causes irritation and hyperesthesia; wash hands thoroughly before and immediately after application	McCarty et al, 1994; PL/PL, 2001, 2002
Magnesium combined with	May relieve pain and improve energy	Magnesium hydroxide, 200-300 mg bid;	Research regarding effectiveness is	www.cc.NIH NIH, 2002 website; PL/PL, 2001,

malic acid	levels	malic acid, 800-1200 mg bid. Adult UL, 350 mg	limited; magnesium can interact with blood pressure medications; avoid if history of renal disease or heart block is present; SE: loose stools, diarrhea	2002; Russell et al, 1995
SAMe	May reduce pain, fatigue, morning stiffness; may improve mood and relieve depression	200 mg tid is recommended	SAMe is a naturally occurring compound, has antidepressant effects, and should not be combined with other antidepressants; SAMe can cause flatulence, vomiting, diarrhea, headache, anxiety, or any combination	Bottiglieri et al, 1994; Horstman, 1999; Jacobsen et al, 1991; PL/PL, 2001, 2002; Rosenbaum et al, 1990
Aromatherapy				
Analgesic or calming essential oils. Analgesic	May help provide comfort	Massage: 2-5 gtts of essential oil in 5 ml carrier oil to make a	Check for allergy; must be diluted in carrier oil such as almond	Buckle, 1997, 2001; PL/PL, 2002

Continued

Table 7-3 Biologic-Based Therapies for Fibromyalgia—cont'd

Intervention	Management	Treatment Regimen	Cautions, Precautions, Interactions	References
Aromatherapy—cont'd				
oils—lemongrass, rosemary, frankincense, juniper, rose, ginger, verbena, spike lavender, peppermint, myrrh, clove bud, ylang ylang, true lavender, sweet marjoram, black pepper. Antispasmodic oils—Roman chamomile, lemon-scented eucalyptus, sage (Salvia officinalis)		2%-5% solution; compress: 1-5 gtts in a bowl of warm water, wring compress, and apply; inhalation: 1-2 gtts on a tissue	oil; allow patients to smell before applying; oils not for ingestion. Caution—regarding topical application effects of sage: sage contains thujone; considered unsafe when taken orally in excess because menstrual stimulation and possible abortifacient effects may result. Read safety issues for all oils	

Bid, Twice daily; gtts, drops; SAMe; S-adenosyl-methionine; SE, side effects; tid, three times daily; UL, upper limits—the maximum level of daily nutrient that is likely to pose no risk of adverse effects. Includes intake from food, water, and supplements; URI, upper respiratory infection.

MANIPULATIVE AND BODY-BASED METHODS AND ENERGY THERAPIES FOR FIBROMYALGIA

Massage therapy (Hirschberg, 1997; Sunshine et al, 1996) and transcutaneous electrical stimulation (Sunshine et al, 1996) may be beneficial in relieving symptoms associated with fibromyalgia. Research indicates that sleeping on a magnetic mattress pad may improve sleep and relieve pain in some patients (Colbert et al, 1999). In addition, micro-current electrical therapy (MET) may be useful (Lichtbroun et al, 2001; Tyers, Smith, 2001) as well as light therapy or laser (Saul, 1999; Longo et al, 1997; Fitzcharles, 1997). Anecdotally, therapeutic touch, healing touch, Reiki, or any combination may provide comfort, relaxation, and relief from anxiety and pain for people with fibromyalgia (Krieger, 1993; Mentgen, 2001; Quinn, 2002; Stein, 1997; Umbreit, 2002). Therapeutic Touch studies have been done on patients with arthritis (Gordon, 1998; Peck, 1997, 1998) and patients with musculoskeletal pain (Lin, Taylor, 1998) showing improvement of symptoms. Table 7-4 presents a selection of body-based and energy therapies that have been used for the treatment of fibromyalgia.

NAC THERAPIES FOR LOW BACK STRAIN

Low back strain (LBS) is "non-radiating low back pain associated with a mechanical stress to the lumbosacral spine" (Borenstein et al, 1995, p. 184). Over 50% of patients with mechanical low back pain are diagnosed with LBS (Borenstein et al, 1995). The cause of LBS is usually related to ligamentous or muscular strain secondary to either a specific traumatic episode or continuous mechanical stress. Acute low back pain is often self-limiting, with 90% of patients spontaneously recovering within 4 to 6 weeks. Therefore the focus of treatment is on prevention of further injury or reinjury.

Symptoms include an aching type of muscular pain or spasm located in the lumbosacral area. The pain may be referred to either the buttocks or anterior thigh but does not radiate to the lower extremities. Neurologic symptoms are absent. Signs include stiff or slow gait, decreased range of motion with increased back pain on flexion, point tenderness, muscle spasm, or any combination. Neurologic signs are absent, including a negative straight-leg and cross-leg raise test. Radiologic studies are not routinely indicated if the history and physical examination clearly indicate a diagnosis of LBS. The goal of using NAC therapies with patients with LBS is to relieve pain and improve function with minimal adverse effects from treatment. Furthermore, assisting the patient in identifying sources of mechanical stress to the lumbosacral area is desirable so that muscle strain can be prevented in the future. The practitioner must obtain a thorough knowledge of conventional therapies that the patient currently uses for LBS to ensure safe introduction of NAC regimens.

Table 7-4 Manipulative and Body-Based and Energy Therapies for Fibromyalgia

Intervention	Management	Treatment Regimen	Cautions, Precautions, Interactions	References
Chiropractic manipulation	May reduce pain and improve range of motion	Varies with individual	Qualified practitioner needed; limited research conducted; a pilot study did not look at specific fibromyalgia outcome measures	Blunt et al, 1997; Ernst, 2001
Connective tissue massage	May relieve pain and depression; improves quality of life; massage also generally increases circulation and mobility	Specific sites are massaged as needed	In the study, relief lasted for 3 months	Brattberg, 1999; Ernst, 2001
Skinrolling massage	Provides long-lasting pain relief	Varies with individual	Technique may be initially painful while adhesions are released from underlying fascia; may be difficult to	Hirschberg, 1997

		locate a skilled practitioner	
Swedish massage	May help decrease pain, fatigue, and anxiety; may improve sleep	Very gentle massage is used; patient sets the tone for amount of pressure and areas to be massaged	Qualified practitioner who is familiar with fibromyalgia needed	Sunshine et al, 1996
Magnetic mattress pad	May improve sleep and relieve pain	Patient sleeps on magnetic mattress for a minimum of 16 wks	Further research is needed to determine long-term benefits or effects; research has been done with pad containing 270 ceramic magnets that deliver a 200-600 G static magnetic field; other types of pads may or may not be effective	Colbert et al, 1999
TENS	May decrease pain, fatigue, and anxiety and improve sleep	Varies with individual	Therapeutic effect may not be demonstrated until several wks of therapy is completed	Guieu, 1991; Sunshine et al, 1996
MET	May reduce pain; promotes sleep	Varies with individual	Use with caution or not at all if patient has	Lichtbroun et al, 2001;

Continued

Table 7-4	Manipulative and Body-Based and Energy Therapies for Fibromyalgia—cont'd			
Intervention	Management	Treatment Regimen	Cautions, Precautions, Interactions	References
MET, cont'd			pacemaker; resuscitation may be required	Tyers et al, 2001
Therapeutic touch, healing touch, Reiki	May help reduce anxiety and pain and promote comfort	Sessions are 30-60 min; first 3 Reiki sessions should be given as close together as possible (e.g., daily for 3 days)	Obtain permission from patient	Krieger, 1993; Mentgen, 2001; Quinn, 2002; Stein, 1997; Umbreit, 2002

G, Gauss (measure of magnet strength); MET, micro-current electrical therapy; TENS, transcutaneous electrical nerve stimulation.

ALTERNATIVE HEALTH CARE SYSTEMS FOR LOW BACK STRAIN

Yoga may help with low back pain (Ernst, 2001). From anecdotal experience, Jones (1998) suggests use of the yoga positions the Cat, Pelvic Lift, Dance of the Legs, and Relaxation poses for back pain and the Tree, Cobra, Backward Bend, and Crocodile poses for "sciatica".

In Traditional Chinese Medicine (TCM), LBS is differentiated into a chronic or acute condition. A chronic condition includes weak and aching muscles interspersed between more intense episodes of muscle spasms or pain and tends to be long term. A deficiency of the Kidney energy (Qi) is the root cause. Acute LBS comes on suddenly, usually with heavy lifting or overwork. The pain is intense, stabbing, and causes rigidity and stiffness of the muscles. The diagnosis is Qi and Blood stagnation in the Urinary Bladder (UB) channel; often some degree of Kidney deficiency is present as well. Acupuncture and Chinese herbs are used for low back pain. In addition, Qi gong may be helpful.

Shiatsu, a form of Eastern massage (Brady et al, 2001), may also provide relief for low back pain. Table 7-5 lists some alternative health care system therapies for LBS.

MIND-BODY-SPIRIT INTERVENTIONS FOR LOW BACK STRAIN

The *2001 Clinical Evidence Handbook* (van Tulder, Koes, 2001) reviews research that supports cognitive-behavioral therapy as an effective means for managing acute low back pain. When compared with biofeedback, risk factor–based cognitive-behavioral therapy reduced pain more in a group of 50 patients with acute low back pain and sciatica. Furthermore, behavioral therapy was more effective in reducing low back pain and perceived disability than were analgesics and back exercises in a group of 107 people after a treatment period of 9 to 12 months (van Tulder, Koes, 2001; Turner, 1996).

Imagery and prayer have been studied as therapeutic modalities for chronic pain; however, limited data are available for treating low back pain specifically. Naparstek (1995a) has developed a guided imagery audiotape designed for pain relief that may be effective with patients who suffer from low back pain. Similarly, patients with back pain may benefit from prayer. In a study that examined religious coping and pain, Bush and colleagues (1999) found that positive religious coping strategies were associated with a positive effect. Affirmation may help promote optimism and hope. Table 7-6 presents mind-body-spirit NAC therapies that may be helpful in treating low back pain.

BIOLOGIC-BASED THERAPIES FOR LOW BACK STRAIN

The herb devil's claw has been used for the treatment of lumbago because of its apparent antiinflammatory effect, although research is

Table 7-5 Alternative Health Care Systems for Low Back Strain

Intervention	Management	Treatment Regimen	Cautions, Precautions, Interactions	References
Ayurveda				
Yoga	Helps relieve back pain "Sciatica"	Cat, Pelvic Lift, Dance of the Legs, Relaxation poses, Tree, Cobra, Backward Bend, Crocodile	Qualified practitioner recommended to teach yoga; some participants may not be able to perform some poses; poses are performed gently and without force	Jones, 1998; Nespor, 1989
Traditional Chinese Medicine				
Acupuncture	Provides pain relief	For chronic conditions: Kidney 3 and UB 23 to support the Kidney; local tender points on the low back; UB 40 or 60 as a distal point to open channel stagnation. For acute conditions: local tender points to relieve	Qualified practitioner needed; inform acupuncturist of pregnancy (certain points are avoided if patient is pregnant); advise acupuncturist of medications, especially anticoagulants,	Cherkin, 2001; Ernst et al, 1998; Maciocia, 1994; NIH, 1997; Smith-Fassler et al, 2001

Continued

		stagnation in channel; Governing Vessel 3, 4, and 8; distal points depending on location of strain; sessions are 2-3 times/wk for acute problem. Wean gradually as condition allows	glucocorticoids, and anticonvulsants; if Kidney deficiency is present, treat 1-2 times/month after condition is stable
Qi gong	Provides pain relief	Daily practice of meditation, physical movement, and breathing exercises is recommended	Promising preliminary results; qualified instructor needed to teach	Berman et al, 1997; Ernst, 2001
Chinese herbs	Helps relieve chronic and acute back strain	Niu Xi (Radix Achyranthis Bidentatae) nourishes Kidney and relieves Blood stagnation; Sang Ji Sheng (Ramus Loranthi) nourishes Kidney and Blood; Du Zhong (Cortex Eucommiae Ulmoidis) tonifies Kidney and promotes circulation. Herbs are combined into a formula for best effect;	Chronic Kidney deficiency requires herbal treatment for several months to a year; an acute strain is treated with a formula to move Qi and Blood for 1-2 wks, followed by a supportive formula for 3-4 wks; use is always dependent on individual	Bensky et al, 1986; Maciocia, 1994

Table 7-5 Alternative Health Care Systems for Low Back Strain—cont'd

Intervention	Management	Treatment Regimen	Cautions, Precautions, Interactions	References
Chinese herbs, cont'd		many other herbs are considered to treat the specific imbalance.	response; an experienced herbalist should be consulted to ensure accurate diagnosis and treatment; use of an inappropriate formula may exacerbate symptoms	
Shiatsu	Decreases pain and anxiety	Multiple sessions over several months are usually recommended	May be uncomfortable initially; sessions may not be covered by insurance, Medicaid, or Medicare	Brady et al, 2001

UB, *Urinary Bladder.*

Table 7-6	Mind-Body-Spirit Interventions for Low Back Strain			
Intervention	Management	Treatment Regimen	Cautions, Precautions, Interactions	References
Affirmation	Helps self-esteem; Hay considers the back as the "support of life" (p. 16)	For the back: "I know that Life always supports me" (p. 16); for low back: "I trust the process of life. All I need is always taken care of. I am safe" (p. 16)	Participant says a positive, personal, present-tense statement	Hay, 2000
Biofeedback	Reduces muscle spasm or teaches patient to relax one set of muscles while strengthening other muscles	EMG biofeedback training; varied sessions and regular sessions are needed	Qualified practitioner needed	Freeman, Lawlis, 2001
Cognitive-behavioral therapy	May reduce pain and perceived disability	Counseling needed. See Chapter 2.	Qualified counselor in cognitive-behavioral therapy and pain management needed	Turner, 1996; van Tulder, Koes, 2001
Hypnosis	May help reduce pain, depression, time to sleep, and medications	Self-hypnosis	Skilled practitioner needed. No driving or operating machinery	McCauley, 1983

Continued

Table 7-6 Mind-Body-Spirit Interventions for Low Back Strain—cont'd

Intervention	Management	Treatment Regimen	Cautions, Precautions, Interactions	References
Imagery	May help reduce pain	Audiotapes for imagery include Naparstek, *Pain* (1995) and *Stress I and Stress II* (1995)	No driving or operating machinery while listening to audiotapes	Naparstek [audiotapes], 1995a, 1995b
Meditation-prayer	May relieve stress and improve affect, quality of life, and optimism; enhances psychologic well being; reduces pain; gives insight; provides positive form of coping	Intercessory (interested person prays for another) or personal prayer as preferred by patient.		Bush, 1999; Dunn et al, 2000; King et al, 1994; Meisenhelder et al, 2000; Shuler et al, 1994; Wirth el al, 1994
Relaxation	Decreases time to fall asleep medication use, and pain	Various techniques may be used	No driving or operating machinery while practicing relaxation	McCauley, 1983

needed to confirm effectiveness (PL/PL, 2002). Another herb, rosemary, has been used topically for joint and musculoskeletal pain. The effectiveness of rosemary in treating low back pain has not been systematically studied; however, low back pain may be somewhat relieved with topical application of rosemary oil because it appears to improve circulation (PL/PL, 2002). Similarly, aromatherapy may be beneficial and comforting for low back pain. Table 7-7 lists a few biologic-based therapies for LBS.

MANIPULATIVE AND BODY-BASED METHODS AND ENERGY THERAPIES FOR LOW BACK STRAIN

Chiropractic manipulation, massage, magnets, MET, and transcutaneous stimulation may provide relief of pain and improved mobility for some patients. Chiropractic manipulation "best evidence synthesis" suggests that "as a treatment of acute or chronic back pain" spinal manipulation "is supported by moderately conclusive evidence" (Ernst, 2001, p. 223). Osteopathic manipulation is probably as effective as is standard care (Ernst, 2001) and in many cases *is* standard care. Massage has not been studied in depth but anecdotally seems to provide comfort, increase circulation, and improve mobility. Similarly, healing touch, Therapeutic Touch, and Reiki may provide comfort. Table 7-8 presents a selection of therapies that may be helpful for treating uncomplicated LBS.

NAC THERAPIES FOR OSTEOARTHRITIS AND RHEUMATOID ARTHRITIS

Osteoarthritis

Osteoarthritis (OA) occurs when ulceration and loss of articular cartilage occur with sclerosis and eburnation (bone becomes dense and hard as ivory) of subchondral bone (Hochberg, 1997).

OA is the most common type of arthritis in the United States and is the second most common cause of long-term disability among adults (Peyron, Altman, 1992; Boh, 1997). The weight-bearing joints, lumbosacral spine, hips, knees, and feet are most commonly affected. Risk factors for the development of OA include the following: (1) middle age to older adult; (2) occupation or sports activity that subjects particular joints to repetitive trauma; (3) obesity; (4) woman after age 55; (5) history of joint trauma or fracture; (6) history of bone or joint disorders; (7) history of inflammatory arthritis, acromegaly, hemochromatosis, ochronosis, or chondrocalcinosis; and (8) presence of rare inherited genetic mutations of collagen (Fife, 1997).

Symptoms include mild-to-moderate localized pain and stiffness surrounding the affected joint, with limitation of function. Pain increases with joint use and decreases with rest. Morning stiffness, usually 30 minutes or less, is present; and symptoms worsen during

Table 7-7 Biologic-Based Therapies for Low Back Strain

A complete prescribing source should be consulted before using biologic therapies. Nutrient doses may be above the recommended daily allowance or tolerable upper limit. In illness or deficiency, such doses may be acceptable; however, long-term use may not be appropriate. Herbs may cause allergic reactions and interactions. Herbs are generally contraindicated or not recommended for women during pregnancy and lactation and for children unless research data or a long history of safe use has been established.

Intervention	Management	Treatment Regimen	Cautions, Precautions, Interactions	References
Devil's claw (*Harpagophytum procumbens*); traditional native African folk remedy	Provides pain relief and antiinflammatory activity comparable to phenylbutazone	Oral use: one study used powdered devil's claw root 2.6 g/day; also 1.0-4.5 g/day; root is used; can make tea with 4.5 g of root in 300 ml boiled water steeped for 8 hrs at room temperature then strained; makes three portions	Should not be used if patient has gastric or duodenal ulcers, heartburn, gastritis, or gallstones because devil's claw promotes secretion of stomach acid; drug interactions may occur	Chrubasik et al, 1996; DerMarderosian, 2001; PL/PL, 2002
Rosemary	Provides pain relief	Topical use: pour 1 c of boiling water over 1-2 tsp of herb, steep	External application may ease muscle pain, sciatica, and	Hoffman, 1994; PL/PL, 2002

		for 10-15 minutes; make poultice and apply to affected area	neuralgia; no controlled studies for back pain identified; the concentrated essential oil of rosemary should not be taken internally	

Aromatherapy

Analgesic or calming essential oils. Analgesic oils—lemongrass, rosemary, frankincense, juniper, rose, ginger, verbena, spike lavender, peppermint, myrrh, clove bud, ylang ylang, true lavender, sweet marjoram, black pepper. Antispasmodic	May provide comfort	For massage: 2-5 gtts of essential oil in 5 ml carrier oil to make a 2%-5% solution. For compress: 1-5 gtts in a bowl of warm water, wring compress, and apply. For inhalation: 1-2 gtts on a tissue	Check for allergy. Oil must be pure essential oil. Must be diluted with carrier oil such as almond oil; allow patients to smell before applying; oils not for ingestion. Caution regarding the topical application effects of sage: sage contains thujone and is considered unsafe when taken orally in excess, since it may cause menstrual	Buckle, 1997, 2001; PL/PL, 2002

Continued

Table 7-7	Biologic-Based Therapies for Low Back Strain—cont'd			
Intervention	Management	Treatment Regimen	Cautions, Precautions, Interactions	References
Aromatherapy—cont'd				
oils—Roman chamomile, lemon-scented eucalyptus, sage (Salvia officinalis)			stimulation and possible abortifacient effects. Read safety issues for other oils	

Gtts, Drops.

Table 7-8 Manipulative and Body-Based Methods and Energy Therapies for Low Back Strain

Intervention	Management	Treatment Regimen	Cautions, Precautions, Interactions	References
Chiropractic manipulation	Provides pain relief	Varies with individual. Appears to be effective for acute low back pain.	Study results are mixed regarding effectiveness of chiropractic manipulation; may be the same as physical therapy	Bonfort, 1999; Cherkin et al, 1998; Waddell, 1999; Weintraub, 2001
Massage	Provides pain relief	Varies with individual; may have Swedish massage for relaxation, or deep-tissue or neuromuscular massage for specific area	May need 1 mo of therapy before pain is resolved; massage is not done immediately after injury	Preyde, 2000
Bipolar permanent magnets and magnets	May reduce pain	Varies. One study treatment: 6 hrs for 3 times for 1 wk, then repeat for 1 more wk	Further research needed; limited studies have been conducted in this area with conflicting results; no substantial scientific data established; treatment has focused on patients with chronic rather than acute low back pain	Collacott et al, 2000 Weintraub, 2001

Continued

Table 7-8 Manipulative and Body-Based Methods and Energy Therapies for Low Back Strain—cont'd

Intervention	Management	Treatment Regimen	Cautions, Precautions, Interactions	References
TENS	Decreases pain; improves mobility	Varies with individual	Study results are mixed regarding the beneficial effects of TENS in relieving acute low back pain; short-term relief has been demonstrated for relief of chronic low back pain; therapeutic effect may not be demonstrated until 6 wks of therapy is completed	Gadsby et al, 2000; Marchand et al, 1993
MET	Reduces pain; promotes healing	Varies with individual	Use with caution or not at all if patient has pacemaker; resuscitation may be required	Meyer et al, 1983
Healing touch, Therapeutic Touch, and Reiki	May help provide comfort	Sessions last for 30-60 min; first 3 Reiki sessions should be close together (e.g., daily for 3 days)	Obtain permission from patient	Krieger, 1993; Mentgen, 2001; Quinn, 2002; Stein, 1997; Umbreit, 2002

MET, Micro-current electrical therapy; TENS, transcutaneous electrical nerve stimulation.

damp, cool, or rainy weather. In addition, joint instability is present, especially the knees. Signs include bony enlargement, tenderness at joint margins, decreased range of motion, and crepitus. Radiographic features include bony proliferation at the joint margin and asymmetric joint space narrowing. Subchondral sclerosis, subchondral cysts, and bone remodeling may become apparent as the disease progresses.

The goal of using NAC therapies for patients with OA is to improve quality of life, minimize joint damage, improve function, relieve pain, and provide comfort. Physical and occupational therapy can have beneficial effects through muscle strengthening, aerobic conditioning, and improvement in range of motion (Farhey, Hess, 2001). Furthermore, appliances and assistive devices such as braces, splints, and canes can reduce inflammation, improve joint alignment, and decrease joint trauma (Farhey, Hess, 2001).

Rheumatoid Arthritis

Rheumatoid arthritis (RA) is a chronic, inflammatory, systemic disease that affects predominately the diarthrodial joints (Goronzy, Weyand, 1997). RA is an inflammatory polyarthritis with a wide spectrum of features and varying degrees of joint destruction (Korn, 2001). Clinical features vary among patients and within individual patients as the disease progresses. A specific cause of the disease is unknown; however, genetic and environmental factors are associated with the extent, progression, and pattern of inflammatory response (Goronzy, Weyand, 1997). Because no unique features of the disease have been identified, symptoms and signs are features of the diagnostic criteria for RA. Diagnosis is based on the following set of criteria (Arnett et al, 1988; Klippel, 1997): (1) morning stiffness for greater than 30 minutes; (2) arthritis of three or more joint areas; (3) arthritis of hand joints; (4) symmetric arthritis; (5) rheumatoid nodules; (6) serum rheumatoid factor; and (7) radiographic changes.

Rheumatoid factor (RF) is detected in serum of 85% of patients with RA. The presence of RF often correlates with severe, unremitting disease, nodules, and extra-articular lesions. The erythrocyte sedimentation rate (ESR) typically correlates with the degree of synovial inflammation (Anderson, 1997). Posteroanterior hand and wrist radiographs indicate erosion and unequivocal bony decalcification, either localized or adjacent to involved joints (Arnett et al, 1988). HCPs are familiar with the use of natural techniques such as physical therapy, occupational therapy, and appliances or devices (braces and splints) in treating RA. These techniques can maintain joint mobility and protect joints from injury and deformity as well.

For treating RA a window of opportunity exists to gain control for a more positive outcome and possibly slow disease progression. *The Prescriber's Letter* (2002) states that patients even with early RA need more than nonsteroidal antiinflammatory drugs (NSAIDs). Thus early conventional intervention is necessary:

> Maintaining normal joint structure and anatomy can only be achieved by controlling the disease before any irreversible damage has occurred. Studies have revealed that DMARD [disease-modifying antirheumatic drug] therapy early in the course of RA slowed disease progression more effectively than did delayed use. This has led to a general agreement that the inflammation of RA should be controlled as completely as possible, as soon as possible, and that this control should be maintained for as long as possible. (Gornisiewicz, Moreland, 2001, p. 93)

A variety of NAC therapies are available that have been beneficial in relieving the symptoms associated with both OA and RA. The purpose of including NAC therapies in the treatment regimen for patients with RA is to reduce inflammation, provide analgesia and comfort, improve joint mobility, provide further protection, and emphasize the prevention of deformity (Kolasinski, 2001). The practitioner must have thorough knowledge of current conventional OA and RA therapies to ensure safe introduction of NAC regimens.

ALTERNATIVE HEALTH CARE SYSTEMS FOR OSTEOARTHRITIS AND RHEUMATOID ARTHRITIS

Ayurveda for Arthritis

Ayurveda distinguishes three types of arthritis that correspond to each of the three primary doshas (vata, pitta, and kapha). All types of arthritis are viewed as originating in the colon when one of the doshas goes out of balance. The resulting slowing down of the digestive fire (agni) leads to the accumulation of toxic by-products of inadequate digestion (ama). This ama travels through the system and lodges in the bone and joint tissues, eventually causing the pain and stiffness characteristic of arthritis. Therefore the overall aim of Ayurvedic treatment of all types of arthritis is to remove the ama from the joints, bring it back into the colon, and eliminate it.

Vata-type arthritis is characterized by dry joints that crack and pop, are cold but not swollen, and are painful at one particularly tender spot, mainly on movement. Any strenuous weight-bearing exercise aggravates the pain. Pitta-type arthritis, in contrast, is associated with inflamed, red, hot joints that are painful even without movement. In kapha-type arthritis, however, the joints are cold, swollen, and stiff, and a little movement decreases the pain. Characteristically, kapha-type arthritis pain, as compared with the other two types, is worse in the morning and decreases as the individual gets up and moves around (Lad, 1998). In addition to the dosha-specific types of arthritis, Ayurvedic practitioners have used measures for the Western medical diagnoses of RA and OA. Ayurvedic treatments for arthritis are listed in Table 7-9.

Table 7-9 Alternative Health Care Systems for Arthritis

A complete prescribing source should be consulted before using biologic therapies. Herbs may cause allergic reactions and interactions. Herbs are generally contraindicated or not recommended for women during pregnancy and lactation and for children unless research data or a long history of safe use has been established.

Intervention	Management	Treatment Regimen	Cautions, Precautions, Interactions	References
Ayurveda				
Diet therapy	For vata-type arthritis	Vata-pacifying (balancing) diet encouraged; warm, easy-to-digest foods are recommended.	Avoid cold foods and drinks, beans, drying grains (e.g., barley and corn), and the nightshades (e.g., tomatoes, potatoes, eggplant)	Lad, 1998
	For pitta-type arthritis	Pitta-pacifying or reducing diet is encouraged; favored foods include most sweet fruits (e.g., figs, grapes, mangos), sweet and bitter vegetables (e.g.,	Avoid hot, spicy, sour, and fermented foods; in particular, avoid sour fruits (e.g., cranberries, oranges), pungent vegetables (e.g., garlic, onions, spinach, tomatoes),	Frawley et al, 1988

Continued

Table 7-9 Alternative Health Care Systems for Arthritis—cont'd

Intervention	Management	Treatment Regimen	Cautions, Precautions, Interactions	References
Ayurveda—cont'd				
Diet therapy, cont'd		broccoli, carrots, peas), soft cheese, white meat chicken or turkey, and freshwater fish	yogurt and sour cream, red meat, seafood, and sour and spicy condiments (e.g., pickles, chili pepper mustard)	
	For kapha-type arthritis	Kapha-reducing diet is encouraged.	Especially avoid dairy products and cold drinks	Lad, 1998
	For osteoarthritis	Use turmeric in cooking (active ingredient: curcumin); curries and similar dishes should be frequently included		Castleman, 2000
	For rheumatoid arthritis	Cook with turmeric and ginger	Avoid ginger if inflammatory skin condition, fever, bleeding, or ulcers are present; avoid turmeric if high-pitta condition, acute	Castleman, 2000; Srivastava, 1992

Continued

Herbal therapy	For all types arthritis: to cleanse colon	Triphala: take 1 tsp in ½-1 c warm water hs Nutritive herbs (e.g., shatavari, ashwagandha): mix with sesame oil, ghee, or milk, and use as a gentle enema	jaundice, or hepatitis is present; avoid during pregnancy	Lad, 1998
	For vata-type arthritis: to cleanse colon	Haritaki: ½ tsp in ½-1 c warm water hs	Not to be used during pregnancy. May cause dehydration, severe exhaustion or emaciation, or excess pitta	Lad, 1998; Frawley et al, 1988
	For vata-type arthritis	Yogaraj guggulu: 1 tab tid		Lad, 1998; Frawley et al, 1988
	For pitta-type arthritis: to cleanse colon	Amalaki: take 5 g powder in 1 c of warm water bid	Can cause acute diarrhea	Lad, 1998; Frawley et al, 1988
	For pitta-type arthritis	Kaishore guggul: 350 mg with warm water tid		Lad, 1998

Table 7-9 Alternative Health Care Systems for Arthritis—cont'd

Intervention	Management	Treatment Regimen	Cautions, Precautions, Interactions	References
Ayurveda—cont'd				
Herbal therapy, cont'd		Sudarshan: ½ tsp with warm water bid		
	For kapha-type arthritis: to cleanse colon	Bibhitaki powder: 250 mg in warm water bid	High vata	Lad, 1998; Frawley et al, 1988
	For kapha-type arthritis	Punarnava guggulu: take one 250-mg tab tid		Lad, 1998; Frawley et al, 1988
	For osteoarthritis	Yogaraj guggulu: 1 tab bid; Gandharva haritaki (herb sautéed in castor oil): ½ tsp hs or 2 tsp castor oil in 1 cup ginger tea hs	Has laxative effect	Kulkarni, 1991; Lad, 1998
		Curcumin: 400 mg tid		
	For rheumatoid arthritis	Simhanada: 350 mg tid; Chitrak adhivati: 200 mg bid; Yogaraj guggulu: ¼ tsp with warm water tid; castor oil with natural steroid	Has laxative effect	Castleman, 2000 Lad, 1998

		precursors: 2 tsp in 1 cup ginger tea hs *Boswellia serrata* (also called Indian Frankincense): Two 150-mg caps tid for 1 month, then 1 cap tid Curcumin: 300 mg tid	Boswellia is leukotriene-B4 inhibitor	Etzel, 1996; PL/PL, 2002
Marma point therapy	For all types of arthritis	Apply pressure to Shanka Marma (temples) and Utek Shepa Marma (just below temples)	Using thumb or fingers, apply firm but not painful pressure and hold it for 3 min, then gently massage area	Castleman, 2000 Frawley et al, 2001
	For vata-type arthritis	Stimulation of points between eyebrows and on crown of head (Sthapani and Adhipati Marmas), or apply stimulating oil (e.g., camphor or eucalyptus) to area and leave on until next shower	Apply firm but not painful thumb pressure for 1-3 min	Frawley et al, 2001
External applications	For vata-type arthritis	Medicated oils and heat; mahanarayan oil; apply to affected joints		Lad, 1998

Continued

Table 7-9 Alternative Health Care Systems for Arthritis—cont'd

Intervention	Management	Treatment Regimen	Cautions, Precautions, Interactions	References
Ayurveda—cont'd				
External applications, cont'd		followed by local application of moist heat		
		Warm sesame oil medicated with herb (e.g., sandalwood, shatavari, or ashwagandha); massage over affected joints		
	For pitta-type arthritis	Cooling external applications. Cool coconut or castor oil; rubbed gently over affected joints bid	Lad, 1998	
		Sandalwood paste: mix 1 tsp powder with enough water to make paste; rubbed gently over affected joints bid		
		Apply ice bag to inflamed painful joints for 20 min tid	Contraindicated if high-kapha condition or lung congestion is present	

	For kapha-type arthritis	Calamus root paste: mix 1 tsp powder in enough water to make a paste, and apply to affected joints	FDA prohibits calamus use in food products because of presence of carcinogenic constituent beta-isoasarone in 3 of the 4 distinct strains; however, content varies widely; not recommended for internal use; likely unsafe	Frawley et al, 1988; Lad, 1998; PL/PL, 2002
		Punarnarva and ginger paste: mix 1 tsp of each herb with small amount water; apply to joints with effusion		Frawley et al, 1988; Lad, 1998
Yoga	Decreases pain and joint tenderness; improves range of motion in patients with RA	Daily practice of various asanas (postures) is recommended	Some movements may need to be modified or avoided depending on individual; use gentle, careful movements	Garfinkel et al, 1994; Hastock et al, 1994

Continued

Table 7-9 Alternative Health Care Systems for Arthritis—cont'd

Intervention	Management	Treatment Regimen	Cautions, Precautions, Interactions	References
Ayurveda—cont'd				
Yoga, cont'd	For vata-type arthritis	Forward Bend, Chest-Knee, Maha Mudra, Half Bridge, simple sitting poses (e.g., Easy Pose) are recommended	Perform gently and consistently without straining	Frawley et al, 2001; Lad, 1998
	For pitta-type arthritis	Boat, Bow, Camel, Cow, and Locust poses, Moon Salutation are recommended	Practice gently for 20-30+ min/day as tolerated; avoid strain on joints	Lad, 1998
	For kapha-type arthritis	Tree, Triangle, Forward Bend, Spinal Twist poses are recommended	Practice 20-30+ min/day as tolerated	Frawley et al, 1988; Lad, 1998
Breathing exercises	For pitta-type arthritis	Cooling breath exercise; Sitali Pranayama; make a tube of tongue, breathe deeply through the mouth, hold a few seconds, then exhale through the nose; do 12 repetitions		Lad, 1998

Traditional Chinese Medicine

Acupuncture	Open meridians to spread Qi and Blood; expels invading pathogens; may help osteoarthritis pain, function; has been used for RA; studies "flawed"	Points are needled in the area of pain and distal to the pain on the same channel to open blockage; points are also chosen to eliminate specific pathogens. To expel wind: UB 12, GB 31, and TW 6. To expel cold: Stomach 36, UB 10 and 23, Ren 6, and Governing Vessel 3 and 14, all with moxibustion. To clear heat: LI 4 and 11 and Stomach 43. To expel damp: Spleen 6 and 9, GB 34, and UB 20	Treat 1-2 times/wk until condition stabilizes; follow-up treatment may be needed every 3-4 wks for several months depending on patient response; acupuncture needles over the chest and upper back are inserted obliquely to avoid puncturing the lungs	Berman et al, 1995; Christensen, 1992; Ernst, 1997; Ezzo et al, 2001; Gaw et al, 1975; Maciocia, 1994; Takeda et al, 1994; see Appendix B for meridians and points
Moxibustion	Warms the channels and improves circulation	Moxibustion is the burning of the mugwort herb on or over the acupuncture needles	Care is taken while using moxibustion to avoid burning the skin	Maciocia, 1994
Acupressure	For OA and RA; may provide pain relief;	Finger or hand pressure is applied to balance Qi;	Qualified practitioner is needed or participant	Gach, 1990; Horstman, 1999

Continued

| Table 7-9 | Alternative Health Care Systems for Arthritis—cont'd |

Intervention	Management	Treatment Regimen	Cautions, Precautions, Interactions	References
Traditional Chinese Medicine—cont'd				
Acupressure, cont'd	increases range of motion and relaxation	uses acupuncture points LI 4 and 11, TW 5, Stomach 36, and GB 20	may learn to do own points. Do not have to use all the points. No studies conducted	Farrell et al, 1999; Horstman, 1999
Qi gong	For OA and RA; improves balance; relieves stress; improves depression	Daily practice of meditation, physical movement, and breathing exercises is recommended	Qualified instructor needed to teach the practice	
Tai chi	For OA and RA; helps build muscle strength; improves balance; relieves stress; improves depression	Daily practice for 12 wks improved quality of life, self-efficacy, and functional mobility among older adults with OA (Hartman study). May reduce risk of falls; can be combined with dance therapy	Need instruction to begin; considered a safe weight-bearing exercise for patients with RA	Farrell et al, 1999; Hartman et al, 2000; Kirsteins et al, 1991; van Deusen et al, 1987; Wolf et al, 1996; Wolfson et al, 1996

Thunder god vine (Tripterygium vilfordii)	For RA (reduces signs and symptoms)	30 mg/day of extract was used in one study; Chinese studies.	SE: GI upset, lymphocyte suppression, infertility, amenorrhea, one incident of death; showed cytotoxicity in cultured mammalian cell lines	DerMarderosian, 2001; Ernst, 2001; PL/PL, 2002
Homeopathy				
Individualized homeopathic remedies	Provides improvement in pain, stiffness, and grip strength in patients with RA; may relieve symptoms of OA	Treatment is designed to fit individual needs	Symptoms may initially worsen dramatically for a brief period before improving	Ernst, 2001; Fisher et al, 1989; Gibson et al, 1980; Jonas et al, 2000

Bid, *Twice daily*; FDA, *U.S. Food and Drug Administration*; GB, *gallbladder*; GI, *gastrointestinal*; hs, *bedtime*; LI, *large intestine*; OA, *osteoarthritis*; RA, *rheumatoid arthritis*; SE, *side effects*; tid, *three times daily*; TW, *triple warmer (also called San Jiao)*; UB, *urinary bladder*.

Traditional Chinese Medicine for Arthritis

Acupuncture and acupressure have been used for thousands of years in Asia with strong overall evidence that these ancient Chinese practices can ease the pain of arthritis (Horstman, 1999). In TCM, arthritis is known as "painful obstruction syndrome." This syndrome refers to the pain, stiffness, or numbness of the joints, muscles, and tendons. The condition occurs when the circulation of Qi and Blood through the acupuncture meridians is "obstructed" by an invasion of wind, cold, heat, or damp conditions. The symptoms differ when each of the following elements invade:

- Wind blockage: the pain in joints is widespread and moves from one area of the body to another.
- Cold blockage: severe pain improves with warmth to the area and is worse with cold weather.
- Heat blockage (similar to rheumatoid arthritis): the area is hot, red, and swollen with limitation of movement and severe pain.
- Damp blockage: pain or soreness is localized and does not move. A feeling of heaviness and numbness of limbs is present. Pain is aggravated by damp weather.
- A combination of the different types of blockage often occur. (Maciocia, 1994)

The treatment strategy is to open meridians to spread Qi and Blood and to expel invading pathogens. Table 7-9 offers alternative health care system modalities for arthritis.

MIND-BODY-SPIRIT INTERVENTIONS FOR OSTEOARTHRITIS AND RHEUMATOID ARTHRITIS

For reducing inflammatory symptoms and pain, research suggests using intercessory prayer. Matthews and colleagues (1998) prospectively studied 40 patients diagnosed with RA. All patients who received direct-contact intercessory prayer showed significant overall improvement during the one year follow-up. Astin and colleagues (2000 in Ernst 2001) published a review of randomized trials of distant healing, and Ernst comments that "the question of whether spiritual healing alleviates arthritic pain more than placebo does not find a uniform answer in these studies" (p. 341). However, because religious or spiritual activities, including prayer, have been significantly related to a positive effect among patients experiencing chronic pain (Bush et al, 1999) and improved quality of life for patients with chronic disease (Flannelly, Inouye, 2001), prayer and other faith-based activities may be beneficial in treating pain for patients with both OA or RA.

Cognitive-behavioral therapy and coping skills may be beneficial for arthritis patients (Keefe et al, 2001). In a randomized, controlled clinical trial, Bradley and colleagues (1987) examined the effects of various psychologic therapies on patients with RA. Relaxation training

> ### Box 7-1
>
> Principles of Joint Protection and Energy Conservation
>
> Respect pain—know what is usual and what is not
> Balance work and rest
> Conserve energy
> Avoid positions of deformity
> Use larger or stronger joints
> Use each joint in its most stable plane
> Avoid staying in one position

Adapted from Luck J: Enhancing functional ability. In Robbins L, ed: Clinical care in the rheumatic diseases, *ed 2, Atlanta, Ga, 2001, Association of Rhemuatology Health Professionals.*

was found to be a significant NAC therapy in reducing pain, disease activity, and anxiety. Imagery, biofeedback, journaling, and hypnosis may also be useful (Achterberg et al, 1981; Day, 2001; Ernst, 2001; Naparstek, 1992; Smyth, 1999; Weissenberg, 1998). Social support may moderate pain, functional ability, and depression levels for people with OA (Blixen, Kippes, 1999; Keefe et al, 2001).

Movement also seems to be an important component of pain management for patients with both OA and RA. Movement techniques such as exercise, Tai chi (Kirsteins et al, 1991) and yoga (Haslock et al, 1994) have been used. The Arthritis Foundation (Klippel, 1997) recognizes the benefits of an exercise program that focuses on range-of-motion activities and muscle strengthening for patients with arthritis. The primary goal of exercise is to focus on maintaining joint function and joint protection. Box 7-1 covers principles of joint protection and energy conservation. Table 7-10 summarizes various mind-body-spirit therapies that may be beneficial in treating patients with OA or RA.

BIOLOGIC-BASED THERAPIES FOR OSTEOARTHRITIS AND RHEUMATOID ARTHRITIS

A growing body of evidence suggests that glucosamine sulfate is an effective disease-modifying agent that can reduce joint narrowing and pain. Reginster and colleagues (2001) conducted a randomized, double-blind, placebo-controlled trial in which 212 patients with OA of the knee were randomly assigned to receive either 1500 mg of oral glucosamine sulfate or placebo daily over a 3-year period. Patients who received the glucosamine sulfate reported pain improvement, and radiologic findings indicated maintenance of joint space during the treatment period. Similarly, Verbruggen and colleagues (1998),

Table 7-10 Mind-Body-Spirit Interventions for OA and RA

Intervention	Management	Treatment Regimen	Cautions, Precautions, Interactions	References
Biofeedback	May help reduce pain and tension; improves sleep	Individual plan is developed; EMG, temperature biofeedback taught to patient. Therapy was combined with relaxation therapy in the RA study		Achterberg et al, 1981
Cognitive-behavioral therapy	For OA and RA: patients with RA have shown decreased pain, pain behavior, anxiety, and depression as compared with social support group	Steps include: (1) rationale for treatment; (2) training in coping skills; (3) training in methods for maintenance of coping skills to prevent setbacks in coping efforts	Practitioner needs knowledge in this area or appropriate referral resources	Bradley et al, 1987; Keefe et al, 2001
Coping skills	Adjustment to chronic disease needed	Teaching is from the easiest to the most difficult strategies: from relaxation, to imagery,	Trained practitioner or referral resources needed	Keefe et al, 2001

		to activity-rest pacing, to cognitive restructuring		
Dance	May increase ROM in RA	Dance program can be combined with Tai chi and imagery	Safety is a concern	van Deusen, 1987
Exercise	Provides pain relief; may need fewer medications; increases walking distance for patients with OA of one or both knees	Fitness walking, aerobic, resistance, and flexibility exercises are used	Safety is a concern; start with easy exercises	Klippel, 1997; Kovar et al, 1992; Pizzorno, 1995
Hypnosis	May help decrease OA and RA symptoms	Several sessions are usually needed	Skilled therapist needed; needs study	Ernst, 2001; Weissenberg, 1998
Imagery	Relieves OA and RA symptoms; gives sense of control; provides relaxation	Naparstek Audiotapes: Pain (1995) and A Guided Meditation to Help You with Rheumatoid Arthritis or Lupus (1992)	No driving or operating machinery while listening to audiotapes	Naparstek [audiotapes], 1992, 1995a
Journaling/writing	Provides a possible way to express when talking is	Writings can be any style: poetry or narrative; Day suggests	Privacy of the journal may be important	Day, 2001; Smyth et al, 1999

Continued

Table 7-10 Mind-Body-Spirit Interventions for OA and RA—cont'd

Intervention	Management	Treatment Regimen	Cautions, Precautions, Interactions	References
Journaling/ writing, cont'd	difficult; provides a means of self-discovery and self-reflection; provides creative outlet; encourages positive coping	"AlphaPoem," captured moments, character sketch, clustering (free association around a central word), dialogue, inner wisdom, list of 100 (e.g., 100 ways to nurture myself), different points of view, unsent letter		
Prayer-spirituality	Provides pain relief and hope and positive method of coping; improves health perception and resourcefulness	May use various ways of praying and expressing spirituality. Regular prayer or meditation is encouraged as is attendance at religious services or other spiritual connection.	HCP needs nonjudgmental approach; respect individual preferences	Astin et al, 2000; Bill-Harvey et al, 1989; Matthews et al, 1998; Mackenzie et al, 2000; Potter et al, 2000; Strawbridge et al, 1997

Psychologic counseling	Provides a means to deal with pain and loss; provides reconciliation; improves coping; provides a means to regain hope	Spiritual healing is encouraged. Appropriate referral for the individual is provided. May need to give several choices of different types of therapists.	Need skilled therapist; HCP needs to have appropriate and varied referrals	Bradley et al, 1987
Relaxation	Decrease OA and RA symptoms; helps relieve pain and tension; improves mood, walking, and bending	Progressive muscle relaxation or other forms such as autogenics. See Chapter 2 and 12 for examples	Special instruction needed; then participant can self-start	Lundgren et al, 1999; Peck, 1998
Rest	Helps relieve RA symptoms; promotes general good health; offsets fatigue	General rest and joint-specific rest is advised; time, place, position techniques are taught; goal is to establish regular night sleep and 30-60 min morning and afternoon rest periods	Approach with a positive attitude	Minor et al, 2001

Continued

Table 7-10 Mind-Body-Spirit Interventions for OA and RA—cont'd

Intervention	Management	Treatment Regimen	Cautions, Precautions, Interactions	References
Social support	Helps relieve OA and RA symptoms; studies of patients with OA reveal long-term improvements in physical disability; may moderate pain, limitation, and depression	Social support is encouraged; help participant find networks, support groups; include informal networks (e.g., family, friends) and hobby groups, as well as formal networks	HCP needs resource base; cultural aspects to consider	Blixen et al, 1999; Keefe et al, 1999, 2001
Stress management	Helps relieve stress; improves coping	Counseling, affirmation, assertiveness, breathing, cognitive restructuring, imagery, meditation, prayer, relaxation are combined		Naparstek [audio tapes], 1995b; Parker et al, 1995; see Chapter 2 and Chapter 12

EMG, *Electromyogram*; HCP, *health care practitioner*; OA, *osteoarthritis*; RA, *rheumatoid arthritis*; ROM, *range of motion*.

who examined the effects of chondroitin sulfate on finger joints affected by OA, found a significant decrease in joint erosion in the patients who received chondroitin sulfate. The combined therapy of glucosamine sulphate, chondroitin, and manganese ascorbate (Das, Hammad, 2000; Leffler et al, 1999) in relieving the symptoms associated with osteoarthritis of the knee was also effective. Many products that have both glucosamine sulfate with chondroitin sulfate are combined to maximize the beneficial effects on joints affected by OA. However, no proof exists that these substances are better together than they are alone. In a metaanalysis of studies, investigating both chondroitin and glucosamine, the authors concluded:

> Trials of glucosamine and chondroitin preparations for OA symptoms demonstrate moderate to large effects, but quality issues and likely publication bias suggest that these effects are exaggerated. Nevertheless, some degree of efficacy appears probable for these preparations. (McAlindon et al, 2000, p. 1469)

Neither glucosamine sulfate nor chondroitin sulfate appears to have a therapeutic effect on joints affected by RA. However, patients with RA may benefit from oral ingestion of the mineral selenium. In a German, double-blind, placebo-controlled study, patients with RA who received selenium had significantly fewer tender points, less swelling, and less morning stiffness when compared with the control group (Heinle et al, 1997). In a study conducted by Kremer and colleagues (1990), patients with RA who ingested dietary fish oil showed significantly reduced joint pain. Ingestion of fish, evening primrose, and borage oils (Belch et al, 1998; Leventhal et al, 1993) may prove beneficial in improving function and reducing pain and inflammation of RA. "Low dietary intakes of copper, calcium, magnesium, zinc, vitamins D, E, and A, pyridoxine, folate, and omege-3 fatty acids have been reported consistently in adult and childhood forms of the disease [rheumatoid arthritis] by many investigators (Morgan et al, 1997; Stone et al, 1997)" (Fillmore et al, 1999; p. 675). Additionally, some evidence suggests that the trace mineral boron can reduce pain associated with OA and RA through antiinflammatory actions (Newnham, 1994). For osteoarthritis, Pizzorno (1995) suggests the supplements yucca; vitamins C and E; methionine; niacinamide; and eliminating from the diet tomatoes, potatoes, eggplant, peppers, and tobacco (Solanaceae family). Table 7-11 presents various biologic-based NAC therapies that may be beneficial in relieving symptoms associated with OA and RA.

MANIPULATIVE AND BODY-BASED METHODS AND ENERGY THERAPIES FOR OSTEOARTHRITIS AND RHEUMATOID ARTHRITIS

Massage therapy and chiropractic manipulation may provide symptom relief for some patients who have arthritis (Horstman, 1999;

Table 7-11 Biologic-Based Therapies for Osteoarthritis and Rheumatoid Arthritis

A complete prescribing source should be consulted before using biologic therapies. Nutrient doses may be above the recommended daily allowance or tolerable upper limit. In illness or deficiency, such doses may be acceptable; however, long-term use may not be appropriate. Herbs may cause allergic reactions and interactions. Herbs are generally contraindicated or not recommended for women during pregnancy and lactation and for children unless research data or a long history of safe use has been established. Patients with RA may be on numerous medications. Drug interactions should be determined with all biologic use.

Intervention	Management	Treatment Regimen	Cautions, Precautions, Interactions	References
Elimination diets	May reduce inflammatory symptoms of RA	Eliminate dairy or suspected offending foods or try a complete elimination diet	Some evidence suggests that when dairy is removed from diet, inflammatory symptoms improve	Panush et al, 1986; Parke, 1981; Ratner, 1985
Fasting followed by vegetarian diet	May provide decrease of symptoms and long-term decrease of pain	Duration will depend on overall condition	Close supervision and supplementation is needed; several trials from Scandinavia have been conducted	Ernst, 2001; Henderson, 1999
Dietary oil: omega-3 fatty acids, EPA, and	May be used with RA; In study, reduced NSAID	Fish oil is recommended; EPA: 3.8 g/day and DHA: 2 g/day; food	SE: GI upset; fish oils can reduce vitamin-E levels; omega-3 fatty	Belch, 1988; Caughey et al, 1996; Ernst,

DHA	consumption; decreased morning stiffness; may decrease inflammation and pain	sources include herring, mackerel, sardines, salmon, tuna. Also flaxseed has conflicting research for benefit with RA.	acids can decrease pulmonary function in aspirin-sensitive individuals; fish oil in doses greater than 6 g/day can increase blood glucose level; fish oils can lower BP; increased risk of bleeding can occur with anticoagulants; see other interactions	2000, 2001; Haggerty, 1999; Kremer et al, 1990; Lau, 1993; Leventhal, 1993; McCarthy, Kenny, 1992; Nordstrom et al, 1995; PL/PL, 2002; Zurier, 1996
Dietary oil: GLA (one of the omega-6 fatty acids)	May reduce RA inflammation	GLA: 1.1 g/day; evening primrose or borage oil is often used as a source of GLA	Might prolong bleeding time, especially if used with other herbs or drugs that increase bleeding potential	Herstman, 1999
ASU	Decreases pain and improves functional measures of patient with OA of the knee; reduces NSAID use	In study, ASU was used for 6 months	Two clinical trials have been reported	Ernst, 2001; Maheu et al, 1998

Continued

Table 7-11 Biologic-Based Therapies for Osteoarthritis and Rheumatoid Arthritis—cont'd

Intervention	Management	Treatment Regimen	Cautions, Precautions, Interactions	References
Type II collagen (oral)	Reduces inflammation and pain	Dosage varies; 20 µg/day is the lowest dose	This product, extracted from animal cartilage, is still under investigation; preliminary studies are promising and show no or few SE	Barnett et al, 1998; Trentham et al, 1993
SAMe	May treat symptoms of OA; may reduce pain, fatigue, morning stiffness; may improve mood and relieve depression	200 mg tid	SE: SAMe can cause flatulence, vomiting, diarrhea, headache, or anxiety. SAMe, a naturally occurring compound, has antidepressant effects and should not be combined with other antidepressants	Berger et al, 1987; Bradley et al, 1994; Konig, 1987; Muller-Fassbender et al, 1987; PL/PL, 2002
Chondroitin sulfate	May treat symptoms of OA; relieve pain; improve function;	200-400 mg bid to tid	SE: GI upset, edema; no evidence that combination of glucosamine and	Ernst, 2001; PL/PL, 2002; Uebelhart, 1998

Glucosamine sulfate (glucosamine hydrochloride, also used usually in combination with chondroitin sulfate and manganese ascorbate)	decrease NSAID consumption; has fewer adverse effects compared with NSAIDs May treat symptoms of OA; relieve pain; improve function; has fewer adverse effects compared with NSAIDs	500 mg tid or 1500 mg/day	chondroitin is any better than either product is alone; do not take with anticoagulants SE: GI upset; may increase insulin resistance. Long-term use is needed for lasting effects. Use caution if combined with manganese—amount may exceed UL for manganese	da Camara et al, 1998; Ernst, 2001; PL/PL, 2002; Reginster et al, 2001
Vitamin E	May treat symptoms of OA; may help relieve pain	400 to 800 IU/day UL is 1000 mg/day		Blakenhorn, 1986; Jordan et al, 1998; Machtey et al, 1978; PL/PL, 2002; Stone, 1997
Minerals				
Boron	May be useful for treating OA	Recommended foods with boron include	Excess can lead to reproductive and	Fracp et al, 1990; NAP, 2002;

Continued

Table 7-11 Biologic-Based Therapies for Osteoarthritis and Rheumatoid Arthritis—cont'd

Intervention	Management	Treatment Regimen	Cautions, Precautions, Interactions	References
Minerals—cont'd				
Boron, cont'd		fruit-based beverages, Newnham, potatoes, legumes, milk, avocado, peanut et al, 1987; butter, and peanuts. Adult UL: 20 mg/day.	observed in animals; estrogen levels	developmental effects 1994; Nielsen may increase serum PL/PL, 2002
Selenium	May help treat symptoms of OA and RA; may reduce number of tender points and morning stiffness	Dose varies: 50-200 μg/day; adult RDA: 55 μg/day; Adult UL: 400 μg/day	Doses greater than 900 μg/day can be toxic; may have improved effect if combined with fish oil supplements	Ernst, 2001; Heinle et al, 1997; NAP, 2002; PL/PL, 2002
Zinc sulfate	Reduces joint swelling and morning stiffness, and improved walking time were reported; however, PL/PL states that zinc is	15 mg bid is recommended; adult RDA: 8 mg/day (women) and 11 mg/day (men); UL: 40mg/day. RA recommendation is high but zinc	UL: increased zinc can lead to depletion of copper, iron, calcium, and magnesium; elevated copper, calcium, or iron can deplete zinc; can	NAP, 2002; PL/PL, 2002; Simkin, 1976

Continued

"possibly ineffective" in treating RA (p.1380)

absorption is reduced in people with RA

interfere with glucocorticoids and immunosuppressants; doses greater than 50 mg/day can lower HDL levels; different salt forms contain different amounts of zinc; vegetarians and people with diarrhea need more zinc. Must have proper zinc/copper ratio. Ratio of zinc to copper that was fed to humans of 2:1, 5:1, and 15:1 had limited effects on copper absorption; thus stay within ratio of 15:1 or less

Table 7-11 Biologic-Based Therapies for Osteoarthritis and Rheumatoid Arthritis—cont'd

Intervention	Management	Treatment Regimen	Cautions, Precautions, Interactions	References
Herbs				
Capsaicin (cayenne or red peppers)	May provide pain relief	Topical use: cream with 0.025%-0.075% capsaicin; apply cream 4-5 times/day for at least 4 wks; use diluted vinegar solution to remove cream; is an FDA-approved OTC preparation	Avoid use on broken skin; do not use with heating pad; has temporary effect; use regularly for best results; initially, application causes irritation and hyperesthesia; wash hands thoroughly immediately after application; avoid eye exposure	McCarthy, Marty, 1992; PL/PL, 2002; Rains et al, 1995
Devil's claw (*Harpagophytum procumbens*), traditional native African folk remedy	May treat symptoms of OA; provides pain relief; antiinflammatory activity comparable to phenylbutazone	1.0-4.5 g/day of root is recommended; one OA study used a specific powdered devil's claw root product (Harpadol) dosed at 2.6 g/day	Should not be used if patient has gastric or duodenal ulcers, heartburn, gastritis, or gallstones because devil's claw promotes secretion of stomach	Chrubasik et al, 1996; DerMarderosian, 2001; PL/PL, 2002

Herb	Use	Notes	Studies	References
Garlic (*Allium sativum*)	May treat symptoms of RA	300 mg/day for 4-6 wks	acid; check for drug interactions in reputable herb source. Small study of 15 patients with RA: 87% showed a good "partial response" to treatment	Ernst, 2001
Ginger (*Zingiber officinale*)	May treat symptoms of OA and RA; to provide pain relief and reduce swelling	PL/PL states that the ginger constituent 6-gingerol seems to have antiinflammatory effects, but the whole ginger preparation may not	Controlled studies needed; in an uncontrolled study with ginger (28 patients with RA), 75% reported pain relief and reduced swelling	Bliddal et al, 2000; Ernst, 2001; PL/PL, 2002
Herbal combination (*Phytodolor*) of common ash bark (*Fraxinus excelsior*), aspen leaves, and bark (*Populus tremula*); goldenrod aerial	May treat symptoms of RA; to relieve arthritic pain; equally effective as NSAIDs	Standardized to contain salicin, salicylic alcohol, isofraxidin, and rutin; brand name: Phytodolor	10 randomized controlled studies showed Phytodolor superior to placebo and equally effective to NSAIDs	Ernst, 2001; PL/PL, 2002

Continued

Table 7-11 Biologic-Based Therapies for Osteoarthritis and Rheumatoid Arthritis—cont'd

Intervention	Management	Treatment Regimen	Cautions, Precautions, Interactions	References
Herbs—cont'd				
(Solidago virgaurea) Willow bark (Salix species)	May treat symptoms of RA and OA of knee or hip	1-3 g dried bark tid to qid or 1 c tea is recommended; a standardized preparation was used in study over a 14-day trial period	Interactions with salicylates and anticoagulants reported	Ernst, 2001; PL/PL, 2002
Aromatherapy				
Analgesic or calming essential oils. Analgesic oils—lemongrass, rosemary, frankincense, juniper, rose, ginger, verbena, spike lavender, peppermint,	May provide comfort	Massage: 2-5 gtts of essential oil in 5 ml carroer oil to make a 2%-5% solution. Compress: 1-5 gtts in a bowl of warm water, wring compress, and apply. Inhalation: 1-2 gtts on a tissue	Check for allergy; must be pure essential oil; oil must be diluted with carrier oil such as almond oil; allow patients to smell oil before applying; oils not for ingestion; read safety issues for all oils	Buckle, 1997, 2001

myrrh, clove bud,
ylang ylang,
true lavender,
sweet marjoram,
black pepper.
Calming oil—
lavender

ASU, Avocado-soybean unsaponifiables; bid, twice daily; BP, blood pressure; DHA, docosahexaenoic acid; EPA, eicosapentaenoic acid; GI, gastrointestinal; GLA, Gamma linolenic acid; gtts, drops; HDL, high-density lipoprotein; IU, international units; NSAID, nonsteroidal antiinflammatory drug; OA, osteoarthritis; OTC, over-the-counter; PL/PL, Pharmacist's Letter/Prescriber's Letter; qid, four times daily; RA, rheumatoid arthritis; RDA, recommended daily allowance; SAMe, S-adenosyl-methionine; SE, side effects; tid, three times daily; UL, upper limits—the maximum level of daily nutrient that is likely to pose no risk of adverse effects. Includes intake from food, water, and supplements; URI, upper respiratory infection.

Dietary recommended intake (DRI) values expands on the RDAs and contain four categories of recommendations (i.e., RDA, AI [Adequate Intake], UL, EAR [Estimated Average Requirement]). Check for the latest data.

Both the AI and the RDA are goals for intakes, but are defined differently.

RDA is the intake at which risk of inadequacy is very small (2%-3%); RDA is expected to meet the nutrient needs of 97%-98% of the individuals in a life stage and gender group.

AI is the observed average or experimentally set intake by a defined population or subgroup that appears to sustain a defined nutritional status, such as growth rate, normal circulating nutrient values, or other functional indicators of health. An AI is used if sufficient scientific evidence is not available to derive an EAR. AN AI IS NOT AN RDA.

EAR is the intake that meets the estimated nutrient needs of half of the individuals in a group.

References from the Food and Nutrition Board National Academy of Sciences Institute of Medicine, www.nap.edu or www4.nationalacademies.org

Berkson, 1991; Field, 1997, 2000). Field showed in a small study with 20 children with juvenile rheumatoid arthritis (JRA) that:

> parents massaging their children with JRA before bedtime each night can help decrease their anxiety and stress hormone levels. After 30 days of massage therapy, the children were also experiencing less pain, thus confirming the pain-relieving effects of massage therapy. Although the underlying mechanism for the relationship between massage therapy and pain reduction is not known, massage seems to be a cost-effective therapy for children with juvenile rheumatoid arthritis. The parents reported that they enjoyed massaging their children and felt that they were "contributing to their treatment." (Field, 2000, p. 67)

Other body-based methods include assistive technology, appliances, and braces that are available to help maintain activities of daily living, joint alignment, and protection. Numerous splints, including resting, functional, corrective, and soft splints, are available. Splints may be used with wrist, wrist-hand, wrist-thumb, fingers, thumbs, and proximal and distal interphalangeal joints (Harrell, 2001). Assistive technology is outlined in Box 7-2.

Promising evidence suggests that various energy-based NAC therapies may improve symptoms associated with both OA and RA. Pulsed electromagnetic field therapy (PEMF) is not approved for use in the United States, but it has been studied in relation to treatment for OA at Yale University. In a double-blind, placebo-controlled study at Yale, the effects of PEMF on OA of the knee revealed that

---

Box 7-2

Examples of Assistive Devices and Technology

Enlarged grips for writing, cushion in front of keyboard, large number phone pad, book holder

Knob and faucet turners, single-lever faucet, lever handles

Enlarged or foam handles for comb, brush, toothbrush, razor

Dressing stick, long-handled shoehorn, buttonhook, zipper pull, Velcro, front-close bra

Cooking or eating utensils with large or long-cushioned handles, angled knives, raised-edge dishes, straws, nonslip matting under plates, jar openers

Trashcan on wheels

Adapted from Luck J: Enhancing functional ability. In Robbins L, ed: Clinical care in the rheumatic diseases, ed 2, Atlanta, Georgia, 2001, Association of Rheumatology Health Professionals.

Table 7-12 Manipulative and Body-Based Methods and Energy Therapies for Osteoarthritis and Rheumatoid Arthritis

Intervention	Management	Treatment Regimen	Cautions, Precautions, Interactions	References
Appliances and assistive techniques and devices	May treat symptoms of OA and RA; to ease mobility; improve coordination and activities of daily living; ABLEDATA: on-line repository of assistive technology products (www.abledata.com)	Braces, splints, canes, eating and kitchen utensils, devices for reaching, opening, and fetching, and other devices are used	Safety is important; physical and occupational therapists can assist selection and use of devices	Farhey et al, 2001; Harrell, 2001; Hillstrom et al, 2001; Luck, 2001; Paget, 1997
Aquatics and exercise	May treat symptoms of OA and RA	Warm water therapy program is recommended	Instructors are certified by the National Arthritis Foundation (i.e., the Arthritis Foundation, YMCA, Aquatics Program)	YMCA, 2001; YWCA, 2003

Continued

Table 7-12 Manipulative and Body-Based Methods and Energy Therapies for Osteoarthritis and Rheumatoid Arthritis—cont'd

Intervention	Management	Treatment Regimen	Cautions, Precautions, Interactions	References
Chiropractic manipulation	May treat symptoms of OA	Varied number and type of treatments are used	Qualified practitioner is needed; no forceful manipulations or work with inflamed joints	Berkson, 1991
Massage	May treat symptoms of OA and RA; may help reduce stiffness and pain; may enhance ability to begin an exercise program	Gentle massage is used; various types are available, such as Swedish massage. Aromatherapy massage increased well being in one study; juvenile RA: parental massage to child decreased anxiety, cortisol level, and pain	No massage with active flare-ups, fever, open sores	Cherkin, 2001; Ernst, 2001; Field, 1997, 2000; Horstman, 1999
Physical and occupational therapy	Encourages optimal joint use, range of motion, and activities of daily	Varied number and type of sessions are used	Experienced practitioners familiar with OA and RA are needed	Paget, 1997

	living; provides joint protection and muscle strengthening			
PES	May treat symptoms of OA and RA; improves function; provides pain relief	4-wk treatment period (6-8 hrs/night) is recommended	Research using PES for RA has demonstrated effective reduction of hand symptoms	Caldwell et al, 1994
Low-frequency magnetic fields; static magnets	In study, less pain and improved functions in OA of the knee	Reduction of pain after treatment is used. One study used pads containing magnets (unipolar neodynmium iron-boron disks) or placebo. Two week time period. Subjects wore pad with pain and took off when no pain.		Hinman, 2002; Jacobson, 2001
PEMF	May improve function; may provide pain relief	Usually, treatment involves nine 1-hour sessions over a 5-day period	At this time, PEMF has not been approved for use in the United States; available in Mexico, British Columbia, Europe, Bahamas	Trock et al, 1993, 1994

Continued

Table 7-12 Manipulative and Body-Based Methods and Energy Therapies for Osteoarthritis and Rheumatoid Arthritis—cont'd

Intervention	Management	Treatment Regimen	Cautions, Precautions, Interactions	References
Therapeutic Touch, healing touch, and Reiki	May promote relaxation and provide pain relief; in study of older adults, hand function improved	Sessions usually last from 30 min-1 hour; number and frequency of treatments depends on condition	Trained practitioner with experience is preferable	Gordon, 1998; Peck, 1997, 1998
Water treatments	May treat symptoms of RA and OA; aids in relaxation; helps relieve pain; provides calming effect	Bath hot packs are used; bath water may include various minerals, salts, and essential oils	May need help in and out of tub; all safety features needed (e.g., grab bars)	Hayes, 2001

PEMF, *Pulsed electromagnetic therapy*; PES, *pulsed electrical stimulation.*

patients who received the PEMF had significantly reduced pain and improved function when compared with the control group (Trock et al, 1993). In another study (N = 176) using low-frequency magnetic fields for OA of the knee, pain reduction was significant after treatment in the magnet-on group compared with the magnet-off group (Jacobson et al, 2001).

A study using pulsed electrical stimulation (PES) was conducted at Johns Hopkins with patients diagnosed with OA of the knee. Patients who received PES also had significant pain reduction and improvement of joint function (Zizic et al, 1995). Caldwell and colleagues (1994) conducted a similar study using PES on patients with RA. After a week-long treatment period, patients in the treatment group had improved function and range of motion and reduced pain and morning stiffness. Table 7-12 presents several energy-based NAC therapies that may be helpful in treating patients with OA or RA.

REFERENCES

Achterberg J, McGraw P, Lawlis GF: Rheumatoid arthritis: a study of relaxation and temperature biofeedback training as an adjunctive therapy, *Biofeedback Self-Regul* 2:207, 1981.

Anderson RJ: Rheumatoid arthritis: clinical and laboratory features. In Klippel JH, editor: *Primer on the rheumatic diseases*, Atlanta, Ga, 1997, Arthritis Foundation.

Arnett FC et al: The American Rheumatism Association 1987 revised criteria for the classification of rheumatoid arthritis, *Arthritis Rheumatol* 31:315, 1988.

Astin J: Why patients use alternative medicine: results of a national study, *JAMA* 279:1548, 1998.

Astin J, Harkness E, Ernst E: The efficacy of "distant" healing: a systematic review of randomized trials, *Ann Intern Med* 132:903, 2000.

Barnett ML et al: Treatment of rheumatoid arthritis with oral type II collagen. Results of a multicenter, double-blind, placebo-controlled trial, *Arthritis Rheumatol* 41:290, 1998.

Belch JJ et al: Effects of altering dietary essential fatty acids on requirements for non-steroidal anti-inflammatory drugs in patients with rheumatoid arthritis: a double-blind placebo-controlled study, *Ann Rheum Dis* 47:96, 1998.

Bennett RM et al: Group treatment of fibromyalgia: a 6-month outpatient program, *J Rheumatol* 23(3):521, 1996.

Bensky D, Gamble A: *Chinese herbal medicine: materia medica*, Seattle, 1986, Eastland Press.

Berger R, Nowak H: A new medical approach to the treatment of osteoarthritis: report of an open phase IV study with ademetionine, *Am J Med* 83(5A):84, 1987.

Berkson DL: Osteoarthritis, chiropractic and nutrition: osteoarthritis considered as a natural part of a three-stage subluxation complex: its reversibility, its relevance and treatability by chiropractic and nutritional correlates, *Med Hypoth* 36:4, 356, 1991.

Berman BM, Sing BB: Chronic low back pain: an outcome analysis of a mind-body intervention, *Compl Ther Med* 5:29, 1997.

Berman BM et al: Efficacy of traditional Chinese acupuncture in the treatment of symptomatic knee osteoarthritis: a pilot study, *Osteoarth Cartilage* 3:139, 1995.

Bill-Harvey D et al: Methods used by urban, low-income minorities to care for their arthritis, *Arthritis Care Res* 2(2):60, 1989.

Blankenhorn G: Clinical effectiveness of vitamin E in activated arthroses: a multi-center placebo-controlled double-blind study, *Z Orthop* 124(3):340, 1986.

Bliddal J et al: A randomized placebo-controlled, cross-over study of ginger extracts and ibuprofen in osteoarthritis, *Osteoarth Cartilage* 8:9, 2000.

Blixen C, Kippes C: Depression, social support, and quality of life in older adults with osteoarthritis, *Image* 31(3):221, 1999.

Blunt KL, Rajwani MH, Guerriero RC: The effectiveness of chiropractic management of fibromyalgia patients: a pilot study, *J Manipulative Physiol Ther* 20:6, 389, 1997.

Boh LE: Osteoarthritis. In DiPiro JT et al, editors: *Pharmacotherapy: a pathophysiologic approach*, Stamford, Conn, 1997, Appleton and Lange.

Bonfort G: Spinal manipulation, current state of research and its indications, *Neurol Clin North Am* 17(1):91, 1999.

Borenstein DL, Wiesel SW, Boden SD: *Low back pain: medical diagnosis and comprehensive management*, ed 2, Philadelphia, 1995, Saunders.

Bottiglieri T, Hyland K, Reynolds EH: The clinical potential of ademetionine (S-adenosylmethionine) in neurological disorders, *Drugs* 48:137, 1994.

Bradley JD et al: A randomized, double-blind placebo-controlled trial of intravenous loading with S-adenosylmethionine (SAM) followed by oral SAM therapy in patients with osteoarthritis, *J Rheumatol* 21(5):905, 1994.

Bradley LA et al: Effects of psychological therapy on pain behavior of rheumatoid arthritis patients. Treatment outcome and six-month follow-up, *Arthritis Rheumatol* 30(10):1105, 1987.

Brady LH et al: The effects of Shiatsu on lower back pain, *J Holistic Nurs* 19(1):57, 2001.

Bramwell B: The use of ascorbigen in the treatment of fibromyalgia patients: a preliminary study, *Alt Med Rev* 5(5):455, 2000.

Brattberg G: connective tissue massage in the treatment of fibromyalgia, *Eur J Pain* 3:235, 1999.

Buckelew S et al: The effects of biofeedback and exercise on fibromyalgia: a controlled trial, *Arch Phys Med Rehabil* 73:980, 1998.

Buckle J : *Clinical aromatherapy in nursing*, San Diego, 1997, Singular Publishing.

Buckle J: The role of aromatherapy in nursing care. In Colbath J, Prawlucki P, editors: *Nurs Clin North Am* 36(1):57, 2001.

Burckhardt C: Fibromyalgia. In Robbins L, ed: *Clinical care in the rheumatic diseases*, ed 2, Atlanta, Ga, 2001, Association of Rheumatology Health Professionals.

Burckhardt C et al: A randomized, controlled clinical trial of education and physical training for women with fibromyalgia. *J Rheumatol* 21, 714, 1994.

Bush E et al: Religious coping with chronic pain, *Appl Psychol Physiol Biofeedback* 24(4):249, 1999.

Caldwell JR et al: Pulsed electrical stimulation in the treatment of rheumatoid arthritis, *Arthritis Rheumatol* 37(9):S338, (supplement), 1994.

Castleman M: *Blended medicine: the best choices in healing*, Emmaus, Pa., 2000, Rodale.

Caughey Ge et al: The effect on human tumor necrosis factor and interleukin-1: Production of diets enriched in omega 3 fatty acids from vegetable oil and fish oil, *Am J Clin Nutr* 63:116, 1996.

Chapman E, Wilson J: Homeopathy in rehabilitation medicine, *Physical Med Rehab Clin North Am* 10(3):705, 1999.

Cherkin DC et al: A randomized trial comparing acupuncture, therapeutic massage and self-care education for chronic low back pain. Abstract based on oral presentation at International Conference on Complementary, Alternative, and Integrative Medicine Research, May 17-19, 2001. Abstract in *Alt Ther Health Med* 7(3):103, 2001.

Cherkin DC et al: A comparison of physical therapy, chiropractic manipulation and provision of an educational booklet for the treatment of patients with low back pain, *N Engl J Med* 339(15):1021, 1998.

Christensen BV: Acupuncture treatment of severe knee osteoarthritis. A long-term study, *Acta Anaesthesiol Scand* 36(6):519, 1992.

Chrubasik S et al: Effectiveness of *Harpagophytum procumbens* (devil's claw) in treatment of acute low back pain, *Phytomed* 3:1, 1996.

Colbert AP et al: Magnetic mattress pad use in patients with fibromyalgia: a randomized double-blind pilot study, *J Back Musculoskel Rehab* 13:19, 1999.

Collacott EA et al: Bipolar permanent magnets for the treatment of chronic low back pain, *JAMA* 283:1322, 2000.

Creamer PB, Singh B, Berman MC: Evidence of sustained improvement from a "mind-body" intervention in patients with fibromyalgia, *Arthritis Rheumatol* 41(suppl):S258, 1998.

da Camara CC, Dowless GV: Glucosamine sulfate for osteoarthritis, *Ann Pharmacother* 32(5):580, 1998.

Das A, Hammad TA: Efficacy of a combination of glucosamine hydrochloride, low molecular weight sodium chondroitin sulfate and manganese ascorbate in the management of knee osteoarthritis, *Osteoarth Cartilage* 8:343, 2000.

Day A: The journal as a guide for the healing journey. In Colbath J, Pawlucki P, editors: *Nurs Clin North Am: Holistic Nurs Care* 36(1):131, 2001.

DeLuze J et al: Electroacupuncture in fibromyalgia: results of a controlled study, *BMJ* 305:1249, 1992.

Devine E: Neural function. In Porth C: *Pathophysiology*, ed 6, Philadelphia, 2002, Lippincott.

Deyo RA: Low-back pain, *Sci Am* 103(8):49, 1998.

Dossey L: *Healing beyond the body*, Boston, 2001, Shambhala.

Dunn K, Horgas A: The prevalence of prayer as a spiritual self-care modality in elders, *J Holistic Nurs* 18(4):337, 2000.

Eisenberg DM et al: Trends in the alternative medicine use in the United States 1990-1997: results of a follow-up national survey, *JAMA* 280:569, 1998.

Ernst E: Acupuncture as a symptomatic treatment of osteoarthritis, *Scand J Rheumatol* 26:444, 1997.

Ernst E, Chrubasik S: Phyto-anti-inflammatories. A systemic review of randomized, placebo-controlled, double-blind trials, *Rheum Dis Clin North Am* 26:13, 2000.

Ernst E, ed: The *desktop guide to complementary and alternative medicine*, St Louis, 2001, Mosby.

Ernst E, White AR: Acupuncture for back pain: a meta-analysis of randomized controlled trials, *Arch Intern Med* 158:2235, 1998.

Etzel R: Special extract of Boswellia serrata (H15) in the treatment of rheumatoid arthritis, *Phytomedicine* 3(1):91, 1996.

Ezzo J et al: Acupuncture for osteoarthritis of the knee: a systematic review, *Arthritis Rheumatol* 44:819, 2001.

Farhey Y, Hess E: Managing rheumatic pain: a body-and-mind approach to osteoarthritis care, *Women's Health Prim Care* 4:335, 2001.

Farrell S, Ross A, Sehgal K: Eastern movement therapy. In *Physical Med Rehab Clin North Am* 10(3):617, 1999.

Ferraccioli G et al: EMG-biofeedback training in fibromyalgia syndrome, *J Rheumatol* 14(4):820, 1987.

Field T: *Touch therapy*, Edinburgh, 2000, Churchill Livingstone.

Field TM et al: Juvenile rheumatoid arthritis: benefits from massage therapy, *J Pediatr Psychol Proceedings* 22:607, 1997.

Fife R: Osteoarthritis: epidemiology, pathology and pathogenesis. In Klippel JH, ed: *Primer on the rheumatic diseases*, Atlanta, Ga, 1997, Arthritis Foundation.

Fillmore C et al: Nutrition and dietary supplements. In Schulman R, Cotter A, Harmon R, editors: *Physical Med Rehab Clin North Am* 10(3):673, 1999.

Fisher P et al: Effect of homeopathic treatment on fibrosis, *BMJ* 299:365, 1989.

Fitzcharles M, Esdaile J: Nonphysician practitioner treatments and fibromyalgia syndrome, *J Rheumatol* 24:937, 1997.

Flannelly L, Inouye: Relationships of religion, health status, and socioeconomic status to the quality of life of individuals who are HIV positive, *Issues Ment Health Nurs* 22(3):253, 2001.

Fracp RL et al: Boron and arthritis: the results of double-blind study, *J Nutritional Med* 1:127, 1990.

Frawley D, Lad V: *The yoga of herbs*, Twin Lakes, Wisc, 1988, Lotus Press.

Frawley D, Ranade S: *Ayurveda: nature's medicine*, Twin Lakes, Wisc, 2001, Lotus Press.

Freeman L, Lawlis G: *Mosby's complementary and alternative medicine*, St Louis, 2001, Mosby.

Freundlich B, Leventhal L: Diffuse pain syndromes. In Klippel JH, ed: *Primer on the rheumatic diseases*, Atlanta, Ga, 1997, Arthritis Foundation.

Gach M: *Acupressure's potent points*, New York, 1990, Bantam.

Gadsby JG, Flowerdew MW: *The effectiveness of transcutaneous electrical nerve stimulation (TENS) and acupuncture-like transcutaneous electrical nerve stimulation (ALTENS) in the treatment of patients with chronic low back pain*, issue 3, Oxford, 2000, The Cochrane Library.

Garfinkel MS et al: Evaluation of a yoga-based regimen for treatment of osteoarthritis in the hands, *J Rheumatol* 21:2341, 1994.

Gaw A, Chang L, Shaw LC: Efficacy of acupuncture on osteoarthritic pain, *N Engl J Med* 293(8):375, 1975.

Gibson RG et al: Homoeopathic therapy in rheumatoid arthritis: evaluation by double-blind clinical therapeutic trial, *Br J Clin Pharmacol* 9(5):453, 1980.

Gordon A: The effects of therapeutic touch on patients with osteoarthritis of the knee, *J Fam Pract* 47(4):271, 1998.

Gornisiewicz M, Moreland L: Rheumatoid arthritis. In Robbins L, ed: *Clinical care in the rheumatic diseases*, ed 2, Atlanta, Ga, 2001, Association of Rheumatology Health Professionals.

Goronzy JJ, Weyand CM: Rheumatoid arthritis: epidemiology, pathology and pathogenesis. In Klippel JH, Ed: *Primer on the rheumatic diseases*, Atlanta, Ga, 1997, Arthritis Foundation.

Guieu R, Tardy-Gevet M, Roll J: Analgesic effects of vibration and transcutaneous electrical nerve stimulation applied separately and simultaneously to patients with chronic pain, *Can J Neurol Sci* 18(2):113, 1991.

Haanen H, Hoenderdos, H, Van Romunde L: Controlled trial of hypnotherapy in the treatment of refractory fibromyalgia, *J Rheumatol* 18:72, 1991.

Haggerty W: Flax: ancient herb and modern medicine, *HerbalGram* 45:51, 1999.

Halcon L: Reiki. In Snyder M, Lindquist R, editors: *Complementary/alternative therapies in nursing*, ed 4, New York, 2002, Springer.

Harrell P: Splinting of the hand. In Robbins L, ed: *Clinical care in the rheumatic diseases*, ed 2, Atlanta, Ga, 2001, Association of Rheumatology Health Professionals.

Hartman C et al: Effects of T'ai chi training on function and quality of life indicators in older adults with osteoarthritis, *J Am Geriatr Soc* 48:1553, 2000.

Haslock I et al: measuring the effects of yoga in rheumatoid arthritis, *Br J Rheumatol* 33:787, 1994.

Hayes K: Physical modalities. In Robbins L et al, ed: *Clinical care in the rheumatic diseases*, ed 2, Atlanta, Ga, 2001, Association of Rheumatology Health Professionals.

Heinle K et al: Selenium concentration in erythrocytes of patients with rheumatoid arthritis. Clinical and laboratory chemistry infection markers during administration of selenium, *Med Klin* 92(suppl 3):29, 1997.

Henderson CJ, Panush RS: Diets, dietary supplements, and nutritional therapies in rheumatic diseases, *Rheum Dis Clin North Am* 25:937, 1999.

Hillstrom H et al: Lower extremity conservative realignment therapies and ambulatory aids. In Robbins L, ed: *Clinical care in the rheumatic diseases*, ed 2, Atlanta, Ga, 2001, Association of Rhemuatology Health Professionals.

Hinman M et al: Effects of static magnets on chronic knee pain and physical function: A double blind study, *Altern Ther Health Med* 8(4):50, 2002.

Hirschberg G: Skinfold tenderness and skinrolling massage in fibromyalgia, *J Orthop Med* 19(3):77, 1997.

Hochberg MC: Osteoarthritis: clinical features and treatment. In Klippel JH, ed: *Primer on the rheumatic diseases*, Atlanta, Ga, 1997, Arthritis Foundation.

Hoffman D: *The new holistic herbal*, Shaftesbury, Dorset, 1994, Element Books Limited.

Horstman J: *The arthritis foundation's guide to alternative therapies*, Atlanta, Ga, 1999, Arthritis Foundation.

Jacobsen S, Danneskiold-Samsoe B, Andersen RB: Oral S-adenosylmethionine in primary fibromyalgia: double-blind clinical evaluation, *Scan J Rheumatol* 20:294, 1991.

Jacobson J et al: Low-amplitude, extremely low frequency magnetic fields for the treatment of osteoarthritic knees: a double-blind clinical study, *Alt Ther Health Med* 7(5):54, 2001.

Jonas W, Linde L, Ramirez G: Homeopathy and rheumatic disease, *Rheum Dis Clin North Am* 26:117, 2000.

Jones A : Yoga : *A step by step guide*, Boston, 1998, Element.

Jordan JM et al: Naturally-occurring anti-oxidants may prevent knee osteoarthritis, *Arthritis Rheumatol* 41(suppl):S133, 1998.

Kaplan KH, Goldenberg DL, Galvin-Nadeau M: The impact of a meditation-based stress reduction program on fibromyalgia, *Gen Hosp Psychiatr* 15(5):284, 1993.

Keefe F, Caldwell D, Aspnes A: Cognitive behavioral interventions. In Robbins L, ed: *Clinical care in the rheumatic diseases*, ed 2, Atlanta, Ga, 2001, Association of Rheumatology Health Professionals.

Keefe F et al: Spouse-assisted coping skills training in the management of knee pain in osteoarthritis: long term follow-up of results, *Arthritis Care Res* 12:101, 1999.

King D et al: Beliefs and attitudes of hospital inpatients about faith, healing and prayer, *J Fam Pract* 39:3349, 1994.

Kirsteins AE, Dietz F, Hwang SM: Evaluating the safety and potential use of a weight-bearing exercise, Tai-chi chuan, for rheumatoid arthritis patients, *Am J Phys Med Rehab* 70(3):136, 1991.

Klippel JH, ed: *Primer on the rheumatic diseases,* ed 11, Atlanta, Ga, 1997, Arthritis Foundation.

Kolasinski S: Complementary and alternative treatments. In Robbins L, ed: *Clinical care in the rheumatic diseases,* ed 2, Atlanta, Ga, 2001, Association of Rheumatology Health Professionals.

Konig B: A long-term (two years) clinical trial with S-adenosylmethionine for the treatment of osteoarthritis, *Am J Med* 83(5A):89, 1987.

Korn JH: Rheumatoid arthritis. In Andreoli T, ed: *Cecil essentials of medicine,* Philadelphia, 2001, Saunders.

Kovar PA et al: Supervised fitness walking in patients with osteoarthritis of the knee: a RCT, *Ann Int Med* 116:529, 1992.

Kremer JM et al: Dietary fish oil and olive oil supplementation in patients with rheumatoid arthritis. Clinical and immunologic effects, *Arthritis Rheumatol* 33:810, 1990.

Krieger D: *Accepting your power to heal,* Santa Fe, NM, 1993, Bear and Co.

Kulkarni R et al: Treatment of osteoarthritis with a herbomineral formulation: a double-blind, placebo-controlled, crossover study, *J Ethnopharmacol* 33(1-2):91, 1991.

Lad V: *The complete book of Ayurvedic home remedies,* New York, 1998, Three Rivers Press.

Lau CS, Morley KD, Belch JJ: Effects of fish oil supplementation on non-steroidal anti-inflammatory drug requirement in patients with mild rheumatoid arthritis: a double-blind placebo-controlled study, *Br J Rheumatol* 32:982, 1993.

La Valle J et al: *Natural therapeutics pocket guide,* Hudson, Ohio, 2000, LexiComp.

Leffler MC et al: Glucosamine, chondroitin and manganese ascorbate for degenerative joint disease of the knee or low back: a randomized, double-blind, placebo-controlled pilot study, *Military Med* 164:85, 1999.

Leventhal LJ, Boyce EG, Zurier RB: Treatment of rheumatoid arthritis with gamma-linolenic acid, *Ann Int Med* 119:867, 1993.

Lichtbroun A, Raicer M, Smith R: The treatment of fibromyalgia with cranial electrotherapy stimulation, *J Clin Rheumatol* 7(2):72, 2001.

Lin Y, Taylor A: Effects of therapeutic touch in reducing pain and anxiety in an elderly population, *Integrat Med* 1(4):155, 1998.

Longo L et al: Laser therapy for fibrocyositic rheumatisms, *J Clin Laser Med Surg* 15:217, 1997.

Luck J: Enhancing functional ability. In Robbins L, ed: *Clinical care in the rheumatic diseases,* ed 2, Atlanta, Ga, 2001, Association of Rheumatology Health Professionals.

Lundgren S, Stenstrom C: Muscle relaxation training and quality of life in rheumatoid arthritis; a randomized controlled clinical trial, *Scand J Rheumatol* 28:47, 1999.

Machtey I, Ouaknine L: Tocopherol in osteoarthritis: a controlled pilot study, *J Am Geriatr Soc* 26:328, 1978.

Maciocia G: *The practice of Chinese medicine,* New York, 1994, Churchill Livingstone.

Mackenzie ER et al: Spiritual support and psychological well-being: older adults' perceptions of the religion and health connection, *Alt Ther Health Med* 6:37, 2000.

Maheu E et al: Symptomatic efficacy of avocado/soybean unsaponifiables in the treatment of osteoarthritis of the knee and hip, *Arthritis Rheumatol* 41:81, 1998.

Marchand S et al: Is TENS a placebo effect? A controlled study on chronic low back pain, *Pain* 54:99, 1993.

Matthews DA, Marlowe SM, McNutt FS: Beneficial effects of intercessory prayer ministry in patients with rheumatoid arthritis, *J Gen Intern Med* 13(suppl):1177, 1998.

McAlindon T et al: Glucosamine and chondroitin for treatment of osteoarthritis, *JAMA* 283(11):1469, 2000.

McCarthy G, Kenny DL: Dietary fish oil and rheumatic diseases, *Semin Arthritis Rheumatol* 21:368, 1992.

McCarthy GM, Marty DJ: Effect of topical capsaicin in the therapy of painful osteoarthritis of the hands, *J Rheumatol* 19:604, 1992.

McCarty DJ et al: Treatment of pain due to fibromyalgia with topical capsaicin: a pilot study, *Semin Arthritis Rheumatol* 23:41, 1994.

McCauley JD et al: Hypnosis compared to relaxation in the outpatient management of chronic low back pain, *Arch Phys Med Rehab* 64:548, 1983.

Meisenhelder J, Chandler E: Prayer and health outcomes in church members, *Alt Ther Health Med* 6:56, 2000.

Mentgen J: Healing touch. In Colbath J, Prawlucki P, editors: *Nurs Clin North Am* 36(1):143, 2001.

Meyer F, Nebrensky A: A double-blind comparative study of micro stimulation and placebo effect in short term treatment of the chronic back pain patient, *Calif Health Rev* 2(1):R1, 1983.

Miller E: Healing Journey, [audiotape], Stanford, Calif, 1980, Source Tapes.

Minor M, Westby M: Rest and exercise. In Robbins L, ed: *Clinical care in the rheumatic diseases*, ed 2, Atlanta, Ga, 2001, Association of Rheumatology Health Professionals.

Morgan S et al: Nutrient intake patterns, body mass index and vitamin levels in patients with rheumatoid arthritis, *Arthritis Care Res* 10:9, 1997.

Muller-Fassbender H et al: Double-blind clinical trial of S-adenosylmethionine versus ibuprofen in the treatment of osteoarthritis, *Am J Med* 83(5A):81, 1987.

Naparstek B: Pain, [audiotape], Akron, Ohio, 1995a, Image Paths.

Naparstek B: Stress I and Stress II, [audiotape], Akron, Ohio, 1995b, Image Paths.

Naparstek B: *Staying well with guided imagery*, Akron, Ohio, 1994, Image Paths.

Naparstek B: A Guided Meditation to Help You with Rheumatoid Arthritis or Lupus, [audiotape], Akron, Ohio, 1992, Image Paths.

National Institutes of Health [NIH]: Consensus Statement, *Acupuncture* 15:1, 1997.

Nespor K: Psychosomatics of back pain and the use of yoga, *Int J Psychosom* 36:72, 1989.

Newnham RE: Essentiality of boron for healthy bones and joints, *Environ health Perspect* 102(7):83, 1994.

Nielsen FH et al: Effect of dietary boron on mineral, estrogen and testosterone metabolism in postmenopausal women, *FASEB J* 1:39, 1987.

Nordstrom DC et al: Alpha-linoleic acid in the treatment of RA. A double-blind, placebo-controlled and randomized study: Flaxseed vs safflower seed, *Rheumatol Int* 14:231, 1995.

Paget SA: Rheumatoid arthritis: treatment. In Klippel JH, ed: *Primer on the rheumatic diseases*, Atlanta, Ga, 1997, Arthritis Foundation.

Panush RS et al: Food-induced (allergic) arthritis, inflammatory arthritis exacerbated by milk, *Arthritis Rheumatol* 29:220, 1986.

Parke AL et al: Rheumatoid arthritis and food: a case study, *BMJ* 282:2027, 1981.

Parker JC et al: Effects of stress management on clinical outcomes in rheumatoid arthritis, *Arthritis Rheumatol* 38(12):1807, 1995.

Peck S: The efficacy of therapeutic touch for improving functional ability in elders with degenerative arthritis, *Nurs Sci Q* 11(3):123, 1998.

Peck S: The effectiveness of therapeutic touch to decrease pain in elders with degenerative arthritis, *J Holistic Nurs* 15(2):176, 1997.

Peyron JG, Altman RD: The epidemiology of osteoarthritis. In Moskowitz RW et al, editors: *Osteoarthritis: diagnosis and medical/surgical management*, ed 2, Philadelphia, 1992, Saunders.

Pharmacist's Letter/Prescriber's Letter [PL/PL]: *Natural medicines comprehensive database*, Stockton, Calif, 2002, Therapeutic Research Faculty.

PL/PL: Fibromyalgia, *Natural Med Clin Manage* 2001:29, 2001. PL/PLCE booklet.

Pizzorno J: Natural medicine approach to treating osteoarthritis, *Altern Compl Ther* 1(2):93, 1995.

Potter M, Zauszniewski J: Spirituality, resourcefulness, and arthritis impact on health perception of elders with rheumatoid arthritis, *J Holistic Nurs* 18(4):311, 2000.

Preyde M: Effectiveness of massage therapy for subacute low-back pain, *CMAJ* 162:1815, 2000.

Quinn J: Therapeutic touch. In Snyder M, Lindquist R, editors: *Complementary/alternative therapies in nursing*, ed 4, New York, 2002, Springer.

Rains C, Bryson HM: Topical capsaicin. A review of its pharmacological properties and therapeutic potential in post-herpetic neuralgia, diabetic neuropathy and osteoarthritis, *Drugs Aging* 7:317, 1995.

Ratner D et al: Juvenile rheumatoid arthritis and milk allergy, *J R Soc Med* 78:410, 1985.

Reginster JY et al: Long-term effects of glucosamine sulphate on osteoarthritis progression: a randomized, placebo-controlled clinical trial, *Lancet* 357:251, 2001.

Rosenbaum JF et al: The antidepressant potential of oral S-adenosyl-l-methionine, *Acta Psychiatr Scand* 81:432, 1990.

Russell IJ et al: Treatment of fibromyalgia syndrome with Super Malic: a randomized, double-blind, placebo-controlled, cross-over pilot study, *J Rheumatol* 22, 953, 1995.

Saul D: Newer treatments for fibromyalgia pain, *Internat J Integr Med* 1(3):27, 1999.

Shuler P et al: The effects of spiritual/religious practices on psychological well-being among inner city homeless women, *NP Forum* 5:106, 1994.

Simkin PA: Oral zinc sulphate in rheumatoid arthritis, *Lancet* 2(7985):539, 1976.

Singh B et al: A pilot study of cognitive behavioral therapy in fibromyalgia, *Alt Ther Health Med* 4:67, 1998.

Smith-Fassler M, Lopez-Bushnell K: Acupuncture as complementary therapy for back pain, *Holistic Nurs Pract* 15(3):35, 2001.

Smyth J et al: Effects of writing about stressful experiences on symptom reduction in patients with asthma or rheumatoid arthritis: a randomized trial, *JAMA* 281:1304, 1999.

Sprott H et al: Pain treatment of fibromyalgia by acupuncture, *Arthritis Rheumatol* 39(suppl):S91, 1996.

Sprott H et al: Pain Treatment of Fibromyalgia by Acupuncture, [letter], *Rheumatol Int* 18:35, 1998.

Stein D: *Essential Reiki, freedom*, Calif, 1997, Crossing Press Inc.

Stone J et al: Inadequate calcium, folic acid, vitamin E, zinc, and selenium intake in rheumatoid arthritis patient, *Semin Arthritis Rheumatol* 27:180, 1997.

Srivastava K: Extracts from two frequently consumed spices—cumin (Cuminum cyminum) and ginger (Zingiber officinale) in rheumatism and musculoskeletal disorders, *Med Hypoth* 39(4):3422, 1992.

Strawbridge WJ et al: Frequent attendance at religious services and mortality over 28 years, *Am J Public Health* 87(6):957, 1997.

Sunshine W et al: Fibromyalgia benefits from massage therapy and transcutaneous electrical stimulation, *J Clin Rheumatol* 2:18, 1996.

Takeda W, Wessel J: Acupuncture for the treatment of pain of osteoarthritic knee, *Arthritis Care Res* 7(3):118, 1994.

Taylor A: Complementary/alternative therapies in the treatment of pain. In Spencer J, Jacobs J, editors: *Complementary/alternative medicine: an evidence-based approach*, St Louis, 1999, Mosby.

Trentham DE et al: Effects of oral administration of type II collagen on rheumatoid arthritis, *Science* 261(5129):1727, 1993.

Trock DH et al: A double-blind trial of the clinical effects of pulsed electromagnetic fields in osteoarthritis, *J Rheumatol* 20:456, 1993.

Trock DH, Bollet AJ, Markoll, R: The effect of pulsed electromagnetic fields in the treatment of osteoarthritis of the knee and cervical spine, *J Rheumatol* 21:1903, 1994.

Turner J: Educational and behavioral interventions for back pain in primary care, *Spine* 4:2851, 1996.

Tyers S, Smith: A comparison of cranial electrotherapy stimulation alone or with chiropractic therapies in the treatment of fibromyalgia, *Am Chiropract* 23(2):39, 2001.

Uebelhart D et al: Effects of oral chondroitin sulfate on the progression of knee osteoarthritis: a pilot study, *Osteoarthritis Cartilage* 6:39, 1998.

Umbreit A: Healing touch. In Snyder M, Lindquist R, editors: *Complementary/alternative therapies in nursing*, ed 4, New York, 2002, Springer.

van Deusen J, Harlowe D: Efficacy of the ROM dance program for adults with rheumatoid arthritis, *Am J Occup Ther* 40:90, 1987.

van Tulder M, Koes B: Low back pain and sciatica. In Barton S, ed: *Clinical evidence*, London, 2001, BMJ Publishing Group.

Verbruggen G, Goemaere S, Veys EM: Chondroitin sulfate: structure/disease modifying antiosteoarthritis in the treatment of finger joint OA, *Osteoarthritis Cartilage* 6:37, 1998.

Waddell G: Chiropractic for low back pain: evidence for manipulation is stronger than that for most orthodox medical treatment, *BMJ* 318(7178):262, 1999.

Weintraub M: *Alternative and complementary treatment in neurologic illness*, New York, 2001, Churchill Livingstone.

Weissenberg M: Cognitive aspects of pain and pain control, *Int J Clin Exper Hypnosis* 46:44, 1998.

Wirth D, Cram J: The psychophysiology of nontraditional prayer, *Int J Psychosm* 41:68, 1994.

Wolf SL et al: Reducing frailty and falls in older persons: an investigation of Tai chi and computerized balance training, *J Am Geriatr Soc* 44:489, 1996.

Wolfson LR et al: Balance and strength training in older adults: intervention gains and Tai chi maintenance, *J Am Geriatr Soc* 44:498, 1996.

www.nap.edu/catalog, Nutrition information 2003. Accessed 1/16/03.

www4.nationalacademies.org. Dietary reference intakes: Elements. Vitamins, 2003. Accessed 1/16/03.

www4.nationalacademies.org/IOM/IOMhome. nsf/pages/food+and+ nutrition+board. Accessed 1/17/03.

www.cc.nih.gov/ccc/supplements:magnesium, 2002. Accessed 1/16/03.

YMCA, 2001, http://www.ymca.org. Accessed 1/16/03.

YWCA, 2003, http//www.ywca.org. Accessed 1/16/03.

Zizic TM et al: The treatment of osteoarthritis of the knee with pulsed electrical stimulation, *J Rheumatol* 22:1757, 1995.

Zurier R et al: Gamma-linolenic acid treatment of rheumatoid arthritis, *Arthritis Rheumatol* 39:1808, 1996.

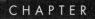

CHAPTER 8

NEUROLOGIC AND PSYCHOLOGIC DISORDERS

Wendy Noble ▪ Roxana Huebscher ▪ Helen Miller ▪ Louise Rauckhorst

NAC THERAPIES FOR NEUROLOGIC AND PSYCHOLOGIC DISORDERS

This chapter reviews natural-alternative-complementary (NAC) therapies in the areas of dementia, Parkinson's disease, eating disorders, addictions, and headaches. These disorders are complex with minimal NAC study. In addition, findings are inconsistent and interpretations are numerous, especially for the biologic therapies for several of the areas. Nonetheless, because these disorders cause much suffering for patient and family alike, modalities that have been tried are presented.

NAC THERAPIES FOR DEMENTIA AND PARKINSON'S DISEASE

Dementia

Dementia is "characterized by global non-reversible impairment of cerebral function with preservation of clear consciousness. It usually results in loss of memory (initially of recent events), loss of executive function (such as the ability to make decisions or sequence complex tasks), and changes in personality" (Barton, 2001, p. 694). People with dementia may have language impairment, apraxia, agnosia, or any combination. Dementia affects 30% to 50% of adults by age 85. Alzheimer's disease (AD) accounts for approximately two thirds of cases, with vascular dementia and a combination of AD and vascular dementia accounting for most of the rest (Lyons et al, 2002). Box 8-1 presents some of the proposed theories related to dementia.

Diagnosing the exact type of dementia is difficult. However, whatever the diagnosis, and even when it is not known, families of patients with dementia may turn to various forms of NAC therapy in an attempt to promote relaxation and sleep, to improve depression and memory, and to stimulate social interaction and expression for their loved ones. Furthermore, more long-term care facilities have recognized the beneficial effects that NAC therapies can have on patients with dementia. Thus some of these modalities are discussed here.

Parkinson's Disease

Parkinson's disease (PD) is a debilitating neurologic disease resulting from a lack of dopamine production in the substantia nigra. The lack

---

Box 8-1

Theories of Alzheimer's Disease and Dementia

- Patients with Alzheimer's disease lack adequate levels of the neurotransmitter acetylcholine, which may account for some of the cognitive defects associated with the disease. Solutions:
    - Supply postsynaptic cholinergic receptor agonists that can be used as acetylcholine analogs.
    - Supply precursors of acetylcholine.
    - Use anticholinesterases to inhibit acetylcholinesterase, the enzyme that breaks down acetylcholine.
- Oxidative stress and inflammation may contribute to Alzheimer's disease and dementia.
- Beta-amyloid protein fibril formation and deposition may lead to neurotoxicity.
- High homocysteine levels may contribute to the development of dementia.
- Hormonal changes may contribute to dementia.
- Cerebral insufficiency may contribute to dementia.

Adapted from PL/PL: Natural medicines in clinical management: Alzheimer's disease, Continuing Education Booklet 2:1, 2000.

of dopamine production results in inadequate dopamine in the motor tracts of the basal ganglia, resulting in dysregulation of smooth muscle coordination. The cardinal signs of PD are tremor, rigidity, and bradykinesia (Lewis et al, 1999). PD is a progressive disease that can lead to severe limitations. A survey of 201 patients with PD (Rajendran et al, 2001) found that 81 (40%) used at least one form of NAC care. The most common therapies were vitamins, herbs, massage, and acupuncture.

ALTERNATIVE HEALTH CARE SYSTEMS FOR DEMENTIA AND PARKINSON'S DISEASE

Ayurveda Perspectives on Nervous System Disorders

Vata (air) energy is considered as the energy that moves through the brain and the nerves that control both voluntary and involuntary functions. Although nervous system disorders always involve some weakness, disturbance, or hypersensitivity, these disorders can also be brought about by excess pitta (that can "burn out" the nervous system, causing disruption in nerve impulses) and excess kapha (that can clog or block impulses). Blockage of energy flow (or prana) through the nervous system causes spasms, rigidity, numbness, or paralysis, while abnormal flow causes tremors and involuntary movements. Nervous system disorders are considered linked with mental disorders; for example, emotional or psychologic blockages may cause nervous system disorders. Therefore mental status is examined carefully when any nervous system disorder is present (Frawley, 2000).

General treatment of blockage conditions includes using herbs such as calamus (to open the flow of nerve impulses) and basil (to cleanse and clear the nervous system). Other herbs that may be taken internally or used as essential oils for aromatherapy include bayberry, guggul, myrrh, turmeric, bay leaves, and mint. Because vata is the underlying dosha behind all nerve function, anti-vata herbs and diet may be used temporarily, even by individuals with pitta- and vata-type nervous disorders. Massage with medicated oils is recommended because it is believed that the nerves can be nourished through the skin. For calming the nerves, application to the head is recommended with an essential oil such as sandalwood. To stimulate the nerves, essential oils such as camphor, musk, myrrh, and frankincense can be applied to the temple. Several nose drops of gotu kola or calamus ghee may also be applied morning and night. Gotu kola (brahmi) is recommended for pitta-type nervous system disorders to clear the nervous system and relieve inflammation, as well as skullcap, bhringaraj, passionflower, hops, and betony. For kapha-type nervous system disorders, equal parts gotu kola with honey is recommended, while in pitta-type disorders, gotu kola alone (with ghee) and in vata-type disorders, calamus alone (with ghee or warm water) is preferable (Frawley, 2000).

Memory problems

Cognitive function is well recognized in Ayurveda. The mind (*manus*) is thought to be the inner instrument for perception. Mind, ego, and intellect together form an internal organ, whose chief function is to receive impulses from the external environment and respond suitably. The system includes sensory and motor organs as accessories. The whole apparatus, consisting of the internal organ and its several accessories, corresponds to the brain and the nervous mechanisms associated with its function, which is similar to concepts in modern psychology. Intelligence is referred to as *Buddhi*; dementia is termed *Cittinasa* (loss of mind). (Manyam, 2001, p. 71)

According to Ayurveda, memory is recorded on the sensitive film of the nerve cells within the brain, which are of a kapha nature. However, memories are recalled by means of vata. Most memory problems are considered as the result of the aggravation of kapha (with its stagnation effects) or of vata (with its light, "spacy" qualities). Therefore, to improve memory, balancing (reducing) kapha and vata becomes necessary. Because pitta qualities are sharp and penetrating, enhancing pitta supports sharpness of recall. Carrots, carrot or beet juice, sweet potatoes, tapioca, okra, and spinach are foods recommended to improve memory. Fresh fruits and vegetables, almonds, oranges, ghee, and milk are also recommended. Heavy meat should be avoided by anyone with memory problems. A 5-day kitchari fast (one-half basmati rice and one-half split yellow mung dal with cilantro and spices added for flavor) or a 3- to 5-day fruit fast (using types of fruits that will help balance the doshas taken with ½ teaspoon triphala steeped in hot water at night) can be used to cleanse the system and help to strengthen memory. A fruit fast should not be attempted with individuals who tend to become hypoglycemic (Lad, 1998).

Specific Ayurvedic herbs used to improve memory include brahmi (gotu kola), jatamamsi, bhringaraj, and shanka pushpi. These herbs may be used separately or mixed in equal proportions to make a tea (1 teaspoon herbs steeped in 1 cup hot water, taken on an empty stomach morning and evening for a 1-month trial and then indefinitely, if benefits are apparent).

Other Ayurvedic recommendations to improve memory include daily walking for 30 minutes five times a week, yoga postures, especially the inverted poses, which help to bring more circulation to the brain (Shoulder Stand, Headstand, Plow, and Camel poses), the rest pose (Savasana), and the Bow and Cobra poses. Twelve cycles of the Sun Salutation are also recommended (Lad, 1998).

Brahmi oil rubbed on the soles of the feet and the scalp is thought to stimulate skin receptors that send messages to the brain cells and activate memory. Five drops of brahmi ghee in each nostril may also help improve memory because the nose is considered as the doorway to the brain.

Alternate nostril breathing is recommended to improve cerebral circulation, and regular meditation is recommended to relieve the anxiety and stress that can exacerbate memory problems. Avoiding toxic substances, such as alcohol and drugs that directly affect the brain, is also considered essential (Lad, 1998).

Parkinson's disease PD (*kampavata*) has been described as early as 1400 AD in written Ayurvedic literature. PD is considered as a vata disease with a pitta component. Pitta is viewed as pushing vata to the point that nerve impulses do not flow properly. For deficiency or degenerative conditions such as multiple sclerosis or PD, tonic herbs such as ashwagandha and shatavari can be combined with gotu kola or calamus. Other good tonic herbs are haritaki, guggul, and bala. Kapikacchu (1 to 3 grams powder twice a day) is used for PD because it is a natural source of levodopa (L-dopa) (Frawley, 2000).

Mucuna pruriens is included in 18 of the 35 different formulations for treatment of PD. L-dopa is present in the herb, and, dose for dose, *Mucuna pruriens* is "twice as effective", in animal studies, as is synthetic L-dopa (Manyam, 2001, p. 72). A human study revealed significant reduction of scores on The Unified Parkinson's Disease Rating Scale (Manyam, 1995).

Because of the close connection between the nervous system and the mind, spiritual therapies such as yoga, breathing exercises (pranayama), mantra meditation, and visualization are important. Yoga may be helpful because it can improve posture and muscle tone, reduce pain, and increase range of motion, balance, stamina, and flexibility. Postures are modified when balance is impaired, and, when necessary, yoga can be performed in a wheelchair (Ross, 2001). For nervous system disorders such as PD, in which rigidity prevails, plugging the left nostril (for days or weeks) is recommended; plugging the right nostril is used for hyperactive conditions such as insomnia. The mantra SOM is good for long-term debilitating disorders. The mantra SHAM calms the nerves, and OM is effective for clearing and calming the nervous system (Frawley, 2000).

Seizure disorder   Although a seizure disorder is most frequently viewed as a kapha disorder (caused by channel blockage), it can also be a manifestation of a pitta disorder (with inflammation of the nerves) or of a vata disorder (caused by hypersensitivity). Ayurvedic treatment includes purgation with castor oil taken with a little ginger juice and honey, and the herbal compound triphala (1 g of powder or tablets with meals). Nerve tonics such as gotu kola are used, as well as calamus, to relieve the channel blockage. Foot massage with sesame oil is used for a general calming effect. The herbal preparation chyavan prash is used as a tonic in between attacks (Frawley, 2000).

Traditional Chinese Medicine for Dementia and Parkinson's Disease

Dementia   An article in *Acupuncture Today* (2002) reviews the research presented at the World Alzheimer's Conference. Two separate studies have shown that acupuncture can increase verbal and motor skills and improve mood and cognitive function in patients with AD. Lombardo (2000) studied 11 patients, 10 with AD and 1 with vascular dementia. Each patient received a minimum of 22 acupuncture treatments over 3 months. Patients took a variety of tests for anxiety, depression, and cognitive function before and after treatment. Lombardo found statistically significant improvements in anxiety and depression scores. Although no control group was used for cognitive function, treatment providers noted subjective improvement in thinking skills of subjects. The second study by Kao (2000) involved eight patients with mild to moderate AD. Patients were graded before and after treatment using the Mini-Mental Status Examination (MMSE) and the Traditional Chinese Medicine

(TCM) Symptoms Checklist for Alzheimer's. Patients were each treated for 21 days, over a 1-month period. Significant improvement was seen in measures of verbal orientation and motor coordination, and higher MMSE scores were produced. Clinical improvement was also noted on the TCM checklist.

In a small study ($n = 10$) using foot acupressure and massage on patients with AD and other dementias, Sutherland and colleagues (1999) reported a decrease in wandering, pulse, and respirations and an increase in quiet time. The authors did not report which acupressure points were used. Although no statistical significance was found (the sample was small), "the 'wandering' mean narrowly missed the $p < .05$" significance level (p. 348).

Parkinson's disease Hsu and Cheng (2001) report that little TCM clinical information about PD has been translated. "However, the rat model has shown that a combination of acupuncture and herbal medicine increases dopamine levels in the midbrain and caudate nucleus" (p. 22).

Qi gong may be helpful for PD. Sancier and Hole (2001) report on a Chinese study of 15 patients who had a course of 60 Qi gong treatments (Chen, 1989). Improvement for most of the group was assessed by diminished "tremble," increased interval between attacks, improved speech, or any combination.

Homeopathy for Parkinson's Disease

To determine the appropriate remedy, case taking would be needed as it would for any homeopathic assessment. Several remedies for PD might include *Cuprum metallicum*, *Mercurius solubilis*, *Thuja occidentalis*, and *Zincum metallicum* (La Valle, 2000). Chapman (2001) reports a double-blind crossover study of 20 individuals with PD who were given a nerve growth factor, neurotrophin, derived from cobra venom, in the potencies 6X, 12X, 30X (see Chapter 11 for information on dilutions in homeopathy). Significant improvement was noted in tremor, bradykinesia, rigidity, confusion, on-off phenomena, and medication dosage. Table 8-1 reviews some alternative health care systems for dementia and PD.

MIND-BODY-SPIRIT INTERVENTIONS FOR DEMENTIA AND PARKINSON'S DISEASE

Music for Dementia

Music is an especially appropriate intervention for patients with dementia because verbal skills are not required, music appeals to the senses rather than requiring cognitive ability, and music facilitates expression in patients who are otherwise nonverbal. Some anecdotal reports showed patients with advanced dementia singing all the words to a familiar song or spontaneously dancing to a familiar tune.

Table 8-1   Alternative Health Care Systems for Dementia and Parkinson's Disease

Intervention	Management	Treatment Regimen	Cautions, Precautions, Interactions	References
Ayurveda				
Diet	Help improve memory and cleanse the system	5-day kitchari fast (one half basmati rice and one half split yellow mung dal with cilantro and spices added for flavor) OR a 3-5 day fruit fast (using types of fruits that will help to balance the doshas taken with ½ tsp triphala steeped in hot water at night)	Individuals who tend to become hypoglycemic should not attempt a fruit fast. Supervision with any fast is advisable	Lad, 1998
Foods	Help improve memory	Carrots, carrot or beet juice, sweet potatoes, tapioca, okra, spinach, fresh fruits and vegetables, almonds, oranges, ghee, and milk are recommended;	Avoid heavy meat	Lad, 1998

Continued

Table 8-1	Alternative Health Care Systems for Dementia and Parkinson's Disease—cont'd			
Intervention	Management	Treatment Regimen	Cautions, Precautions, Interactions	References
Ayurveda—cont'd				
Herbs	Help improve memory	Brahmi (gotu kola), jatamamsi, bhringaraj, and shanka pushpi may be consumed separately or mixed in equal proportions to make a tea (1 tsp herbs steeped in 1 c hot water, taken on an empty stomach morning and evening for a 1-mo trial and then indefinitely if it seems beneficial)	Should observe all herbal precautions before using	Lad, 1998
	For deficiency or degenerative conditions, such as multiple sclerosis or PD	Tonic herbs: ashwagandha and shatavari can be combined with gotu kola or calamus; other good tonic herbs are haritaki, guggul, and bala Kapikacchu: 1-3 g powder bid for PD (natural source of L-dopa)	All herbal precautions should be observed before using	Frawley, 2000

Oils	Stimulates skin receptors that send messages to the brain cells; activates memory	Brahmi oil rubbed on the soles of the feet and the scalp		Lad, 1998
	Help improve memory	5 drops of brahmi ghee in each nostril		Lad, 1998
Movement	Help improve memory	Exercise: daily walking for ½ hr 5 times/wk		Lad, 1998
Yoga	Help improve memory	Yoga postures: Shoulder Stand, Headstand, Plow, and Camel poses; the rest pose (Savasana), Bow, and Cobra poses; twelve cycles of the Sun Salutation	Some yoga poses are not recommend when people have certain chronic conditions; no inverted poses with certain conditions such as glaucoma, neck problems or weak back, obesity, menstruation, pregnancy, hypertension, etc.	
	For PD; may improve posture and muscle tone, reduce pain, increase range of motion, balance, stamina, and flexibility	Various modified postures.	Postures are modified when balance is impaired and when necessary; yoga can be performed in a wheelchair	Ross, 2001

Continued

Table 8-1 Alternative Health Care Systems for Dementia and Parkinson's Disease—cont'd

Intervention	Management	Treatment Regimen	Cautions, Precautions, Interactions	References
Ayurveda—cont'd				
Breathing	Help improve memory For PD	Alternate nostril breathing recommended When rigidity prevails, plugging the left nostril (for days or weeks) is recommended		Lad, 1998 Frawley, 2000
Meditation	For PD and other neurological conditions	Mantra SOM is good for long-term debilitating disorders; the mantra SHAM calms the nerves, and OM is effective for clearing and calming the nervous system		Frawley, 2000
Traditional Chinese Medicine				
Acupuncture	For dementia; may improve anxiety, depression, verbal orientation, motor coordination, thinking skills	Qualified acupuncturist and individualized treatment recommended	Qualified practitioner needed	Acupuncture Today, 2000; Bensky, 1981; Emerson, Lombardo, 2000; Kao, 2000; O'Connor,

	For PD; in rat model, acupuncture increased dopamine levels	Needs human study	Qualified practitioner needed	Hsu et al, 2001
Acupressure	May decrease wandering in patients with AD and increase quiet time	Foot acupressure (4 points) and massage 5 min on each foot for 10 days	5 in experimental group and 5 in control group; must know technique for foot massage	Gach, 1990; Snyder, Tseng, 2002; Sutherland et al, 1999
Qi gong	For PD; One study showed diminished "tremble," increased interval between attacks, and improved speech	Awareness, breathing, meditation, movement self-practice recommended; or practitioner used if too ill	Qualified practitioner needed	Chen, 1989; Sancier et al, 2001
Homeopathic remedies	In one study there was reduced tremor, bradykinesia, rigidity, confusion, on-off phenomena, and medication dosage	*Neurotrophin* or other remedies as appropriate; case-taking must occur, and patient must fit profile for the remedy	Qualified practitioner needed	Chapman, 2001; LaValle, 2000; Lockie, Geddes, 1995

AD, *Alzheimer's disease*; L-dopa, *levodopa*; PD, *Parkinson's disease*; tid, *three times daily.*

Campbell (1997) describes one woman who had not spoken or interacted with others for 2 years but suddenly started singing aloud in a beautiful voice when she heard the tune, "You Made Me Love You." Following this incident, she continued to sing and to be more social. Music has no adverse effects or interactions with other treatments, can be used in any setting, and is an inexpensive intervention. In two studies, patients with AD who participated in music therapy demonstrated increased blood flow and activity as measured by positron emission tomography (PET) and electroencephalogram (EEG) studies; patients also showed improvement in spatial task performance (Adams et al, 2001; Nakamura et al, 1999; Rideout, Laubach, 1996). Music decreased problem behaviors, promoted social interaction, and enhanced memory (Adams et al, 2001). In one study, the researchers noted that the patients were better able to remember new information when it was presented in the form of music rather than the spoken word (Brotons et al, 1997).

Kumar and colleagues (1999) found that music therapy produced significantly elevated levels of melatonin, norepinephrine, and epinephrine in patients with AD. The authors note that most AD patients have significant disruption in melatonin secretion, disturbing the normal circadian rhythms. Twenty male patients with a probable diagnosis of AD had daily music therapy sessions for 4 weeks in groups of four or five patients. The therapy included 10 minutes of singing familiar songs and 10 minutes of drumming. Between the songs and the drumming, the patients were encouraged to create musical sounds on xylophones in response to the music therapist's direction. The serum melatonin in the music therapy subjects continued to increase even after the study was discontinued. In addition, behavioral changes were noted, including increased social interaction, increased ability to follow direction and learn new songs, and improved ability to anticipate endings and changes in the music.

Campbell (1997) suggests using songs that are easy to sing, well known, and relevant to the background of the patients, such as religious hymns or other familiar music. When planning music activities, health care providers (HCPs) need to consider the attention span of the patients, as well as to avoid music with complicated phrasing or too many verses. Some patients enjoy having simple rhythm instruments such as shakers or tambourines with which to keep time. Building reminiscing activity around old familiar tunes is an activity that is especially important in early-stage AD. Music may be combined with other NAC therapies to promote relaxation.

One nursing home in New Jersey has created a special room to promote relaxation. The room is called a "Snoezelen Room" after the Dutch words for "to sniff" and "to snooze." The room has soft-colored lights, calming music, and soothing aromatherapy. This approach, originating in Holland, is being introduced in more long-term care facilities in the United States (Diskin, 1999).

Music for Parkinson's Disease

Other case studies describe the usefulness of music for patients with PD:

> Randall (1991) described several cases of people with PD who were aphasic but could sing words of previously known songs. Another woman with an advanced case of the disease would sit stiff and motionless for long periods of time, yet play the piano for hours. (Adams et al, 2001, p. 60)

While listening to music, some patients with PD are able to regain some rhythmic movements they have lost, such as walking. Pachetti and colleagues (2000) conducted a 3-month study of the benefits of music therapy for patients with PD. Thirty-two patients were divided into two groups, one receiving music therapy and one receiving physical therapy. The music therapy group participated in choral singing, voice exercises, rhythmic and free body movements, and group music invention. The other group focused on stretching, balance and gait, and specific motor tasks. At 3 months, the music therapy group had a significant improvement in bradykinesia, as measured on the Unified Parkinson's Disease Rating Scale; they also demonstrated positive emotional changes on the Happiness Measure.

Campbell (1997) describes a music professor whose PD symptoms disappeared when he played the harp, only to return after several days of not playing. Campbell demonstrates that brain waves can be modulated by music. He postulates that music affects coordination through a direct connection between the auditory nerve and the body's muscles. Gardner (1990) describes the experience of playing music for her father who had both AD and PD. Though he was rarely lucid for more than a few seconds, he was able to carry on a normal conversation after listening to one of Campbell's compositions.

The HCP should select music that evokes both an emotional and a physiologic response from the patient. Researchers at Beth Israel Hospital suggest using stimulating music that will facilitate a particular movement but that is also familiar enough so that the patient may continue to benefit outside of the music session (Family Caregiver Alliance, 2001).

Exercise for Parkinson's Disease

Because movement and coordination are the functions that PD affects most significantly, exercise is a logical intervention and often recommended as part of an overall treatment program. However, many forms of exercise are frightening for these patients because of the fear of falling, losing balance, or both. Argue (2001) suggests a series of progressive exercises designed to help maintain flexibility and function. The focus is on the need to make movement *conscious*, because unconscious control of movement is lost in this disease. By practicing the exercises, the patient uses the body to train the mind. Besides the physical practice of the exercise, patients are encouraged to cultivate a quiet mind, a state of relaxed alertness, and focused attention. Patients are instructed to stop one action before starting another, promoting a sense of completion that decreases impatience and frustration (Argue, 2001).

Before starting any exercise program, patients should consult with their HCP. HCPs can consult available references and recommend simple chair exercises for flexibility and strengthening. An exercise therapist who is familiar with PD can be consulted before starting a more ambitious program. Dance therapy may also be appropriate.

Other Mind-Body-Spirit Interventions for Dementia and Parkinson's Disease

For dementia and PD, art therapy and other creative arts may support expression, improve coordination, and focus attention (Leslie, 2001; Sandrick, 1995; Sanzotta, 1996; Sterrett, Pokorney, 1994). *The Brown University Long-Term Care Quality Advisor* (1998) discusses techniques that benefit patients with AD. Techniques include a 16-week program of relaxation music and aromatherapy (flowers, smells from the kitchen, spices) paired with reminiscing (for nursing home residents with problematic behaviors related to dementia). Residents are able to redirect nervous energy and recapture past memories. In addition, social support and stress-management interventions are needed for both the patient and the caregiver. These measures include support groups, individual or group counseling, respite and day care services, skills training, and specific programs (Freeman, Lawlis, 2001). Caregivers and patients may also benefit from affirmations, journaling, imagery, reminiscence, meditation, and prayer (Luckoff, 2000; Geidt, 1997; Hay, 2000; MacKenzie, 2000). Table 8-2 provides an overview of mind-body-spirit interventions for dementia and PD.

BIOLOGIC-BASED THERAPIES FOR DEMENTIA AND PARKINSON'S DISEASE

Diet, Vitamins, and Minerals for Dementia

The role of diet and supplements on dementia and AD has had increased research focus (Burns et al, 1990; Cunha, 1995; Franchi et al, 1998; Khalsa, 1998; Kleinjnen et al, 1991; LaRue et al, 1997; Sano et al, 1997). Adams and colleagues (2001) state that "many studies have been fraught with methodologic problems. Nevertheless, investigators are seeking to identify key variables and improve methodologies for investigating the clinical utility of vitamins" (p. 56).

Table 8-2 Mind-Body-Spirit Interventions for Dementia and Parkinson's Disease

Intervention	Management	Treatment Regimen	Cautions, Precautions, Interactions	References
Snoezelen room	Calms and soothes; promotes relaxation	Long-term care alternative	Ensure safety	Diskin, 1999
Innovative programs	Arizona Model and other models and principles of care	Example: Arizona Model. Social activity-based, homelike environment emphasizing safety and activities designed to maintain the residents' highest level of function. Career ladder and mandatory continuing education for caregivers. Family and volunteer education. Risk reduction/prevention program. NP makes rounds 5 days/wk and on 24-hr call for emergencies. Also had recommended levels for each patient's functional level, including cooking cleaning, painting for highest level 1 of function to		Cesarotti et al, 2001; Jelinek, 2001; Mc Andrew et al, 2001; Rauckhorst 2001

Continued

Intervention	Management	Treatment Regimen	Cautions, Precautions, Interactions	References
Innovative programs, cont'd		5 min/hr, one on one or companionship, hugs, being read to as tolerated at level 5 and 6, the lowest level of function		
Alzheimer's Disease and Related Disorders Association	Provides videotapes, audiotapes, brochures, books, information	Individual preference. www.alz.org		
Alzheimer's Association Safe Return Program	For patient with AD and dementia who wanders; operated by Alzheimer's Association and National Center for Missing Persons	Program provides identification products such as wallet cards, identification bracelets, necklaces, clothing tags; patient is registered; national photo database and a 24-hr toll-free emergency crisis line is available		Safe Return, Box A-3956, Chicago, IL 60690, 800-572-1122 to report a lost patient
ADEAR Center; clearinghouse	Drug treatment, research, support	Sponsored by the National Institute on Aging (ADEAR);		

		www.alzheimers.org; adear@alzheimers.org		
for information on AD	services, literary searches for professionals, educational materials, information available			
Exercise	For PD; improves flexibility, coordination, and muscle control	Patient strength and coordination is assessed; HCP clearance if needed; ascertain appropriate exercises for PD; involve PT or activity therapist; yoga may also be helpful	Coordinate exercise program with other disciplines if unfamiliar with exercise physiology	Argue, 2001; Ross, 2001
Imagery	For PD and caregivers; helps increase confidence and reduce stress and pain	Recommended: *Healing Journey* (Miller); *Pain* (Naparstek); *Stress I and Stress II* (Naparstek)	No driving or operating machinery while using audiotapes	Geidt, 1997; Miller, 1980; Naparstek, 1995a, 1995b
Journaling or writing	For PD and caregivers; A possible way to express when cannot talk; facilitates self-discovery, self-	Journal can be any style: poetry, narrative, etc.; Day suggests AlphaPoem, captured moments, character sketch, clustering (free association around a central word), dialogue, inner wisdom, list of 100 (e.g., 100		Day, 2001; Snyder, 2002a

Continued

Intervention	Management	Treatment Regimen	Cautions, Precautions, Interactions	References
Journaling or writing, cont'd	reflection; provides creative outlet; enhances positive coping	ways to nurture myself), different points of view, unsent letter; Snyder suggests free flow, topical, and intensive		
Meditation	May improve cognitive and behavioral flexibility and associative learning in people with mild to moderate cognitive impairment	TM	In study, people doing TM had highest 3-yr survival when compared with relaxation and mindfulness group	Alexander et al, 1989; Rauckhorst, 2001
Music therapy	For dementia; may improve cognitive function, social interaction, and expression	Select familiar music that is pleasing to patient; provide structured listening; provide rhythm instruments	None	Adams et al, 2001; Brotons et al, 1997; Campbell, 1997; Kumar et al, 1999
	For PD; improves coordination and	Select music that is familiar and pleasing; focus on physiologic	Balance and safety are concerns	Adams, 2001; Campbell,

	facilitates smooth movements; may help aphasia	response to music-stimulated movement		1997; Family Caregiver Alliance, 2001; Gardner, 1990; Pacchetti et al, 2000; Randall, 1991
Prayer	For patient and caregivers	Personal preference		Dossey, 1993, 1999; Meisenhelder et al, 2000; Snyder et al, 2002; Stolley et al, 1999
Relaxation	For caregiver as support	Numerous modalities		Davis et al, 2000
Reminiscing	For AD or PD; redirects energy; recaptures past memories	Is combined with relaxation, aromatherapy		Brown University, 1998
Social support and caregiver strategies	For early-stage AD and caregivers; provides emotional support, offers modeling, enhances coping,	Consists of services, skills training, special programs. Caregiver skills and counseling include how to create safe environment; emphasis on importance of flexibility for	Support is crucial for caregivers; HCP must have large base of resources	Davies, Robinson, 1995; Freeman, Lawlis, 2001; Geldmacher et al, 2001;

Continued

Table 8-2	Mind-Body-Spirit Interventions for Dementia and Parkinson's Disease—cont'd			
Intervention	**Management**	**Treatment Regimen**	**Cautions, Precautions, Interactions**	**References**
Social support, cont'd	provides a sense of belonging	feeding, ADL, handling difficult behaviors, community services, respite care, day care, tending to caregiver's health		Luskin et al, 1999
Art therapy	For dementia, AD, and PD for self-expression and diversion; drawings may be revealing. Also for caregivers	Externalize emotions is the goal	Safety concerns	Leslie, 2001; Sandrick, 1995; Sanzotta, 1996; Sterrett et al, 1994
Dance therapy	For dementia and AD to improve and maintain mobility and flexibility and social interaction; possibly reduce stress	Excess energy dissipation; exercise; to help with balance and mobility	Safety concerns	Andrews et al, 1999

AD, Alzheimer's disease; ADEAR, Alzheimer's Disease Education and Referral; ADL, activities of daily living; HCP, health care provider; PD, Parkinson's disease; PT, physical therapist; TM, Transcendental meditation.

516

Grant (1997) reviewed studies examining the links between diet and AD, stating that fat consumption and total caloric intake are apparent dietary risk factors. Countries in which the diets are the lowest in fats (Nigeria or China, for example) also have the lowest incidence of AD (Hendrie et al, 1995; Graves et al, 1996). Khalsa (1998) cites a study in which low levels of omega-3 fatty acids have been implicated in memory loss among the aged and AD patient (Soderberg et al, 1991).

Several sources recommend a diet rich in antioxidants to prevent and treat AD (Behl et al, 1992; Fricker, 1997; La Valle, 2000; Sano et al, 1997). Antioxidant and free-radical scavenger nutrients include vitamin A, vitamin C, vitamin E, selenium, and beta-carotene, lycopene, and lutein. Weil (1998) and Murray and Pizzorno (1998) suggest supplements such as folic acid, thiamin, vitamin B12, vitamin C, vitamin E, and flaxseed oil as part of the nutritional treatment of early-stage AD.

Adams and colleagues (2001) discuss vitamin B complex, vitamin E, niacin, and lecithin among the nutrients most associated with dementia:

> Vitamin B12 serves as a coenzyme in the synthesis of serotonin and catecholamine neurotransmitters, whereas vitamin B6 acts as a cofactor in the production of a variety of neurotransmitters and acts on receptors in the glutamatergic neurotransmitter system, which plays an important role in learning and memory. Low levels of vitamins B12 and B6 may lead to blood vessel damage and increased risk of localized cerebrovascular disease, whereas vitamin B12 deficiency may spur a series of reactions that interfere with the DNA replication needed for optimal functioning of neurons. Finally, vitamin E serves to trap free radicals that threaten nerve cell membranes, thereby protecting against cell damage. (Adams et al, 2001, p. 56)

In addition, lecithin (a phospholipid) increases levels of choline, necessary for synthesis of acetylcholine, a neurotransmitter for memory and learning (Adams et al, 2001; Holford, Peace, 1994); in the normal older person, lecithin has helped increase memory (Safford, Baumel, 1994). Niacin (vitamin B3) is taken for many functions: to decrease lipids, improve memory loss, increase circulation, and treat chronic brain syndrome (*Pharmacist's Letter/Prescriber's Letter* [PL/PL], 2000).

Another nutritional supplement that has shown promising results is L-acetylcarnitine (LAC). Carnitine is a combination of the amino acids lysine and methionine. LAC is a combination of carnitine and acetic acid and is naturally produced in the brain. LAC acts as an antioxidant and mimics the action of acetylcholine, which is deficient in the brains of patients with AD. Because they are structurally similar to acetylcholine, both LAC and carnitine have been evaluated as to their efficacy in slowing the progression of AD. In a multicenter year-long study of 130 patients, the patients who received LAC scored significantly better on cognitive tests than did the placebo group (Thal et al,1996).

PL/PL (2002) states that both choline and lecithin are "likely ineffective" when used for memory loss, AD, and dementia and that 5-hydroxytryptophan (5-HTP) is possibly ineffective. The authors do say that vitamin E is possibly effective in slowing cognitive decline in AD and that a combination of vitamin C and E showed a decreased risk of developing vascular or other dementias, but not AD; they also say that LAC is:

> possibly effective when used orally for improving memory and slowing the rate of decline in Alzheimer's disease. [LAC] might slow the rate of disease progression and improve some measures of cognitive function and behavioral performance in people with Alzheimer's disease. It is most likely to be effective in those with early onset Alzheimer's disease who are less than 66 years of age and have a faster rate of disease progression and mental decline...may not be beneficial for patients with early onset Alzheimer's disease who do not have rapid disease progression and rapid rate of cognitive decline. (PL/PL, 2002, p. 18)

LAC may take up to 6 months to work. Ernst (2001) says the evidence for alpha-tocopherol, LAC, lecithin, and phosphatidylserine is "encouraging," although the effect size is small.

Herbals for Dementia

Gingko biloba Gingko biloba has been promoted for its ability to enhance memory in patients with dementia. Gingko has several mechanisms of action that help explain its usefulness in both Alzheimer's and multiinfarct dementia. Gingko biloba relaxes smooth vascular muscle and exerts a vasorelaxation effect in the cerebral arteries; it is an antagonist of platelet activating factor; and it has antioxidant properties. Gingko scavenges free-radical anions, molecules that play a role in cerebral ischemia and cell damage in AD (Kleinjnen et al, 1992; Adams et al, 2001).

A randomized, double-blind study assessed the efficacy and safety of gingko biloba in patients with dementia. Three hundred nine subjects who received the gingko showed stabilization and, in most cases, demonstrated marked improvement of cognitive function based on the Alzheimer's Disease Assessment Scale, the Geriatric Evaluation by Relative's Rating Scale, and the Clinical Global Rating Instrument. The benefits lasted from 6 months to a year. In addition to improvement in cognitive function, caregivers noted positive changes in the subjects' daily living skills and social behavior (Le Bars et al, 1997 in Adams et al, 2001). McKenna and colleagues (2001) outlined the studies that have been done on ginkgo, stating that, in a meta-analysis (Oken et al, 1998), only 4 of 50 studies met the essential inclusion criteria, leaving only 212 subjects. Nonetheless, a significant modest effect size from the gingko treatment was reported.

Most authors recommend gingko biloba that is standardized to contain 24% flavone glycosides. Murray and Pizzorno (1998) recommend that gingko biloba extract be taken for at least 12 weeks to determine its efficacy. The recommended dosage is from 120 to 240 mg a day in divided doses (Fetrow, Avila, 1999; Murray, Pizzorno 1998; PL/PL, 2002). Patients who have bleeding disorders or who are taking anticoagulants should avoid gingko or consult their HCP. Rare side effects include mild gastrointestinal irritation, headache, and skin rash. Gingko is contraindicated for children and for women during pregnancy.

Ginseng (Panax) Although research is limited, *Panax* ginseng has also been studied for patients with AD because of its action as an acetylcholine agonist; it has shown benefits comparable to gingko (Adams et al, 2001). In one study (Zhao, McDaniel, 1998), rats with prefrontal cortex lesions were given a 0-mg, 40-mg, or 80-mg dose of ginseng. After 30 days, the rats that had received the higher dose of ginseng performed better on learning and memory tasks than did the lower dose group and the control group. In normal rats, ginseng improved learning, memory, and task performance. In another study (Beneshin, 1991), the brains of rats that had received ginseng showed a significant increase in acetylcholine activity in the hippocampus, the region of the brain responsible for memory (Adams et al, 2001). Fetrow and Avila (1999) give an overview of several human studies with ginseng.

Aromatherapy for Dementia
Camarius (2001), a nurse who worked with AD patients in a Colorado nursing home, gave aromatherapy massages to patients with late-stage AD. All of these patients required antipsychotic medications to control their behavior. Camarius administered the massages twice a week in 40-minute sessions. After 5 weeks, none of the patients required medication for behavior control. When Camarius moved to another nursing home, she expanded her use of aromatherapy to include room diffusers. Camarius used lemon in the morning to wake people up and calming scents such as ylang ylang in the afternoon. As her interest grew, Camarius began teaching massage therapy students how to use essential oils in massages with AD patients; she also has developed an aromatherapy massage kit for nurses. Camarius offers suggestions for the aromatherapy with patients with AD, including discussion of oils, on her web site (www.nana.org/alz2.html).

Uplifting essential oils include clary sage, peppermint, lemon, bergamot, and rosemary. Relaxing oils include lavender, German chamomile, rose, geranium, and ylang ylang. Guidelines for the use of essential oils should be followed, especially considering age and skin sensitivities. Buckle (1993, 1997, 1999) also has essential oil recommendations for specific conditions.

Dietary Supplements for Parkinson's Disease

A low-protein diet with supplemental vitamins and minerals is recommended for patients with PD (Bradford, 1996). Patients who are taking L-dopa should avoid high-protein foods because the L-dopa must compete with the dietary protein for absorption in the small intestine. Patients should maintain an adequate intake of calcium and vitamin D to minimize their risk of bone fractures with falls. Patients with PD are prone to constipation from their medications and need to monitor their intake of fluids and fiber; a diet high in fresh fruits and vegetables and whole grains is beneficial. Vitamin B6 interferes with the action of L-dopa, thus it should not be supplemented for patients on this medication, nor should any of the B vitamins without consulting with a HCP (Spratto, Woods, 2002).

Research interest in the role of antioxidants in PD has increased. The central nervous system is rich in saturated fats and is metabolically very active, making it susceptible to neuronal damage from oxidative stress (Dawson, Dawson, 1996; Fahn, Cohen, 1992). Fahn (1991) found that patients with PD who received large daily doses of vitamin C (3000 mg) and vitamin E (3200 international units [IU]) over a period of 7 years showed a delayed progression in the illness compared with patients who did not receive the antioxidants. The antioxidant group was able to delay the onset of drug therapy for up to 3 years longer than did the other group. Another antioxidant found to be beneficial in PD is glutathione. A decline in the antioxidant molecule glutathione has been shown to be a factor in the development of PD, as well as several other neurodegenerative disorders (Schulz et al, 2000; Bains, Shaw, 1997; Kidd, 2000). Perlmutter (2000b) found that intravenous administration of glutathione almost completely reversed the symptoms of PD for up to 4 months. Glutathione must be administered intravenously and works by potentiating the effects of dopamine and increasing sensitivity to serotonin. The standard dose Perlmutter uses is 400 to 1000 mg of glutathione in saline given over 10 minutes three times a week (Perlmutter, 2000b). Perlmutter reports no significant side effects associated with glutathione therapy.

Coenzyme Q10, an antioxidant, has potential benefit in reducing the damage to the mitochondria of nerve cells in the substantia nigra, the area of the brain affected by PD. Both mitochondrial dysfunction and damage from free radicals have been demonstrated in

PD. Shults (2001) found that the level of coenzyme Q10 was significantly lower in PD patients than it was in normal controls.

The Perlmutter regimen (2000) for PD includes glutathione; coenzyme Q10; nicotinamide adenine dinucleotide (NADH); phosphatidylserine; vitamins C, D, and E; alpha lipoic acid; N-acetylcysteine; LAC; and ginkgo biloba. Kidd (2000) recommends management of PD with glutathione, LAC, coenzyme Q10, and NADH. NADH is essential to intracellular adenosine triphosphate (ATP) production. The heart and the brain, both organs that require large amounts of energy, contain the greatest amounts of NADH. Clinical trials in Europe have demonstrated that NADH may help relieve symptoms of PD. Birkmayer (1993) gave 885 patients with PD different doses and forms of NADH. One half of the patients received 12.5 mg of NADH in normal saline administered intravenously over 30 minutes. The other one half received an oral dose of 5 mg of NADH. The NADH was administered over 14 days: 19.3% showed a significant decrease in disability, and 21.8% showed a moderate improvement. The benefits of the oral dose were similar to those of the parenteral dose. NADH is also being studied for use in depression, AD, and for possible use in boosting athletic performance. No toxic effects have been noted.

Herbals for Parkinson's Disease

Herbs that have mention for PD include ginkgo, grape seed, and passionflower (La Valle, 2000; Fetrow, Avila, 1999). Gingko has neuroprotective effects and peripheral circulatory benefits, while passionflower (*Passiflora incarnata*) is an antispasmodic, anxiolytic, and sedative. Grape seed is an antioxidant that is used for neurologic, vascular, and visual problems (La Valle, 2000; PL/PL, 2000); however, German Commission E has no specific Parkinson's recommendation for these herbs (Blumenthal et al, 2000). Table 8-3 reviews biologic-based therapies for dementia and PD.

MANIPULATIVE AND BODY-BASED METHODS AND ENERGY THERAPIES FOR DEMENTIA AND PARKINSON'S DISEASE

Massage for Dementia and Parkinson's Disease

Massage has been demonstrated to benefit patients with AD by producing relaxation and a sense of well being; it may also decrease agitation and anxiety, increase circulation, promote comfort, and strengthen the relationship between caregiver and patient, as well as reduce wandering and withdrawal. Dementia patients who received a hand massage showed improved relationships with family members and care providers, as well as decreased agitation and withdrawal (Kilstoff, Chenoweth, 1998; Snyder et al, 1995, 2002). Even when brief massages are given for only a few days, patients demonstrate improvement in behavior. Massage provides caring touch, muscle

Table 8-3 Biologic-Based Therapies for Dementia and Parkinson's Disease

A complete prescribing source should be consulted before using biologic therapies. Nutrient doses may be above the recommended daily allowance or tolerable upper limit. In illness or deficiency, such doses may be acceptable; however, long-term use may not be appropriate. Herbs may cause allergic reactions and interactions. Herbs are generally contraindicated or not recommended for women during pregnancy and lactation and for children unless research data or a long history of safe use has been established. Information regarding dementia and biologic-based therapies is conflicting.

Intervention	Management	Treatment Regimen	Cautions, Precautions, Interactions	References
Diet	For dementia; may slow onset or progression of cognitive decline	Omega-3 and -6 essential fatty acids; fish oil (has EPA, DHA [omega-3s]); flaxseed (has ALA [an omega-3]); take 1 tbsp flaxseed oil/day; evening primrose (has GLA [an omega-6])	May have increased bleeding with evening primrose, fish oil; evening primrose may lower seizure level; fish oil may alter glucose regulation	Grant, 1997; PL/PL, 2000, 2002; Murray, Pizzorno, 1998; Soderberg et al, 1991; Weil, 1998
	For PD; protein may compete with L-dopa for absorption in small intestine	Low-protein diet recommended if on L-dopa	Watch nutritional status to ensure nutrient intake	Bradford, 1996

Vitamins			
	For dementia; may slow onset or progression of cognitive decline; vitamins C and E together may protect against vascular and mixed dementias	Murray and Pizzorno recommended antioxidant dose for dementia: vitamin C, 500-1000 mg tid; vitamin E, 400-800 IU/day. Adult RDA: vitamin C, 75 mg (female), 90 mg (male). Adult UL for vitamin C: 2000 mg/day. Vitamin E RDA 15 mg/day. UL for vitamin E, 1000 mg/day.	Vitamin A, beta carotene, lutein, lycopene also have mention for dementia	Murray, Pizzorno, 1998; PL/PL, 2000, 2002; Weil, 1998
	For PD; may slow progression in patients not yet on medication and delay need for medications up to 2 to 3 yrs longer	Vitamin C, 250-1000 mg qd; vitamin D, 400 IU qd; vitamin E, 800-1200 IU qd. High doses (vitamin C, 3000 mg/day, vitamin E, 3200 IU/day) were given in the study	See UL and RDA above; all patients on study eventually required PD medications	Fahn, 1991; Fahn et al, 1992; Murray, Pizzorno, 1999
	For dementia	Vitamin B complex: includes folate, thiamine, niacin (B3), pyridoxine (B6), cobalamin (B12); inositol varied specific	Doses for dementia and AD will be more than RDA; check sources	Adams, 2001; Murray, Pizzorno, 1998, 1999; PL/PL 2002

Continued

Table 8-3 Biologic-Based Therapies for Dementia and Parkinson's Disease—cont'd

Intervention	Management	Treatment Regimen	Cautions, Precautions, Interactions	References
Vitamins, cont'd		recommended doses for dementia. Adult RDAs and ULs: Folate, 400 µg/day. adult UL: Folate, 1000 µg/day. Thiamine, 11 mg/day (female), 12 mg/day (male). Thiamine UL not determined. Niacin, 14 mg/day (female), 16 mg/day (male). Niacin UL 35 mg/day. Pyridoxine, 13-17 mg/day; Pyridoxine UL 100 mg/day. Vitamin B12, 24 µg/day; vitamin B12 UL not determined. Pantothenic acid (B5) RDA: 5 mg. UL: none given. Inositol (B8) PL/PL says "possibly ineffective."		

	For PD; NAD may produce short-term relief of symptoms	NAD: 5 mg/day PO given in study and compared with IV administration; oral results similar to parenteral; PL/PL: vitamin B3 includes niacin (nicotinic acid) and niacinamide (nicotinamide); niacinamide is incorporated into coenzymes NAD and NADP		Kidd, 2000; Perlmutter, 2001; PL/PL, 2002
Minerals	For PD: Minerals that regulate muscle and nerve function; ensures bone strength	Adult RDA: calcium, 1000-1200 mg/day; adult UL: calcium, 2500 mg/day. Magnesium RDA 310-420 mg/day; magnesium UL 350 mg/day	UL for Mg represents intake from a pharmacologic agent only and does not include intake from food and water	NAP, 2002
	For dementia; modest slowing of cognitive decline in AD. Zinc is neurotoxic at high levels but is	Adult RDA: zinc, 8 mg (female), 11 mg (male); UL: 40 mg/day. Must have proper zinc/copper ratio; ratio of zinc to copper fed to humans of	Increased zinc can lead to depletion of copper, iron, calcium, and magnesium. Elevated copper, calcium, or iron can deplete zinc.	NAP, 2002; PL/PL, 2002

Continued

Table 8-3 Biologic-Based Therapies for Dementia and Parkinson's Disease—cont'd

Intervention	Management	Treatment Regimen	Cautions, Precautions, Interactions	References
Minerals, cont'd	markedly reduced in brains of patients with AD	2:1, 5:1, and 15:1 had limited effects on copper absorption, thus stay within that range; vegetarians and people with diarrhea need more zinc; different salt forms contain different amounts of zinc	Interferes with glucocorticoids and immunosuppressants; doses greater than 50 mg/day can lower HDL levels	
Other	For PD; glutathione potentiates effects of dopamine	Glutathione: 400-1000 mg IV 3 times a week; does not seem to absorb well orally	Glutathione must be diluted in normal saline and given IV	Bains, Shaw, 1997; Kidd, 2000; Perlmutter, 2000, 2001; PL/PL, 2002; Schulz et al, 2000
	For PD; part of the Perlmutter supplement regimen	Coenzyme Q10; alpha lipoic acid; N-acetyl-cysteine; LAC; phosphatidylserine		Perlmutter, 2001; Shults, 2001

For dementia; LAC may improve memory and slow rate of cognitive decline in patients with AD; may supply postsynaptic cholinergic-receptor agonists that may be used as acetylcholine analogs	LAC for AD: 1500-4000 mg/daily (usually divided in 2 or 3 doses). For memory impairment: 1500-2000 daily		PL/PL, 2000, 2002; Spagnoli, 1991; Thal et al, 1996
For dementia; acetylcholine precursors. AD suggests cholinergic deficit, thus a theoretical basis for prescription with choline (a precursor) and lecithin (lecithin increases choline)	Possibly lecithin, choline, phosphatidylcholine (a constituent of lecithin; if no improvement in 2 wks with phosphatidylcholine, discontinue use	PL/PL state benefit of lecithin, phosphatidylcholine, or choline not apparent in patients with AD because increases in central cholinergic activity are not apparent	Murray, Pizzorno, 1998; PL/PL, 2002

Continued

Table 8-3 Biologic-Based Therapies for Dementia and Parkinson's Disease—cont'd

Intervention	Management	Treatment Regimen	Cautions, Precautions, Interactions	References
Other, cont'd	For dementia; possibly effective when used for AD and senile dementia in the short-term; constituent of lecithin (but not acetylcholine precursor) has shown benefit	Phosphatidylserine 100 mg tid (not a precursor but helps short-term memory and cognition)		PL/PL, 2002; Rauckhorst, 2001
Herbals				
Gingko (Gingko biloba)	For AD and vascular and mixed dementias; gingko enhances cerebral circulation through anticoagulant properties and reduces damage	Gingko dosage: 120-240 mg/day divided in 2 or 3 doses; take at least 12 wks to determine benefits. Start at 120 mg/day and titrate up if needed to reduce GI side effects and	SE: may cause rash, GI irritation, headache; numerous potential interactions; gingko has anticoagulant properties; do not give to patients on anticoagulant therapy	Adams et al, 2001; Fetrow, Avila, 1999; Kleinjnin et al, 1992; LeBars et al, 1997; McKenna et al, 2001;

	from free radicals; acts as antiinflammatory		potential bleeding.	Oken, 1998; PL/PL, 2000, 2002
	For PD	Ginkgo biloba, grape seed, passionflower (Passiflora incarnata), varying doses	Read prescribing data	Fetrow, Avila, 1999; La Valle, 2000
Ginseng (Panax ginseng)	Improves cognitive function (for loss of concentration)	0.6-3.0 g (cut or powdered root) 1-3 times/day or 1 c of tea 1-3 times/day; tea made with 3 g of root in 150 ml boiling water, steeped for 10-15 minutes, and strained. Use for 3-4 weeks.	Numerous interactions; do not combine ginseng with estrogen therapy; ginseng may interfere with antiepileptic medications. Take from 3 weeks to 3 months. A Panax-free period of 2 weeks is recommended between consecutive courses.	Blumenthal et al, 2000; PL/PL, 2002
Cat's claw (Uncaria tomentosa or Uncaria guianensis)	For dementia (memory and cognition); may possibly block formation or deposition of beta-amyloid protein	PTI-00703 (a specific cat's claw extract); no specific dementia dose given	May lower BP; may inhibit cytochrome P450 system	PL/PL, 2000, 2002

Continued

Table 8-3 Biologic-Based Therapies for Dementia and Parkinson's Disease—cont'd

Intervention	Management	Treatment Regimen	Cautions, Precautions, Interactions	References
Chinese club moss (Huperzia serrata)	Possibly improves memory; inhibits acetylcholinesterase (the enzyme that breaks down acetylcholine)	Huperzine A (an alkaloid isolate of Chinese club moss): 50-200 µg bid	Must be Chinese club moss, which contains huperizine A (reversible and crosses blood-brain barrier). Various interactions with asthma, COPD, cardiovascular or GI disease.	Ernst, 2001; Murray, Pizzorno, 1999; PL/PL, 2000, 2002
Gotu kola (Centella asiatica)	For dementia; possibly effective in improving memory and intelligence; early evidence only in efficacy for AD	No dementia dose given	SE: elevation of BP, glucose, triglycerides, cholesterol levels	PL/PL, 2000, 2002
Aromatherapy	Reduces agitated behavior in patients with dementia; may help in PD	Select oils for their properties. Uplifting essential oils include: clary sage, peppermint, lemon, bergamot, and rosemary. Relaxing oils	Do not apply essential oils directly to skin; assess for sensitivities; caution with patients who have respiratory conditions or allergies;	Buckle, 1993, 1997; Camarius, 2001; Cesarotti, Stern, 2001;

include: lavender, German chamomile, rose, geranium, and ylang ylang. Pine, eucalyptus, peppermint are used to trigger conversation and memory. Dilute in carrier oil; assess patient response; use with massage or diffuser	do not apply over broken skin	Rauckhorst, 2001; Robins, 1999

ALA, Alpha-linolenic acid; bid, twice daily; BP, blood pressure; DHA, docosahexaenoic acid; EPA, eicosapentaenoic acid; GI, gastrointestinal; GLA, gamma linolenic acid; HDL, high-density lipoprotein; IU, international units; IV, intravenous; LAC, L-acetylcarnitine; L-dopa, levodopa; NAD, nicotinamide adenine dinucleotide; NADP, nicotinamide adenine dinucleotide phosphate; NAP, National Academy Press; PL/PL, Pharmacist's Letter/Prescriber's Letter; PO, by mouth; qd, daily; RDA, Recommended Daily Allowance; SE, side effects; tid, three times daily; UL, upper limits—the maximum level of daily nutrient that is likely to pose no risk of adverse effects. Includes intake from food, water, and supplements.
Dietary recommended intake (DRI) values expand on the RDAs and contain four categories of recommendations (i.e., RDA, AI [adequate intake], UL, EAR [estimated average requirement]). Check for the latest data.
Both the AI and the RDA are goals for intakes, but are defined differently.
RDA is the intake at which risk of inadequacy is very small (2% to 3%); RDA is expected to meet the nutrient needs of 97% to 98% of the individuals in a life stage and gender group.
AI is the observed average or experimentally set intake by a defined population or subgroup that appears to sustain a defined nutritional status, such as growth rate, normal circulating nutrient values, or other functional indicators of health. An AI is used if sufficient scientific evidence is not available to derive an EAR. AN AI IS NOT AN RDA.
EAR is the intake that meets the estimated nutrient needs of one half of the individuals in a group.
From the Food and Nutrition Board, National Academy of Sciences, Institute of Medicine (www.nap.edu).

relaxation, and meaningful sensory stimulation. Patients with late-stage AD are especially touch-deprived other than what they receive during custodial care. With patients who are agitated, starting with a simple hand massage to avoid over-stimulation may be best. The patient's response should be monitored; if the patient seems confused or agitated by the touch, the massage should be discontinued. Family members can be taught to give simple massages as a way of promoting emotional connection and physical contact. The HCP needs to continue assessing patient tolerance for touch and provide privacy, as well as assessing the skin condition and following the usual massage precautions.

Massage can be relaxing to the stiff muscles and joints of patients with PD. Gentle massage promotes circulation and lymphatic flow, provides relaxation and relief from joint and muscle stiffness, may help decrease rigidity, and enhances a sense of well being, as well as providing stress relief for patients with PD (Brandabur, 2001). Gottlieb (1995) suggests gentle massage of muscles above and below stiff joints. Effleurage and gentle friction may be helpful, although Brandabur suggests that the type of massage (e.g., shiatsu, Swedish massage) is a matter of personal preference and recommends that patients seek a licensed massage therapist.

Koryo hand therapy (KHT) is based on a "systematic relationship between the body and the hand" and works on the same principles as those of acupuncture, except that pressure instead of needles are used. KHT has been promoted for use with neurologic disorders, including PD (Hole, 2001, p. 296). KHT was developed by a Korean physician, Tae Woo Yoo, in 1971. The several levels of treatment include the "Correspondence," "Basic," and "Formulary":

> Correspondence: This approach uses the corresponding or sensitive points on the hand to treat the affected target body area. This is the "aspirin" level of treatment; it is the simplest to learn and usually gives immediate and effective results.
>
> Basic: The Basic approach energized the upper, middle, and lower "heaters" or "burners." This set of points should be used in support of all other KHT treatments.
>
> Formulary: Formularies are specific KHT point prescriptions formulated by Dr. Yoo for different conditions. This "cookbook" approach, based on Dr. Yoo's years of experience, is especially useful for those who are new to KHT. (Hole, 2001, p. 299)

In addition, more complex levels are used for more complex conditions. These levels are called "Three Constitutions," "Five Elements," or "Birth Constitution Biorhythmic."

KHT has been used with blepharospasm, cerebellar ataxia, neuropathy, headache, herpetic neuralgia, visual disturbances, and herniated disc. Case examples are given in Hole's chapter (Hole, 2001).

Energy Therapies for Dementia and Parkinson's Disease

Because Reiki, Therapeutic Touch (TT), and healing touch (HT) may help alleviate pain and anxiety and improve functional ability (Halcon, 2002; Kreiger, 1993; Quinn, 2002; Umbreit, 2002), these therapies may be useful for patients with dementia or PD. Woods and colleagues (1996), using a three-group design (n = 57) with Therapeutic Touch, mimic touch, and a control group, report that:

> residents receiving therapeutic touch exhibited a marked decrease in vocalization after intervention when compared with the control group.., as well as a decrease in manual manipulation. A difference approaching significance for searching and wandering was ascertained for the mimic group after intervention, compared with the control group. Post-intervention decreases in disruptive behavior coincided with the times the intervention was administered. (Woods et al, 1996, p. 96)

The TT was performed twice daily for 5 to 7 minutes for only 3 days. Residents were from a special care unit for patients with AD. In addition, Griffin and Vitro (1998 in Rauckhorst, 2001) found that TT relaxed patients and put them at ease, slowing respiration and decreasing agitated behavior.

Light therapy may also be helpful. Studies have shown a decrease in nighttime restlessness with daytime or early evening use of light boxes (Lovell et al, 1995; Satlin, 1992 in Rauckhorst, 2001). Light therapy may be an inexpensive and an easy way to decrease agitated behaviors.

NAC PRACTICES FOR EATING DISORDERS AND ADDICTIONS

Eating Disorders

The eating disorders include anorexia nervosa, bulimia nervosa, and binge-eating disorder. Anorexia nervosa is characterized by self-inflicted starvation or severe caloric restriction resulting in emaciation, severe electrolyte and endocrine imbalances, and potential death caused by hypokalemic-induced cardiac dysrhythmias. Bulimia nervosa is characterized by episodes of binge eating followed by purging through self-induced vomiting, laxatives, and diuretic abuse. Patients with binge-eating disorder consume large quantities of food without any attempt to lose weight or prevent weight loss (Stuart, Laraia, 2001). Because patients with these disorders tend to have problems with body image, modalities that focus on the self and body awareness may be helpful.

Addictions

Drug and alcohol addiction is a chronic health problem with a poor record of treatment success. However, some forms of NAC, particularly auricular acupuncture, have shown positive results in terms of treatment response and decreased rates of recidivism.

ALTERNATIVE HEALTH CARE SYSTEMS FOR ADDICTION

Acupuncture for Addiction

Acupuncture, which was used in Hong Kong in 1972 to treat acute drug withdrawal (Brumbaugh, 1993), was used in a few settings in the United States in the 1970s, primarily in drug treatment facilities. Since then, acupuncture has been increasingly studied and used as an adjunctive therapy in a variety of addictive disorders. Brumbaugh (1993) describes one of the first residential treatment settings (in Portland, Oregon) where acupuncture was used. Patients in this facility who received acupuncture as part of their treatment were six times less likely to return within the following 6 months than were the patients who had been treated before the introduction of acupuncture. The rate of program completion went from 60% to 92%. Patients withdrawing from heroin were better able to tolerate the withdrawal symptoms, and the depression and cravings associated with crack cocaine withdrawal were easier to tolerate. Brambaugh (1993) cites studies of the successful use of acupuncture in jails and homeless programs. In the Santa Barbara County Jail Women's Honor Farm, a 13-month acupuncture treatment program was carried out with 29 inmates who had a history of substance abuse. All of the subjects received at least 10 treatments, with an average number of 31.2 treatments each. At the end of the study, the women who had received the acupuncture treatments had a 17% lower reincarceration rate than did the controls. A positive correlation was found between the number of treatments and the reincarceration rates. Subjects who received 32 or more treatments over the 13 months had a 26% lower reincarceration rate than did controls and a 17% lower reincarceration rate than did subjects who received fewer than 32 treatments (Brumbaugh 1993).

In Minnesota, acupuncture has been integrated into four state prison chemical dependency treatment programs. In 1994 the Minneapolis Medical Research Foundation received a National Center for Complementary and Alternative Medicine (NCCAM) grant to study the use of acupuncture in addiction. The programs have been successfully treating a wide range of addictive behaviors with higher success rates compared with conventional treatment programs.

Lincoln Hospital in New York has developed protocols for using acupuncture in treating chemical dependency. The hospital protocols include a "sleep mix" herbal tea, 45-minute group acupuncture treatments during which talking is discouraged and promotion of responsibility and empowerment is encouraged (Margolin, 1993). Acupuncture is also used to treat chemically dependent pregnant women and babies at Lincoln Hospital. Because many of the commonly abused substances are teratogenic to the fetus, and because the process of withdrawal can be traumatic to both the mother and the fetus, acupuncture provides a safe way to withdraw gradually without the discomfort of withdrawal or the use of benzodiazepines (Smith, 1990).

Part of the success of acupuncture programs is that their approach is nonpunitive and that relapse is accepted as part of the disorder rather than being met with sanctions (Brumbaugh, 1993). The most successful programs have used acupuncture as part of a comprehensive program of group support, counseling, and 12-step programs. The main contraindication to acupuncture is clotting irregularities. Otherwise, the procedure is low risk and well tolerated. Ernst (2001) reports on both success and failure with several acupuncture programs.

Qi Gong for Addiction

Sancier and Hole (2001) report on Qi gong for heroin addicts. Three groups (n = 86), one with Qi gong for 2 to 2½ hours a day, one with medication (lofexidine), and one with basic care but not medications, participated in the study. The Qi gong group had lower withdrawal syndrome scores and less morphine-positive urines at 3 days (negative tests: Qi gong—50%; control group—23%, and medication group—8%). In addition, the medication and the Qi gong group had less anxiety symptoms.

Yoga for Addiction

Another study comparing *hatha* yoga with dynamic group psychotherapy (Shaffer et al, 1997) as treatment in a methadone maintenance program showed that both therapies worked approximately the same. Both therapies contributed to a clinical regimen that reduced drug and criminal activity. However, "some clients may benefit more from alternative methadone treatment than from conventional methadone treatment. During this study, for example, a number of patients reported that the practice of yoga was pivotal in their recovery" (p. 64).

MIND-BODY-SPIRIT INTERVENTIONS FOR EATING DISORDERS AND ADDICTION

Affirmation for Eating Disorders and Addictions

Over the years, Louise Hay (2000), a Science of Mind minister, has compiled healing affirmations for various conditions. For alcoholism, Hay says there is a "feeling of futility, guilt, inadequacy. Self-rejection" (p. 11). Hay recommends the affirmations: "I live in the now. Each moment is new. I choose to see my self-worth. I love and approve of myself."

For addictions, there is "Running from the self. Fear. Not knowing how to love the self" (p. 10). Hay recommends: "I now discover how wonderful I am. I choose to love and enjoy myself."

For anorexia, Hay states that there is "denying the self life. Extreme fear, self-hatred and rejection" (p. 13). Hay recommends the following affirmations: "It is safe to be me. I am wonderful just as I am. I choose to live. I choose joy and self-acceptance." For bulimia, Hay describes "hopeless terror. A frantic stuffing and purging of self-hatred" (p. 22). Affirmations are: "I am loved and nourished and supported by Life itself. It is safe for me to be alive."

For the overweight person, Hay talks of "fear, need for protection. Running away from feelings. Insecurity, self-rejection. Seeking fulfillment" (p. 54). Affirmations are: "I am at peace with my own feelings. I am safe where I am. I create my own security. I love and approve of myself" (p. 54).

Biofeedback and Hypnotherapy for Addiction

Ernst (2001) reports on biofeedback studies, two of which showed improvement over placebo. One of the studies included transcendental meditation (with training) that also showed improvement. Hypnotherapy has had minimal study, and Ernst (2001) reports one study with a negative outcome. In addition, self-hypnosis has been used for smoking cessation and other habits.

Cognitive-Behavioral Therapy and Journaling for Eating Disorders

Frisch and Frisch (1998) suggest cognitive-behavioral therapy as a useful structured treatment strategy for bulimia. Hall and Ostroff (1999) recommend a journal as a useful healing tool for patients with anorexia. These authors suggest that the journal may become a guide to help patients explore their feelings, family, and personal journey. Some of the applications of the journal might include writing a life story, telling the patient's family story, or developing a healing timeline. The authors suggest answering important questions about the anorexia in the journal, such as:

> What will replace the anorexia?
> What am I recovering to?
> What are the myths and rules that I have developed about eating?
> (Hall, Ostroff, 1999, p. 114)

The important shift that occurs in the process of this self-exploration is that the patient may begin to focus on the self, not the body image.

Guided Imagery for Addiction

Achterburg, Dossey, and Kolkmeier (1994) have a guided imagery script for overcoming addictions. Patients repeat positive affirmations of no longer craving the substance and visualize situations in which the substance is being used, but they are abstinent. The imagery focuses on releasing old habits and recovering power. Rehearsal of an exercise such as this one can be used in conjunction with other approaches to help change thought patterns and visualize benefits of abstinence. In addition, Naparstek (1994) has imagery audiotapes that can help overcome addictions. *Alcohol and Drug Recovery* (1997), *Stop Smoking* (1997), and *Weight Loss* (1997) are three of these audiotapes. Guided imagery empowers patients to feel a greater sense of control over themselves and helps them visualize a positive lifestyle without chemicals. Imagery may also be used for improving body image and anxiety (Geidt, 1997).

Prayer for Eating Disorders and Addiction

Shuler and colleagues examined the relationship between prayer and the use of alcohol or street drugs among inner-city homeless women (1994). In their study, women who reported personal prayer as an effective coping mechanism reported a lower use of alcohol or cocaine than did women who did not use prayer for psychologic support. Similarly, in a recent study conducted by Baetz and colleagues (2002) among hospitalized psychiatric patients in Canada, the use of private spirituality or prayer was associated significantly with less current alcohol use. Prayer may also benefit people with eating disorders.

Twelve-Step Programs for Eating Disorders and Addictions

In addition, 12-step programs have helped many individuals and their families regain sanity through working a program and through social support. These programs are not religious but rather spiritually based. Programs are available in most communities and include Alcoholics Anonymous (AA), AlAnon (for friends and relatives of alcoholics), Narcotics Anonymous and Overeaters Anonymous.

BIOLOGIC-BASED THERAPIES FOR EATING DISORDERS AND ADDICTION

Diet Therapy for Addiction and Eating Disorders

Chemically dependent people are often deficient in a number of nutrients resulting from a combination of drug effects and poor eating habits. Alcoholics are frequently deficient in B vitamins and may have decreased vitamin absorption because of damage to the lining of the gastrointestinal tract. Chemically dependent patients should have supplementation of vitamin B6, thiamine, riboflavin, and niacin. These patients should also have an adequate intake of minerals and antioxidants to offset some of the damage from chronic substance abuse (Gottlieb, 1995). For example, alcoholism is associated with zinc deficiency (NIH, 2002). Health promotion and self-care strategies should be an important part of the nursing care of the chemically dependent patient. The HCP can emphasize the importance of a healthy diet and adequate nutrition as part of the recovery program and as a way for the patient to restore self-respect and overall health as well.

Dietary factors are obviously a major concern with anorexia and bulimia. Individual consideration is needed because many patients may have nutrient deficiencies, and some will need hospitalization. Numerous psychosocial factors are intertwined with eating disorders, and appropriate referral is needed. Consultation with a nutritionist is recommended. Anorexia has been treated with zinc gluconate (100 mg daily) with a resultant 10% increase in body mass index at twice the rate of placebo (Birmingham et al, 1994). Studies of the relationship of zinc to anorexia go back to the 1980s. Some research suggests that zinc deficiency both results from and contributes to the anorexia and that zinc supplementation should be considered part of standard treatment for anorexia nervosa.

Herbal Therapy for Addiction

The National Acupuncture Detoxification Association suggests a "sleep mix tea" for addicts. The tea is a combination of chamomile, hops, valerian or catnip, skullcap, peppermint, and yarrow. The patients drink the tea during their treatments to promote relaxation and at home as a sleep aid (Smith, 1979).

Other herbals are a combination of plants that have been used in TCM to treat alcohol addiction. In 2000 the Center for Addiction and Alternative Medicine Research, a branch of the Minneapolis Medical Research Foundation, began human trials comparing the effects of an herbal compound with a placebo. One of the main ingredients in the compound is kudzu, a weed is considered a nuisance in the Southeastern United States. Kudzu is used to treat alcohol abuse in China (per Marderosian, 2000). However, a recent small study (n = 38) did not support kudzu's effect on sobriety or craving (Shebek, Rindone, 2000).

MANIPULATIVE AND BODY-BASED METHODS AND ENERGY THERAPIES FOR EATING DISORDERS AND ADDICTIONS

Massage for Eating Disorders and Addictions

Massage is often a comforting therapy in which the body may be experienced as a source of pleasure and sensation. For patients with anorexia, who view their bodies as a "foreign enemy," something to be defeated rather than enjoyed, massage can be one way to rediscover and reconnect with their own physical sensations. Massage can decrease stress and anxiety, improve body image, decrease cortisol levels, and increase dopamine and norepinephrine levels. Field,

Schonbern, and Kuhn (1997) have had success using massage for adolescent patients with bulimia and anorexia. In one study, bulimic adolescents received a massage twice a week for 5 weeks. At the end of this time, the participants demonstrated a more positive body image, a decrease in depression and anxiety, a decrease in serum cortisol, and an elevation in serum serotonin levels (Field et al, 1997). In another study, women with anorexia nervosa were divided into two groups. One group received massage therapy twice a week, and the other group received standard treatment. After 5 weeks, the women who received massage therapy reported decreases in stress and anxiety and increased satisfaction with body image. The women in the massage group also had lower cortisol levels and higher dopamine and norepinephrine levels than did the control group (Hart et al, 2001). The massage treatment includes the usual massage precautions.

Massage may also be helpful in people who are trying to break addictive behavior, largely because massage provides relaxation, and it can help produce sleep and increase well being (Snyder, Tseng 2002). Although no studies were found regarding people discontinuing substances, anxious patients who are going through withdrawal may nonetheless benefit from massage.

Light Therapy for Eating Disorders

Castleman (1996) describes a study of 14 subjects with bulimia who spent 30 minutes a day in front of either a 500-lux light or a 10,000-lux light. The subjects who sat in front of the 500-lux light showed a decrease of 12% in binging and purging episodes. The subjects who sat in front of the 10,000-lux light had a 42% decrease in these behaviors. Bulimia seems to be more prevalent during the winter months (Rosenthal, 1985), and bulimia shares some symptoms with seasonal affective disorder: dysphoric mood, carbohydrate craving, and decreased serotonin and norepinephrine activity (Stuart, Laraia, 2001). Light therapy requires the purchase of a light and the investment of time (approximately 30 minutes per day); it is not contraindicated in conjunction with any other treatment for eating disorders. Light therapy may cause eyestrain or headache, and the participant is not to look directly into the light.

NAC THERAPIES FOR HEADACHE AND PAIN

Headache is a common symptom, with diagnoses ranging from tension headache, migraine and temporal arteritis to such things as brain tumor and intracranial bleeding. Headache can originate from structures such as sinuses, teeth, eyes, ears, and cranial nerves or be a consequence of anemia, infection, endocrine processes, or constipation. Headache is ubiquitous. However, after the cause of headache or any pain is ascertained, and appropriate testing and treatments applied, the *pain* may still be present and require treatment. NAC therapies may be appropriate for headache and for pain.

ALTERNATIVE HEALTH CARE SYSTEMS FOR HEADACHE AND PAIN

Traditional Chinese Medicine for Headache

Herbs, acupuncture, and acupressure (Gach, 1990; Weiss, 2002) can be used for pain and headache. The course of treatment for headaches with acupuncture will depend on the type of headache and the strength of the patient. Many people require regular treatments for several months to a year. A person need not be suffering a headache when he or she comes for treatment. In fact, treating the root cause when people are pain-free, and treating more symptomatically when they have a headache, is desirable. Both approaches are necessary to relieve the pain and correct the underlying imbalance. Table 8-4 outlines some research that has been done using acupuncture for headache.

Between 50 and 60 types of headache have been described in Chinese medical texts, necessitating categorization for differentiation and diagnosis. Three of the most common perspectives are (a) diagnosis according to location of the headache, (b) diagnosis according to type of pain, and (c) diagnosis by root or internal cause. The third category, root or internal cause, includes a consideration of aggravation and lessening of pain that can be extremely important in diagnosing the root cause (Scott, 1984; Maciocia, 1994).

Diagnosis According to Location

Location of headache is an important perspective for the acupuncturist. Location indicates which acupuncture channels are involved. Table 8-5 demonstrates examples of location of pain and related channels.

Diagnosis According to Type of Pain

The two main categories of pain are excess and deficient. Excess is a full, intense type of pain that worsens with pressure to the scalp. The pain can be acute in nature, such as a sinus infection, or an internal condition involving heat and stagnation. Deficient is a dull type of pain that is chronic and improves with pressure to the scalp. This headache is caused by weakness of Qi and Blood in the body. These substances have a difficult time reaching the upper body, and a diffuse headache results (Scott, 1984). Table 8-6 describes the category of excess and deficient headache pain and indications.

Diagnosis by Internal or Root Cause

Because so many conditions can produce a headache, discussion is limited to some of the most common and more chronic types. These conditions include Liver Yang Rising, Phlegm-Damp, Stagnant

Table 8-4   Acupuncture Headache Research

Study	Type	Number	Measure	Outcome
Baischer, 1995	Treatment and 3-yr follow-up	31 patients	Patient diary pretreatment and posttreatment and in 3 yrs	Improvement more than 33% for 18 patients after treatment, 15 patients at 3 yrs
Carlsson et al, 1990	Comparison of acupuncture vs. physiotherapy	31 acupuncture patients, 31 PT patients, control group of 30	Patient rating for HA intensity and muscle tenderness; measurement of neck mobility with inclinometer	Intensity of HA and muscle tenderness improved in acupuncture and PT; greater improvement in PT group; neck mobility unchanged in either group
Dowson et al, 1985	Acupuncture vs. placebo (mock transcutaneous nerve stimulator)	48 patients divided equally	Patient diary and pain scale ratings	Acupuncture 20% more effective than placebo but not statistically significant
Hansen et al, 1985	Acupuncture vs. placebo acupuncture; with crossover	18 patients	Patient diary	Acupuncture pain reduction 31% better than placebo
Liguori et al, 2000	Acupuncture vs. drug therapy; follow-up for 1 yr	120 patients divided equally	Patient time sheets; researcher assigned units of	At 6 mos, acupuncture patients had 80% decrease in values

Continued

Table 8-4	Acupuncture Headache Research—cont'd			
Study	**Type**	**Number**	**Measure**	**Outcome**
Liguori et al, 2000, cont'd			value/hr and quality of life changes caused by pain	compared with 46% decrease for drug therapy; no side effects with acupuncture compared with 75% of patients reporting side effects with drug therapy
Loh et al, 1984	Acupuncture vs. drug therapy; crossover attempted	48 patients total; 29 had both forms of treatment	Patient diary and benefit rating	24 of 41 patients improved with acupuncture; 9 of 36 patients improved with drug therapy
Melchart et al, 1999	Review of controlled trials	22 studies	Compared acupuncture with: (1) no treatment; (2) sham acupuncture; (3) other interventions	9 of 14 sham trials showed greater improvement with "real" acupuncture; discussed problems of consistent research techniques and sample size

Tavola et al, 1992	Acupuncture vs. sham acupuncture	30 patients, divided equally	Patient diary and pain rating	Decrease in frequency of HA, drug consumption, and HA index in both groups, but no significant difference between 2 groups
Vincent, 1989	Real acupuncture vs. sham acupuncture	30 patients divided equally	Patient HA and medication diaries; anxiety and pain behavior tests given	Pain scores after treatment reduced by 43% in real acupuncture group; 14% in sham group; maintained reduction at 4-mo and 1-yr follow-up

HA, *Headache*; PT, *physiotherapy*.

Blood, and Kidney Deficiency conditions. Treatment strategy is included with the pathology. The following section describes the conditions, and Table 8-7 lists the Chinese herbal therapies commonly used for each of these conditions.

Liver Yang Rising headache Liver Yang Rising is an excess type of headache known as a migraine, because it usually manifests as a uni-lateral headache in the temple or eye area. The pain can also be in both temples. The pain comes to this part of the head via the

Table 8-5	Headache According to Location of Pain and Related Channels
Location	**Relates to Channel**
Top of the head (vertex)	Nourished by Governing Vessel; relates to Liver organ
Both sides of head	Gallbladder channel
One side of head	Gallbladder channel
Forehead	Stomach channel
Back of head (occipital)	Urinary Bladder channel
Whole head	No particular channel because many cross the head; are excess or deficient in nature (see next section)

Maciocia G: The practice of Chinese medicine, New York, 1994, Churchill Livingstone; Scott J: The diagnosis and treatment of headaches by acupuncture, J Chin Med 15:5, 1984.

Table 8-6	Excess and Deficiency Headache Pain and Indications
Excess Headache Pain	**Indication**
Throbbing, full	Heat, as in infection, or with Liver Yang rising to head
Stabbing, sharp	Blood stagnation
Continuous	Blood stagnation
Heavy	Damp stagnation
Deficient Headache Pain	**Indication**
Dull	Too little Qi and Blood rising to head
Empty	Deficiency of Kidney Yin or Yang

Maciocia G: The practice of Chinese medicine, New York, 1994, Churchill Livingstone.

Table 8-7	Chinese Herbal Therapy for Headaches

Chinese Herbal Therapy for Liver Yang Rising Headache

Chinese Name	Latin Name	Function
Tian Ma	Rhizoma Gastrodiae elatae	Calms the Liver, clears head, and stops pain
Ju Hua	Flos Chrysanthemum	Subdues Liver Yang, relieves pain in head
Bai Shao	Radix Paeoniae albae	Harmonizes Liver, nourishes blood
Suan Zao Ren	Semen Ziziphi spinosae	Calms the mind, promotes sleep

Chinese Herbal Therapy for Phlegm-Damp Headache

Chinese Name	Latin Name	Function
Chuan Xiong	Rhizoma Ligustici wallichii	Relieves pain in head
Qiang Huo	Radix et Rhizoma Notopterygii	Eliminates dampness in head
Bai Zhu	Rhizoma Atractylodis macrocephalae	Tonifies Spleen and resolves dampness
Chen Pi	Pericarpium Citri reticulatae	Moves Qi and resolves dampness

Chinese Herbal Therapy for Stagnant Blood Headache

Chinese Name	Latin Name	Function
Chuan Xiong	Rhizoma Ligustici wallichii	Moves Blood and relieves pain in head
Tao Ren	Semen Persica	Moves Blood
Hong Hua	Flos Carthami tinctorii	Moves Blood

Other herbs are added to treat underlying conditions.

Chinese Herbal Therapy for Kidney Deficiency Headache

Chinese Name	Latin Name	Function
Shu Di Huang	Radix Rehmanniae praeparata	Nourishes Kidney
Du Zhong	Radix Eucommiae	Nourishes Kidney Yang
Sang Ji Sheng	Ramus Loranthi	Nourishes Kidney and expels wind-damp

Continued

Table 8-7	Chinese Herbal Therapy for Headaches —cont'd
Many herbs would be used in combination to support the Kidneys, Qi, and Blood. The herbalist needs to differentiate whether the imbalance is more Yin or Yang deficient because the herbs are quite different in nature for each.	

Bensky D, Gamble A: Chinese herbal medicine materia medica, *Seattle, 1986, Eastland Press; Maciocia G:* The practice of Chinese medicine, *New York, 1994, Churchill Livingstone.*

Gallbladder channel. The headache is intense, throbbing, and severe in character.

The pain arises when the Yang, or warming energy, which should rise naturally and normally to the head, becomes excessive and creates pain in the head. The origin of this excess can be emotional, stemming from long-term anger or frustration. Liver Yang Rising headache is usually accompanied by a deficient condition in the lower part of the body that allows the Yang to rise out of control. When, for instance, headache coincides with the menstrual cycle, contributing conditions of Blood deficiency and Blood stagnation can produce the headache. Kidney deficiency may also be a factor in allowing the Yang to lose control and become symptomatic.

When the Liver Yang ascends, it may also move sideways and invade the Stomach, which produces the nausea and vomiting common with this type of headache. Other symptoms may include irritability, dizziness, tinnitus, or insomnia. The vision may be blurred, or photophobia may be present (Maciocia, 1989).

Treatment strategy for Liver Yang Rising headache: calm the Liver and control the Yang energy. Acupuncture points include Large Intestine 4, Liver 3, Triple Warmer (San Jiao) 5, and Gallbladder 41. Underlying deficient conditions including Blood or Kidney deficiency must be supported using points such as Stomach 36, Spleen 6, Kidney 3 or 6, and Urinary Bladder 18, 20, and 23. If nausea or vomiting were present, Pericardium 6 and Conception Vessel (Ren mo) 12 would be used (Blackwell, 1991). Chinese herbal therapy is also used. An experienced herbalist must be consulted to verify diagnosis and for use of specific herbal formulas. (See Table 8-7 for a list of the herbs for each imbalance as examples of herbs to be included for treatment.)

Phlegm-Damp headache This type of headache manifests as a dull, heavy sensation in the head and may be accompanied by difficulty in thinking or concentrating. Sinus drainage or a feeling of blockage in the sinus passages may be present. The pain may cover the whole head or be more specific to the forehead; it may also affect only one side of the head if the Gallbladder channel is primarily affected. The symptoms are usually worse in the morning; the dampness will drain downward as the day progresses and as activity increases. Nausea, loss of appetite, and vomiting of clear phlegm may occur. A phlegm-damp headache arises out of a chronic weakness of the Spleen, preventing the Spleen from adequately processing fluids. Gradually, the fluids change into phlegm that obstructs the Middle Burner and eventually spreads upward to block the head (Maciocia, 1994; Blackwell, 1991).

Treatment strategy for Phlegm-Damp headache: transform Phlegm-Damp and support function of the Spleen. Acupuncture points include Stomach 40 and 36, Spleen 3 and 6, Conception Vessel (Ren mo) 12, Urinary Bladder 20, Pericardium 6, and Stomach 8 (Maciocia, 1994).

Stagnant Blood headache   This type is a chronic but severe type of headache. Characteristic manifestation is an intense, stabbing, continuous pain that is fixed in one location. Stagnant Blood headache derives from local stasis of Blood, either from a fall or accident (even many years before) or from chronic deficiency and dryness of the Blood contributing to pain in the head. Diagnosis of the underlying conditions is essential in treating this pain. Stagnant Blood headache is more common in older people compared with the general population. The pain may be worse at night. Other signs of Blood stagnation, such as a dark complexion or purple spots on the tongue, may be present.

Treatment strategy for Stagnant Blood headache: move the Blood and correct underlying conditions. Acupuncture points include Large Intestine 4 and 11, Spleen 6 and 10, Liver 3, and local points on the head.

Kidney Deficiency headache   A deficiency headache is characterized by a dull ache that comes and goes. The ache is relieved by rest and worsened by excessive work. If the Kidney Yin or Yang is deficient, the head is not nourished properly, and pain results. The pain may be felt at the vertex, more at the occiput, or it may cover the whole head. Dizziness, a general feeling of fatigue, and low backache may be present (Blackwell, 1991).

Treatment strategy for Kidney Deficiency headache: nourish the Kidney Yin, Yang, or both. Acupuncture points include Kidney 3 and 6, Conception Vessel (Ren mo) 4, Governing Vessel (Du mo) 4 and 20, Urinary Bladder 23 and 62, and Gallbladder 19.

Homeopathy for Headaches

In a double-blind study with migraine (Brigo, Serpelloni, 1991; Chapman, 2001), a significant reduction in intensity, duration, and frequency of headache was found. The study used a classic homeopathy remedy of 30C (see Chapter 11 for dilution explanation) potency, four times, at 2-week intervals for 6 weeks. Patients were followed for a total of 4 months. Attempted replications of this study did not show success; however, chronic headache instead of specific migraine was studied, and different methodology confounded the attempt.

MIND-BODY-SPIRIT INTERVENTIONS FOR HEADACHE AND PAIN

Therapies for headache and pain include biofeedback, hypnotherapy, imagery, music, relaxation, autogenic training, prayer, and meditation. Taylor (1999) provides an overview of both acute and chronic pain outcomes research, including for postoperative pain, pain after dental surgery, renal colic, low back pain, headache, fibromyalgia, temporomandibular joint disorders, and bone marrow transplant pain. The mind-body-spirit interventions that showed success for some types of pain included relaxation, biofeedback, cognitive-behavioral therapy, and hypnosis. (Transcutaneous electrical nerve stimulation [TENS] and acupuncture also showed success.)

Electromyographic (EMG) biofeedback, relaxation therapy, and hypnosis are effective for tension headache, and thermal biofeedback assists with migraine headaches. In addition, biofeedback can help with musculoskeletal pain (Hammond, Kabbani, 2001; McGrady, 2001). A meta-analysis of 18 studies using hypnosis showed a large positive effect in pain management (Ernst, 2001; Montgomery et al, 2000). Hammond and Kabbani (2001) state that an estimated 70% to 80% of patients can "obtain some degree of analgesia and a few patients can block all perception of pain and create an anesthesia" (p. 287). Although more research is needed with most of these therapies, they may provide some level of comfort and are generally noninvasive.

Imagery may be helpful for pain, anxiety, and stress (Geidt, 1997). Naparstek (1994) has imagery scripts, audiotapes, and compact discs (CDs) for arthritis, headache, pain, multiple sclerosis, cancer, chemotherapy, radiation therapy, and trauma or grief. Box 8-2 and Box 8-3 present imagery headache and pain scripts. The Diamond Headache Clinic uses biofeedback for their patients; Box 8-4 presents a brief sample of a script that is used with thermal biofeedback (Diamond, Myers, 2000).

BIOLOGIC-BASED THERAPIES FOR HEADACHE AND OTHER PAIN

Dietary Measures for Headache

Hypoglycemia can be a cause of headache, and people with poor or irregular eating patterns may have headaches. Thus setting a regular eating pattern may be helpful, as well as keeping a headache diary, including intake of foods and other substances so that any relationships can be ascertained. Decreasing headache-producing foods can then be accomplished. Withdrawal from some substances is also a common

Box 8-2

Imagery Script for Headache (approximately 10 minutes)

To begin with, see if you can position yourself as comfortably as you can, shifting your weight so that you're allowing your body to be fully supported. After you take a nice, full breath, try to slowly and gently turn your head to the right, as far as it will go...and then breathe out, slowly bringing your head back forward...and now, breathing in again, turn your head as far as it will go to the left...and as you breathe out, gently turn your head back to looking straight in front of you...and now, still very gently, take another breath and lift your chin as far up as it will comfortably go...and breathe out, returning your chin to its normal position...and taking another breath in slowly let your chin drop to your chest...and breathe out, returning your chin to its normal position...

And now...see if you can align your head with your neck and spine...so they are all in a straight line...and your energy can move freely and easily all the way up and down your spine....

And gently allowing yourself to turn your attention inward...focusing inside for just this next while...to see how your body feels...taking a gentle, curious inventory...

Noticing how your body is feeling...continuing to breathe fully and deeply...and sensing your energy level...your mood...just looking inward with the neutral, honest eye of a camera....

Seeing where your body might be tense or tight or sore...and where it feels loose and soft and open...so just letting your awareness move around inside your body...friendly and detached....

Starting with your head...checking to see what it feels like inside your head...noting any tension or tightness that might be there...perhaps just a congestion of thoughts and worries...or an excess of energy, a busyness in there...and on the exhale, seeing yourself breathing it all out...fully and easily...and again...noting in a detached way any tightness in your scalp...along the top or at the base of your skull...and feeling it begin to soften and release...as you breathe it out of your body....

Noting with each breath a gentle softening all through your head...a loosening and stretching of the muscle sheath...like smoothing soft, friendly sheets over a bed...and perhaps even feeling the blood vessels soften, relax, and open...returning to their normal width...as the tiny muscle bands around them soften and release...allowing them to return to their pliable soft texture....

Continued

Box 8-2

Imagery Script for Headache (approximately
10 minutes)—cont'd

Continuing to breathe...deeply and easily...as you move your awareness down into your neck and shoulders...perhaps gently rotating your neck...over to your right...(pause)...and over to your left...(pause)...breathing into any tight, tense places...and feeling the warm energy of the breath...warming, loosening, and softening them...and gathering up all the tension...and breathing it out...so that, more and more, you can feel relaxed and easy...sensing the subtle stretch and release of muscle and tissue....

And taking another deep, full breath...as you gently lift your shoulders as high up along your neck as they will comfortably go...and as you breathe out...rotating them back, softly and slowly...letting them settle in place...letting them drop into a comfortable, balanced position of their own accord...and again...breathing in deeply...and gently lifting your shoulders as high up on your neck as they will comfortably go...and as you breathe out...rotating them forward, slowly and easily...and again letting them settle softly in place at their most comfortable level...so just taking a moment to feel the shift...sensing the release of energy all through your neck and across your shoulders....

And moving your awareness down into your heart...continuing to breathe fully and deeply...sensing how it feels around your heart...(pause)...noticing any heaviness or tightness there...as you continue to let the breath warm and loosen and soften any discomfort...and sending it out with the exhale....

And checking to see how your whole chest feels...(pause)...moving your awareness around to your back...(pause)...checking out the entire length of your back...(pause)...and moving around to the belly...looking to see what it feels like in there...continuing to breathe deeply and easily...noting with friendly but detached interest any tension or tightness in the belly....

Breathing into the center of your body...wherever you sense that to be...(pause)...and breathing out...(pause)...and again...deep into the very center of your body...(pause)...and exhaling fully and easily...(pause)....

Grateful for your body's ingenious methods of cleansing and clearing itself...its filtering of unwanted particles from the blood...and sensing the liver and kidneys removing any irritants that might contribute to your discomfort...flushing them out...efficiently and easily...leaving your tissue free and clear...light and strong....

Continued

Box 8-2

Imagery Script for Headache (approximately 10 minutes)—cont'd

And continuing to move your awareness down into your bottom...seeing how it feels along your whole pelvic floor...(pause)...noting any tension or discomfort...continuing to breathe, deeply and easily...maintaining your curious but neutral interest in how your body feels to you....

And down into your legs...feeling any tightness or rigidity in the legs...all the way down to the feet...all the way down to the tips of the toes....

Just doing this gentle, curious inventory of the inside of your body...no praise, no blame...just noting where it might feel denser, heavier...and where it feels looser and lighter...knowing you can use the intelligence of the breath to disperse tension...and balance your energy...breathing into the core of the tightness...letting the breath warm and loosen and soften all around and through it...and them breathing the discomfort out, deeply and fully....

So just taking this space to reacquaint yourself with this body of yours...your steadiest companion...your oldest friend...and listening to it...tuning into it...acknowledging it...

And letting your awareness sink down into it...allowing your spirit to settle all the way down into your body...gently and easily letting it float into all your inner spaces...all the way down to the tips of your fingers and toes...with the soft, easy rolling motion of a thick, rich, misty fog....

And just letting yourself feel the fullness of it...softly nodding to yourself...acknowledging how good it feels to connect back into yourself...your energy balanced and even and steady....

And so...whenever you are ready...taking another full, deep breath...and gently, with soft eyes...coming back into the room whenever you are ready...knowing you are better for this....

And so you are....

From Naparstek B: Staying well with guided imagery, *New York, 1994, Warner.*

cause of headache; coffee, tea, alcohol, and certain drugs are examples. Other headache triggers may be chocolate, garlic, onions, monosodium glutamate (MSG), sulfites, and aged or fermented products.

Herbal Therapies for Headache and Pain

Feverfew (*Tanacetum parthenium* or *Chrysanthemum parthenium* and several other names) is an old remedy used as a prophylaxis and

Box 8-3

Imagery Script for Pain (approximately 11 minutes)

To begin with...see if you can position yourself as comfortably as you can. Shifting your weight so that you're allowing your body to be well supported.* You might even want to take a moment to feel the support beneath you as you adjust your body. Try to arrange it so that your head, neck, and spine are all in alignment.

And taking a deep, full, cleansing breath...(pause)...exhaling as fully as you comfortably can...breathing deep into the belly if you can...(pause) and breathing all the way out....

And again...breathing in...and any unwelcome thoughts that come to mind...those, too, can be sent out with the breath... released with the exhale...so that for just a moment, the mind is empty...for just a split second, it is free and clear space, and you are blessed with stillness....

And any emotions that are rocking around inside...those, too can be noted and acknowledged, and sent out with the breath... so that your emotional self can be still and quiet...like a lake with no ripples....

And now, imagining a place where you feel safe and peaceful and easy...a place either real or imaginary...a place from your past... or somewhere you've always wanted to go...it doesn't matter...just so it's a place that feels good and safe and peaceful to you....

And allowing the place to become real to you...looking around you...taking the place in with your eyes...enjoying the colors...the scenery...taking in every detail with your eyes...over to your right...and over to your left....

And listening to the sounds of the place...whatever they might be...the music of moving wind or water...birds or crickets...just so your ears can become familiar with the sounds of your place...that is so safe and peaceful to you....

And feeling whatever you're sitting against or lying upon... whether it's sand or pine needles or grass...you might be in a cozy armchair...or maybe sitting on a nice, warm rock in the sun....

And feeling the air on your skin...either brisk and breezy...or soft and still...crisp and dry...or balmy and wet...perhaps you are inside, feeling the warmth of a cozy fire on your face and hands...or maybe you are outdoors, and there's just the subtlest caress of a fragrant, gentle breeze...so just enjoying the feel of the place on your skin....

And smelling its rich fragrance...whether it's the soft, full scent of flowers...or sharp, salt sea air...sweet meadow grass...or maybe the pungent smell of peat moss in the woods....

Continued

Box 8-3

Imagery Script for Pain (approximately 11 minutes)—cont'd

So just taking it all in...soaking up the richness of it...with all of your senses...becoming more and more attuned to your special place...feeling thankful and happy to be there....

Letting your body take in the healing vibrance of the place...feeling it penetrate all the way into you soaking into your skin...all the way down through muscle and bone...all the way to each and every cell....

Softly soaking into the places that are tight or tense or sore...places where pain is stored...and feeling the beginnings of subtle shift deep inside...a softening around the pain....

And breathing into the pain, you can feel the soft energy of the breath moving all around and through it...the warmth of the breath massaging and opening tight, trapped energy...and breathing it out...(pause)....

And again, breathing into the pain...with care and concern for that part of your body...soft and easy...letting the gentle energy of the breath caress and release some of the pain...and breathing it out...(pause)....

And again...breathing in and perhaps this time, if it feels right, and you can, putting your hands over the place that hurts...letting the warmth of your hands move softly and easily into the pain...encouraging your body to open to it...to loosen around it...so it can move more freely...and again, breathing it out...(pause)....

Watching the intelligence of the body...as it softens and opens around the pain...giving it more room to shift and move...easing the jagged places...softening constricted muscle...dispersing the heaviness of what aches...dissolving the boundaries of the pain...and watching its edges disappear...floating out with the breath....

Feeling the warm, vibrating softness from your hands...gently softening and loosening tension and tightness...slowly and steadily...moving deeper and deeper into the core of the pain...gently releasing as it goes...sensing the density of the pain getting thinner and lighter as its energy expands and floats free....

Continuing to breathe deeply and easily...feeling a kind and gentle softness toward yourself...a compassion for each and every aching, weary place in your body...respect for your forbearance...gratitude for your steady courage...taking deep satisfaction in your ability to be present, even under these trying circumstances...focused, aware, and fully alive....

Knowing you can always travel with the breath as it moves into the pain on the inhale...softening and releasing it...(pause)...and then feel it carrying the pain out of the body with the exhale....

Continued

Box 8-3

Imagery Script for Pain (approximately 11 minutes)—cont'd

Always able to touch into the peaceful stillness at your center...safe and grounded and connected into yourself...steady and centered...no longer at odds with any part of you...but accepting and allowing it all...your body attuned and humming with its own vibrant, healing energy....

And so...feeling peaceful and easy...you see very clearly that you can call forth this place...and the healing power of your breath and your hands...whenever you choose to again....

And so...wishing your special place goodbye for now...you can once again feel yourself sitting in your chair...or lying down...breathing in and out, very rhythmically and easily....

So gently with soft eyes...coming back into the room whenever you are ready...pleased with the powerful resources that are yours to use whenever you wish...and knowing you are better for this....

And so you are....

From Naparstek B: Staying well with guided imagery, New York, 1994, Warner.

*If you are using this imagery for muscular low back pain, you might want to lie on the floor with your legs over the seat of a chair, thighs at right angles with your body, and your shins parallel to the floor. This position gives your lower back maximal support while you "breathe into it" with the imagery.

treatment in migraine; it also has been used for menstrual pain and arthritis. The plant consists of at least 39 constituents but how it works in not known (PL/PL, 2002). Feverfew has several physiologic pathways: it appears to inhibit prostaglandin synthesis; prevent release of arachidonic acid; inhibit serotonin release; inhibit phagocytosis, deposition of platelets on collagen surfaces, and mast cell release of histamine; and exhibit antithrombotic potential (Facts and Comparisons, 2001; Fetrow, Avila, 1999). Other herbs for headache include willow bark and devil's claw. Topical treatments include tiger balm, peppermint, and rosemary.

Aromatherapy for Headache and Pain
Aromatherapy may be helpful for many types of pain. Buckle (1997, 1999) suggests various remedies for the treatment of pain. The author reviews current research and suggests that aromatherapy works at both a relaxation and a physiologic level (1999). Table 8-8 gives an overview of biologic-based therapies for headache and pain.

Box 8-4

Sample Instructions Used in Biofeedback Thermal Training

Let all your muscles become loose and heavy. Settle back quietly and comfortably. As you breathe in, imagine clean, fresh air cleansing your body. Your stomach rises as you breathe in and falls as you breathe out. Let all the tension and pain melt out of your body as you exhale. Let the breath out of your mouth slowly, making a blowing sound. Blow your breath out and away. Your tummy is simply rising and falling as you breathe in and out. Allow your body to pause as you exhale all of the air in your lungs. Start up again only when you need to. Notice that the tone on the machine is getting lower and lower. That means you are doing well.

Now imagine warmth and heaviness spreading over your scalp. Your scalp feels loose and heavy. Let your forehead become loose and heavy. Allow all the muscles in your temples to become heavy and warm. Release your lower jaw. All of your facial muscles feel smooth and heavy, as your tummy rises and falls with each breath. You are starting to feel warm and heavy all over, all over your head and face. You feel quiet and calm but are still alert. Notice the sound on the machine has turned off; it only beeps once in a while. Now let's relax the throat muscles....

From Diamond S, Myers L: Headache of the month: biofeedback for young migraine sufferers, Consultant 40(8):1500, 2000.

MANIPULATIVE AND BODY-BASED THERAPIES AND ENERGY THERAPIES FOR HEADACHE AND PAIN

Chiropractic treatments have been used with good effect on tension, cervicogenic, and posttraumatic headaches (Ernst, 2001). Massage, including soft tissue or neuromuscular massage, can help relieve headaches. Head and neck, shoulders, and upper back massage may be relaxing and help decrease pain. In addition, facial exercises and massage techniques may relieve symptoms of temporomandibular joint syndrome (Stevens, 2001).

Therapeutic Touch (TT) has been used in tension headache. Keller (1986) compared noncontact TT with placebo simulation on 60 volunteers with tension headache. The author found a significant reduction in headache pain as measured on the McGill-Melzack Pain Questionnaire, and relief was sustained after 4 hours. In addition, Reiki and healing touch (HT) and TT may be helpful for other types of pain as well (Krieger, 1993; Easter, 1997).

Table 8-8 Biologic-Based Therapies for Headache and Other Pain

A complete prescribing source should be consulted before using biologic therapies. Nutrient doses may be above the recommended daily allowance or tolerable upper limit. In illness or deficiency, such doses may be acceptable; however, long-term use may not be appropriate. Herbs may cause allergic reactions and interactions. Herbs are generally contraindicated or not recommended for women during pregnancy and lactation and for children unless research data or a long history of safe use has been established.

Intervention	Management	Treatment Regimen	Cautions, Precautions, Interactions	References
Dietary measures	Regular eating patterns; Find triggers	Eat at regular intervals; reduce sugars; keep food diary; eliminate caffeine or other triggers		
Vitamins	Migraine headache prevention	Riboflavin (B₂) 400 mg qd Adult RDA: 1.1 to 1.3 mg Adult UL: none given Migraine prevention Dose is very high compared to RDA	Maintain balance of B vitamins by taking B complex. Maximum benefit may take up to 3 mos.	PL/PL, 2002
Minerals	Premenstrual Migraine reduction and migraine prophylaxis and	Magnesium in study, 360 mg/day of Mg pyrrolidine carboxylic acid was given from	Diarrhea Numerous drug interactions	PL/PL, 2002

	cluster and acute migraine.	15th day of cycle of menses. 1 Gm IV has been given for cluster and acute migraine Adult RDA: 320-420 mg Adult UL: 350 mg		
Herbal therapy	For rheumatic conditions, musculoskeletal pain, headache	Devil's claw (Harpagophytum procumbens), decoction, extract, infusion	Contraindicated with peptic ulcer; CAUTION with gallstones	Blumenthal et al, 2000; Ernst, 2001 ; PL/PL, 2002
	For migraine headache, prophylaxis, and treatment	Feverfew (Chrysanthemum parthenium or Tanacetum parthenium), pure leaf, extract, infusion, teas, liquid, tablets. PL/PL states "possibly effective" for preventing migraine and "possibly ineffective" to treat or abort acute migraine (p. 528). For prophylaxis, 50-100 mg of feverfew extract daily or freeze-dried leaf	SE: mouth ulcers, fast heart rate. Post-feverfew syndrome: withdrawal symptoms of discontinuing drug (pain, joint and muscle stiffness) Not intended for children or for women during pregnancy or lactation. May inhibit platelet aggregation.	Facts and Comparisons, 2001; Fetrow, Avila, 1999; PL/PL, 2002

Continued

Table 8-8 Biologic-Based Therapies for Headache and Other Pain —cont'd

Intervention	Management	Treatment Regimen	Cautions, Precautions, Interactions	References
Herbal therapy, cont'd		50-125 mg/day with food, or fresh leaf		
	For headache, low back pain, rheumatic and arthritic conditions, toothache, fever	2.5 leaves/day with food. Willow bark (Salix alba, S. purpurea, S. fragili), dried bark, decoction, extract, tincture	Interactions with salicylates	Blumenthal et al, 2000; PL/PL, 2002
	For headache, myalgia, and neuralgia	Peppermint oil (Mentha x piperita), liniment, ointment, or ethanol solutions. Rub across forehead and temples.	EXTERNAL use only	Blumenthal et al, 2000; PL/PL, 2002
	For rheumatic diseases, muscle aches	Rosemary leaf (Rosmarinum officinalis), bath, soaks, ointment. For bath, 50 g of crude leaf in 1 L hot water and add to bath.	EXTERNAL use only	Blumenthal et al, 2000
Aromatherapy	For pain, including arthritis, cancer, headache	Analgesic essential oils: lemongrass, rosemary, frankincense, juniper,	Check for allergy and be sure patient likes the essential oil smell	Buckle 1993, 1997, 1999

	rose, ginger, verbena, spike lavender, peppermint, myrrh, clove bud, ylang ylang, true lavender, sweet marjoram, black pepper. Various applications used (topical or inhalation) depending on oil, but always dilute. Topical use: 1-5 gtts diluted for a compress or in carrier oil for topical massage or 2 gtts on cotton ball inhaled for 5-10 min	before using; Buckle says oils can enhance orthodox analgesia and does not suggest that they be used in place of conventional analgesia medications; avoid spike lavender or rosemary in hypertension and seizures; see individual cautions; check for dermatologic problems	Buckle, 1997
Sickle cell pain	Essential oil: geranium. Prepare as above.	Same as above, and see individual precautions	Buckle, 1999
Particularly suitable for children	Essential oil: Roman chamomile, geranium, mandarin, neroli, palma rosa, sandalwood; either inhaled or topical for all of these	See individual precautions for each	
Headache	Tiger balm applied locally to temples, forehead, etc.	Avoid eyes	Ernst, 2001

gtts, *Drops*; SE, *side effects*.

REFERENCES

Achterberg J, Dossey B, Kalkmeier L: *Rituals of healing: Using imagery for health and wellness*, New York, 1994, Bantam Books.

Adams L, Gatchel R, Gentry C: Complementary and alternative medicine: applications and implications for cognitive functioning in elderly populations, *Alt Ther Health Med* 7(2):52, 2001.

Alexander CN et al: Transcendental meditation, mindfulness and longevity: An experimental study with the elderly, *J Personality Soc Psychol* 57:950, 1989.

Allen M: Alzheimer's disease and acupuncture, *Acupuncture Today* (editorial) 1(9):1, 2000. URL: www.acupuncturetoday.com/archives/sep/09alzheimers.html

Andrews M et al: *Nurses handbook of alternative and complementary therapies*, Springhouse, Pa., 1999, Springhouse.

Argue J: *Parkinson's disease and the art of moving*, Oakland, Calif, 2000, New Harbinger Publications Inc.

Baetz M et al: Canadian psychiatric inpatient religious commitment: an association with mental health, *Can J Psychiatr* 47(2):159, 2002.

Bains J, Shaw C: Neurodegenerative disorders in humans: the role of glutathione in oxidative stress-mediated neuronal death, *Brain Res Rev* 3:335, 1997.

Baischer W: Acupuncture in migraine: long-term outcome and predicting factors, *Headache* 35:472, 1995.

Barton S, ed: *Clinical evidence*, ed 6, London, 2001, BMJ Publishing.

Behl C et al: Vitamin E protects nerve cells from beta-amyloid protein toxicity, *Biochem Biophys Res Comm* 186:944, 1992.

Beneshin C et al: Effects of ginsenoside Rb1 on central cholinergic metabolism, *Pharmacol* 42:223, 1991.

Bensky D, Gamble A: *Chinese herbal medicine materia medica*, Seattle, 1986, Eastland Press.

Birmingham C et al: A controlled study of zinc supplementation in anorexia nervosa, *In J Eating Dis* 15(3):251, 1994.

Blackwell R: The treatment of headache and migraine by acupuncture, *J Chin Med* 35:20, 1991.

Blumenthal M, Goldberg A, Brinckmann J: *Herbal medicine: expanded commission E monographs*, Newton, Mass, 2000, Integrative Medicine Communications.

Bradford N, ed: *The one spirit encyclopedia of complementary health*, London, 1996, Hamlyn.

Brandabur M: Complementary therapies and Parkinson's disease, 2001. Retrieved 9/28/01. URL: http://www.parkinson.org/therapies.htm.

Brigo B, Serpelloni G: Homeopathic treatment of migraines: a randomized double-blind controlled study of sixty cases, *Berl J Res Homeo* 1:98, 1991.

Brotons M, Koger M, Pickett-Cooper P: Music and dementia: a review of literature, *J Music Ther* 24:204, 1997.

Brown University: Relaxation techniques benefit AD residents, *The Brown University Long-Term Care Quality Advisor* 10(10):5, 1998.

Brumbaugh A: Acupuncture: new perspectives in chemical dependency treatment [electronic version], *J Subst Abuse Treat* 10(1):35, 1993.

Buckle J: Use of aromatherapy as a complementary treatment for chronic pain, *Alt Ther Health Med* 5(5):42, 1999.

Buckle J: *Clinical aromatherapy in nursing*, San Diego, Calif, 1997, Singular.

Buckle J: Aromatherapy: does it matter which lavender essential oil is used? *Nurs Times* 89:32, 1993.

Burns A, Marsh A, Bender DA: A trial of vitamin supplementation in senile dementia, *Int J Feriatr Psychiatr* 4:333, 1990.

Bush M: Dementia: Current research and future hopes, *NP Forum* 12(1):56, 2001.

Camarius M: Aromatherapy massage, 2001. Retrieved 2/11/01. URL: http://www.alzheimers.com/health_library/treatment/treatment_07_aromatherapy.html

Campbell D: *The Mozart effect: tapping the power of music to heal the body, strengthen the mind, and unlock the creative spirit*, New York, 1997, Avon Books.

Carlsson J, Fahlcrantz A, Augustinsson LE: Muscle tenderness in tension headache treated with acupuncture or physiotherapy, *Cephalalgia* 10:131, 1990.

Castleman M: *Nature's cures*, Emmaus, Penn, 1996, Rodale Press.

Cesarotti E, Farris S : The Arizona Model : An innovative nurse practitioner model for Alzheimer's care, *NP Forum* 12(1):23, 2001.

Chapman E: Homeopathy. In Weintraub M, ed: *Alternative and complementary treatment in neurologic illness*, Philadelphia, 2001, Churchill Livingstone.

Chen X: Exploration of using emitted Qi of Qi gong for curing parkinsonism. Second International Conference on Qi gong, Xian, China, 1989.

Cunha UG et al: Vitamin B12 deficiency and dementia, *Int Psychogeriatr* 7(1):85, 1995.

Davies H, Robinson D: Supportive group experiences for patients with early-stage Alzheimer's disease, *J Am Geriatr Soc* 43(9):1068, 1995.

Davis M, Eshelman E, McKay M: *The relaxation and stress workbook*, ed 5, Oakland, Calif, 2000, New Harbinger Publications, Inc.

Dawson KL, Dawson TM: Nitric acid neurotoxicity, *J Chem Neuroanat* 3(4):179, 1996.

DerMarderosian A: *The review of natural products*, St Louis, 2002, Facts and Comparisons.

Diamond S, Myers L: Headache of the month: biofeedback for young migraine sufferers, *Consultant* 40(8):1500, 2000.

Diskin C: Nursing homes turning to alternative therapies, 1999, Bergen Record. Retrieved 6/25/2001. URL: http://bergen.com/region/therapycd/199908181.htm

Dossey L: Healing and the non-local mind, *Alt Ther Health Med* 5(6):4, 1999.

Dossey L: *Healing words*, San Francisco, 1993, Harper.

Dowson D et al: The effects of acupuncture versus placebo in the treatment of headache, *Pain* 21:35, 1985.

Easter A: The state of research on the effects of therapeutic touch, *J Holistic Nurs* 15:158, 1997.

Emerson LN: *Acupuncture to treat anxiety and depression in Alzheimer's disease and vascular dementia: A pilot feasibility and effectiveness trial*, Presented at the World Alzheimer's Conferences, Washington, DC, July 9-18, 2000.

Ernst E, ed: *The desktop guide to complementary and alternative medicine*, St Louis, 2001, Mosby.

Facts and Comparisons: *The review of natural products*, St Louis, 2001, Facts and Comparisons.

Fahn S: An open trial of high dosage antioxidants in early Parkinson's disease, *Am J Clin Nutrition* 53:380S, 1991.

Fahn S, Cohen G: The oxidant stress underlying Parkinson's disease: evidence supporting it, *Ann Neurol* 6:804, 1992.

Family Caregiver Alliance: Music therapy for Parkinson's and dementia, 2001. Retrieved 6/25/2001. URL: http://www.caregiver.org.ca/cgcihidmmt.html

Fetrow C, Avila J: *Complementary and alternative medicines*, Springhouse, Penn, 1999, Springhouse.

Field T et al: Elder retired volunteers benefit from giving massage therapy to infants, J Appl Gerontol 17:229, 1997.

Field T, Schanberg S, Kuhn C: Bulimic adolescents benefit from massage therapy, Adolescence 33:555, 1997.

Franchi F et al: A review on the relations between the vitamin status and cognitive performances, Arch Gerontol Geriatr 6:207, 1998.

Frawley D: Ayurvedic healing: a comprehensive guide, ed 2, Twin Lakes, Wisc, 2000, Lotus Press.

Freeman L, Lawlis F: Complementary and alternative medicine: a research based approach, St Louis, 2001, Mosby.

Fricker J: Antioxidants may slow AD progression, Lancet 9061:1300, 1997.

Frisch N, Frisch L: Psychiatric mental health nursing, Albany, New York, 1998, Delmar.

Gach M: Acupressure's potent points: a guide to self-care for common ailments, New York, 1990, Bantam Books.

Gardner K: Sounding the inner landscape: Music as medicine, Stonington, Maine, 1990, Caduceus.

Geldmacher D, Heck E, Otoole E: Providing care for the caregiver, Patient Care Nurs Pract Feb:36, 2001.

Giedt J: Guided imagery: a psychoneuroimmunological intervention in nursing practice, J Holistic Nurs 15:112, 1997.

Gottlieb B, ed: New choices in natural healing, Emmaus, Penn, 1995, Rodale Books.

Grant W: Dietary links to Alzheimer's disease, Alzheimer Dis Rev 2:42, 1997.

Graves A et al: Prevalence of dementia and its subtypes in the Japanese American population of King's County Washington state, Am J Epidemiol 144:760, 1996.

Griffin R, Vitro E: An overview of therapeutic touch and its application to patients with AD, Am J Alzheimer Dis 13:211, 1998.

Halcon L: Reiki. In Snyder M, Lindquist R, editors: Complementary/alternative therapies in nursing, ed 4, New York, 2002, Springer.

Hall L, Ostroff M: Anorexia nervosa: a guide to recovery, Carlsbad, Calif, 1999, Gurze Books.

Hammond DC, Kabbani S: Neurohypnosis. In Weintraub M, ed: Alternative & complementary treatment in neurologic illness, Philadelphia, 2001, Churchill Livingstone.

Hansen PE, Hansen J: Acupuncture treatment of chronic tension headache: a controlled cross-over trial, Cephalalgia 5:137, 1985.

Hart S et al: Anorexia nervosa symptoms are reduced by massage therapy, Eating Disorders: J Treat Prevent 9:217, 2001.

Hay L: Heal your body, Carlsbad, Calif, 2000, Hay House (www.hayhouse.com).

Hendrie H et al: Prevalence of Alzheimer's disease and dementia in two communities: Nigerian Africans and African Americans, Am J Psychiatr 152:1485, 1996.

Hole L: Koryo hand therapy: acupuncture to go. In Weintraub M, ed: Alternative and complementary treatment in neurologic illness, Philadelphia, 2001, Churchill Livingstone.

Holford N, Peace K: The effect of tacrine and lecithin in Alzheimer's disease: a population pharmacodynamic analysis of five clinical trials, Eur J Clin Pharmacol 47(1):17, 1994.

Hsu D, Cheng R: Acupuncture. In Weintraub M, ed: Alternative and complementary treatment in neurologic illness, Philadelphia, 2001, Churchill Livingstone.

Hughes P, Meize-Grochowski R, Harris C: Therapeutic touch with adolescent psychiatric patients, J Holistic Nurs 14(1):6, 1996.

Jelinek D: Unique/proactive methods to change the paradigm of care for Alzheimer's disease and other dementias: Developing and operating a business to address unmet needs, *NP Forum* 12(1):71, 2001.

Kao H et al: *Acupuncture enhancement in clinical symptoms and cognitive-motor abilities of the Alzheimer's disease patients*, Presented at the World Alzheimer's Conference, Washington, DC, July 9-18, 2000.

Keller E, Bzdek V: Effects of therapeutic touch on tension headache pain, *Nurs Res* 35(2):101, 1986.

Khalsa DS: Integrated medicine and the prevention and reversal of memory loss, *Alt Ther Heath Med* 4(6):38, 1998.

Kidd PM: Parkinson's disease as multifactorial oxidative neurodegeneration: implications for integrative management, comment in *Alt Med Rev* 6:501, 2000.

Kilstoff K, Chenoweth L: New approaches to health and well-being for dementia day-care clients, family carers and day-care staff, *Int J Nurs Pract* 4(2):70, 1998.

Kleinjnen J, Knipschild P: Niacin and vitamin B6 in mental functioning: a review of controlled trials in humans, *Biol Psychiatr* 29:931, 1991.

Kleinjnen J, Knipschild P: Gingko biloba, *Lancet* 340:1136, 1992.

Krieger D: *Accepting your power to heal: the personal practice of therapeutic touch*, Santa Fe, NM, 1993, Bear and Co.

Kumar A et al: Music therapy increases serum melatonin levels in patients with Alzheimer's disease, *Alt Ther Health Med* 5(6):49, 1999.

Lad V: *The complete book of Ayurvedic home remedies*, New York, 1998, Three Rivers Press.

LaRue A et al: Nutritional status and cognitive functioning in a normally aging sample: a 6-y reassessment, *Am J Clin Nutr* 65(1):20, 1997.

La Valle J et al: *Natural therapeutic pocket guide*, Hudson, Ohio, 2000, LexiComp.

LeBars P et al: A placebo-controlled, double-blind randomized trial of an extract of gingko biloba for dementia, *JAMA* 278:1327, 1997.

Leslie H: Dementia and art, *Nursing older people* 13(7):10, 2001.

Lewis S et al: *Medical-surgical nursing: assessment and management of clinical problems*, St Louis, 1999, Mosby.

Liguori A et al: Comparison of pharmacological treatment versus acupuncture treatment for migraines without aura—analysis of sociomedical parameters, *J Tradit Chin Med* 20(3):231, 2000.

Lockie A, Geddes N: *Homeopathy: the principles and practice of treatment*, London, 1995, Dorling Kindersley Limited.

Loh L et al: Acupuncture versus medical treatment for migraine and muscle tension headaches, *J Neurol Neurosurg Psychiatr* 47:333, 1984.

Lovell B, Ancoli-Israel S, Gevertz R: Effect of bright light treatment on agitated behavior in institutionalized elderly subjects, *Psychol Res* 57:7, 1995.

Luckoff D: The importance of spirituality in mental health, *Alt Ther Health Med* 6:80, 2000.

Luskin F et al: Complementary/alternative therapies in select populations: elderly persons. In Spencer J, Jacobs J, editors: *Complementary/alternative medicine*, St Louis, 1999, Mosby.

Maciocia G: *The foundations of Chinese medicine*, New York, 1989, Churchill Livingstone.

Maciocia G: *The practice of Chinese medicine*, New York, 1994, Churchill Livingstone.

Mackenzie E et al: Spiritual support and psychological well-being: older adults' perceptions of the religion and health connection, *Alt Ther Health Med* 6:37, 2000.

Manyam B: Ayurvedic approach to neurologic illness. In Weintraub M, ed: *Alternative and complementary treatment in neurologic illness*, London, 2001, Churchill Livingstone.

Manyam BV et al: An alternative medicine treatment for Parkinson's disease, *J Alt Complem Med* 1:249, 1995.

Margolin A: Acupuncture for the treatment of cocaine dependence in methadone-maintained patients, *Am J Addictions* 3:194, 1993.

McAndrew C, Vandivort M: The six principles of excellent clinical care for dementia: Nurse practitioners and physicians working together, *NP Forum* 12(1):12, 2001.

McGrady A: Biofeedback in the neurologic disorders. In Weintraub M, ed: *Alternative and complementary treatment in neurologic illness*, New York, 2001, Churchill Livingstone.

McKenna D, Jones K, Hughes K: Efficacy, safety and use of gingko biloba in clinical and preclinical applications, *Alt Ther Health Med* 7(5):70, 2001.

Meisenhelder J, Chandler E: Prayer and health outcomes in church members, *Alt Ther Health Med* 6:56, 2000.

Melchart D et al: Acupuncture for recurrent headaches: a systematic review of randomized controlled trials, *Cephalalgia* 19:779, 1999.

Miller E: Healing Journey (1980) and other stress-relief tapes, 1-800-52-TAPES.

Montgomery G, DuHamel K, Redd W: A meta-analysis of hypnotically induced analgesia: how effective is hypnosis? *Int J Clin Exp Hypn* 48:138, 2000.

Murray M, Pizzorno J: Alzheimer's disease. In Pizzorno J, Murray M, editors: *Textbook of natural medicine*, London, 1999, Churchill Livingstone.

Murray M, Pizzorno J: *Encyclopedia of natural medicine*, ed 2, Rocklin, Calif, 1998, Prima Publishing.

Nakamura S et al: Analysis of music-brain interaction with simultaneous measurement of regional cerebral blood flow and EEG beta rhythm in human subjects, *Neuroscience Letters* 275:222, 1999.

Naparstek B: CDs and audiotapes, 1997, (www.healthjourneys.com).

Naparstek B: *Staying well with guided imagery*, Akron, Ohio, 1994, Image Paths.

Naparstek B: *Pain* [audiotape], Akron, Ohio, 1995a, Image Paths.

National Institutes of Health (NIH): Zinc, www.cc.nih.gov/ccc/supplements/zinc.html, 2002. Accessed 1/17/03.

O'Connor J, Bensky D: *Acupuncture: a comprehensive text*, Seattle, 1981, Eastland Press.

Oken B, Storzbach D, Kaye J: The efficacy of gingko biloba on cognitive function in Alzheimer's disease, *Arch Neurol* 55:1409, 1998.

Pachetti C et al: Active music therapy in Parkinson's disease: an integrative method for motor and emotional rehabilitation, *Psychosom Med* 3:386, 2000.

Perlmutter D: Perlmutter health center newsletter, 2000a. Retrieved 9/17/01. URL: http://www.perlhealth.com.vol5no.1.htm.

Perlmutter D: Brainrecovery.com, Naples, Fla, 2000b, Perlmutter Health Center.

Pharmacist's Letter/Prescriber's Letter (PL/PL): *Natural medicines comprehensive database*, Stockton, Calif, 2002, Therapeutic Research Faculty.

PL/PL: Natural medicines in clinical management: Alzheimer's disease, *Continuing Education Booklet* 2:1, 2000.

Quinn J: Therapeutic touch. In Snyder M, Lindquist R editors: *Complementary/alternative therapies in nursing*, ed 4, New York, 2002, Springer.

Rajendran P, Thompson R, Reich S: The use of alternative therapies by patients with Parkinson's disease, *Neurol* 5:790, 2001.

Randall T: Music not only has charms to soothe, but also to aid elderly coping with various disabilities, *JAMA* 266:1323, 1991.

Rauckhorst L: Integration of complementary and conventional health care in Alzheimer's disease and other dementias, *NP Forum* 12(1):44, 2001.

Rideout B, Laubeck C: EEG correlates of enhanced spatial performance following exposure to music, *Perceptual Motor Skills* 82:427, 1996.

Robins J: The science and art of aromatherapy, *J Holistic Nurs* 17(1):5, 1999.

Rosenthal N: *Seasons of the mind*, New York, 1985, Bantam.

Ross R: Yoga as a therapeutic modality. In Weintraub M, ed: *Alternative and complementary treatment in neurologic illness*, New York, 2001, Churchill Livingstone.

Safford F, Baumel B: Testing the effects of dietary lecithin on memory in the elderly: an example of social work/medical research collaboration, *Res Soc Work Pract* 4:349, 1994.

Sancier K, Hole L: Qi gong and neurologic illness. In Weintraub M, ed: *Alternative and complementary treatment in neurologic illness*, New York, 2001, Churchill Livingstone.

Sandrick K: Art therapy: passage into their past, *Hosp Health Net* 60(14):155, 1995.

Sano M et al: A controlled trial of selegiline, alpha-tocopherol, or both as treatment for Alzheimer's disease, *N Engl J Med* 336(17):1216, 1997.

Sanzotta M: The magic of three-dimensional interactive art, *J Long-Term Care Admin* 23(4):41, 1996.

Satlin A et al: Bright light treatment of behavior and sleep disturbances in patients with Alzheimer's disease, *Am J Psychiatr* 149:1028, 1992.

Schulz J et al: Glutathione, oxidative stress and neurodegeneration, *Eur J Biochem* 16:4904, 2000.

Scott J: The diagnosis and treatment of headaches by acupuncture, *J Chin Med* 15:5, 1984.

Shaffer H, LaSalvia T, Stein JP: Comparing hatha yoga with dynamic group psychotherapy for enhancing methadone maintenance treatment: a randomized clinical trial, *Alt Ther Health Med* 3(4):57, 1997.

Shebek J, Rindone J: A pilot study exploring the effect of kudzu root on the drinking habits of patients with chronic alcoholism, *J Alt Compl Med* 6:45, 2000.

Shuler P et al: The effects of spiritual/religious practices on psychological well-being among inner city homeless women, *NP Forum* 5:106, 1994.

Shults C: Mitochondrial function and coenzyme Q10 in Parkinson's disease, 2001. Retrieved 9/28/01. URL: http://www.parkinson.org/mitochon.htm

Smith M: Raising healthy babies for the 90s. Available through Lincoln Hospital, Maternal Substance Abuse System, 349 East 140th Street, Bronx, NY, 10454, 1990.

Smith M: Acupuncture and natural healing in drug detoxification, *Am J Acupuncture* 7:97, 1979.

Snyder M: Journaling. In Snyder M, Lindquist R, editors: *Complementary/alternative therapies in nursing*, ed 4, New York, 2002a, Springer,

Snyder M: Prayer. In Snyder M, Lindquist R, editors: *Complementary/alternative therapies in nursing*, ed 4, New York, 2002b, Springer.

Snyder M, Egan E, Burns K: Efficacy of hard massage in decreasing agitation behaviors associated with care activities in persons with dementia, *Geriatr Nurs* 16(2):60, 1995.

Snyder M, Tseng Y: Massage. In Snyder M, Lindquist R, editors: *Complementary/alternative therapies in nursing*, ed 4, New York, 2002, Springer.

Soderberg M et al: Fatty acid composition of brain phospholipids in aging and Alzheimer's disease, *Lipids* 26:421, 1991.

Spagnoli A et al: Long-term acetyl-L-carnitine treatment in Alzheimer's disease, *Neurol* 41:1726, 1991.

Spratto G, Woods A: *PDR nurse's drug handbook,* Montvale, NJ, 2002, Delmar.

Stevens S: Chasing the dragon: beauty, anti-aging, and jaw tension, *Massage and Bodywork* 15(6):60, 2001.

Sterrett P, Pokorney M: Art for patients with Alzheimer's and related disorders, *Geriatr Nurs* 15(3):155, 1994.

Stuart G, Laraia M: *Principles and practice of psychiatric nursing,* St Louis, 2001, Mosby.

Sutherland J, Reakes J, Bridges C: Food, acupressure and massage for patients with Alzheimer's disease and related dementias, *Image* 31(4):347, 1999.

Tavola T et al: Traditional Chinese acupuncture in tension-type headache: a controlled study, *Pain* 48:325, 1992.

Taylor A: Complementary/alternative therapies in the treatment of pain. In Spencer J, Jacobs J, editors: *Complementary/alternative medicine: an evidence-based approach,* St Louis, 1999, Mosby.

Thal L, Carta A, Clarke W: A 1-year multicenter placebo-controlled study of acetyl-L-carnitine in patients with Alzheimer's disease, *Neurol* 47:705, 1996.

Umbreit A: Healing touch. In Snyder M, Lindquist R, editors: *Complementary/alternative therapies in nursing,* ed 4, New York, 2002, Springer.

Vincent CA: A controlled trial of the treatment of migraine by acupuncture, *Clin J Pain* 5:305, 1989.

Weil A: Alzheimer's update, *Self-Healing* [newsletter], August, 1998, p. 3.

Weiss P: Acupressure. In Snyder M, Lindquist R, editors: *Complementary/alternative therapies in nursing,* ed 4, New York, 2002, Springer.

Woods D, Craven R, Whitney J: The effect of therapeutic touch on disruptive behaviours of individuals with dementia of the Alzheimer type [conference abstract], *Alt Ther Health Med* 2(4):95, 1996.

Zhao R, McDaniel W: Ginseng improves strategic learning by normal and brain-damaged rats, *Neuroreport* 9:1619, 1998.

CHAPTER 9

GENITOURINARY CONCERNS

Pamela Shuler ▪ Roxana Huebscher ▪ Helen Miller ▪ Louise Rauckhorst

WOMEN'S HEALTH

Women's health concerns cover a wide range of diagnoses, including serious as well as minor disease; thus an accurate diagnosis is necessary before instituting any conventional or natural-alternative-complementary (NAC) treatment. However, many women choose to know about or use NAC therapies for less serious female conditions. The beginning of this chapter provides two NAC views on female function, giving examples of Ayurvedic and Traditional Chinese Medicine theory. After this discussion, NAC treatments for the common women's concerns of benign breast symptoms, premenstrual symptoms and syndrome, dysmenorrhea, vaginitis, and menopause are presented. The second part of the chapter gives NAC therapies for urinary incontinence and male concerns regarding the prostate.

ALTERNATIVE HEALTH CARE SYSTEMS FOR WOMEN'S HEALTH

Ayurvedic Perspectives on Women's Health

Unlike western society, which tends to view female physiologic functioning negatively (e.g., calling menstruation "the curse" and menopause the dreaded "change of life"), Ayurveda views the menstrual cycle positively as a monthly purification through elimination of waste products (ama) that have the potential of creating illness and the opportunity for body-mind renewal that keeps women healthy. Ayurvedic prescriptions for menstruation include: (1) keeping to a lighter schedule and resting more during the heavy days of flow but not sleeping during the day; (2) reducing one's exercise workout to no more than a 15- to 30-minute walk during the period; (3) allowing one's awareness to turn inward so as to pay attention to one's own body and individual needs and happiness; (4) drinking a few sips to a cup of plain, pure hot water every 30 to 60 minutes during the period to help regulate flow and reduce cramping; and (5) eating light, warm foods in less amounts than usual, especially in the evening, and avoiding carbonated beverages, as well as very sour, very spicy, fermented, or cold foods and waste-product (ama) producers, such as cheese, yogurt, red meat, chocolate, and fried foods. A more easily digested liquid diet (including juices, soups, or blended solid foods made from vegetables and whole grains) is beneficial on the first day of the period. If salt and sweet cravings are experienced, recommendations are to satisfy the salt craving first and, if the sweet craving persists, substitute fresh whipped cream or warm milk sweetened with honey for ice cream, cake, pastries, or other highly sweet foods (Lonsdorf et al, 1995).

Menorrhagia The prolonged and excessive menstrual bleeding that characterizes menorrhagia is usually a result of excessive pitta. According to Ayurveda, causes include overeating hot, spicy, sour, or salty food; smoking or drinking; unresolved anger, resentment, and hostility; or any combination. Treatment includes a pitta-reducing diet and avoiding all hot (both temperature- and spice-wise) and oily food, keeping cool, and avoiding exercise, as well as heat and sunlight exposure. Astringent and hemostatic herbs such as manjishta, ashok, lodhra, ashwagandha, arjuna, aloe, and bhringaraj may be used. Once the bleeding is over, or if the condition has persisted for some time, tonic herbs such as amalaki and shatavari are given as well. Shatavari and manjishta in equal proportions or ashok herbal wine are especially recommended (Frawley, 2000).

Amenorrhea Long-term amenorrhea is viewed mainly as a deficiency disorder caused by excessive vata and by exposure to cold, poor nutrition, dehydration, and anemia. A moist vata-reducing diet, including primarily dairy foods, nuts, oils, whole grains, and other nourishing foods, is indicated, along with iron supplements. Herbs to promote menstruation and reduce pain, such as myrrh (10 to 30 drops of tincture every 3 to 4 hours), and spicy herbs to counteract cold, such as ginger, black pepper, cinnamon, and rosemary, are indicated, along with tonics such as shatavari or ashwagandha compounds to rejuvenate the reproductive system. A simple formula is two parts each shatavari and ashwagandha and one part each of turmeric and ginger (take 1 teaspoon powder mix per cup of warm water). Warm sesame oil applied to the abdomen or used as a douche and mild laxatives such as triphala or aloe gel or low doses of castor oil may also be used (Frawley, 2000).

Traditional Chinese Medicine Theory of Women's Growth and Reproduction

The process of growth and reproduction as described in Chinese medicine depends on many factors. Qi (pronounced "chee"), Blood, and a substance called Jing must be in adequate supply and circulating normally for normal growth to occur during childhood and for sexual maturation to occur at puberty. Jing is housed in the Kidney and is said to have a fluidlike nature. Jing, or "essence," has no equivalent in Western medical physiology; the closest substance to it is semen for men and vaginal fluids or menstrual blood for women. Jing is also an essential part of the "marrow," which includes bone marrow, the brain, and the spinal column. Humans receive Jing from parents (prenatal Jing) and produce Jing from the foods that are eaten (postnatal Jing). Besides the reproductive function, Jing also controls the development of bones, teeth, hair, and the brain (Martucci, 1989; Maciocia, 1989; Wolfe, 1990).

A combination of several organ functions produces the menstrual cycle. For the monthly flow to occur, an overabundance of Blood must be present. Blood is created by the combined work of three organs: the Spleen, Heart, and Kidney. The Spleen distills food and fluids and sends the purified remnants to the Heart. The Kidney provides Jing to the Heart as a substrate, and the Heart "creates" Blood. The Heart then pumps the Blood to the rest of the body (Wolfe, 1990). The Spleen and Kidneys are mature enough at puberty to produce excess Blood to nourish the uterus and the fetus, if pregnancy occurs.

The Liver plays a vital role in the menstrual cycle because it has the function of storing the Blood and regulating the Qi necessary to produce the menses. The Liver disperses a specific volume of Blood and regulates the frequency of the flow. The Liver is responsible for the unobstructed flow of Qi throughout the body, thus any symptoms of pain, clotting, or irregularity associated with the period are a result of Liver Qi stagnation. This imbalance is also the major component in any premenstrual discomfort (Wolfe, 1990).

In the grid of acupuncture meridians, 12 main meridians are related to the internal organs. Additionally, eight "extraordinary" meridians are present; two of these are essential to proper functioning of the female organs. These meridians are the Ren Mo, or Conception Vessel, and the Chong Mai, or Penetrating Vessel. The Ren Mo circulates mostly Qi in the abdomen, while the Chong Mai circulates blood through the central core of the pelvis. The Chong Mai is also called the "Sea of Blood." Points from the 12 main meridians are used to regulate the Chong Mai channel (Spleen and Pericardium, for example). Proper nourishment and circulation of these meridians ensures regular menstrual cycles and normal amount of menstrual blood (Lyttleton, 1990; Wolfe, 1990). See Appendix B for a diagram of the meridians.

Although women's symptoms and signs may be similar in various cultures, theoretical, physiologic, and clinical points of view to women's care may be different. Alternative health care systems have many therapies for women's conditions. To be well informed and to provide a breadth and depth of care, the reader is encouraged to become acquainted with the many NAC therapies available for women's care.

NAC THERAPIES FOR BENIGN BREAST SYMPTOMS

Benign breast symptoms (BBS) refer to benign breast conditions that include breast pain, tenderness, fullness or lumpiness (or both) that are often cyclic in nature (Johnson, 1999; Love, 2000; Northrup, 1998). These symptoms are sometimes grouped together and called fibrocystic breast disease (FBD); however, a controversy regarding use of the term FBD exists (Love, 2000). During the 1970s and early 1980s, several studies suggested that women with FBD had an increased risk for breast cancer (Northrup, 1998). On further investigation, the National Cancer Association Consensus Committee (NCACC) and the Cancer Committee of the American College of Pathologists (CCACP) determined that on microscopic examination, the breast tissue in 70% to 80% of the women diagnosed with FBD actually demonstrated normal changes in breast anatomy (Love, 2000; Northrup, 1998). Only a small percentage of women with FBD had cellular breast changes that potentially increased their risk for developing breast cancer. These cellular changes, called hyperplasia atypia, seem to be more problematic if the woman has a positive family history of breast cancer (Harris et al, 2000; Love, 2000). In light of the controversy, and for the purposes of this book, the term fibrocystic breast disease will not be used. NAC therapies for BBS will be presented and discussed.

Symptoms and signs of BBS include breast pain, tenderness, engorgement, increased density, increased nodularity, enlargement of cystic lumps, and thickened, nodular breast tissue or a cystic lump noted on palpation. Cystic lumps are usually mobile, round or oval, varied in size, and are soft to firm. Clear (or serous) nipple discharge may be present (Harris et al, 2000; Love, 2000; Northrup, 1998).

Often, no diagnostic tests are warranted. However, if a discrete lump is detected, a fine needle aspiration (FNA) or stereotactic core biopsy should be done, along with an ultrasound to differentiate a cyst from a solid mass (Johnson, 1999). A diagnostic mammogram may be ordered for women, as warranted; age 35 is a guideline, and generally not recommended before age 25 (Padden, 2000), although a mammogram "should be offered to any woman who has a distinct lump, or to any woman with a strong family history of breast cancer" (Johnson, 1999, p. 144). If the lump is a cyst, the FNA should return benign fluid, the excisional or core biopsy should be negative for cancer cells, the ultrasound should indicate the presence of a cyst, and the mammography, if indicated, should be negative for cancer. Other newer diagnostic and screening tests include digital mammography, magnetic resonance imaging (MRI), radiopharmaceuticals, positron emitting tomography (PET) scans, and elastography (Cole, Coleman, 1999).

ALTERNATIVE HEALTH CARE SYSTEMS FOR BENIGN BREAST SYMPTOMS

The regular practice of yoga may tone breast tissue and improve circulation to the breast area (Weed, 1996). In addition, acupuncture and Chinese herbs may provide relief. Table 9-1 outlines alternative health care systems for BBS.

MIND-BODY-SPIRIT INTERVENTIONS FOR BENIGN BREAST SYMPTOMS

Several NAC therapies have been used successfully to relieve specific BBS. Having the woman keep a daily breast pain and symptom chart can be helpful in evaluating both the cause of symptoms and the form of treatment (Padden, 2000). In addition, prayer, meditation, and counseling may provide relief of mind-spirit issues that may accompany breast symptoms. Table 9-2 outlines some mind-body-spirit interventions for BBS.

BIOLOGIC-BASED THERAPIES FOR BENIGN BREAST SYMPTOMS

Women who experience symptoms of pain, tenderness, or inflammation associated with BBS should examine their nutritional status (Shuler, 1993; Padden, 2000). Although research results show conflicting evidence, some women experience a decrease in breast pain after following a caffeine-free diet (Johnson, 1999; Northrup, 1998). For optimal benefit, products containing methylxanthine compounds (cola, chocolate, root beer, and decaffeinated coffee) should be avoided, especially 1 to 2 weeks before menses (Northrup, 1998; Padden, 2000).

Oral vitamin E (Abrams, 1965; London et al, 1982; Northrup, 1998), oral gamma linolenic acid (Johnson, 1999; Northup, 1998; Padden, 2000; Pye et al, 1985; Weed, 1996), and iodine supplementation (Eskin et al, 1967) may reduce inflammation and breast pain. Table 9-3 lists some biologic-based therapies for BBS.

MANIPULATIVE AND BODY-BASED METHODS AND ENERGY THERAPIES FOR BENIGN BREAST SYMPTOMS

Women who experience premenstrual congestion or fullness to a point of discomfort may benefit from breast massage or breast self-massage (Mowen, 2001; Chikly, 2001; Curties, 2001; Northrup, 1998; Weed, 1996), while castor oil packs (Northrup, 1998; Weed, 1996) may reduce inflammation and breast pain.

The health care provider should acquire a thorough knowledge of conventional therapies that the patient currently uses to ensure safe introduction of NAC regimens. Tables 9-4 lists body-based and energy interventions for BBS.

Table 9-1 Alternative Health Care Systems for Benign Breast Symptoms

Intervention	Management	Treatment Regimen	Cautions, Precautions, Interactions	References
Ayurveda, Yoga	Can tone breasts and improve circulation to the breast area	Regular weekly intervals at least 3 times/wk	Yoga instructor needed who is familiar with the following positions: the Bow, Camel, and Cobra	Weed, 1996
Traditional Chinese Medicine, acupuncture, Chinese herbs	May be effective in relieving cyclic and noncyclic breast pain	Varies, depending on condition of participant	May be combined with Chinese herbs; most of the research has been done in the area of breast cancer	Love, 2000

Table 9-2   Mind-Body-Spirit Interventions for Benign Breast Symptoms

Intervention	Management	Treatment Regimen	Cautions, Precautions, Interactions	References
Meditation	Help strengthen immune system; relieves tension	Varies, usually daily	Should be practiced regularly to receive full benefits	Weed, 1996
Personal prayer and intercessory prayer	Help strengthen immune system; relieve tension; can enhance the healing process	Varies, usually daily	Research indicates the power of intercessory prayer in the healing process; further research is needed to explore preventative influences of prayer	Byrd, 1993; Northrup, 1998; Weed, 1996
Mind-body therapy (psychologic counseling, relaxation, and stress management)	May reduce breast pain	Individualized treatment plan developed	Women with history of emotional and psychologic trauma often have breast pain; these patients may have difficulty developing nurturing relationships and need support	Northrup, 1998
Visualization	May be effective in relieving cyclic and noncyclic breast pain	Varies, usually daily	Often combined with prayer or meditation for enhanced effect; most of the research has been done in the area of breast cancer	Love, 2000

Table 9-3 Biologic-Based Therapies for Benign Breast Symptoms

Intervention	Management	Treatment Regimen	Cautions, Precautions, Interactions	References
Gamma linolenic acid (found in evening primrose oil, black currant seed oil, borage oil) and Alpha linolenic acid (flaxseed)	Helps reduce inflammation and pain	500 mg qid of GLA or 1 tbsp of ground flaxseed bid with a full glass (6 oz) of water	GLA supplements might prolong bleeding time; caution with anticoagulant drugs and herbs; flax must be taken with sufficient water to avoid intestinal blockage	Northrup, 1998; PL/PL, 2002; Pye et al, 1985; Weed, 1996
Iodine	Helps reduce pain; resolves some breast cysts	Adult RDA: 150 µg/day; adult UL: 1100 µg/day; for "fibrocystic breast disease." Per PL/PL: 80 µg/kg of molecular iodine. Note: this dose is well above the UL. Iodine can be increased in diet by eating a small amount of softened wakame or kombu (sea vegetables) or seaweed, iodized salt, or marine life	Caution used for patients with thyroid disorders; iodine supplements can cause sore throat or sore neck glands; interacts with drugs and lab tests. Can cause hypersensitivity. See all precautions.	Eskin et al 1967; Ghent, 1993; Northrup, 1998, 2002; PL/PL, 2002; Weed, 1996
Selenium	Helps strengthen immune system;	200 µg/day. Adult RDA: 55 µg/day; adult UL:	CAUTION: different varieties of selenium	Clark et al, 1996; NRC,

	Benefits	Dose	Precautions	References
	used as a breast cancer preventative; has antioxidant effects	400 µg/day; selenium can be increased in diet by eating onions, garlic, fish, wheat poultry regularly	are available; selenium can be toxic; research indicates that low levels of selenium have been associated with some forms of cancer, including breast cancer. Interacts with cisplatin.	1989; Northrup, 1998; PL/PL, 2002; Weed, 1996
Vitamin A; 1 µg of vitamin A = 3.33 units of vitamin A	Helps strengthen and activate the immune system; may help reduce cancer risk including breast cancer	10,000 IU/day maximum betacarotene; if more than that taken, needs to be for a limited time; adult RDA vitamin A: 700 µg/day (2300 IU); adult UL: 3000 µg/day (3 mg, 10,000 IU); vitamin A foods are liver, whole milk and fortified fat-reduced milk, cheese, whole egg, darkly colored fruits and vegetables (carrots, sweet potatoes, broccoli)	Large doses can cause dry lips, dry nails, alopecia. Fat-soluble vitamin, thus toxicity can occur; liver damage, birth defects can occur; people with high alcohol intake, liver disease, hyper-lipidemia, or protein malnutrition are susceptible to adverse effects; women of child-bearing age should not take more than 10,000 IU/day	Love, 2000; Northrup, 1998; Weed, 1996
Vitamin C	Helps strengthen and activate the immune system;	500 mg bid; Adult RDA: 75 mg (women) and 90 mg (men). Adult UL:	High doses of vitamin C (ascorbic acid) can cause diarrhea; vitamin	Love, 2000; Northrup, 1998;

Continued

Table 9-3 Biologic-Based Therapies for Benign Breast Symptoms—cont'd

Intervention	Management	Treatment Regimen	Cautions, Precautions, Interactions	References
Vitamin C, cont'd	used as a cancer preventative	2000 mg/day.	C is optimally absorbed when obtained through fresh fruits and vegetables	Weed, 1996
Vitamin E RRR alpha tocopherol; natural vitamin E	Helps reduce inflammation and pain; may resolve some breast cysts. However PL/PL say it is "likely ineffective when used for benign breast disease" (p. 1294)	200-800 IU/day. Adult RDA: 15 mg/day. Adult UL: 1000 mg/day. To convert IUs of RRR alpha tocopherol (natural vitamin E) to mg, multiply IUs × 0.67. Example: 30 IUs = 20 mg.	Must be in the form of d'alpha tocopherol to have a biologic effect; vitamin E can increase the risk of bleeding (inhibition of platelet aggregation and antagonism of vitamin K–dependent clotting factors); caution used for patients on warfarin; vitamin E can reduce effectiveness of chemotherapy	Abrams, 1965; London et al, 1982; Northrup, 1998; PL/PL, 2002; Weed, 1996

bid, Twice daily; GLA, gamma linolenic acid; IU, international units; NRC, National Research Council; PL/PL, Pharmacist's Letter/Prescriber's Letter; qid, four times daily; RDA, recommended daily allowance; UL, upper limits—the maximum level of daily nutrient that is likely to pose no risk of adverse effects. Includes intake from food, water, and supplements.

Table 9-4 Manipulative and Body-Based Methods and Energy Therapies for Benign Breast Symptoms

Intervention	Management	Treatment Regimen	Cautions, Precautions, Interactions	References
Breast massage	Helps relieve premenstrual breast tenderness and congestion; tenderness and pain related to benign conditions, discomforts of pregnancy, breast-feeding, and weaning	Varies with patient and condition	Massage therapist who is experienced with breast massage needed; contraindications for breast massage: lactational mastitis, postsurgical infection, abscess, undiagnosed lump present (not known whether massage can possibly spread cancer cells), presence of lateral and subscapular pain with implanted breasts; professional boundaries must be clear; patient must feel comfortable with procedure and therapist; patient must give consent	Mowen, 2001; Chikly, 2001; Curties, 2001; Northrup, 1998

Continued

Table 9-4 Manipulative and Body-Based Methods and Energy Therapies for Benign Breast Symptoms—cont'd

Intervention	Management	Treatment Regimen	Cautions, Precautions, Interactions	References
Breast self-massage (can make patients feel more comfortable monitoring breast changes during breast self-examination)	Helps relieve breast premenstrual tenderness and congestion; tenderness and pain related to benign conditions, discomforts of pregnancy, breast-feeding, and weaning	Varies with condition and patient, but at least monthly is recommended (anytime is permissible; after menses, breasts are less tender and "lumpy")	Some type of oil such as olive oil is recommended; herbal oils for breast massage can be used; breast massage oil blends can be ordered from Avena Botanicals (207) 594-0694, Natura-Sacred Play (505) 535-2255, Red Moon Herbs (828) 669-1310; see above contraindications	Weed, 1996

| Castor oil packs with heat application | Reduces inflammation and pain | Packs applied 3 times/wk for 1 hr for 2-3 months, then 1 time/wk | Classic application: wool flannel soaked in castor oil, applied directly to skin; on the outer side, plastic and a heat source placed; kits can be ordered from Women to Women (207) 846-6163, Phillips Products and Services (800) 705-5559, Home Health Inc. (800) 468-7313, Home Health Products (800) 284-9123. Take burn precautions with any heat source | Northrup, 1998; Weed, 1996 |

NAC THERAPIES FOR DYSMENORRHEA AND PREMENSTRUAL SYNDROME

Dysmenorrhea

Dysmenorrhea refers to painful menstruation or menstrual cramps (Northrup, 1998). The release of high levels of the hormone prostaglandin F2 alpha (PGF2 alpha) into the bloodstream as the endometrial lining breaks down causes the uterus to spasm, which results in "cramps" (Northrup, 1998; Rees et al, 1984). Dysmenorrhea affects over 50% of menstruating women monthly (Northrup, 1998). The pain associated with menstruation is classified as either primary or secondary. Primary dysmenorrhea usually begins within the first few years of the first menstrual cycle. The classic cramping usually improves with age and often resolves after childbirth. Secondary dysmenorrhea may be associated with endometriosis or other pelvic disease (Northrup, 1998). Menstrual cramps may or may not be associated with premenstrual syndrome.

Primary dysmenorrhea usually occurs during the first few days of menstruation and is characterized by suprapubic, "cramping" pain that may radiate to the back, thighs, or both. Associated symptoms may include nausea, diarrhea, and vomiting. Secondary dysmenorrhea may occur during menstruation or at other points in the cycle. The symptoms are usually reflective of the underlying pathologic condition, which can be gynecologic (e.g., endometriosis, leiomyomas, infection) or nongynecologic (e.g., gastrointestinal, urinary tract) in nature (Copeland, 2000; Northrup, 1998).

Premenstrual Syndrome

Premenstrual syndrome (PMS) is a group of somatic and affective symptoms occurring during the luteal phase of the menstrual cycle. Symptoms decrease shortly after onset of menstruation (Copeland, 2000; Dalton, 1999; Scott et al, 1999). Estimates are that over 50% of all women experience some degree of PMS (Northrup, 1998; Varney, 1997). More than 100 different symptoms have been reported, ranging from mild fatigue, anxiety, or depression to life-threatening situations that include self-inflicted injuries and suicidal ideation (Varney, 1997). The cause of PMS is unknown, although postulated etiologic factors include insufficient progesterone, fluid retention, nutritional problems, glucose metabolism disorders, vitamin deficiencies, ovarian infections, altered serotonin and endorphin levels, and elevated prolactin levels (Copeland, 2000; Scott et al, 1999). The more common symptoms of PMS include abdominal bloating, irritability, crying episodes, feeling of being "out of control," change in libido, depression, weight gain, breast tenderness, headache, fatigue, hot flushes, mood swings, change in bowel habits, loss of concentration, aggression, and hostility (Copeland, 2000; Dalton, 1999; Scott et al, 1999; Varney, 1997). Peak prevalence for

PMS is in the thirties with a decline noted in the forties. Symptoms are considered diagnostic for PMS if they are cyclic or worsen premenstrually. If physical examination and imaging findings are unremarkable, the diagnosis is made by the history. If conventional lab tests are normal, however, adrenal function testing may be helpful. Salivary testing is a convenient and relatively easy way to assess adrenal function. The patient collects four specimens over a 24-hour period (8:00 AM, 12:00 PM, 4:00 PM, and 12:00 AM) (Great Smokies Diagnostic Lab [GSDL], 1999). Furthermore, similar testing of other hormonal status may be warranted.

ALTERNATIVE HEALTH CARE SYSTEMS FOR DYSMENORRHEA AND PREMENSTRUAL SYNDROME

Ayurveda for Dysmenorrhea

Dysmenorrhea occurs more commonly in vata types because of the lack of proper uterine and vaginal secretions or spasms of the uterine smooth muscles and is associated with severe, colicky pain, headache, anxiety, palpitations, bloating, gas, constipation, or any combination. Treatment includes a vata-reducing diet (see previous section on amenorrhea), application of heat or warm sesame oil to the lower abdomen, and herbs such as turmeric, nutmeg, asafetida, ginger, valerian, and jatamamsi taken along with demulcent herbs such as shatavari or licorice, which possess a soothing effect (Frawley, 2000).

Ayurveda for Premenstrual Syndrome

Ayurveda proposes that PMS and other menstrual cycle problems happen when women experience any or all of three interdependent conditions during their child-bearing years: (1) diurnal biologic rhythms are off kilter, thus destabilizing the monthly menstrual cycle rhythm; (2) one or more of the doshas is out of balance; or (3) a build-up of excess metabolic by-products during the month has occurred caused by poor eating, not exercising, and going to bed late. Vata is responsible for downward flow; pitta for blood, hormones, and cleansing; and kapha for the mucus, fluids, and tissues. Modern medicine has found PMS difficult to manage because of the wide variety of symptoms for which there is no one universal treatment. However, Ayurveda views each symptom as the expression of an imbalance at deeper levels of the mind-body system, and therapies at that deeper level are able to treat all symptoms at once (Lonsdorf et al, 1995).

Vata-type PMS is characterized by anxiety, depression, rapid mood shifts, insomnia, constipation, headache, and severe cramping pain. The pain is worse at sunrise or sunset (times of the day when vata is most active). The woman may also experience agitation, feeling spaced out, fainting, vertigo with tinnitus, and even suicidal feelings. Most of the symptoms disappear once the period starts to flow according to the usual vata pattern—delayed, irregular, scanty brown flow that lasts only a few days. Treatment of vata-type PMS includes a vata-reducing diet with tonic foods such as garlic and cooked onions. Spices to promote menstruation such as turmeric and ginger combined with antispasmodic spices such as nutmeg are taken in warm milk at bedtime. Warm sesame oil can be applied to the head and lower abdomen. All stimulants, especially caffeine, tobacco, alcohol, and drugs must be avoided. Herbal treatment includes aloe gel, shatavari, ashwagandha, licorice, turmeric, dill, fennel, valerian, jatamamsi, and asafetida. A simple herbal formula for vata-type PMS consists of a mixture of thee parts shatavari with one part each of turmeric, cinnamon, valerian, or licorice (take 2 to 5 grams with honey before meals) (Frawley, 2000). Helpful lifestyle measures include rest, regular bedtime, and meditation (Lonsdorf et al, 1995).

Pitta-type PMS is characterized by anger, irritability, and argumentativeness, along with the upper one half of the body feeling hot, thirst, skin rashes, and diarrhea. Symptoms are worst at noon and midnight (times of the day when the pitta dosha is most active). The period tends to come early, and the blood flow is usually heavy and may contain clots. Treatment of pitta-type PMS includes a pitta-reducing diet combined with menstruation-promoting herbs such as turmeric, coriander, fennel, saffron, and safflower. Hot spices should be avoided. Aromatherapy with jasmine, rose, sandalwood, and gardenia essential oils is also helpful. Ayurvedic herbal therapy includes aloe gel, shatavari, turmeric, cyperus, saffron, gotu kola, and bhringaraj. A simple herbal formula for pitta-type PMS consists of a mixture of three parts shatavari and one part each of turmeric, cyperus, and gotu kola (take 2 to 5 grams of the powder before meals with warm water and natural sugar) (Frawley, 2000).

Kapha-type PMS is characterized by tiredness, heavy feeling, crying, and feeling sentimental or needing to be loved, as well as lack of appetite, mild nausea, and breast swelling. Emotional changes are not as severe as are those in the other types of PMS, but susceptibility to colds or influenza and mucous discharges will increase. Symptoms will be worst in early morning or early evening (times of the day when kapha dosha is most active). The period will tend to be late, and the flow will be pale, thick, and mixed with clots or mucous. Treatment includes a kapha-reducing diet, with an emphasis on hot spices and light vegetables and avoidance of heavy and oily foods. Short-term fasting or skipping the evening meal may be helpful. Other recommendations include increasing physical activity, deep-breathing exercises, and spending time outdoors. Herbal therapy includes aloe gel, turmeric, cyperus, cinnamon, black pepper, pippali, ginger, calamus, and the Ayurvedic trikatu or clove compound. A simple remedy is to take 1 tablespoon of aloe gel with ¼ teaspoon of dry ginger before meals (Frawley, 2000).

Traditional Chinese Medicine for Dysmenorrhea and Premenstrual Syndrome

Acupuncture (Helms, 1987) may have benefit for patients suffering from the varied symptoms associated with PMS. In addition, various acupuncture and herbal remedies are used for dysmenorrhea. Some of the herbal names for dysmenorrhea remedies include *Free and Easy Wanderer* variation and *Women's Treasure* remedy. Herbal combinations may include dang gui (Maciocia, 1998). Table 9-5 lists alternative health care systems for dysmenorrhea and PMS.

MIND-BODY-SPIRIT INTERVENTIONS FOR DYSMENORRHEA AND PREMENSTRUAL SYNDROME

The symptoms associated with dysmenorrhea and PMS are intensified by stress and unresolved emotional problems (Northrup, 1998; Varney, 1997). Therefore a thorough psychologic and social history must be included in the patient evaluation. Furthermore, because the range of symptoms associated with PMS are so varied, concomitant physical and psychologic problems should be ruled out or identified, especially if the symptoms are not completely cyclic. Patients with PMS are often frustrated by their symptoms and relieved when a diagnosis of PMS is made. After diagnosis, the patient has a reason for the feelings that have made her feel "out of control" (Varney, 1997). The goal of treatment is to identify underlying imbalances that led to the PMS and then treat the imbalances to relieve the symptoms (Northrup, 1998). The literature suggests an increase in aerobic exercise (Bolomb et al, 1998; Prior et al, 1987). An evaluation of dietary preferences, exercise, stresses, and stress-management behaviors can uncover patterns that are contributing to PMS. Table 9-6 examines mind-body-spirit interventions for dysmenorrhea and PMS.

BIOLOGIC-BASED THERAPIES FOR DYSMENORRHEA AND PREMENSTRUAL SYNDROME

For PMS, reducing or eliminating dairy products (Northrup, 1998), caffeine (in the form of soft drinks, coffee, tea, or chocolate) (Rossignol, 1985), refined sugar (Dirke et al, 1985), and partially hydrogenated oils that contain trans-fatty acids (Northrup, 1998) may decrease or even eliminate the symptoms associated with PMS. Therefore diet modification is often included in the treatment plan for PMS.

Vitamin and herbal therapy has also been used successfully with some patients with PMS. Vitamin E may reduce breast tenderness,

Table 9-5 Alternative Health Care Systems for Dysmenorrhea and Premenstrual Syndrome

Intervention	Management	Treatment Regimen	Cautions, Precautions, Interactions	References
Ayurveda				
Diet	For vata-type PMS	Vata-reducing diet with tonic foods such as garlic and cooked onions. Spices to promote menstruation such as turmeric and ginger combined with antispasmodic spices such as nutmeg, are taken in warm milk at bedtime	All stimulants, especially caffeine, tobacco, alcohol, and drugs, must be avoided	Frawley, 2000
	For pitta-type PMS	Pitta-reducing diet	Hot spices should be avoided	Frawley, 2000
	For kapha-type PMS	Kapha-reducing diet with an emphasis on hot spices and light vegetables; short-term fasting or skipping the evening meal may be	Avoid heavy and oily foods	Frawley, 2000

Herbs			
	For vata-type PMS	helpful; other recommendations include increasing physical activity, deep-breathing exercises, and spending time outdoors Herbal treatment includes aloe gel, shatavari, ashwagandha, licorice, turmeric, dill, fennel, valerian, jatamamsi, and asafetida; formula for vata-type PMS consists of a mixture of 3 parts shatavari with 1 part each of turmeric, cinnamon, valerian or licorice (take 2-5 g with honey before meals)	For aloe gel, be aware of the "potential contamination with the anthraquinone constituent" (PL/PL, p. 41)	Frawley, 2000; PL/PL, 2002
	For pitta-type PMS	Diet with menstruation-promoting herbs such as turmeric, coriander, fennel, saffron, and safflower; Ayurvedic herbal therapy includes aloe gel, shatavari,	Aloe gel precaution as above	Frawley, 2000

Continued

Table 9-5 Alternative Health Care Systems for Dysmenorrhea and Premenstrual Syndrome—cont'd

Intervention	Management	Treatment Regimen	Cautions, Precautions, Interactions	References
Ayurveda—cont'd				
Herbs, cont'd		turmeric, cyperus, saffron, gotu kola, and bhringaraj; a simple herbal formula for pitta-type PMS consists of a mixture of 3 parts shatavari and 1 part each turmeric, cyperus, and gotu kola (2-5 g of the powder is taken before meals with warm water and natural sugar)		
	For kapha-type PMS	Herbal therapy includes aloe gel, turmeric, cyperus, cinnamon, black pepper, pippali, ginger, calamus and the Ayurvedic trikatu or clove compound;	Aloe gel precaution as above	Frawley, 2000

Oils	For vata-type PMS	a simple remedy is to take 1 tbsp aloe gel with ¼ tsp dry ginger before meals		Frawley, 2000
	For pitta-type PMS	Warm sesame oil can be applied to the head and lower abdomen. Aromatherapy with jasmine, rose, sandalwood, and gardenia essential oils is also helpful		Frawley, 2000
Traditional Chinese Medicine				
Acupuncture	Relieves menstrual cramps	Number and frequency of treatments depend on patient's condition	Use of sterile disposable needles a must; practitioner must be informed of use of medications, especially anticoagulants, glucocorticoids, and anticonvulsants	Helms, 1987

PMS, *Premenstrual syndrome.*

Table 9-6 Mind-Body-Spirit Interventions for Dysmenorrhea and Premenstrual Syndrome

Intervention	Management	Treatment Regimen	Cautions, Precautions, Interactions	References
Guided imagery	May help menstrual symptoms, reduces mood swings	Guided imagery and visualization audiotape for 5 min 3 times/wk or Naparstek's Stress I and Stress II audiotapes	Most effective if combined with progressive relaxation; technique must be practiced at least 3 times/wk for best results	Groer et al, 1993; Naparstek, 1994, 1995
Hypnosis	May help relieve PMS, dysmenorrhea, menstrual disorders	Several sessions are usually required or may purchase self-hypnosis recordings	Trained therapist with knowledge of the pathophysiologic factors needed	Temes, 1999
Journaling	Provides distraction; promotes the expression of	See Chapter 2; AlphaPoem, general journaling, captured moments,		Day, 2001; Snyder, 2002

	feelings	dialogue, affirmations, unsent letters		
Meditation or PR	Helps relieve dysmenorrhea and various PMS symptoms	Meditation: technique practiced 1-2 times/day for 15-20 min; PR: practice 7-10 min at least 3 times/wk	For best results, meditation should be practiced daily, and PR methods at least 3 times/wk; results may not be evident for several wks to mos	Ben-Menachem, 1980; Goodale et al, 1990; Groer et al, 1993
Support groups	Provides emotional support, sharing of experiences, resources	Self-help groups, hobby groups	See Dalton for a list of support groups by state; it may be necessary to develop a support group	Dalton, 1999

PMS, *Premenstrual syndrome*; PR, *progressive relaxation*.

anxiety, food cravings, and depression (Butler et al, 1955; Landau et al, 1983; London et al, 1983, 1987; Northrup, 1998), while chasteberry and magnesium may relieve irritability, mood swings, and headaches (Abraham, 1983; Facchinetti et al, 1991; Hoffman, 1994; McCaleb et al, 2000; Schellenberg, 2001; Walker et al, 1998). Natural progesterone therapy (Northrup, 1998) may be beneficial for some patients with PMS.

Calcium supplements and the herbals black cohosh, cramp bark, dong quai, and false unicorn have been used for relief of dysmenorrhea (Castleman, 1991; Foster, 1996; Foster et al, 1990; Greunwald et al, 1998a,b; Hoffman, 1994; Jones et al, 1998; Mills, 1991; Newall et al, 1996, Nicholson et al, 1972; Northrup, 1998; *Pharmacist's Letter/Prescriber's Letter* [PL/PL], 2001). Table 9-7 lists biologic-based therapies for dysmenorrhea and PMS.

MANIPULATIVE AND BODY-BASED METHODS AND ENERGY THERAPIES FOR DYSMENORRHEA AND PREMENSTRUAL SYNDROME

Several body-based and energy methods may be appropriate for PMS. These methods include chiropractic care (Radler, 1984), massage (Field, 2000), micro-current therapy (Radler, 1984), and reflexology (Oleson, Flocco, 1993; Blum, 1995). Table 9-8 reviews manipulative and body-based and energy therapies for dysmenorrhea and PMS. Oleson and Flocco (1993) used foot, hand, and ear reflexology in a randomized control trial (n = 35), reporting a significant decrease in PMS symptoms in the reflexology group. Similarly, Field (2000), in a randomized study of 24 women with PMS (mean age 33) used massage for 30 minutes, two times a week, for 5 weeks. Subjects were facing up for the first 15 minutes and facing down for the last. The women received massage of the neck, forehead, shoulder, hand, arm, stomach, leg, ankle, calf, thigh, and back. Women in the control group received written relaxation instruction and training and were told to perform relaxation on the same schedule as those who were massaged. Symptoms were measured on the Menstrual Distress Questionnaire, Profile of Mood States, Visual Analogue Scale for Pain, and the *State Trait Anxiety Inventory*. The massaged group showed decreased anxiety levels, improved mood, and a reduction in pain, as well as improvement in the overall PMS symptom profile. The relaxation group showed decreased anxiety on the first day.

NAC THERAPIES FOR VAGINITIS

Vaginitis refers to infection or inflammation of the vagina and surrounding tissues. Causes include irritants, virus, bacteria, and fungus. Many types of vaginitis, such as sexually transmitted infections, are best treated with conventional therapy. However, for recurrent candidiasis and bacterial vaginosis, providers are sometimes baffled by the inability to cure the problem. Table 9-9 lists

Table 9-7   Biologic-Based Therapies for Dysmenorrhea and Premenstrual Syndrome

A complete prescribing source should be consulted before using biologic therapies. Nutrient doses may be above the recommended daily allowance or tolerable upper limit. In illness or deficiency, such doses may be acceptable; however, long-term use may not be appropriate. Herbs may cause allergic reactions and interactions. Herbs are generally contraindicated or not recommended for women during pregnancy and lactation and for children unless research data or a long history of safe use has been established.

Intervention	Management	Treatment Regimen	Cautions, Precautions, Interactions	References
Diet modification	May relieve various PMS symptoms	Caffeine, refined sugar, refined flour products and trans-fatty acids eliminated; intake of dairy products reduced	Must adhere to strict elimination of products in diet to fully benefit; may want to eliminate one food type at a time	Northrup, 1998; Rossignol, 1985; Dirke et al, 1985
Fish oil or flaxseed oil	May relieve dysmenorrhea	Fish oil: 500 mg tid-qid; flaxseed oil: 15-30 ml/day	Supplement labels must be read carefully to ensure correct dose	Harel et al, 1996; Northrup, 1998; PL/PL, 2002
Vitamin B6 in combination with B complex vitamins	May relieve symptoms of dysmenorrhea and depression	50 mg of B complex bid. Adult RDA: Folate, 400 µg/day; adult UL folate, 1000 µg/day. Adult RDA thiamine, 1.1 mg/day	Must be taken within the B complex to maintain a balance of all B vitamins; doses higher than 100 mg/day must	Abraham, 1983; Bernstein, 1990; PL/PL, 2001;

Continued

Table 9-7 Biologic-Based Therapies for Dysmenorrhea and Premenstrual Syndrome—cont'd

Intervention	Management	Treatment Regimen	Cautions, Precautions, Interactions	References
Vitamin B6, cont'd		(women), 1.2 mg/day (men); adult UL thiamine not determined. Adult RDA niacin, 14 mg/day (women), 16 mg/day (men); adult UL: niacin, 35 mg/day. Adult RDA pyridoxine (B6), 1.3-1.7 mg/day; adult UL: pyridoxine, 100 mg/day. Adult RDA riboflavin, 1.1 mg/day (women), 1.3 mg/day (men); adult UL riboflavin not determined. Adult RDA vitamin B12, 2.4 µg/day; adult UL B12 not determined.	be avoided because peripheral neuropathy can occur; can decrease serum levels of phenytoin and Phenobarbital. Biotin, choline, inositol, and pantothenic acid (vitamin B5) are often included in B vitamin complex.	Stewart et al, 1984
Vitamin C	May relieve various PMS symptoms	500-1000 mg/day; adult RDA: 75 mg/day (women), 90 mg/day (men); adult UL: 2000 mg/day	The natural rather than synthetic form must be taken to maximize absorption or eat foods high in Vitamin C.	Landau et al, 1983; Northrup, 1998

Vitamin E	For dysmenorrhea, breast tenderness, anxiety, food cravings, depression	400 IU/day of d'alpha tocopherol. Adult RDA: 15 mg/day (22 IU of the RRR alpha tocopherol); adult UL 1000 mg/day; must be in the form of d'alpha tocopherol for it to have a biologic effect	Vitamin E can increase the risk of bleeding (inhibition of platelet aggregation and antagonism of vitamin K–dependent clotting factors); caution for patients on warfarin; vitamin E can reduce effectiveness of chemotherapy and cause intolerance to nitrates	Butler et al, 1955; Landau et al, 1983; London et al, 1983, 1987; Northrup, 1998; Petit, 2001; PL/PL, 2001, 2002
Calcium	Decreases mood swings, bloating, food cravings, dysmenorrhea; helps prevent osteoporosis	1000-1200 mg of elemental calcium daily. Adult RDA: 1000-1200 mg/day; adult UL 2500 mg/day	Also 400-800 IU vitamin D daily (may be included in multiple vitamin); caution used for patients with hyperparathyroidism, hyperphosphatemia, hypothyroidism, renal insufficiency, sarcoidosis	Northrup, 1998; PL/PL, 2001; NAP, 2002; Thys-Jacobs et al, 1998
Magnesium	Improves mood; helps relieve headache,	200-360 mg magnesium. Adult RDA: 310-420	UL represents intake from a pharmacologic	Abraham, 1983;

Continued

Table 9-7 Biologic-Based Therapies for Dysmenorrhea and Premenstrual Syndrome—cont'd

Intervention	Management	Treatment Regimen	Cautions, Precautions, Interactions	References
Magnesium, cont'd	tension, dysmenorrhea; fluid retention	mg/day; adult UL magnesium 350 mg/day. Northrup (2001) recommends a calcium/magnesium ratio of 1:1 or 2:1	agent only and does not include daily intake from food and water; best when taken with a multiple vitamin and mineral supplement that includes calcium and selenium; for best absorption, a chelated form is used	Facchinetti et al, 1991; PL/PL, 2002; Walker et al, 1998
Black cohosh (Cimicifuga racemosa)	Helps relieve dysmenorrhea and PMS	Black cohosh extract tablets 40-80 mg bid; should be standardized to 1 mg of triterpene glycoside per 20-mg tablet	SHOULD NOT be taken by pregnant or breast-feeding women; caution used for women on estrogen	Foster, 1996; Hoffman, 1994; Greunwald et al, 1998a,b; PL/PL, 2002
Chasteberry (Vitex agnus-castus)	May relieve irritability, mood swings, anger, headaches, breast tenderness	Dose depends on formulation: tea, tinctures, capsules; extracts standardized to contain	Takes 4-12 wks for benefits to be noticeable; not used during pregnancy or if history	Hoffman, 1994; McCaleb et al, 2000; PL/PL,

Continued

				2001, 2002
Cramp bark (Viburnum opulus)	Helps relieve menstrual pain and associated nausea, vomiting, sweating	2-4 g of dried bark simmered in boiling water for 10-15 min. Drink mixture tid OR 5-10 ml tincture can be taken tid	of uterine, ovarian, or breast cancer, endometriosis uterine fibroids, or ovarian cysts. Cramp bark berries are considered potentially poisonous. Avoid using in pregnancy	Foster et al, 1990; Hoffman, 1994; Nicholson et al, 1972; PL/PL, 2002
False unicorn (Chamaelirium luteum)	Helps relieve dysmenorrhea	1-2 g of dried root tid, or tea: steep 1-2 g dried root in 150 ml boiling water and strain	SE: GI upset; unsafe during pregnancy	Mills, 1991; PL/PL, 2002
Natural Hormones				
Natural progesterone therapy	May relieve mood swings, depression, headache	2% natural progesterone cream (400 mg per oz): ¼-½ tsp applied topically bid on days 14-28 of menstrual cycle	Must use for at least 3 mos to see full effects; applied to soft areas of skin (abdomen, inner arms, thighs, neck), and sites rotated; must not use synthetic progesterones (prog-estins);	Dalton, 1999; Northrup, 1998

Table 9-7 Biologic-Based Therapies for Dysmenorrhea and Premenstrual Syndrome—cont'd

Intervention	Management	Treatment Regimen	Cautions, Precautions, Interactions	References
Natural Hormones—cont'd				
	Natural progesterone therapy, cont'd		patient must have stable blood sugar, and any candida infections must be treated before starting progesterone therapy	

bid, Twice a day; GI, gastrointestinal; IU, international units; NAP, National Academy Press; PL/PL, Pharmacist's Letter/Prescriber's Letter; PMS, premenstrual syndrome; qid, four times daily; RDA, Recommended Daily Allowance; SE, side effects; tid, three times daily; UL, upper limits—the maximum level of daily nutrient that is likely to pose no risk of adverse effects. Includes intake from food, water, and supplements.

Dietary Recommended Intake (DRI) values expand on the RDAs and contain four categories of recommendations (i.e., RDA, AI [Adequate Intake], UL, EAR [Estimated Average Requirement]). Check for the latest data.

Both the AI and the RDA are goals for intakes, but are defined differently.

RDA is the intake at which risk of inadequacy is very small (2% to 3%); RDA is expected to meet the nutrient needs of 97% to 98% of the individuals in a life stage and gender group.

AI is the observed average or experimentally set intake by a defined population or subgroup that appears to sustain a defined nutritional status, such as growth rate, normal circulating nutrient values, or other functional indicators of health. An AI is used if sufficient scientific evidence is not available to derive an EAR. AN AI IS NOT AN RDA.

EAR is the intake that meets the estimated nutrient needs of half of the individuals in a group.

References from the Food and Nutrition Board, National Academy of Sciences, Institute of Medicine (www.nap.edu).

Table 9-8   Manipulative and Body-Based Methods and Energy Therapies for Dysmenorrhea and Premenstrual Syndrome

Intervention	Management	Treatment Regimen	Cautions, Precautions, Interactions	References
Chiropractic Massage	May reduce pain Helps reduce anxiety and pain; improve mood	Varies with individual 30-min massage twice/wk for 5 wks from one premenstrual week to the following cycle's premenstrual week	In a field study, control group received relaxation	Radler, 1984; Field, 2000
Reflexology	For dysmenorrhea and various PMS symptoms	Usual treatment: 30-60-min/wk sessions for 8 wks; massage of hand, foot, and ear. See Appendix E for foot reflexology chart.	A practitioner familiar with treating women's health issues needed	Blum, 1995; Oleson, Flocco, 1993
Full-spectrum light therapy	Helps reduce irritability, carbo-hydrate cravings, fatigue, depression, social withdrawal, weight gain; also for SAD	2 hrs of light exposure/day for individualized period depending on the condition; light boxes for SAD treatment have 2500-10,000 lux; used at eye level (thought to	Can use natural light or a full-spectrum light source; light box must filter out potentially harmful ultraviolet rays; light visors produce lower levels than do	Parry et al, 1991; Singer, 2001

Continued

Table 9-8 Manipulative and Body-Based Methods and Energy Therapies for Dysmenorrhea and Premenstrual Syndrome—cont'd

Intervention	Management	Treatment Regimen	Cautions, Precautions, Interactions	References
Full-spectrum light therapy, cont'd		be the eyes and retina that mediates effect of light); typical SAD treatment is 30 min/day at 10,000 lux	standard light boxes; staring at light avoided; bright morning light exposure is preferable; contraindicated if taking photosensitive drugs	
Micro-current therapy	May reduce pain by making nerves less sensitive to effects of prostaglandins	Varies with individual	Qualified practitioner familiar with women's concerns needed	Radler, 1984

lux, *Units of illumination;* PMS, *premenstrual syndrome;* SAD, *seasonal affected disorder;* tid, *three times daily.*

Table 9-9 Biologic-Based Therapies for Vulvovaginal Candidiasis

The following is a brief overview; full-prescribing text should be consulted before using these therapies. Most therapies do not have research validation. Douching may introduce bacteria into the uterus; in general, patients should avoid douching. Many herbs are contraindicated for women during pregnancy and lactation. These herbs should not be used during pregnancy and lactation unless they have been shown to be safe.

Intervention	Management	Treatment Regimen	Cautions, Precautions, Interactions	References
Dietary measures	For recurrent infections	Refined sugars eliminated; must test for and control diabetes	May need to rule out diabetes	
Acidophilus (Lactobacillus)	For recurrent infections (PO)	4-6 acidophilus capsules (40 million-1 billion units)/day (especially 2-3 days before menses)	May use concurrently with patients who are also on antibiotics; can cause flatulence	Carcia, Secor, 1992; PL/PL, 2002
Yogurt (plain, lactobacillus-containing)	For recurrent infections (PO or vaginal)	8 oz/day of lactobacillus, unsweetened, unflavored, nonprocessed yogurt po 1-2 tsp inserted into vagina with vaginal applicator		Carcia, Secor, 1992
Boric acid	Has been used in the past vaginally; for recurrent infections	Boric acid capsules (600 mg intravaginally each night for 2 wks) or 1 tbsp boric acid powder in 1 q warm water as douche	Boric acid is TOXIC systemically, and potentially POISONOUS. Read safety precautions, use cautiously. NEVER TAKE ORALLY	Carica, Secor, 1992

Continued

Table 9-9 Biologic-Based Therapies for Vulvovaginal Candidiasis—cont'd

Intervention	Management	Treatment Regimen	Cautions, Precautions, Interactions	References
Echinacea (Echinacea augustifolia, pallida, purpurea)	For recurrent vaginal infections (tincture or decoction)	Dose varies; orally can be used in combination with topical antifungal cream to lower recurrence of vaginal infection. See interactions. Decoction: 1-2 tsp of root mixed with 1 c water; boiled for 10-15 min tid	Allergy may result; not to be used in patients with HIV; not for long-term use	PL/PL, 2002; Williams, 1999
Garlic (Allium sativum)	For recurrent infections (PO as beverage, or vaginal suppository or douche); also used for tinea cruris	PO: beverage is 1 dozen chopped raw cloves mixed in juice (can blend with carrots for taste); consumed in 2-3 servings Vaginal suppository: clove peeled and wrapped in unbleached gauze; for 6 nights inserted vaginally each night and removed in morning	SE with oral use: GI upset, flatulence, odor; platelet dysfunction may occur; interacts with anticoagulants, hypoglycemic medications (can lower blood glucose level); lowers BP	PL/PL, 2002; Williams, 1999

Gentian violet 1%	An old remedy. For recurrent infections: topical application to vagina; NOT FOR INGESTION; not to be confused with plain gentian root (they are unrelated)	Vaginal douche: 1 tsp of fresh garlic juice with 3 tsp of plain unsweetened, unflavored, unprocessed yogurt. Painted on the vagina by the provider once a wk for 4 wks or monthly after menses for months	Can cause severe irritant reaction (epithelial exfoliation); stains clothing violet color because of dye properties	Carcia, Secor, 1992
Goldenseal or goldenseal-myrrh (Hydrastis canadensis)	For recurrent infections (PO or douche)	PO: tincture 2-4 ml tid. PO: tea: infused for 10 to 15 min. Drink tid. Douches of goldenseal-myrrh (1 tbsp-3 c water, cooled and strained)	SE: GI upset, constipation, hallucinations; short-term use only; may cause vitamin-B deficiency. Goldenseal is an endangered species. Commonly adulterated. Contraindicated in hypertension, cardiovascular disease, pregnancy. Interacts with anticoagulants, antihypertensives, CNS depressants	Carica, Secor, 1992; DerMarderosian, 2001; Fetrow, Avila, 1999; PL/PL, 2002; Williams, 1999

Continued

Table 9-9 Biologic-Based Therapies for Vulvovaginal Candidiasis—cont'd

Intervention	Management	Treatment Regimen	Cautions, Precautions, Interactions	References
Honey and apple cider vinegar	For recurrent infections (PO)	A daily drink of a mixture of 1 tbsp honey to 1 c apple cider vinegar		Carcia, Secor, 1992
Tea tree (Melaleuca alternifolia)	For recurrent infections; topical only; tampon, douche, suppository; comes in various concentrations from 5%-100%; weaker strengths used for vaginal applications. The essential oil is diluted	Tampon: 1-2 gtts of tea tree blended with 1 tsp of plain yogurt; a tampon is soaked and inserted vaginally nightly, for 6 nights Douche: 40% concentration is the strongest to be used Suppository: size "00" capsules filled with 1-2 gtts of Tea Tree oil; the rest of the capsule filled with calendula oil; 2 capsules inserted vaginally each night for 6 nights	Can cause dermatitis, allergy; NOT FOR INGESTION; tea tree is TOXIC ORALLY	DerMardero-sian, 2001; La Valle et al; PL/PL, 2002; Williams, 1999

BP, Blood pressure; CNS, central nervous system; GI, gastrointestinal; gtts, drops; HIV, human immunodeficiency virus; PL/PL, Pharmacist's Letter/Prescriber's Letter; PO, by mouth; SE, side effects; tid, three times daily.

numerous therapies that have been used for candidiasis. Appropriate diagnosis is necessary before using these treatments. Although little to no research has been done, many of these therapies have persisted over the years. Thus some experiential evidence may exist for their use.

In addition, for problem bacterial vaginosis, remedies that have been used include:

Plain unsweetened acidophilus yogurt douches

Garlic suppositories for 6 nights

Goldenseal douches—1 tablespoon of herb to 3 cups of water, simmered, strained, and cooled

Tea tree oil vaginal suppositories—1 to 2 drops of tea tree oil mixed with calendula oil and placed in gelatin capsules

Boric acid vaginal suppositories—600 mg of boric acid placed in gelatin capsules (Williams, 1999)

Boric acid, which is difficult to obtain (purchaser must sign for the purchase because it is a poison), needs to be used cautiously. Nonetheless, boric acid is an old-time remedy. (See Table 9-9 for biologic-based therapies for vulvovaginal candidiasis.)

NAC THERAPIES FOR MENOPAUSE

Menopause refers to the last menstrual period that a woman experiences. A woman is said to have gone through menopause if she has had 1 year of amenorrhea (excluding pregnancy, breastfeeding, and certain conditions). In addition, the term perimenopause includes both the years before and the years after the time of last menses. Climacteric refers to the years surrounding menopause but is not a term used commonly. Menopause and perimenopause generally are the commonly used terms for the transition time when a woman passes from the reproductive phase. Appendix C outlines a NAC menopausal/perimenopausal treatment plan.

During perimenopause, a woman's body is passing through many hormonal changes:

> The physiologic changes include a series of hormonal and clinical alterations that reflect changing ovarian function. In the 7-10 year period prior to the final menses, serum follicle-stimulating hormone (FSH) levels rise as the time of menopause approaches. At the time of the menopause transition, women often experience menstrual cycle irregularity due to marked fluctuations in the gonadotropins, FSH and luteinizing hormones (LH), and the ovarian hormone, estradiol. (Rousseau, 1998, p. 208)

Women may experience various degrees of symptoms from the simple cessation of menses to several years of severe symptoms. Common symptoms may include hot flushes, night sweats, moodiness, anxiety, irritability, depression, changes in libido, sleep difficulties, memory problems, bladder and urethral symptoms, and vaginal dryness. Diagnostic tests include a routine Pap smear, breast examination, and mammography, as well as follicle-stimulating hormone, thyroid testing, and possibly salivary or serum hormone testing (estrone, estradiol, estriol, progesterone, DHEA, and testosterone). In addition, adrenal function may need to be evaluated, particularly if the woman expresses symptoms such as:

> Weakness, lack of libido, allergies, dark circles under eyes, muscle and joint pain, dizziness, low blood pressure, low blood sugar, food and salt cravings, poor sleep, dry skin, cystic breasts, lines of dark pigment in nails, difficulty recuperating from stresses such as colds or jet lag, no stamina for confrontation, tendency to startle easily, lowered immune function, anxiety, depression, and premature aging. (Shames et al, 2001, p. 133)

Salivary testing is a convenient and relatively easy way to assess adrenal function. The patient collects four specimens over a 24-hour period (8:00 AM, 12:00 PM, 4:00 PM, and 12:00 AM) (GSDL, 1999). Cortisol and dehydroepiandrosterone (DHEA) levels are usually examined in salivary specimens. In addition, with amenorrhea and irregular menses, a pregnancy test is prudent, and with irregular bleeding patterns, a transvaginal or pelvic ultrasound or an endometrial biopsy (or both) may be needed.

ALTERNATIVE HEALTH CARE SYSTEMS FOR MENOPAUSE

Ayurvedic Perspective on Menopause

According to Ayurveda, menopause is associated with the transition from the pitta stage of life into the vata stage of old age, and thus the symptoms are predominantly those of high vata, including increased nervousness, anxiety, thinner and drier skin and mucous membranes, thinning of hair and bones, decreased libido, insomnia, and depression. However, pitta is usually involved as well, because of this dosha's regulation of hormonal balance, which is demonstrated in frequent and pronounced hot flashes, irritability, short temper, heavy bleeding, and skin problems. According to Ayurveda (Lonsdorf et al, 1995), these changes can be largely avoided by keeping the vata dosha in balance. The general treatment includes a vata-reducing diet and lifestyle changes. Herbs that tonify the female reproductive system such as aloe gel, shatavari, saffron, kapikacchu, and ashwagandha taken in milk decoctions or shatavari compound formulas are recommended. Aloe gel is used to maintain the youthfulness of the female reproductive system and is particularly effective for heat sensitivity and night sweats. Sandalwood oil applied to the forehead also helps with the night sweats. Chyavan prash provides a general rejuvenating effect, and shatavari nourishes the female organs and lubricates the mucous membranes and skin. If kapha-type symptoms of heaviness, sleepiness, lack of motivation, weight gain, or water retention are present, kapha-reducing hot spices (e.g., trikatu formula) along with aloe gel, myrrh, or saffron may be used (Frawley, 2000).

Traditional Chinese Medicine Viewpoint on Menopause

During the midlife, which for women is considered the age between 45 and 60, the Jing declines, producing the changes in the sexual organs, bones, teeth, and hair that are considered normal aging. The menstrual periods gradually stop as a way to preserve Blood that is no longer abundant. If a woman is fairly balanced in her health, these changes will occur gradually and asymptomatically. If deficiency or stagnation of Qi and Blood occur over a long time, symptoms reflecting these imbalances may be present. These symptoms are known as the menopausal syndrome (Wolfe, 1990, Martucci, 1989). Menopausal women display four main patterns of imbalance, although these patterns may overlap, and other patterns may be part of the picture as well. These patterns are Kidney Yin deficiency, deficient Yin of Kidney and Heart, Kidney and Spleen Yang deficiency, and deficient Yin and Yang of Kidney.

Kidney Yin deficiency, which usually includes Liver Blood deficiency and Liver Yang rising, has symptoms that include flushing and heat (especially in the upper body), night sweating, insomnia, irritability and temper, headache, dizziness, blurred vision, tinnitus, weakness and soreness of the low back and legs, and dry mouth. The treatment strategy is to nourish Kidney Yin and Liver Blood and to subdue Liver Yang. Acupuncture points are Kidney 3 and 10, Liver 3 and 8, Spleen 6, Ren 4, Gallbladder 20, and Urinary Bladder 18 and 23 (Martucci, 1989, Lyttleton, 1990). Herbal therapy is discussed after the description of all the imbalance patterns. See Appendix B for the meridians and points.

Deficient Yin of Kidney and Heart means that the Kidney and Heart are not communicating. Symptoms include palpitations, anxiety, insomnia, evening fever, night sweats, dream-disturbed sleep, emotional lability, poor memory, and urinary incontinence. The treatment strategy is to nourish Heart and Kidney Yin and subdue Heart fire. The acupuncture points are Heart 5 and 7, Pericardium 6, Urinary Bladder 15 and 23, Kidney 3, and Ren 4 (Martucci, 1989; Wolfe, 1990).

Kidney and Spleen Yang deficiency is a third patten of imbalance. The symptoms are pallor, cold body and limbs, physical and mental fatigue, weakness of legs and lower back, abdominal distention, loose stools, and edema. The treatment strategy is to support and warm the Kidney and Spleen. Acupuncture points are Spleen 6, Stomach 36, Urinary Bladder 20 and 23, Governing Vessel 4, and Ren 6 and 12.

Moxibustion would include Ren 4 and 6 points (Lyttleton, 1990; Martucci, 1989).

Deficient Yin and Yang of Kidney is a fourth pattern. Symptoms include headache and vertigo, dry burning eyes, a hot feeling in the palms and soles, night sweating, fear of cold, cold limbs, uterine hemorrhage, and backache. The treatment strategy is to nourish Kidney Yin and warm Kidney Yang. Acupuncture points are Kidney 3 and 6, Urinary Bladder 23, Ren 4, Governing Vessel 4, and Spleen 6 (Lyttleton, 1990; Maciocia, 1998; Martucci, 1989).

Herbal therapy is essential to moderating and eliminating symptoms of menopause. Treating the Kidney imbalance is part of the strategy for each of these patterns. The principal herbs required will be part of one or more formulas to reestablish harmony in body and spirit.

General herbs to support the Kidney Yin include:
Shu Di Huang—Radix Rehmanniae glutinosae praeparata
Shan Yao—Radix Dioscoreae oppositae
Shan Zhu Yu—Fructus Corni officinalis
Table 9-10 describes Chinese herbal therapy for menopause; Table 9-11 reviews the research conducted on menopause; and Table 9-12 lists alternative health care practices for menopause.

MIND-BODY-SPIRIT INTERVENTIONS FOR MENOPAUSE

Numerous therapies are available for the time surrounding menopause. Modalities are available to help with hot flushes and the psychosocial changes that occur. Because this time is one of transition for women, general well being is also covered. This transition time is for considering what will happen at retirement and when that retirement will be. This time is for creativity and expression and a special time for caring for the self. Furthermore, osteoporosis prevention is important at this time, thus exercise that stresses the long bones is needed. Table 9-13 describes various interventions that practitioners can use.

BIOLOGIC-BASED THERAPIES FOR MENOPAUSE

Dietary considerations for menopause include increased consumption of phytoestrogens. Phytoestrogens are plant-based substances that have weak estrogenic-receptor activity (PL/PL, 1999) and thus exert mild estrogenic effect but are nonsteroidal (Ernst, 2001). Examples are isoflavones, phytosterols, and lignans (Low Dog et al, 2001). Phytoestrogens such as isoflavones are found in many foods, including legumes (soy, chickpeas, pinto beans, lima beans, and alfalfa).

Lignans and lignins are present in seeds, fruits, vegetables, and whole grains. Gut bacteria break down lignin precursors in food to entero-

Table 9-10	Menopause Chinese Herbal Therapy	
Deficient Kidney Yin, Deficient Liver Blood and Liver Yang Rising	Gou Qi Zi—Fructus Lycii chinensis	Tonifies Liver and Kidney Yin and Blood
	Bai Shao—Radix Paeoniae lactiflorae	Tonifies Blood and relaxes stagnant Liver Qi
	Gou Teng—Ramulus Uncariae	Clears Liver heat and lowers Liver Yang
Deficient Kidney Yin and deficient Heart Yin with empty heat	Suan Zao Ren—Semen Zizyphis spinosae	Calms heart and astringes Yin
	Bai He—Bulbus Lilii	Tonifies Yin; clears heat from Heart
Deficient Kidney and Spleen Yang	Rou Gui—Cortex Cinnamomi	Warms Kidney and Spleen, strengthens Yang
	Tu Si Zi—Semen Cuscutae	Tonifies Kidney Yang; strengthens Spleen
Deficient Kidney Yin and Yang	Bai Ji Tian—Radix Morindae officinalis	Tonifies Kidney Yang
	Yin Yang Huo—Herba epimedii	

Bensky D, Gamble A: Chinese herbal medicine materia medica, *Seattle, 1986, Eastland Press; Maciocia G:* Obstetrics and gynecology in Chinese medicine, *New York, 1998, Churchill Livingstone.*

Table 9-11	Alternative Therapies Menopause Research			
Study	**Type**	**Number**	**Measure**	**Outcome**
Seidl, Stewart, 1998a	Qualitative study using interviews and focus group	13 women interviewed who were using alternative therapies for symptoms of menopause	Perception and use of alternative therapies	Perceived as safe and somewhat effective; offered control over health
Seidl, Stewart, 1998b	Literature review from 1966-1997	85 references reviewed	Safety and efficacy of alternative treatments, categorized as nutritional supplements, herbal remedies, homeopathic remedies, and physical approaches	Phytoestrogens most effective for reducing symptoms of menopause; more research needed

Wu Lianzhong et al, 1998	Review of cases	300 women with menopausal syndrome treated with acupuncture	Reduction of symptoms	153 participants cured; 84 markedly improved; 54 improved; 9 ineffective
Wyon et al, 1994	Comparison of EA effects to SNP acupuncture	24 total; 12 in each treatment group	Individual logbooks; Kupperman Index; PGWB Index	Frequency of hot flushes decreased by more than 50% in both groups; EA effects lasted longer; Kupperman Index decreased in both groups; PGWB Index did not change in either group

EA, *Electroacupuncture*; PGWB, *Psychological General Well-Being*; SNP, *superficial needle position.*

Table 9-12 Alternative Health Care Systems for Menopause

Intervention	Management	Treatment Regimen	Cautions, Precautions, Interactions	References
Ayurveda				
Diet	For balancing vata dosha	Vata-reducing diet and lifestyle changes		Lonsdorf et al, 1995
Herbs	For balancing vata dosha and tonifying the female reproductive system	Aloe gel (maintains the youthfulness of the female reproductive system; for heat sensitivity and night sweats), shatavari, saffron, kapikacchu, and ashwagandha taken in milk decoctions or shatavari compound formulas; sandalwood oil applied to the forehead also helps with the night sweats; Chyavan Prash provides a general rejuvenative effect and shatavari nourishes the female organs and lubricates the mucous membranes and skin	All herbal precautions should be followed	Frawley, 2000; Lonsdorf et al, 1995
	For menopausal kapha-type symp-	Kapha-reducing diet includes hot spices (e.g.,		Frawley, 2000

	toms of heaviness, sleepiness, lack of motivation, weight gain, water retention	trikatu formula) along with aloe gel, myrrh, and saffron	
Yoga	For balance and harmony; relieves hot flashes, vaginal and bladder changes, insomnia	Poses: the Locust; the Wide Angle; the Pump	Lark, 1990; Willeford, 1995
Traditional Chinese Medicine			
	Acupuncture and herbs for menopause	See Tables 9-10 and 9-11 for herbal therapy and research information. See text for management meridians and points of menopause patterns.	Need a skilled practitioner	Lyttleton, 1990; Maciocia, 1998; Martucci, 1989
Homeopathy			
	For menopausal symptoms based on case-taking	Common single remedies used for menopause: Amyl nitrosum, Calcarea carbonica, Ignatia amara, Lachesis mutus, Pilocarpus, Sanguinaria canadensis, Sepia, Sulphur, Ustilago maidis	Qualified homeopathic practitioner needed	Skinner, 2001

Table 9-13 Mind-Body-Spirit Interventions for Menopause

Intervention	Management	Treatment Regimen	Cautions, Precautions, Interactions	References
Bibliotherapy	Provides a way to gain knowledge and insight, feeling a sense of control; provides a form of distraction; enhances positive coping; increases relaxation	Reading recommendations: self-help books, health care, fiction, poetry, personal preference literature; health care provider can have a lending shelf of popular works		Numerous authors
Creative and expressive arts, hobbies	Provides general relaxation; promotes well being; people who have increased self-complexity and like to explore the many facets of personality are less prone to stress, depression, illness	Painting, sculpting, crafting and other art forms; creative skills developed; reading recommendations: *The Artist's Way* (Cameron) or *Drawing on the Right Side of the Brain* (Edwards) for inspiration		Dreher, 1995; Linville, 1985; Cameron, 1992; Edwards, 1979

Exercise	Improves mood; increases bone mass	Walking practiced most days of the week, or other exercise preference chosen	Routine should be individualized to patient's capabilities; may need physical and cardiovascular work-up prior to beginning exercise depending on health status	Dell, Stewart, 2000
Imagery	Promotes general well being	Numerous compact discs, audiotapes, and videotapes from many authors available; Miller's *Healing Journey* (1980) and Naparstek's *Stress I and II* (1995), *Healthful Sleep* (2000), and *General Wellness* (1991) recommended	No driving or operating machinery while listening to audiotapes	Miller recording (800) 52-TAPES; Naparstek recordings: (800) 800-8661
Journaling, reflection	Promotes general well being	See Chapter 2; AlphaPoem, general journaling, captured moments, dialogue, affirmations, unsent letters, or writing topic examples		Day, 2001; Snyder, 2002

Continued

Table 9-13 Mind-Body-Spirit Interventions for Menopause

Intervention	Management	Treatment Regimen	Cautions, Precautions, Interactions	References
Meditation/prayer	Promotes general well being	Mindfulness meditation or walking-movement meditation on a regular basis recommended; tapes available Personal prayer on regular basis available	Respect personal preferences	Kornfield, 1996; Northrup, 1998; Pettinati, 2001
Music	Promotes general well being; decreases anxiety	Music usually has to be individualized		White, 2001
Pet therapy	Promotes well being	Pet of choice. Keep in mind the care that a pet needs and patient's lifestyle	Be sure patient desires a pet. Patient needs to want this option; gifts of pets are not always appreciated and not healthy for the animal.	Huebscher, 2000

Relaxation	Promotes general well being; may help relieve hot flashes	Progressive muscle relaxation recommended; general stress management and preferred relaxation techniques also used	See Chapter 2 for stress-management techniques	Dell, Stewart, 2000; Ernst, 2001
Support resources	Provides social support	Help patient find resources. Health care provider can keep a list of groups, networks, hobby groups, etc.		www.menopause.org; www.power-surge.com; www.menopause-online.com
Volunteering	Provides a "Helper's High"; helping is associated with improved health and well being	Any activity in which patient has interest is recommended: church activities, tutoring, reading to a shut-in, local library, social agencies		Dreher, 1995; Luks, 1992

lactone and enterodiol to form the active isoflavones genestein, daidzein, and equol. The high intake of soy and other dietary phytoestrogens is believed partially to explain why hot flashes and other menopausal symptoms do not occur with the same frequency in cultures that eat a primarily plant-based diet. (Low Dog et al, 2001, p. 50)

Isoflavones showed significant reduction of hot flushes in comparison to placebo in only one of eight studies done between 1995 and 1999 (Albertazzi et al, 1999; Baber et al, 1999; Low Dog et al, 2001). However, PL/PL (2002) states that soy is possibly effective in decreasing hot flashes: "Asian women who eat a high-soy diet have fewer hot flashes. Soy protein 20-60 grams providing 34-76 mg isoflavones daily modestly decreased the frequency and severity of hot flashes in menopausal women" (p. 1165). Perhaps the whole soybean needs to be consumed instead of individual isoflavones. Soy also is known to be beneficial for bone density, for lowering low-density lipoprotein (LDL) cholesterol, and for heart health (Albertazzi et al, 1999; PL/PL, 1999, 2002). In addition, wild yams and soybeans are the source of several commercial estrogen prescription products for oral, transdermal and creams (Low Dog et al, 2001).

Colon health also is important in menopause; thus a diet high in fruits and vegetables and fiber is encouraged. Furthermore, B vitamins may be helpful since they help lower homocysteine levels, a potential risk factor for depression and cardiovascular disease.

With respect to herbal therapy, black cohosh (*Cimicifuga racemosa*) has been used for years as a remedy for menopause and women's problems (Foster, 1999). Foster (1999) provides an overview of eight clinical studies researching menopausal symptoms. PL/PL (2002) rates black cohosh as possibly effective when taken orally for symptoms of menopause. Some side effects include gastrointestinal (GI) upset, headache, dizziness, weight gain, heavy feeling in the legs and cramping.

Three popular kinds of ginseng have been used to manage various menopausal symptoms; however, there is no menopause research to confirm their effectiveness:

American ginseng (*Panax quinquefolius*), also called Canadian, North American, Ontario, or Wisconsin Ginseng.

Asian ginseng (*Panax ginseng*), also called Chinese, Japanese, Korean, Oriental, or Red Ginseng.

Siberian ginseng (*Eleutherococcus senticosus*), also called Ci Wu Jia, Devil's Shrub, Thorny Bearer of Free Berries, Untouchable, or Wild Pepper.

American ginseng is considered "possibly effective" for reducing postprandial blood glucose in type 2 diabetes. Asian ginseng (*Panax*) is considered "possibly effective" for numerous concerns, including improving cognitive function, decreasing fasting blood glucose and hemoglobin A1c levels in type 2 diabetes, improving resistance to stress, and it may also decrease the incidence of cancer, in general, and for stomach, lung, liver, ovary, and skin conditions in particular. Siberian ginseng also has numerous "possibly effectives," including for increasing speed, quality, and capacity for physical work; for adapting to high temperatures, hypoxemia, and conditions that cause motion sickness; for preventing atherosclerosis; for pyelonephritis, diabetes, and craniocerebral trauma; as a tonic for invigoration during times of fatigue; and for herpes type 2 infections (PL/PL, 2002, pp. 592, 594, 597).

Numerous other herbs have women's care indications. Chasteberry, red clover, and wild yam are examples. In addition for heart health, guggul *(Commiphora mukul)*, garlic *(Allium sativum)*, and red yeast rice *(Monascus purpureus)* may help reduce cholesterol and triglyceride levels (Low Dog et al, 2001).

Bioidentical hormone replacement therapy (B-HRT) may be beneficial for menopausal women. Before initiating B-HRT, determining hormone levels through either serum or salivary methods is helpful. Based on the woman's hormone profile, a B-HRT plan can be developed using oral substances or compounded lotions and creams or both (Wepfer, 2001). Triple-estrogen (tri-est) and double estrogen (bi-est) therapies are popular estrogen combinations. Tri-est, containing 80% estriol, 10% estradiol, and 10% estrone, is usually compounded as a lotion and applied daily for transdermal absorption. Bi-est is also compounded and consists of 80% to 90% estriol and 10% to 20% estradiol (Wepfer, 2001). Additional hormones including progesterone, testosterone, and DHEA can be added to either of the estrogen preparations as indicated by the patient B-HRT profile. Table 9-14 lists biologic-based therapies used in menopause. Table 9-15 presents a comparison of NAC perimenopause support programs from three perspectives: a physician (Northrup, 2001), a naturopath with a specialty in herbal medicine and iridology (Sharon, 1995), and a nutrition scientist (Lieberman, 2001). In addition, McIntyre (1994) has written a text on women's herbals, *(Woman's Herbal)*, with photographs of the herbs and simple explanations of the female path of life.

MANIPULATIVE AND BODY-BASED METHODS AND ENERGY THERAPIES FOR MENOPAUSE

Various body and energy work can be used to help symptoms of menopause. Cool compresses help hot flashes. Massage can provide stress reduction and relaxation, and Therapeutic Touch, healing touch, or Reiki can also promote a sense of well being or decreased

Table 9-14 Biologic-Based Therapies for Menopause

A complete prescribing source should be consulted before using biologic therapies. Nutrient doses may be above the recommended daily allowance or tolerable upper limit.

In illness or deficiency, such doses may be acceptable; however, long-term use may not be appropriate. Herbs may cause allergic reactions and interactions. Herbs are generally contraindicated or not recommended for women during pregnancy and lactation and for children unless research data or a long history of safe use has been established.

Intervention	Management	Treatment Regimen	Cautions, Precautions, Interactions	References
Diet and Food				
Dietary phytoestrogens, including isoflavones and lignans	Reduces vasomotor and menopausal symptoms; may also reduce LDL and risk of cardiovascular disease and certain cancers; soy helps increase bone density	Patient increases foods high in isoflavones and lignans: soy, legumes, grains, fruits, vegetables. Soy: 60 g/day for reducing hot flashes; 40 g/day for preventing osteoporosis; 25 g/day for lowering cholesterol. Soy foods: tofu, tempeh, soy milk, roasted soy nuts, soy flour, soy bean sprouts	Phytoestrogens bind estrogen sites; effect on tumor growth not studied. Avoid supplements in women with breast or endometrial cancer. Soy can inhibit thyroid hormone synthesis	Dell, Stewart, 2000; PL/PL, 1999, 2002; Low Dog et al, 2001; Weil et al, 2000

Vitamins

B vitamins, including vitamin B6 (pyridoxine), folate, and B12	Improves mood; lowers homocysteine levels	Combined with other B vitamins in a 25- or 50-mg B complex qd-bid. Adult RDA: folate, 400 μg/day; adult UL: folate, 1000 μg/day. Adult RDA thiamine, 1.1 mg/day (women), 1.2 mg/day (men); adult UL thiamine not determined. Adult RDA niacin, 14 mg/day (women), 16 mg/day (men); adult UL niacin, 35 mg/day. Adult RDA pyridoxine, 1.3-1.7 mg; adult UL: pyridoxine, 100 mg/day. Adult RDA vitamin B12, 2.4 μg/day; adult UL vitamin B12 not determined	No studies; excess can cause nerve damage; B complex also usually has choline, inositol, pantothenic acid, biotin in the formulation	Dell, Stewart, 2000; La Valle et al, 2000; PL/PL, 2002
Vitamin E (antioxidant)	May help reduce hot flashes; also, hot flashes are a symptom of vitamin-E deficiency	RDA for Vitamin E: 15 mg (22 IU is based on the alpha tocopherol form); adult UL 1000 mg (1500 IU). Many practi-	Has drug interactions; iron can bind and inactivate vitamin E; the RDA is quite low compared with dosing	Dell, Stewart, 2000; Ernst, 2001; La Valle et al, 2000; Low

Continued

Table 9-14 Biologic-Based Therapies for Menopause—cont'd

Intervention	Management	Treatment Regimen	Cautions, Precautions, Interactions	References
Vitamins—cont'd				
Vitamin E, cont'd		tioners recommend 800 IU for hot flashes	for studies; the HOPE study used 400 IU/day; vitamin E may produce positive effects with heart disease, cancer, and cataracts	Dog et al, 2001; nih.gov/ ccc/ supplements
Minerals				
Calcium and magnesium	Promotes bone health; helps prevent osteoporosis; may be cardioprotective	Adult RDA of calcium, 1000-1200 mg/day; adult UL for calcium, 2500 mg/day; calcium-rich foods also recommended. Adult RDA of magnesium, 310-420 mg/day; adult UL for magnesium, 350 mg/day; UL for magnesium represents intake from a pharmacologic agent	Note that magnesium UL is lower than highest RDA	NAP, 2002; Northrup, 2001

Herbals			
Black cohosh (*Cimicifuga racemosa*)	Decreases hot flashes; may help strengthen vaginal epithelium	40 mg bid of standardized extract; is also a dried rhizome or root tincture; dose form should be verified; black cohosh safely used for 6 mos; was the ingredient in the old "Lydia Pinkham's Vegetable Compound"	SE: GI upset; black cohosh has salicylate constituents; may take 4 wks to feel effect; no data for long-term effects; does not appear to stimulate estrogen receptor–positive breast cancer cells, but no long-term studies done; contraindicated in pregnancy and lactation and people sensitive to salicylates; theoretical interactions with other hormones	Foster, 1999; Ernst, 2001; Low Dog et al, 2001; PL/PL, 1999, 2002
Chasteberry (*Vitex agnus-castus*)	For irregularities in menstrual cycle	Teas, tinctures, capsules; dose varies depending	SE: itching, GI upset, headache; theoretical	Blumenthal et al, 2000; La

(top of prior column) only and does not include intake from food and water; Northrup recommends a calcium/magnesium ratio of 1:1 or 2:1

Continued

Table 9-14 Biologic-Based Therapies for Menopause—cont'd

Intervention	Management	Treatment Regimen	Cautions, Precautions, Interactions	References
Herbals—cont'd				
Chasteberry, cont'd		on formulation; standardized to contain 0.5% agnuside and 0.6% aucubin per dose	interaction with other hormones. Although a study for PMS was done, no data for menopause	Valle et al, 2000; Low Dog et al, 2001; PL/PL, 2002
Dong quai (Angelica sinensis)	For menopausal symptoms	Varying dose forms; may work because generally several herbs are mixed in a formula designed specifically for the individual (PL/PL considers Don quai "possibly ineffective due to the need to look at the combination effect.")	SE: photosensitivity, diarrhea, fever, bleeding; well-documented use in Chinese medicine; research data poor; can double the prothrombin time; contraindicated if on warfarin or ASA or if increased bleeding occurs; theoretical interaction with other hormones	Dell, Stewart, 2000; Fetrow, Avila, 1999; La Valle et al, 2000; Low Dog et al, 2001; PL/PL, 1999, 2002
Ginkgo (Ginkgo biloba)	Improves cognitive function; may treat cerebral insufficiency; helps reduce anxiety and stress	60-120 mg/day; standardized extract that contains 24% flavonoids and 6% terpenes	SE: headache, allergy; affects blood clotting; contraindicated in women on anticoagulants	DerMardrosian, 2001; PL/PL, 2002

Continued

| Ginseng [Asian] (Panax ginseng) | May improve cognitive function; reduce stress | 0.6-3.0 g of cut or powdered root 1-3 times/ day; Panax Ginseng tea bags usually have 1500 mg of ginseng root. To make a tea: 3 g of root soaked in 150 ml boiling water for 10-15 min. A panax-free period is needed between courses (e.g., a regimen of 4 wks on and 2 wks off) is recommended | SE: many reported; nervousness, insomnia, hypertension; thought to compete with estrogen-binding sites; not for use with people who have cardiovascular disease; contraindicated in renal failure, infection, pregnancy, and other health conditions; drug interactions; all prescribing data should be consulted | Dell, Stewart, 2000; DerMardero-sian, 2001; La Valle et al, 2000; PL/PL, 2002; Tesch, 2001 |
| Ginseng [Siberian] (Eleutherococcus senticosus) | Help increase speed and capacity for physical work; is a tonic for invig-oration during times of fatigue and debility; builds strength during convalescence | Dry root 0.6-3.0 g/day for up to 3 mos; a 2-3-wk ginseng-free period used after 30-60 days of treatment with Siberian ginseng; should not be used long term | SE: drowsiness, anxiety, irritability; mastalgia has been reported; caution with cardio-vascular disorders; can cause palpitations, tachycardia, hyperten-sion; long-term use associated with inflamed nerves (sciatica); drug interac- | PL/PL, 2002 |

Table 9-14 Biologic-Based Therapies for Menopause—cont'd

Intervention	Management	Treatment Regimen	Cautions, Precautions, Interactions	References
Herbals—cont'd				
Ginseng [Siberian], cont'd			tions; all prescribing data should be consulted	
Kava (Piper methysticum)	Alleviates anxiety, menopause symptoms; promotes sleep; Ernst reports 2 RCTs (n = 40)	See current recommendations; USE SHOULD BE LIMITED TO AVOID HABITUATION; source of herb must be known; perhaps better to take actual root; CAUTION: recent reports of at least 30 cases of liver toxicity and failure reported	SE: numbness of mouth and tongue, skin rash, visual disturbances, muscle weakness; abuse potential of kava; not to be used in patients with depression. Additive with alcohol and benzodiazepines	DerMardero-sian, 2001; Ernst, 2001; La Valle et al, 2000; PL/PL, 2002
Passionflower (Passiflora incarnata)	For sleep disorders, nervousness	Dried herb: 0.25-2.0 g of dried aboveground parts tid or 1 c tea bid-tid and 30 min before bedtime; various dose forms: dried herb, extract, teas	SE: none reported; no driving or operating machinery; no research data on passionflower	Blumenthal et al, 2000; DerMardero-sian, 2001; Fetrow, Avila, 1999; PL/PL, 1999, 2002

Red clover (*Trifolium pratense*); contains isoflavones, including genistein, daidzein, biochanin A, and formononetin	For menopausal symptoms (hot flashes and night sweats). Help improve systemic arterial compliance	4 g of flower tops tid; some standardized to contain 40 mg isoflavones per dose. Dose forms: drops, infusion, or liquid extract; active part is flower top	SE: breast tenderness, weight gain, infertility in animals; may alter platelet aggregation; interacts with anticoagulants; should be discontinued 14 days before surgery; contraindicated in bleeding conditions	Fetrow, Avila, 1999; La Valle et al, 2000; PL/PL, 1999, 2002
St. John's wort (*Hypericum perforatum*)	For mild to moderate depression	300 mg tid standardized extract to 0.3% hypericin. Abrupt discontinuation should be avoided	SE: GI upset, dizziness, confusion, sedation, dry mouth, hypomania, photosensitivity; serotonin syndrome when used with SSRIs; contraindicated with HIV protease-inhibitor use. Numerous interactions, including with hormonal contraception Tyramine foods avoided: since this may cause hypertensive crisis	Fetrow, Avila, 1999; PL/PL, 2002; Tesch, 2001

Continued

Table 9-14 Biologic-Based Therapies for Menopause—cont'd

Intervention	Management	Treatment Regimen	Cautions, Precautions, Interactions	References
Herbals—cont'd				
Valerian (*Valeriana officinalis* and others)	Help relieve sleep problems, restlessness	400-900 mg up to 2 hrs before bedtime for as long as 28 days; or tea: 2-3 g of the root steeped in 150 ml boiling water for 5-10 min and strained; maximum doses 15 g of root/day	SE: impaired alertness, headache; no driving or operating machinery when taking; can interact with other sedatives	DerMarderosian, 2001; Fetrow, Avila, 1999; PL/PL, 2000a
Wild yam (*Discorea composita* or *floribunda* or others); contains DHEA, a steroid hormone produced in the adrenal gland and the most abundant adrenocorticoid hormone in the body	For menopausal symptoms; may help vaginal dryness	No typical dose given. Standardized to contain 10% diosgenin per dose; some natural hormones are made from wild yam or soy	SE: acne, oily skin, hair loss or hirsutism, headache, menstrual irregularities; potential for stimulating growth of prostate cancer; data lacking for dose and long-term effects; theoretical interactions with other hormones	Fetrow, Avila, 1999; La Valle et al, 2000; PL/PL, 1999, 2002

Aromatherapy, including rose (sedating) and lavender (calming); must be pure oils	Promotes well being; helps relieve depression	Rose aroma: 2 gtts on facial tissue inhaled qid; lavender aroma: 1-5 gtts on a tissue inhaled for about 10 min; can also be added to a carrier oil or base for massage	SE: allergy; true essential oils are steam distillates of aromatic plants and should be 100% pure; oils are highly concentrated, and only 1-5 gtts are used at a time; oils are always diluted if used on the skin	Buckle, 2001
Other				
B-HRT	May help reduce hot flashes and vaginal dryness; improves mood; promotes sleep	Tri-est or bi-est compounded transdermal preparation recommended; may have added progesterone, testosterone, and DHEA as needed	Should not be used in patient with history of breast cancer. Note: follow current information on HRT and cardiovascular status prior to use.	Northrup, 2001; Wepfer, 2001
Natural progesterone cream	May help alleviate vasomotor symptoms	Topical application of topical wild yam and progesterone products; can be compounded	May be for women who do not want to take estrogen; no evidence for increase of bone density or that they affect lipids; may need oral progesterone or medroxyprogesterone	Low Dog et al, 2001

Continued

Table 9-14 Biologic-Based Therapies for Menopause—cont'd

Intervention	Management	Treatment Regimen	Cautions, Precautions, Interactions	References
Other—cont'd				
Natural proges-terone cream, cont'd			if taking oral estrogen. Note: follow current information on HRT and cardiovascular status prior to use.	

ASA, Acetylsalicylic acid; B-HRT, bioidentical hormone replacement therapy; bid, twice daily; DHEA, dehydroepiandrosterone; GI, gastrointestinal; gtts, drops; HIV, human immunodeficiency virus; HOPE, Heart Outcomes Prevention Evaluation; IU, international units; LDL, low-density lipoprotein; PL/PL, Pharmacist's Letter/Prescriber's Letter; PMS, premenstrual syndrome; qd, daily; qid, four times daily; RCTs, randomized controlled trials; RDA, recommended daily allowance; SE, side effects; SSRIs, selective serotonin reuptake inhibitors; tid, three times daily; UL, upper limits—the maximum level of daily nutrient that is likely to pose no risk of adverse effects. Includes intake from food, water, and supplements. Intake (DRI) values expands on the RDAs and contain four categories of recommendations (i.e., RDA, AI [Adequate Intake], UL, EAR [Estimated Average Requirement]). Check for the latest data.

Both the AI and the RDA are goals for intakes, but are defined differently.

RDA is the intake at which risk of inadequacy is very small (2% to 3%); RDA is expected to meet the nutrient needs of 97% to 98% of the individuals in a life stage and gender group.

AI is the observed average or experimentally set intake by a defined population or subgroup that appears to sustain a defined nutritional status, such as growth rate, normal circulating nutrient values, or other functional indicators of health. An AI is used if sufficient scientific evidence is not available to derive an EAR. AN AI IS NOT AN RDA.

EAR is the intake that meets the estimated nutrient needs of half of the individuals in a group.

References from the Food and Nutrition Board, National Academy of Sciences, Institute of Medicine (www.nap.edu)

Table 9-15   Comparison of Perimenopause Supplement Programs

The following provides three examples of supplement programs for menopause. The list is not all-inclusive, and rationale is not given for specific nutrients, although the authors provide these in their writings. Not all supplements are given to everyone. All prescribing data for individual supplements should be reviewed, and a qualified herbal specialist should be consulted.

Suggested Nutritional Supplement	Lieberman, 2001	Northrup, 2001	Sharon, 1994, 1995
Vitamins	Vitamin A and beta carotene, B vitamins, vitamins C, D, E	Vitamin A as beta carotene; B vitamins, including biotin, pantothenic acid, inositol, choline; vitamin C, D, E	Vitamin A and beta carotene; B1, B2, B6, and other B vitamins; vitamins C, D, E; some of these are discussed as coming from herbals
Minerals	Calcium, chromium, iron, magnesium, selenium	Calcium, magnesium, boron, chromium, copper, iron manganese, zinc, selenium, potassium, molybdenum, vanadium, trace minerals (usually from marine mineral complex)	Calcium, iron, manganese, "trace minerals"; some of these are discussed as coming from herbals
Other		Soy foods, omega-3 fatty acids, including flax; glutathione, alpha-lipoic acid, coenzyme Q10	Evening primrose oil (GLA), black current, or borage; bee pollen; seaweed, spirulina

Continued

Table 9-15 Comparison of Perimenopause Supplement Programs—cont'd

Suggested Nutritional Supplement	Lieberman, 2001	Northrup, 2001	Sharon, 1994, 1995
Herbs and herbal formulas	Black cohosh, chasteberry, garlic, ginkgo; American, Asian, and Siberian ginseng; kava kava; St. John's wort	Black cohosh, chasteberry, dong quai, ginkgo, grape seed, licorice root, pine bark, St. John's Wort; Chinese herb formulas: Joyful Change; Yunnan Bai Yao; Tian Wang Bu Xin Wang; Chai Hu Long Gu Muli Wang	Adrenal: borage, mullein, lobelia, ginseng, gotu kola, hawthorn berries, parsley root Herbal formulas: read all prescribing information. Multivitamin, minerals naturally: alfalfa, alkaline formula, anemia formula, calcium formula, spirulina, rosehips Body building: comfrey root, comfrey leaves (comfrey can be liver toxic), Irish moss, marshmallow root, mullein, plantain, white oak bark

Bowel rejuvenator: cascara sagrada, ginger root, golden seal or thyme, slippery elm, turkey rhubarb, wahoo ("likely unstable," PL/PL, 2002, p. 1304), Culver's root

Calcium: horsetail, oat straw, lobelia, marshmallow root, kelp, parsley root

Exhaustion: Gentian root, gotu kola, chondrus crispus, cetraria, cloves, alfalfa, calumba root

Heart: Hawthorn berries, motherwort, ginseng, ginger root, comfrey root, lily of the valley, broom, lime blossoms, bugleweed

Hormone balance: black cohosh, sarsaparilla, ginseng, holy thistle, licorice root, false unicorn, squaw vine, chasteberry

Kidney/bladder: buchu, clivers, gravel root, juniper berries, marshmallow root, parsley root, uva ursi

Continued

Table 9-15 Comparison of Perimenopause Supplement Programs—cont'd

Suggested Nutritional Supplement	Lieberman, 2001	Northrup, 2001	Sharon, 1994, 1995
Herbs and herbal formulas, cont'd			Liver/gallbladder: barberry bark, wild yam root, cramp bark, fennel, catnip, peppermint, dandelion, meadowsweet, wahoo, black root Lymphatic: Echinacea, lobelia, mullein, poke root, burdock, cayenne, chaparral ("likely unsafe," PL/PL, 2002, p. 311) Menopause: alfalfa, chickweed, dandelion, dong quai, fenugreek, horsetail, motherwort, nettles, red clover blossoms, red raspberry leaves, violet leaves, wild yam root Nerve rejuvenator: gotu kola, valerian, kava kava, Irish moss, lady slipper

GLA, *Gamma linolenic acid.*

anxiety. Table 9-16 reviews modalities that may help women through their perimenopausal time.

NAC THERAPIES FOR URINARY INCONTINENCE

Urinary incontinence (UI), as defined by the International Continence Society, is the "involuntary loss of urine that is objectively demonstrable and is a social or hygienic problem" (Hendrix, 2001, p. 162). UI occurs in both men and women but is more common in women. Estimates are that 13 million Americans are incontinent, with 11 million being women. Prevalence is from 13% to 45% of the population.

Types of UI include:

1. Stress—losing urine with coughing, sneezing, laughing, running, or other physical activity
2. Urge—strong and abrupt urge to void with loss of urine often on the way to bathroom
3. Overflow—bladder overdistention with dribbling, urgency, or urge or stress UI
4. Functional—mental or chronic functional disabilities associated with loss of urine, such as inability to get to bathroom or unfasten clothing
5. Reflex—neurologic dysfunction
6. Mixed—combination of urge and stress (Burkhart, 2000; Fantl et al, 1996)

Additionally, the condition of overactive bladder is characterized by frequency, urgency, and, at times, urge incontinence; approximately 40% of people with overactive bladder have urge incontinence (Wein, 1999). Symptoms vary with the type of UI. Common diagnostics include urinalysis, urine culture, postvoid residual volume (PVR) or bladder ultrasound, and possible blood-urea-nitrogen (BUN) and creatinine assessment. Other tests include special pads that stain with urine loss, the visual observation by the examiner of the patient's loss of urine, and a positive Marshall Test, which means that the health care provider can stop the flow of urine by manually elevating and supporting the anterior vaginal wall (Burkhart, 2000). Many natural therapies are available, as well as some alternative treatments. Appropriate diagnosis is necessary before conventional or NAC treatment.

MIND-BODY-SPIRIT INTERVENTIONS FOR URINARY INCONTINENCE

Table 9-17 reviews a few mind-body-spirit interventions for urinary incontinence. These include biofeedback, hypnosis and imagery, and toileting programs.

BIOLOGIC-BASED THERAPIES FOR URINARY INCONTINENCE

First and foremost, preexisting conditions must be treated, and substances that irritate or can cause UI should be avoided. Box 9-1 lists

Table 9-16 Manipulative and Body Based Methods and Energy Therapies for Menopause

Intervention	Management	Treatment Regimen	Cautions, Precautions, Interactions	References
Osteopathic treatment	May help relieve menopausal symptoms, including depression and hot flashes	Once/wk for 10 wks. In study, N = 30; had sham treatment as control	Needs skilled practitioner	Cleary, Fox, 1994; Ernst, 2001
General massage	Promotes relaxation; improves circulation; decreases tension	Patient preference and as budget will allow determines timing and method used; can choose from various types: Swedish for relaxation or deep-tissue or neuromuscular for tension areas; also specialty type massages available	Cost can be a concern	AMTA, ABMP
Therapeutic Touch, healing touch, Reiki	Helps decrease anxiety; promotes relaxation	Sessions usually approximately 30 minutes	Ask permission from participant	

ABMP, *Associated Bodywork and Massage Professionals*; AMTA, *American Massage Therapy Association.*

Table 9-17   Mind-Body-Spirit Interventions for Urinary Incontinence

Intervention	Management	Treatment Regimen	Cautions, Precautions, Interactions	References
Biofeedback, behavioral training, pelvic floor therapy	For overactive bladder or stress, urge or mixed UI with urge-predominant pattern; can be used for men after prostate surgery	4 sessions of biofeedback-assisted behavioral treatment; over 4-8 wks time frame; used together with Kegel's; may have electrical stimulation in second phase of treatment	Biofeedback specialist needed; biofeedback-behavioral training worked better than placebo or drug in study; can also have home therapy	Burgio et al, 1998; Hendrix, 2001
Clothing and hygiene	For all types of UI	Cotton underwear recommended; scented products avoided; white unscented toilet tissue; water-soluble lubricants for intercourse recommended		Bates, 2000
Hypnosis and imagery	For general relaxation with imagery; may work with hypnosis; hypnosis may work well for	Several sessions are usually needed, or participant may purchase imagery recordings	Must be appropriate candidate and have skilled professional help; hypnosis has worked for children	Temes, 1999; Miller, 1980

Continued

Table 9-17 Mind-Body-Spirit Interventions for Urinary Incontinence—cont'd

Intervention	Management	Treatment Regimen	Cautions, Precautions, Interactions	References
Hypnosis and imagery, cont'd	urinary retention, particularly after surgery		and adolescents with enuresis. With anatomic block, hypnosis does not work well	Burkhart, 2000; Hendrix, 2001; Maloney, 2001; Roberts, 2001
Toileting programs	For overactive bladder, urge, functional, overflow UI	Habit retraining: time interval is set that is shorter than the patient's normal voiding, and patient is encouraged to void only at that time		
		Prompted voiding: caregivers check patients on hourly or regular basis; voiding is encouraged q2h from 7:00 AM to 7:00 PM	For the cognitively impaired and extended care facilities	

Timed voiding: established schedule for voiding based on a voiding diary	Need bladder diary; good for people who have tendency to wait too long
Bladder retraining (bladder drill): has a cure rate of about 78% for overactive bladder; voiding at set times regardless of urge; interval increased from about 1 hr the first wk to interval of about 3-4 hrs; increased in 15-min increments	Most successful in people who are motivated and physically and mentally capable

q2h, *Every 2 hours*; UI, *urinary incontinence*.

Box 9-1

Urinary Incontinence Offenders

The following substances may cause stress, urge, or overflow urinary incontinence or cause the person to have overactive bladder symptoms.
Adrenergic agonists*
Adrenergic antagonists
Alcohol
Angiotensin converting enzyme inhibitors
Anticholinergics*
Antidepressants
Antihistamines
Anti-Parkinson
Antipsychotics
Antispasmodics
Caffeine
Diuretics
Narcotics
Sedatives and hypnotics

---

*Also used as treatment for some urinary incontinence.

some UI offenders. In addition, increasing fluid intake and mobility can help prevent some incontinence. People sometimes decrease fluids, thinking this will decrease UI; but instead, the urine becomes concentrated and more irritating. Fecal impaction and constipation also are implicated in UI and thus need care. Making sure the bathroom is convenient and clothing can be easily managed are two more remedies (Burkhart, 2000). Table 9-18 lists biologic-based therapies for UI.

MANIPULATIVE AND BODY-BASED METHODS AND ENERGY THERAPIES FOR URINARY INCONTINENCE

Several options other than surgery are available for UI. Kegel's exercises, when done on a regular basis for an extended period, can bring good results for women with stress, urge, mixed incontinence, and overactive bladder (Bates, 2000; Burkhart, 2000; Hendrix, 2001; Johnson, 2000; Maloney, 2001; Roberts, 2001). In addition, numerous pessaries are available, as well as vaginal weights and electrical stimulation. Table 9-19 outlines body-based and energy therapies for UI.

Table 9-18 Biologic-Based Therapies for Urinary Incontinence

Intervention	Management	Treatment Regimen	Cautions, Precautions, Interactions	References
Increased fluids	Maintains more dilute urine, thus cuts down on irritation from concentrated urine	Maintaining adequate water and nonirritant fluid intake recommended; ½ oz/lb of body weight each day; cranberry juice helps decrease urinary tract infections		Bates, 2000; Burkhart, 2000
Dietary modifications	Decrease irritants	Irritants: caffeine (coffee, tea, chocolate), alcohol, aspartame and artificial sweeteners, spicy foods, acid drinks, soda, tomato-based sauces; not every food will irritate every person; may need to discover which food is an irritant		Bates, 2000

Continued

Table 9-18	Biologic-Based Therapies for Urinary Incontinence—cont'd			
Intervention	**Management**	**Treatment Regimen**	**Cautions, Precautions, Interactions**	**References**
Dietary modifications, cont'd	For constipation	Fiber increased; "power pudding" (see gastrointestinal chapter), fluids increased; hemorrhoids and fissures attended; "the urge" is complied with; that is, the patient is not to put off having a bowel movement		

Table 9-19 Manipulative and Body-Based Methods and Energy Therapies for Urinary Incontinence

Intervention	Management	Treatment Regimen	Cautions, Precautions, Interactions	References
Kegel's exercises	For stress, urge, mixed UI or overactive bladder; strengthens pelvic floor muscles; improvement of from 45%-75% when done correctly	10 min 2-3 times/day; hold for 10 sec; OR 10 contractions every hr; OR 30-80 times/day for at least 8 wks	Must isolate the correct muscles; patient is taught during pelvic examination	Bates, 2000; Burkhart, 2000; Hendrix, 2001; Johnson, 2000; Maloney, 2001; Roberts, 2001
Pessaries	Used when organ prolapse is underlying cause of stress UI; especially helpful when surgery is not an option	Over 200 styles and types are available; health care provider fits client; styles include Cube, Donut, Gehrung, Gellhorn, Hodge, Incontinence dish, Inflatoball, Regula, Ring, Risser, Shaatz, Smith, Tandem cube, Trimo-san; pessaries are made from	Pessary should be cleaned regularly; some need daily cleaning (e.g., Inflatoball, cube); most pessaries difficult for patient to reinsert correctly, especially if older adult has mobility problems, thus provider may change pes-latex,	Burkhart, 2000; Maloney, 2001; Milex Products, 2003

Continued

Table 9-19 Manipulative and Body-Based Methods and Energy Therapies for Urinary Incontinence—cont'd

Intervention	Management	Treatment Regimen	Cautions, Precautions, Interactions	References
Pessaries, cont'd		silicone, or acrylic; several fittings are necessary; important to see client within 24 hrs of fitting and again in 72 hrs; then reexamine every 4-6 wks; refittings often are necessary	sary; can pose transportation and financial difficulties or means the pessary may not be cleaned as often as appropriate; some pessaries have metal components and need to be removed before MRI or x-ray; a "noncompliant" patient should not be fit with any pessary	
Vaginal weight inserts and cones	For stress, urge, or mixed UI	Progressive weights used; works on theories underlying body-building; weights are held in vagina by tightening vaginal muscles; causes or stimulates pelvic floor	Sustained contraction at a given weight increases the strength of the pelvic floor; increase weights progressively by 5 g	Bates, 2000; Burkhart, 2000; Hendrix, 2001; Charon Pierson,

		contraction; 15 min twice/day for 4-6 wks; is often used in conjunction with pelvic floor exercises	2002 personal communication
Electrical stimulation	Improves pelvic muscle tone	Mild electrical pulses stimulate muscle contraction of pelvic floor; done in conjunction with Kegel's exercises and biofeedback equipment	Hendrix, 2001; Hollister, 2003
Ex-MI	For stress, urge, and overflow UI	Extracorporeal magnet produces a pulsing magnetic field; creates brief depolarization potential; produces muscle contractions similar to Kegel's exercises only at a rate of up to 20 times/sec; this is a new treatment. Participant is fully clothed; sits in a treatment chair	Burkhart, 2000

Ex-MI, Extracorporeal magnetic innervation; MRI, magnetic resonance imaging; UI, urinary incontinence.

NAC THERAPIES FOR MALE GENITOURINARY CONCERNS

Prostate Health

Prostate cancer is the most common cancer in American men, thus prostate health is a concern. The clinical incidence of prostate cancer is not as high, however, as the prevalence found at autopsy:

> more than 40% of men over 50 years of age are found to have prostatic carcinoma. Most such occult cancers are small and contained within the prostate gland. Few are associated with regional or distant disease. The incidence of prostatic cancer increases with age. Whereas 30% of men age 60-69 will have the disease, autopsy incidence increases to 67% in men aged 80-89 years. Although the prevalence of prostatic cancer in autopsy specimens around the world varies little, the clinical incidence is considerably different (high in North America and European countries, intermediate in South America, and low in the Far East), suggesting that environmental or dietary differences among populations may be important for prostatic cancer growth. (Stoller et al, 2001, pp. 956-957)

Benign Prostatic Hyperplasia

Benign prostatic hyperplasia (BPH) refers to a nonmalignant enlargement of the prostate gland resulting from an increase in cell numbers (from proliferation of stromal and epithelial elements). BPH can be microscopic, macroscopic, or clinical. The cause seems to be multifactorial and under endocrine control. BPH is a frequent occurrence, representing the most common benign tumor in men. At least 50% of men over age 50, and approximately 80% by age 70, have BPH. Symptoms are both obstructive and irritative. The obstructive symptoms include hesitancy, decreased force and caliber of the stream, a feeling of incomplete emptying, voiding twice, straining, and dribbling. The irritative symptoms include nocturia, frequency, and urgency. Prostate size does not correlate with the patient's symptoms. Patient history, neurologic and digital-rectal examination, serum prostate-specific antigen, urinalysis, creatinine, and the American Urological Association (AUA) symptom score are initial diagnostic tools (Beduschi et al, 1998; Stoller et al, 2001).

MIND-BODY-SPIRIT INTERVENTIONS FOR PROSTATE HEALTH AND BENIGN PROSTATIC HYPERPLASIA

Men may help decrease their risk of prostate cancer by exercising. A brisk walk 20 to 30 minutes most days of the week or other aerobic exercise 3 to 4 days a week are general exercise recommendations (American Cancer Society [ACS], 2001). In addition, imagery may help for general well being. Tapes are available, including Miller's *Healing Journey* (1980), Naparstek's stress-management tapes, *Stress I and Stress II* (1995), or smoking cessation (1997).

BIOLOGIC-BASED THERAPIES FOR PROSTATE HEALTH AND BENIGN PROSTATIC HYPERPLASIA

Dietary factors have been studied and play a role in prostate disease, thus men can take dietary measures to help decrease the risk of prostate cancer. These factors include a low-fat diet and increased consumption of fruits, vegetables, and soy products. With the increased consumption of fruits and vegetables, more of the vitamins and minerals needed for prostate health will be included in the diet. Prostate cancer decreases for men between the ages of 40 and 64 if they use vitamin A, vitamin C, and zinc supplements. The findings for vitamin E are mixed (PL/PL, 2000b). Selenium and boron also seem to play a role in decreasing prostate cancer risk (PL/PL, 2000b; ACT, 2001). Numerous herbs are available for maintaining prostate health and for BPH. For prostate cancer, estrogenic herbs might have an effect. Herbs with estrogenic effects are alfalfa, anise seed, black cohosh, ginseng, licorice, pleurisy root, red clover, saw palmetto, soy, and wild carrot. These herbs contain phytoestrogens. Other natural products that have demonstrated *in vitro* antineoplastic effects are astragalus, cat's claw, garlic, shark cartilage, green tea, St John's wort, milk thistle, and mushroom species, including maitake and shiitake (which contains lentinan) (DerMarderosian, 2001; PL/PL, 2000b). Ernst (2001) reports on a formula PC-SPES that was shown to reduce prostate-specific antigen in patients with prostate cancer and inhibit growth *in vitro*. The formula contains *Chrysanthemum morifolium*, *Gandoderma lucidum* (Reishi mushroom), *Glycyrrhiza glabra*, *Isatis indigotica* (a Chinese herb), *Panax pseudoginseng*, *Robdosia rubesceus*, *Scutellaria baicalensis* and *Serenoa repens* (saw palmetto). This formula has ingredients that have hormonal effects (PL/PL, 2000b). Murray (1999) rates the effectiveness of herbs for BPH, starting with *Serenoa*, then Cernilton, *Pygeum*, and *Uritica*, stating, however, that "in certain situations one herbal approach may be more effective than another" (p. 1149).

Table 9-20 delineates biologic-based therapies for prostate health and BPH. Table 9-21 lists herbs and supplements that can interact with the prostate and are contraindicated in people with prostate cancer or other prostate conditions.

Table 9-20 Biologic-Based Therapies for Prostate Concerns

Intervention	Management	Treatment Regimen	Cautions, Precautions, Interactions	References
Diet	Decrease risk of prostate cancer and helps with prostate health; men who have increased fat in diet have greater risk of developing prostate cancer	Fat in diet decreased to less than 30%; saturated fat and meat in diet reduced. Essential fatty acids, fruits, and vegetables increased; spices, lemon substituted for fat		ACS, 2001; Gupta, 1999; Murray, 1999; PL/PL, 2000b
Cruciferous vegetables and beta-carotene foods	Helps reduce risk of prostate cancer	3 servings of cruciferous vegetables/wk: Brussels sprouts, broccoli, cauliflower, cabbage; deep green and yellow vegetables recommended		PL/PL, 2000b
	Green tea may help prevent bladder cancer	Typical dose: 3 c green tea/day; contains 240-320 mg of polyphenols	Has drug and laboratory interactions; no studies have evaluated tablet formulations	PL/PL, 2002
Antioxidants		Lutein: 2 mg (2000 μg)/day; increase in lutein foods recommended: spinach, kiwi, squash, corn, orange pepper		PL/PL, 2000b

	Clinical Use	Dosage/Recommendation	Cautions	Reference
		Lycopenes: 5-10 mg/day; increase in lycopene foods recommended: tomatoes (raw, cooked or in tomato products [e.g., sauces, ketchup]), grapefruit, watermelon. Heat releases high concentrations of free lycopene, thus cooked tomatoes may be better than raw		PL/PL, 2000b
Soy (contains the isoflavones genistein and daidzein; exerts estrogen effect)		2 or more glasses of soy milk daily or other soy-based products	Allergy to soy; soy can inhibit thyroid hormone synthesis	PL/PL, 2000b
Vitamins				
Vitamin A	For prostate cancer; risk is lower between ages 40-64 with men who use vitamin-A supplements	Vitamin A RDA: 700-900 µg/day; adult UL: 3000 µg (3 mg)/day; vitamin A foods are liver, whole milk and fortified fat-reduced milk, cheese, whole egg,	Is fat-soluble vitamin, thus toxicity can occur; liver damage, birth defects may occur; people with high alcohol intake, liver disease, hyperlipidemia, or protein	PL/PL, 2000b; NAP, 2003; www.nationalacademies.org/news, 2001

Continued

Table 9-20 Biologic-Based Therapies for Prostate Concerns—cont'd

Intervention	Management	Treatment Regimen	Cautions, Precautions, Interactions	References
Vitamins—cont'd				
Vitamin A, cont'd		darkly colored fruits and vegetables (carrots, sweet potatoes, broccoli)	malnutrition are susceptible to adverse effects	
Vitamin C	For prostate cancer (antioxidant form); risk is lower between ages 40 to 64 with men who use vitamin C	RDA: 90 mg/day; adult UL: 2000 mg/day; many researchers recommend more C than the RDA; vitamin-C foods include citrus fruits	SE: diarrhea when bowel tolerance reached; vitamin C enhances the effects of vitamin E	NAP, 2002; PL/PL, 2000b, 2002, www.cc.nih.gov, 2001
Vitamin E	May possibly reduce risk of prostate cancer	59-100 IU/day; RDA is 15 mg/day (22 IU based on alpha tocopherol form); adult UL: 1000 mg/day (1500 IU); vitamin E foods include wheat germ, almonds, safflower, corn and soybean oil, mango, peanuts	Can act as anticoagulant and increase bleeding risk	ACS, 2001; NAP, 2002 PL/PL, 2000b, 2002, www.cc.nih.gov, 2001

Continued

Minerals

Boron	May reduce risk of prostate cancer; in a recent study, 64% lower risk with the highest consumption of boron	Adult UL: 20 mg/day; boron-rich foods recommended: red wine, coffee, fruits, almonds and other nuts; no established daily value for boron	Study of 76 men with prostate cancer compared with 7751 healthy men	ACT, 2001; www.national-academies.org/news, 2001
Selenium	May reduce risk of prostate cancer	PL/PL recommends 200 μg/day. Adult UL: 400 μg/day; RDA: 55 μg/day; Brazil nuts good source of selenium; also, tuna, cod, noodles (pasta), bread	Acute toxicity can occur; selenosis symptoms: GI upset, hair loss, blotchy nails, mild nerve damage	ACS, 2001; PL/PL, 2000b
Zinc	For prostate cancer; risk is lower between ages 40-64 with men who use zinc; zinc is cofactor in many enzymatic reactions; used for BPH	Adult RDA (men) is 11 mg/day; adult UL: 40 mg/day. Oysters, meats, sardines, seafood, fish, egg yolk, Brewer's yeast, spinach, kelp, mushrooms, whole grains, soy, legumes, pecans, pumpkin and sunflower seeds are sources of zinc. Must have proper zinc/copper ratio	Copper, calcium, and iron compete with zinc for protein-binding sites; elevated calcium, copper, or iron can cause depletion of zinc; coffee can inhibit absorption; zinc may reduce HDL; oral contraceptives, diuretics, H2-receptor antagonists can deplete zinc	La Valle et al, 1999; PL/PL, 2000b; 2002; www.cc.nih.gov, 2001; www.national-academies.org/news, 2001

Table 9-20 Biologic-Based Therapies for Prostate Concerns—cont'd

Intervention	Management	Treatment Regimen	Cautions, Precautions, Interactions	References
Herbs				
African wild potato (Hypoxis rooperi)	For BPH; improves urine flow and increases volume of urine; plant is high in beta-sitosterol; may affect prostate growth	Oral beta-sitosterol dose of 60 to 130 mg/day seems to reduce symptoms of BPH by about 50%	Originally a South African plant; is related to asparagus	PL/PL, 2002, 2000b
Pumpkin seed (Cucurbita pepo)	For BPH; irritable bladder, and micturition problems	5 g ground seed bid with fluid	None known	Blumenthal et al, 2000; PL/PL, 2002
Pygeum (Pygeum africana)	For BPH; limits testosterone synthesis by inhibiting intestinal absorption of cholesterol	100-200 mg standardized lipophilic extract/day in 6-8-wk cycles	SE: GI upset. More expensive than saw palmetto. Also plant species survival is threatened.	PL/PL, 2000b, 2002
Rye grass pollen (Secale cereale)	Relieves BPH symptom, including frequency, nocturia, urgency, decreased	Rye grass pollen 126 mg tid recommended. Clinical studies have used Cerniltin	SE: GI upset, allergy; limited research	Murray, 1999; PL/PL, 2000b, 2002

Herb	Actions/Uses	Dosing	Side Effects	References
Saw palmetto (*Serenoa repens*)	rate, dribbling, painful urination, residual urine; possibly shrinks prostate size. For BPH; reduces urinary frequency and nocturia; increases urinary flow; inhibits 5-alpha reductase; antagonizes androgen receptors; has antiinflammatory and estrogenic effects	Various dose extracts recommended; usually 160 mg bid standardized to 85%-95% fatty acids and sterols; check labeling for dose; effects occur in 4 to 6 wks	SE: GI upset, headache; avoid taking with hormone therapy avoided	Blumenthal et al, 2000; DerMarderosian, 2001; PL/PL, 2000b
Stinging nettle root (*Urtica dioica*)	For BPH, difficulty in urination	Used as infusion, decoction, extract, tincture; read labeling for doses	SE: GI upset, allergy, sweating	Blumenthal, 2000; PL/PL, 2000b, 2002

ACS, American Cancer Society; ACT, *Alternative and Complementary Therapies*; bid, *twice daily*; BPH, *benign prostatic hypertrophy*; GI, *gastrointestinal*; HDL, *high-density lipoprotein*; IU, *international units*; NAP, *National Academy Press*; PL/PL, *Pharmacist's Letter/Prescriber's Letter*; RDA, *recommended daily allowance*; SE, *side effects*; UL, *upper limits*—*the maximum level of daily nutrient that is likely to pose no risk of adverse effects. Includes intake from food, water, and supplements.*

Table 9-21 Herbs and Supplements that Can Interact with Prostate Conditions

Product	Interaction with Prostate Conditions
Androstenediol	Should be avoided in men with prostate conditions; might aggravate prostate conditions because of its androgenic activity
Androstenedione	Should be avoided in men with prostate conditions; can stimulate prostate tumor cell growth
Belladonna	Contraindicated in prostate adenoma with residual urine retention because of its anticholinergic effects
Ephedra	Contraindicated in prostate adenoma with residual urine retention because of its sympathetic nervous system effects
Henbane	Contraindicated in prostate adenoma with residual urine retention because of its anticholinergic effects
Jimson weed	Contraindicated in prostate adenoma with residual urine retention because of its anticholinergic effects
Scopolia	Contraindicated in prostate adenoma with residual urine retention because of its anticholinergic effects
Wild lettuce	Contraindicated in men with BPH; the fresh form contains hyoscyamine, which has anticholinergic effects
Yohimbe	Contraindicated in cases of chronic prostate or related sex organ inflammation

BPH, Benign prostatic hypertrophy.

From Pharmacist's Letter/Prescriber's Letter, Continuing Education Booklet: Natural medicines in clinical management: Alzheimer's disease, diabetes, men's health, vol 2000, no 2, Stockton, Calif, 2000, Therapeutic Research Center.
Prescriber's Letter Copyright 2001 by Therapeutic Research Center Pharmacist's Letter/Prescriber's Letter, PO Box 8190, Stockton, Calif 95208, Phone: 209-472-2240; FAX: 209-472-2249

REFERENCES

Abraham GE: Nutritional factors in the etiology of the premenstrual tension syndromes, *J Reproductive Med* 28:446, 1983.

Abrams A: Use of vitamin E for chronic cystic mastitis, *N Eng J Med* 272:1080, 1965.

Albertazzi P et al: The effect of dietary soy supplementation on serum lipoproteins, blood pressure and menopausal symptoms in perimenopausal women, *Menopause* 6:7, 1999.

Alternative and Complementary Therapies [ACT]: News you can use, *ACT* 7(3):125, 2001.

American Cancer Society [ASC]: Prostate cancer: prevention and risk factors, *Cancer Resource Center–Main*, 2001. URL: www3.cancer.org. Accessed 4/17/01.

American Massage Therapy Association [AMTA]: About massage therapy, 2003. URL: www.amtama.org. Accessed 1/22/03.

Associated Bodywork and Massage Professionals [ABMP]: ABMP massage finder, 2000, URL: www.abmp.com. Accessed 1/22/03.

Baber RJ et al: Randomized placebo-controlled trial of an isoflavone supplement and menopausal symptoms in women, *Climacteric* 2:85, 1999.

Bates P: Sharing the secret: talking about urinary incontinence: a guide to women's health: supplement to nursing 2000, *Nurs Manag, Nurs Pract*, October 8, 2000.

Beduschi R, Beduschi M, Oesterling J: Benign prostatic hyperplasia: use of drug therapy in primary care, *Geriatr* 53:24, 1998.

Ben-Menachem M: Treatment of dysmenorrhea: a relaxation therapy program, *Int J Gynaecol Obstet* 17:340, 1980.

Bensky D, Gamble A: *Chinese herbal medicine materia medica*, Seattle, 1986, Eastland Press.

Bernstein AL: Vitamin B6 in clinical neurology, *Ann NY Acad Sci* 585:250, 1990.

Blum J: *Woman heal thyself: an ancient healing system for contemporary women*, Boston, 1995, Charles E. Tuttle.

Blumenthal M, Goldberg A, Brinckmann J: *Herbal medicine: expanded commission E monographs*, Austin, Tex, 2000, Integrative Medicine.

Bolomb LM et al: Primary dysmenorrhea and physical activity, *Med Sci Sports Exerc* 30:906, 1998.

Buckle J: The role of aromatherapy in nursing care. In Colbath J, Prawlucki P, editors: *Nurs Cin North Am* 36(1):57, 2001.

Burgio K et al: Behavioral vs drug treatment for urge urinary incontinence in older women, *JAMA* 280(23):1995, 1998.

Burkhart K: Urinary incontinence in women: assessment and management in the primary care setting, *NP Forum* 11(4):192, 2000.

Butler EB, McKnight E: Vitamin E in the treatment of primary dysmenorrhea, *Lancet* 1:844, 1955.

Byrd R: Positive therapeutic effects of intercessory prayer in a coronary care unit population, *South Med J* 8:826, 1993.

Cameron J: *The artist's way*, New York, 1992, Tarcher Putnam.

Carcia H, Secor RM: Vulvovaginal candidiasis: a current update, *NP Forum* 3(3):135, 1992.

Castleman M: *The healing herbs*, New York, 1991, Bantam Books.

Chikly B: Lymph drainage therapy: an effective complement to breast care, *Massage and Bodywork* 16:32, 2001.

Clark LC et al: Effects of selenium supplementation for cancer prevention in patients with carcinoma of the skin, *JAMA* 276:1957, 1996.

Cleary C, Fox JP: Menopausal symptoms: an osteopathic investigation, *Compl Ther Med* 2:181, 1994.

Cole C, Coleman C: Breast imaging today and tomorrow, *NP Forum* 10(3):129, 1999.

Copeland LJ, editor: *Textbook of gynecology*, Philadelphia, 2000, WB Saunders.

Curties D: Breast wellness: massage deserves attention, *Massage and Bodywork* 16:18, 2001.

Dalton K: *Once a month*, ed 6, Alameda, Calif, 1999, Hunter House.

Day A: The journal as a guide for the healing journey. In Colbath J, Prawlucki P, editors: *Nurs Clin North Am* 36(1):131, 2001.

Dell D, Stewart D: Menopause and mood, *PGM* 108(3):34, 2000.

DerMarderosian A: *The review of natural products*, St Louis, 2001, Facts and Comparisons.

Dirke K et al: The influence of dieting on the menstrual cycle of healthy young women, *J Clin Endocrinol Metab* 60:1174, 1985.

Dreher H: *The immune power personality*, New York, 1995, Dutton Penguin.

Edwards B: *Drawing on the right side of your brain*, New York, 1979, Tarcher.

Ernst E: *The desktop guide to complementary and alternative medicine*, St Louis, 2001, Mosby.

Eskin BA et al: Mammary gland dysplasia in iodine deficiency, *JAMA* 200:115, 1967.

Facchinetti F et al: Oral magnesium successfully relieves premenstrual mood changes, *Obstet Gynecol* 78:177, 1991.

Fantl JA et al: *Managing acute and chronic urinary incontinence. Clinical practice guidelines quick reference guide for clinicians*, no 2, AHCPR Publication #96-0686, 1996 (update), Rockville, MD, 1996, Agency for Health Care Policy and Research.

Fetrow C, Avila J: *Complementary and alternative medicines*, Springhouse, Penn, 1999, Springhouse.

Field T: *Touch therapy*, Edinburgh, 2000, Churchill Livingstone.

Foster S: Black cohosh (Cimicifuga racemosa): a literature review, *HerbalGram* 45:35, 1999.

Foster S: *Herbs for your health*, Loveland, Colo, 1996, Interweave Press.

Foster S, Foster JA: *Eastern/central medicinal plants*, Boston, 1990, Houghton Mifflin Co.

Frawley D: *Ayurvedic healing: a comprehensive guide*, ed 2, Twin Lakes, Wisc, 2000, Lotus Press.

Goodale E, Domar A, Benson H: Alleviation of premenstrual syndrome symptoms with the relaxation response, *Obstet Gynecol* 75:649, 1990.

Great Smokies Diagnostic Lab [GSDL]: *Functional assessment resource manual*, Asheville, NC, 1999, GSDL.

Greunwald J et al, editors: *PDR for herbal medicines*, Montvale, NJ, 1998a, Medical Economics.

Greunwald J et al: Standardized black cohosh (Cimicifuga) extract clinical monograph, *Q Rev Nat Med* Summer:117, 1998b.

Groer M, Ohnesorge C: Menstrual-cycle lengthening and reduction in premenstrual distress through guided imagery, *J Holistic Nurs* 11:286, 1993.

Gupta S et al: Prostate cancer prevention by green tea, *Semin Urol Oncol* 17(2):70, 1999.

Harel Z et al: Supplementation with omega-3 fatty acids in the management of dysmenorrhea in adolescents, *Am J Obstet Gynecol* 174:1335, 1996.

Harris JR et al: *Diseases of the breast*, Philadelphia, 2000, Lippincott Williams and Wilkins.

Helms JM: Acupuncture for the management of primary dysmenorrhea, *Obstet Gynecol* 69:1, 1987.

Hendrix S: Urinary incontinence and menopause: an evidence-based treatment approach, *Clin J Women's Health* 1(3):162, 2001.

Hoffman D: *The new holistic herbal*, Rockport, Mass, 1994, Element.

Holister Company: Continence care products: Urinary incontinence, *Hollister Informational Brochure* 2003. URL: www.hollister.com/us/products/continence. Accessed 1/22/03.

Huebscher R: Pet and animal-assisted therapy, *NP Forum* 11(1):1, 2000.

Johnson C: Benign breast disease, *NP Forum* 10(3):137, 1999.

Johnson S: From incontinence to confidence, *Am J Nurs* 100:6, 2000.

Jones TK et al: Profound neonatal congestive heart failure caused by maternal consumption of blue cohosh herbal medication, *J Pediatr* 132:550, 1998.

Kornfield J: *The inner art of meditation* [videotape], Boulder, Colo, 1996, Sounds True.

Landau RS et al: The effect of alpha-tocopherol in premenstrual symptomatology: a double-blind trial, *J Am Coll Nutrit* 2:115, 1983.

Lark S: *The menopause self-help book*, Berkeley, Calif, 1990, Celestial Books.

La Valle J et al: *Natural therapeutics pocket guide*, Hudson, Ohio, 2000, LexiComp.

Lieberman S: Natural supports for healthy menopause, *Alt Complem Ther* 7(2):96, 2001.

Linville P: Self-complexity and affective extremity: don't put all your eggs in one cognitive basket, *Soc Cognit* 3(1):94, 1985.

London RS et al: The role of vitamin E in fibrocystic breast disease, *Obstet Gynecol* 65:104, 1982.

London RS et al: The effect of alpha-tocopherol on premenstrual symptomology: a double-blind study, *J Am Coll Nutr* 2:115, 1983.

London RS et al: Efficacy of alpha-tocopherol in the treatment of the premenstrual syndrome, *J Reprod Med* 32:400, 1987.

Lonsdorf N, Butler V, Brown M: *A woman's best medicine: health happiness and long life through Maharishi Ayur-Veda*, New York, 1995, Penguin Putnam, Inc.

Love SM: *Dr. Susan Love's breast book*, Cambridge, Mass, 2000, Perseus Publishing.

Low Dog T, Riley D, Carter T: An integrative approach to menopause, *Alt Ther Health Med* 7(4):45, 2001.

Luks A: *The healing power of doing good*, New York, 1992, Fawcett.

Lyttleton J: Topics in gynecology—part one: menopause, *J Chin Med* 33:5, 1990.

Maciocia G: *Obstetrics and gynecology in Chinese medicine*, New York, 1998, Churchill Livingstone.

Maloney C: Noninvasive Evaluation and Treatment of Urinary Incontinence in the Primary Care Setting. Presented at the 2001 Nurse Practitioner Symposium, Keystone, Colo, July 13, 2001.

Martucci CL: The menopause: measures of hygiene and treatment according to Chinese medicine, *J Chinese Med* 30:14, 1989.

McCaleb RS, Leigh E, Morien K: *The encyclopedia of popular herbs*, Roseville, Calif, 2000, Prima Health.

McIntyre A: *The complete woman's herbal*, New York, 1994, Henry Holt.

Milex Products: *Frequently asked questions, Pessaries*, 2003. URL: www.milexproducts. com/products/pessaries. Accessed 3/27/03.

Miller E: Healing from Within [audiotape], Stanford, Calif, 1980, Source Tapes, 1-800-52-TAPES. (Numerous other tapes are available.)

Mills SY: *Out of the earth: the essential book of herbal medicine*, Middlesex, UK, 1991, Viking Arkana.

Mowen K: Breast massage: on the brink of understanding? *Massage and Bodywork* 16:14, 2001.

Murray M: Benign prostatic hyperplasia. In Pizzorno J, Murray M, editors: *Textbook of natural medicine*, Edinburgh, 1999, Churchill Livingstone.

NAP: fruits and vegetables yield less Vitamin A than previously thought; upper limit set for daily intake of Vitamin A and nine other nutrients, 2001. URL: www.nationalacademies.org/news. Accessed 7/28/01.

NAP: *Nutrient information*, 2003. URL: www.nap.edu. Accessed 1/23/2003.

Naparstek B: *A meditation to help you stop smoking* (audiotape), Akron, Ohio, 1997, Image Paths. URL: www.healthjourneys.com.

Naparstek B: *Staying well with guided imagery*, Akron, Ohio, 1994, Image Paths.

Naparstek B: *Stress I and Stress II* (audiotape), Akron, Ohio, 1995, Image Paths. URL: www.healthjourneys.com. (Numerous other tapes and CDs are available: 1-800-800-8661.)

NIH: *Facts about dietary supplements: vitamin E*, 2001. URL: www.nih.gov/ccc/supplements/vite.html. Accessed 8/10/2001.

Northrup C: *The wisdom of menopause*, New York, 2001, Bantam.

Northrup C: *Women's bodies, women's wisdom*, New York, 1998, Bantam Books.

Oleson T, Flocco W: Randomized controlled study of premenstrual symptoms treated with ear, hand and foot reflexology, *Obstet Gynecol* 82:906, 1993.

Padden D: Mastalgia: evaluation and management, *NP Forum* 11(4):213, 2000.

Parry BL et al: Morning vs. evening bright light treatment of late luteal phase dysphoric disorder, *Am J Psychiatr* 146:9, 1991.

Petit JL: Alternative medicine: vitamin E, *Clin Rev* 11:31, 2001.

Pettinati P: Meditation, yoga, and guided imagery. In Colbath J, Prawlucki P, editors: *Nurs Clin North Am: Holistic Nurs Care* 36(1);47, 2001.

Pharmacist's Letter/Prescriber's Letter [PL/PL]: Menopausal symptoms, *Natural Med Clin Manag* 99(4):34, 1999.

PL/PL: Insomnia, *Natural Med Clin Manag* 2000(4):13, 2000a.

PL/PL: Men's health, *Natural Med Clin Manag* 2000(2):38, 2000b.

PL/PL: Premenstrual syndrome, *Natural Med Clin Manag* 2001(2):13, 2001.

PL/PL: *Natural medicines comprehensive database*, ed 3, Stockton, Calif, 2002, Natural Medicines Comprehensive Database.

Prior J et al: Conditioning exercise decreases premenstrual symptoms: a prospective controlled six-month trial, *Fertil Steril* 47:402, 1987.

Pye JK et al: Clinical experience of drug treatments for mastalgia, *Lancet* 2:373, 1985.

Radler M: Dysmenorrhea: chiropractic application, *Am Chiropract* March/April:29, 1984.

Rees MC et al: Prostaglandins in menstrual fluid in menorrhagia and dysmenorrhea, *Br J Obstet Gynecol* 91:673, 1984.

Roberts R: Current management strategies for overactive bladder, *Supplem Patient Care Nurs Pract* Spring, 2001:22, 2001.

Rossignol AM: Caffeine-containing beverages and premenstrual syndrome in young women, *Ame J Publ Health* 75:11, 1985.

Rousseau M: Women's midlife health: reframing menopause, *J Nurs-Midwif* 43(3):208, 1998.

Schellenberg R: Treatment of the premenstrual syndrome with agnus castus fruit extract: prospective, randomized, placebo-controlled study, *BMJ* 322:134, 2001.

Scott JR et al, editors: *Danforth's obstetrics and gynecology*, Philadelphia, 1999, Lippincott Williams and Wilkins.

Seidl M, Stewart D: Alternative treatments for menopausal symptoms: qualitative study of women's experiences, *Can Fam Physician* 44:1271, 1998a.

Seidl M, Stewart D: Alternative treatments for menopausal symptoms: systematic review of scientific and lay literature, *Can Fam Physician* 44:1299, 1998b.

Shames R, Shames K: *Thyroid power*, New York, 2001, Harper Resource.

Sharon F: Natural treatment of menopause using herbs, *Alt Complem Ther* 1(3):147, 1995.

Sharon F: *Creative menopause*, Boulder, Colo, 1994, Wisdom Press.

Shuler P: *Breast disease in women and men: a clinician's handbook*, Durant, Okla, 1993, Essential Medical Information Systems.

Singer E: Seasonal affective disorder, *Clin Rev* 11(11):49, 2001.

Skinner S: *An introduction to homeopathic medicine in primary care*, Gaithersburg, MD, 2001, Aspen.

Snyder M: Journaling. In Snyder M, Lindquist R, editors: *Complementary/alternative therapies in nursing*, New York, 2002, Springer.

Stewart JW et al: Low B6 levels in depressed outpatients, *Biol Psychiatr* 19:613, 1984.

Stoller M, Presti J, Carroll P: Urology. In Tierney L, McPhee S, Papakakis M, editors: *Current medical diagnosis and treatment*, New York, 2001, McGraw-Hill.

Temes R: *Medical hypnosis*, Philadelphia, 1999, Churchill Livingstone.

Tesch B: Herbs commonly used by women: an evidence-based review, *Clin J Women's Health* 1(2):89, 2001.

Thys-Jacobs S et al: Calcium carbonate and the premenstrual syndrome: effects on premenstrual and menstrual symptoms (premenstrual study group), *Am J Obstet Gynecol* 179:444, 1998.

Varney H: *Varney's midwifery*, ed 3, Sudbury, Mass, 1997, Jones and Bartlett Publishers.

Walker AF et al: Magnesium supplementation alleviates premenstrual symptoms of fluid retention, *J Women's Health* 7:1157, 1998.

Weed S: *Breast cancer? Breast health! The wise woman way*, Woodstock, New York, 1996, Ash Tree Publishing.

Weil V, Cirigliano M, Battistini M: Herbal treatments for symptoms of menopause, *Hosp Physician* November:35, 2000.

Wein A, Rovner ES: The overactive bladder: An overview for primary care health providers, *Internat J Fertil Women* 44(2):56, 1999.

Wepfer S: The science behind bioidentical hormone replacement therapy, *Int J Pharmaceutic Compounding* 5(6):10, 2001.

White J: Music as intervention. In Colbath J, Prawlucki P, editors: *Nurs Clin North Am: Holistic Nurs Care* 36(1):83, 2001.

Willeford L: Menopause naturally, *New Age J* Sept/Oct:8, 150, 1995.

Williams P: Nonscientifically validated herbal treatments for vaginitis, *NP Forum* 24(8):101, 1999.

Wolfe H: *Second spring: a guide to healthy menopause through traditional Chinese medicine*, Boulder, Colo, 1990, Blue Poppy Press.

Wu Lianzhong et al: 300 cases of menopausal syndrome treated by acupuncture, *J Trad Chinese Med* 18(4):259, 1998.

Wyon Y et al: Acupuncture against climacteric disorders? Lower number of symptoms after menopause, *Lakartidningen* 91(23):2318, 1994.

CHAPTER 10

ENDOCRINE CONCERNS

Diana Guthrie ▪ Roxana Huebscher ▪ Pamela Shuler ▪ Louise Rauckhorst ▪ Helen Miller

NAC THERAPIES FOR DIABETES MELLITUS TYPE 1 AND TYPE 2

The American Diabetes Association (ADA) defines diabetes as "a group of metabolic diseases characterized by hyperglycemia resulting from defects in insulin secretion, insulin action, or both (ADA, 2003a, p. S5). The criteria for diagnosis are a fasting blood sugar equal to or greater than 126 mg/dl or a random or 2-hour postprandial blood sugar equal to or greater than 200 mg/dl. The criteria for gestational diabetes diagnosis is:

> blood glucose levels equal to or greater than 95 mg/dl fasting or greater than 140 mg/dl one hour after a 50 g glucose load. (ADA, 2003b, p. 103)

Guidelines for diabetes management include a glycosylated hemoglobin less than 7% (indicative of average blood glucose levels less than 150 mg/dl or preferably less than 135 mg/dl); blood pressure less than 130/80 mm Hg; low-density lipoprotein (LDL) level less than 100 mg; and high-density lipoproteins (HDL) more than 45 mg, without the presence of significant low blood sugar occurrences (ADA, 2003c).

Individuals with type 1 diabetes are treated with insulin. Individuals who have type 2 diabetes are treated with diet and exercise; diet, exercise, and one or more oral agents; or diet, exercise, oral agents, insulin, or any combination. People with gestational diabetes are treated with insulin if diet alone is not sufficient (ADA, 2003b). Tightly controlled blood glucose levels result in less complications (DCCT, 1993, 1996) but also a greater chance of becoming hypoglycemic. Therefore frequent monitoring of blood glucose levels is imperative, especially when the patient uses oral hypoglycemic agents, insulin, or a continuous insulin infusion pump. In addition, numerous medications and herbs have the potential to raise and lower blood glucose levels (Guthrie, Guthrie, 2002). (See biologic-based therapies.)

The ADA has concern about natural-alternative-complementary (NAC) therapy use, especially for people with diabetes who are not monitored for side effects related to individual responses. "Natural" does not necessarily mean safe; NAC treatments might interact with conventional medications and affect blood glucose levels. In addition, people who have concomitant complications from diabetes are at extra risk. Therefore special care must be taken to maintain blood glucose levels within normal limits (Boullata, Nace, 2000; Gill et al, 1999; Sabo et al, 1999; Ziegler et al, 1994).

The ADA classifies therapies as: "clearly effective; somewhat/sometimes effective or effective for certain categories of patients; unknown/unproven but possibly promising; or clearly ineffective." Categorization is based on the "effectiveness of the modalities including the number and quality of studies performed, the degree to which independent validation has been accomplished, and the potential risk of harm to patients associated with the modalities." If a therapeutic modality is considered safe and effective, it is or has been approved for use by the U.S. Food and Drug Administration (FDA) or is supported by "data obtained in at least two independent well-controlled studies that have been published in peer-reviewed scientific publications, or endorsed or recommended by the ADA professional practice committee, or endorsed by a relevant or appropriate medical specialty organization" (ADA, 2003d, S142). If the modality fits these criteria, it can still cause harm if used improperly. Not all the modalities in this chapter have been reviewed by the ADA.

ALTERNATIVE HEALTH CARE SYSTEMS FOR DIABETES

Ayurveda for Diabetes

Approximately 4000 years ago, a great Ayurvedic sage named Sushruta described type 1 diabetes as: "Drinking, but always thirsty, eating, but always hungry, the poor patient watches his flesh melt away in a stream of sugary urine." This is an amazingly accurate and vivid description of the triad of symptoms (polyuria, polydipsia, and polyphasia) that modern biomedically trained clinicians have learned are the main symptoms associated with uncontrolled hyperglycemia. The insulin deficiency that is the hallmark of type 1 diabetes is considered to be the result of a long-standing vata disorder. Ayurvedic texts describe patients with this disease, which has its onset more frequently in childhood and adolescence, as being weak and emaciated resulting from tissue depletion. Although the kapha form of diabetes mellitus (type 2) is considered as a disease that is usually able to be healed, Ayurveda recognizes the vata form (type 1) as a condition that cannot be healed but only ameliorated by natural remedies (Tirtha, 1998).

Ayurvedic texts include the clinical syndromes that Western clinicians call type 1 and type 2 diabetes within the category of "obstinate urinary diseases," all of which are related to imbalances in one or other of the three biologic energies (doshas) that comprise each person's individual makeup or constitution. Ten types of adult-onset diabetes have been identified in which the kapha dosha is aggravated or increased, (characterized by obesity and excess consumption of sweet, kaphagenic foods), six forms that represent an imbalance of pitta dosha, including juvenile-onset diabetes (characterized by fever, acidity, ulcerations, irritability, and hypertension), and four that are caused by vata dosha imbalance (characterized by emaciation, dehydration, thirst, extreme hunger, low energy, and insomnia). All forms of diabetes, from the Ayurvedic perspective, have in common an increased quantity and turbidity of urine. *Mahdu* (or "honeylike" because of the sweet and astringent urine) diabetes is equivalent to type 1 diabetes and is considered to be the result of excessive vata depleting the tissues. The *Ikshumeha* and *Sikata* forms of diabetes, also characterized by sweet urination, are equivalent to type 2 diabetes and are considered to be the result of excessive kapha dosha. The *Udaka* form of diabetes, which is similar in description to diabetes insipidus and is characterized by the excretion of large quantities of pale, clear urine, is also a kapha disorder (Tirtha, 1998; Frawley, 2000).

General treatment of all types of diabetes The main goals of therapy are to improve glucose metabolism, provide nourishment, and to pacify or reduce the dosha that is out of balance. In early stages, turmeric powder (1 to 3 grams) is mixed with aloe juice and taken two to three times a day, before meals, to regulate pancreatic and liver function (Frawley, 2000).

Chopra (1999) recommends a diet that includes high fiber with the use of complex carbohydrates, varied fruit intake, and a vegetarian or low-protein dietary modification. Long-term herbal therapy includes shilajit compound with gurmar (Gymnema sylvestre) to improve glucose metabolism and counter sugar cravings. Most bitter herbs and spices such as ginger and cardamom can help with glucose metabolism (Frawley, 2000).

Yoga postures include the Sun Salutation, Peacock, Locust, Leg Lift, and Chest-Knee poses, as well as alternate nostril breathing (Lad, 1998). Shirodhara treatments (an Ayurvedic application of continuous drops of warm sesame oil to the forehead) two nights per week also are part of therapy (Frawley, 2000).

Specific treatment for dosha-type diabetes For vata-type diabetes, a vata-pacifying diet with complex carbohydrates, in place of sugar and sweet foods, is taken as well as calamus or ashwagandha ghee (1 to 2 teaspoons two to three times a day). In addition, tonifying herbs such as shilajit, ashwagandha, shatavari, and chyavan prash are used.

For pitta-type diabetes, bitter herbs, and cooling, demulcent tonics such as shatavari with aloe gel are used as well as Brahmi (gotu kola) ghee, and a liver tonic formula. Other treatments include purgation.

For kapha-type diabetes, patients are on a long-term anti-kapha diet and bitter herbs such as aloe, turmeric and myrrh to control sugar and fat metabolism and liver-pancreas function. Also taken are pungent herbs such as black pepper, cayenne, and ginger to assist weight reduction. Other treatments include periods of fasting (Frawley, 2000; Tirtha, 1998).

Gymnema sylvestra, an herb used for centuries in India and a member of the milkweed family, has been found to increase the endogenous release of insulin and decrease cravings for sweets, due to its mile emetic effect. This herb has been a useful adjunct to overweight individuals who report having difficulty staying away from sweets (Duke, 2002; Baskaran et al, 1990; Persaud et al, 1999; Pharmacist's Letter/Prescriber's Letter [PL/PL], 2000). Anecdotally, people who are obese and choose to use Gymnema may find that they have a lessened tendency to eat candy, which may help them to lose weight. Two Gymnema studies (Shanmugasundaram et al, 1990; Baskaran et al, 1990), one for type 1 and one for type 2 diabetes, did show decreased hemoglobin (Hgb) A_{1C}s and blood sugars, and a few people in the type 2 group were able to discontinue sulfonylureas. Some design details were not delineated in the studies, however (Kapoor, 1990; Shane-McWhorter, 2001).

Homeopathy

Homeopathy has no definite alternative to insulin. However, other medical problems may respond favorably to some of the therapies for colds or mild health concerns. The key offering of homeopathy is the intensive history taking, education, and guidance in self-care. Few, if any, side effects to the use of a homeopathic remedy are known. In one study, 17% of patients with diabetes used homeopathy as a form of therapy, along with herbal therapy and acupuncture (Leese et al, 1997).

Naturopathy

Naturopathy incorporates homeopathy and many other natural therapies as well, such as nutrition and exercise. Murray and Pizzorno (1999), two naturopaths, recommend the diet high in complex carbohydrates and plant fibers popularized by Anderson (1988). The diet is high in cereal grains, legumes, and root vegetables, and it restricts simple sugars and fats. The intake is approximately 70% to 75% complex carbohydrate, 15% to 20% protein, and 10% to 25% fat. Murray and Pizzorno (1999) also recommend at least 200 micrograms a day of chromium; vitamin C–rich foods and supplementation; and other nutrients such as biotin, flavonoids, carnitine, inositol, B vitamins, vitamin E, magnesium, potassium, manganese, zinc, and essential fatty acids.

Traditional Chinese Medicine

Diabetes in Traditional Chinese Medicine (TCM) is described as "thirsting and wasting" disease. The main symptoms are insatiable thirst, loss of weight, and excessive urination. The main organs involved in pathology are the Lungs, Spleen, and Kidney. Often one of these organs will predominate as the prime root of illness. The primary diagnosis is Yin deficiency, which creates thirst. The heat generated in the digestive system creates hunger and loss of weight, as well as thirst. The Kidneys are eventually injured to the extent that urine flows through indiscriminately as the patient drinks more fluids to assuage thirst (Mao-liang, 1984, Haines, 1993).

Acupuncture treatment is directed toward regulating the Lung, Spleen, and Kidney energies to restore proper functioning. An area along the spine at T8 (the 8th thoracic vertebrae on the Bladder channel) is related to the pancreas that may be useful in treatment (Mao-liang, 1984; Haines, 1993). Any other symptoms the patient is experiencing such as pain will also be addressed by the TCM practitioner as part of a holistic approach (Griffith, 1999; Haines, 1993). Pain and accompanying anxiety will influence blood sugar levels.

As a rule, if a patient receiving acupuncture is already insulin-dependant, he or she will continue to require insulin, though the dose may need adjustment. A patient on oral medication may require a lower dose and may possibly discontinue medication with acupuncture treatment, with the cooperation and approval of their health care provider (Haines, 1993).

A study using electroacupuncture on rodents appeared to have a hypoglycemic effect in type 2 but not type 1–induced diabetic animals. Electroacupuncture did not appear to affect insulin resistance in type 2 animals, but electroacupuncture reduced plasma glucose concentration as might occur in the use of biologically administered insulin. Such studies are yet to be done in humans (Chang et al, 1999).

Acupuncture has been used for many types of pain (Sims, 1997). Acupuncture may also be indicated for the diabetic patient with neuropathy (McGrady, Horner, 1999). Abuaisha, Constanzi, & Boulton (1998) studied 44 diabetic patients with chronic painful peripheral neuropathy, including 29 who were on standard medical treatment. Subjects received up to six courses of classical acupuncture over a period of 10 weeks. Thirty four (77%) showed significant improvement. The subjects then were followed for 18-52 weeks, eight (24%) required further acupuncture treatment. Seven (21%) noted that their symptoms cleared completely. (Huebscher, 2000, p. 76)

Xuan seng and di huang are two Chinese herbs used to treat diabetes. No particular side effects are noted for di huang, but bradycardia has been noted with the use of xuan seng (O'Connell, 1999).

Qi gong and Tai chi have long been used in China and other Asian countries. These types of movements relate to focus, flexibility, activity, and exercise, and may help delay the onset of type 2 diabetes or the need for treatment. In one study, Qi gong was found useful in type 2 diabetes (Zhizhou et al, 1987). Table 10-1 lists alternative health care systems for diabetes.

MIND-BODY-SPIRIT INTERVENTIONS FOR DIABETES

Art, music, and dance allow participants to express themselves, allowing for individual emotional responses and assisting in relieving stress; when the body is calm, glucose levels may remain low. A recent study with patients who have type 2 diabetes showed a 0.5% reduction in Hgb A_{1C} with a 30-minute educational sessions plus stress-management training. By the end of 1 year, 32% of the treatment group had dropped more than 1% with their Hgb A_{1C}, although only 12% of the control group (education only) dropped more than 1% (Surwit et al, 2002). The stress management consisted of progressive muscle relaxation (PMR), education on the health consequences of stress, and instruction on cognitive and behavioral skills (recognition of major stressors, guided imagery, thought-stopping, and deep breathing) (Surwit et al, 2002). See Chapters 2 and 11 for information on these techniques.

With the use of relaxation (Monahan et al, 1992), deep breathing, fasting (Suzuki et al, 1976), meditation (Maras et al, 1984), or prayer (Hunt et al, 2000), the body may be able to relax in a way that allows healthier functioning. Monahan and colleagues (1992) had 33 adolescents with type 1 diabetes participate in and listen to a recorded muscle relaxation program 12 times over a 4-week period. The adolescents' anxiety and fructosamine levels showed a significant decrease. Suzuki and colleagues (1976), in a classic paper, focused on individuals who had mild type 2 diabetes and obesity. The subjects used a program that incorporated fasting. Maras and colleagues (1984) mention the effect of meditation on individuals' type 2 diabetes. Meditation also has an effect on people with type 1 diabetes (Hunt et al, 2000). Naparstek (1991, 1995) developed imagery recordings to lower stress levels. Meditation and prayer have resulted in lower blood pressure, lower pulse rate, and the more efficient use of oxygen (Benson, Stuart, 1992). In a recent study at Duke University, patients with type 2 diabetes who took part in five stress management–training sessions lowered their Hgb A_{1C} by an average of 0.5% (ADA, 2002). Mind-body-spirit modalities may thus be useful for the person with diabetes.

Biofeedback increases the temperature of the hands and feet and thus increases circulation. Rice and Shindler (1992) studied thermal biofeedback in 40 patients with diabetes showing an increase in lower extremity temperature. In addition, Good (1998) reports on biofeedback studies (McGrady, Bailey, Good, 1992; Surwit, Feinglos, 1983):

> biofeedback-assisted relaxation has been useful in reducing blood glucose in both insulin-dependent and non-insulin dependent diabetes

Table 10-1 Alternative Health Care Systems for Diabetes

Intervention	Management	Treatment Regimen	Cautions, Precautions, Interactions	References
Ayurveda	For vata-type diabetes	Vata-pacifying diet with complex carbohydrates in place of sugar and sweet foods. Calamus or ashwagandha ghee (1-2 tsp bid-tid); tonifying herbs such as shilajit, ashwagandha, shatavari, and chyavan prash	An herbal prescribing source should be consulted before using Ayurvedic herbs Monitor glucose levels	Frawley, 2000; Tirtha, 1998
	For pitta-type diabetes	Bitter herbs, cooling, demulcent tonics such as shatavari with aloe gel; brahmi (gotu kola) ghee, and a liver tonic formula; other treatments include purgation		Frawley, 2000; Tirtha, 1998
	For kapha-type diabetes	Long-term anti-kapha diet; bitter herbs such as		Frawley, 2000; Tirtha, 1998

Naturopathy	Uses as diabetes regimen	Diet high in complex carbohydrates and plant fiber (high in cereal grains, legumes, root vegetables); approximately 70%-75% complex carbohydrate, 15%-20% protein, and 10%-25% fat; at least 200 µg/day chromium; vitamin C-rich foods and supplementation; and other nutrients such as biotin, flavonoids, carnitine, inositol, B	Simple sugars and fats should be restricted	Murray, Pizzorno, 1999; Anderson, 1988

aloe, turmeric, and myrrh to control sugar and fat metabolism and liver and pancreas function; pungent herbs such as black pepper, cayenne and ginger to assist weight reduction; other treatments include periods of fasting

Continued

Table 10-1	Alternative Health Care Systems for Diabetes—cont'd			
Intervention	**Management**	**Treatment Regimen**	**Cautions, Precautions, Interactions**	**References**
Naturopathy, cont'd		vitamins, vitamin E, magnesium, potassium, manganese, zinc, and essential fatty acids.		
Traditional Chinese Medicine	For diabetes	Chinese herbs Xuan seng and Di huang	Herbal prescribing source should be consulted; SE: Xuan seng, bradycardia	O'Connell, 1999
	For diabetes and peripheral neuropathy	Acupuncture Thoracic vertebrae and along Bladder meridian is one point. See Appendix B.		Abuaisha et al, 1998
	For focus and flexibility, balance	Qi gong and Tai chi	Has had positive effect in a type 2 diabetes study	Zhizhou et al, 1987

bid, Twice daily; SE, side effects; tid, three times daily.

mellitus" and "reduced average blood glucose, glycosylated hemoglobin and fasting values." (Good, 1998, p. 82)

Three studies (Guthrie, 1983; Guthrie et al, 1990, 1995) demonstrated improved peripheral temperature with short-term concentrated
biofeedback. The studies were done on hospitalized patients who had
diabetes and on children who showed improved glycemic indices
when parents were taught relaxation techniques. In addition, lowered
anxiety occurred when biofeedback-enhanced relaxation techniques
was given to parents who were primary care givers for chronically ill
children (Hernandez, Kolb, 1998). Anecdotally, children and adults
with type 1 or type 2 diabetes have had lowered blood glucose levels
when taught biofeedback-assisted relaxation techniques.

Hypnosis is also a modality to consider. Hypnosis has been used
for weight loss, smoking cessation, and for general well being, all of
which are useful for people with diabetes. Hypnotic-type trance is
probably involved in many types of activities, especially those requiring a deep level of concentration. Self-hypnosis training and techniques may help patients through stressful times, as well as help
relieve physical discomfort such as peripheral neuropathy.

BIOLOGIC-BASED THERAPIES FOR DIABETES

Boxes 10-1 and 10-2 list herbs, substances, and medications that
affect blood glucose.

Nutrition

Maintaining glycemic control is the best practice for reducing the risk
of diabetic complications (Diabetes Control and Complications Trial
[DCCT] Research Group, 1993, 1996). Nutritious food and healthy
lifestyle habits, such as regular exercise and no smoking, are always recommended. Dietary options or alternatives for glycemic control have
included Pritikin (*The Diet Advisor,* 2000), Ornish (*The Diet Advisor,*
2000), the Mediterranean diet (Jossa, 1996), macrobiotic diet (Kushi,
1979), vegetarian diets (Snowdon, Phillips, 1985), and the Zone diet
(*The Diet Advisor,* 2000). A variety of other diets have some effect on
blood glucose levels, because of either the fiber content or the protein
content or the total caloric intake and type of carbohydrate intake.

The Pritikin diet, largely vegetarian and high in complex carbohydrates and fiber, contains less than 10% fat. People with type 2
diabetes who followed a Pritikin diet showed significant improvements in blood glucose levels and decreases in required hypoglycemic medication. Patients with newly diagnosed diabetes were
the best responders. These people were able to decrease or eliminate
the need for oral agents. For individuals requiring insulin, results
were less striking. Nonetheless, decreased glucose levels were achieved
in more than one third of these patients (McGrady, Horner, 1999).

Box 10-1

Herbs and Substances with Potential to Decrease or Increase Effect of Medications

Herbs and Substances with Potential Hyperglycemic Effect	Herbs and Substances with Potential Hypoglycemic Effect	
Bee pollen	Ackee	Ginseng, Eleutherococcus
Elecampane	Alfalfa	Ginseng, Panax
Ephedra	Aloe vera	Guar gum
Figwort	Basil	Gymnema
Gotu kola	Bilberry leaf	Horehound
Hydrocotyle	Bitter melon	Horse chestnut seed
Licorice	Burdock	Juniper
St. John's wort	Celandine	Marshmallow
	Celery	Melatonin
	Coriander	Myrrh
	Cornsilk	Myrtle
	Damiana	Nettle
	Dandelion	Night-blooming cereus
	Devil's claw	Onion
	Eucalyptus	Psyllium
	Fenugreek	Sage
	Garcinia	Stinging nettle
	Garlic	Tansy
	Ginger	

Sources: Blumenthal M et al: Herbal medicine: expanded commission E monographs, *Newton, Mass, 2000, Integrative Medicine; Ernst E:* The desktop guide to complementary & alternative medicine: an evidence-based approach, *St Louis, 2001, Mosby; Fetrow C, Avila J:* Complementary & alternative medicine, *Springhouse, Pa, 1999, Springhouse; La Valle et al:* Natural therapeutics pocket guide, *Hudson, Ohio, 2000, LexiComp; PL/PL:* Natural medicine's comprehensive database, *Stockton, Calif, 2002, Therapeutic Research.*

Low-calorie diets and behavior modification also have been shown to lower blood sugar. The recommendation is that total caloric daily intake not be lower than 1000 calories and preferably not less than 1200 calories because a person is unable to obtain recommended nutrients with a daily intake of less than 1200 calories. With low-calorie diets, metabolic conservation may occur. When people have caloric intakes of less than 1000 calories, they have a tendency to metabolize the food as would a person who is starving. Furthermore, weight gain then becomes easier if the person eats just slightly more without adequate activity to balance the food intake.

Box 10-2

Medications that Raise and Lower Blood Sugar

Raise Blood Sugar
Thiazide diuretics and other diuretics
Beta-adrenergic receptor agonists
Calcium channel blockers
Central alpha-agonists
Diazoxide
Glucocorticoids
Oral contraceptives
Phenytoin
Sympathomimetics
Other agents that raise blood glucose levels: 1-asparaginase, nicotinic acid, pentamidine, amiodarone, salmon calcitonin, cimetidine, colchicines, levodopa, lithium, morphine, neuroleptic agents.

Lower Blood Sugar
Ethanol
Salicylates
Beta-blockers
Other agents that lower blood sugar levels: disopyramide, anabolic steroids, clofibrate, monamine oxidase inhibitors, pentamidine, sulfonamide antibiotics, quinine, amphetamine, guanethidine, imipramine, oxytetracycline, penicillamine, pyridoxine.

The Ornish diet (a low-fat, high-fiber diet) was originally designed for people with cardiovascular disease. The Ornish diet is basically a vegetarian diet with 75% of the calories from carbohydrates. Exercise, relaxation, meditation, and social support are part of the regimen. Sixty percent of patients with type 2 diabetes on insulin regimens who adhered to the Ornish plan no longer required insulin (McGrady, Horner, 1999; Ornish, 1990).

The Mediterranean diet has been found useful in people with cardiovascular disease (Giugliano, 2001). The basics of this diet include whole foods, pastas, olive oil, chicken, and fish. Some of the antioxidants in the diet include wine, grapes, and artichokes. This type of eating, especially with olive oil, helps lower LDL levels.

The macrobiotic diet is based on balancing of yin and yang. Diabetes is more often associated with the excessive use of yin foods such as high-fat foods, sweets, and some fruits and nuts (Heidenry,

1991). The diet is 50% to 60% whole-grain cereals, 20% to 30% vegetables, 5% to 10% beans and sea vegetables, and 5% to 10% soups. In addition, occasional fish and seafood, seasonal fruits, nuts and seeds, seasonings, condiments, pickles and garnishes, naturally sweetened snacks and desserts, and natural nonaromatic and nonstimulant beverages are included (Kushi, 1996). The macrobiotic diet is basically vegetarian but does include small amounts of fish and other seafoods. If the seafood is omitted, getting adequate protein might be a problem. Some soups, such as miso, have a high-sodium content and therefore might be a problem if cardiovascular disease is present or other sodium restriction is needed. Such a diet has been found useful for people with cancer (Lerner, 1994). Low vitamin B12, vitamin D, protein, and iron are of concern, but the American version is higher in these nutraceuticals than is the traditional Japanese diet (Kuhn, 1999), and several versions of the diet are available. Kushi (1979) found this diet resulted in lowered blood glucose levels in people who would now be classified as having type 2 diabetes.

Good vegetarian diets need to contain the essential amino acids. With education and careful planning, and, including a variety of foods over the course of a day (corn, beans, nuts, rice, and other grains), many people can follow such a meal plan. Foods appear to absorb rapidly and transverse the colon quickly so blood glucose levels are lower, thus checks for hypoglycemia need to be done. In addition, beans provide zinc, calcium, and iron, as do nuts and seeds. Cereals should be fortified with vitamin B12 (Rosensweig, 1994). In a study that followed 25,000 Seventh-Day Adventists (traditionally vegetarian) for over 20 years, the death rate from diabetes was 45% less than for all Caucasian Americans, and the rate of diabetes development was less (Snowdon, Phillips, 1985). In this study, vegetarian was defined as eating meat less than one time per week. Vegetarians define themselves in many ways, including lacto-ovo, who do not eat meat of any kind but do consume milk and egg products, and vegan vegetarians, who eat no animal products at all.

The Zone diet has been used by diabetics but is not specifically designed for diabetes (Sears, 1995, 2000). The diet is referred to as the 40-30-30 program (www.zonediet.com, accessed June 15, 2002). The protein (30%) is higher than that recommended by nutritionists at this particular time, and this may be a concern if the patient has compromised kidneys. With its 40% carbohydrate content, the Zone diet is less challenging to the insulin secretion of the beta cells (so people stay in "the zone"), and less insulin secretion often means easier weight loss. The Zone diet focuses on a basic set of "rules" to reach the specific percentage of carbohydrate, protein, and fat intake. The rules are:

Always eat a Zone meal within 1 hour after waking.

Try to eat five times per day: three Zone meals and two Zone snacks.

Never let more than 5 hours go by without eating a Zone meal or
  snack—regardless of whether you are hungry or not. In fact, the
  best time to eat is when you aren't hungry because that means
  you have stabilized your insulin levels. Afternoon and late
  evening snacks (which are really mini-Zone meals) are important to keep you in the Zone throughout the day.
Eat more fruits and vegetables (yes, these are carbohydrates) and
  ease off the bread, pasta, grains, and other starches. Treat breads,
  pasta, grains, and other starches like condiments.
Drink at least eight 8-ounce glasses of water every day. That's about
  a [half gallon] of water.
If you make a mistake at a meal, don't worry about it. There's no
  guilt in the Zone. Just make your next meal a Zone meal to get
  you back where you (and your hormones) belong. (Sears, 2000,
  pp. 5-6)

Some diets have been reported useful for normalizing blood glucose levels, and also for weight control. Inadequate education and
support in using such approaches has resulted in some cases of hypoglycemia, especially when the diabetes medication was not lowered
when the body weight decreased, thus careful monitoring is needed.

Vitamins and Minerals

The most recent update of the dietary reference intakes (Trumbo
et al, 2001) for the general population has increased intake and
changes of several nutrients. However, these recommendations are
based on research completed on subjects who are free from chronic
illnesses; people with diabetes or other chronic conditions may have
different needs. Thus determining appropriate vitamin and mineral
levels is difficult. An example of this concept is vitamin C. The level
beyond which the healthy person gets little benefit is estimated to be
200 to 250 mg per day. For the polyuric patient, more vitamin C than
normal is lost in the urine, and therefore, intake logically should be
higher. Research is necessary to determine the best dose for chronic
conditions. The present guidelines, however, do give the health care
provider and the person with diabetes some idea as to where to start
with daily food and nutrient intake. A person who is polyuric, no
matter the cause, would lose multiple water-soluble vitamins and
minerals and may need replacement therapy. In addition, if a person
has developed nephropathy, elimination of the fat-soluble vitamins
might be impaired. Thus the total assessment of the person with diabetes, related to the nutritional status, must take into account blood
glucose levels, rate and amount of kidney function (creatinine
clearance or serum creatinine and total protein), and interfering
stressors that might affect glucose levels. Other individual physiologic variations and whether nutrient content in specific foods is
appropriate are additional issues. Moreover, cultural traditions,

weight (body mass index), and likes and dislikes influence levels of vitamins and minerals.

B vitamins have been controversial regarding the role they may play in diabetic neuropathy. Because people with diabetes may have polyuria, this water-soluble vitamin may be deficient:

> An abstract from the East African Medical Journal (Abbas, Swai, 1997) reported that the severity of symptomatic peripheral neuropathy in clients with diabetes decreased in 48.9% of 100 patients treated with 25 mg/day of thiamine (vitamin B1) and 50 mg/day of pyridoxine (vitamin B6). This was compared to a decrease of 11.4% in a placebo group of 100 patients, who were given one mg/day of thiamine and one mg/day of pyridoxine. Pain, numbness, parasthesia and impairment of sensation were some of the items graded into none, mild, moderate, or severe. In addition, the mean pre-treatment blood thiamine levels were lower in those with the most severe symptoms. Symptoms may have been from B deficiency itself; however, diabetics may be low in this vitamin and need supplementation. (Huebscher, 2000, p. 75)

The question remains as to whether it was the thiamine, the pyridoxine, or the combination that was most effective.

Vitamin B3 has two forms: niacinamide (or nicotinamide) and niacin (or nicotinic acid). Niacin has a negative effect on glycemic control, and nicotinamide appears to help blood glucose levels and insulin release, especially early in the diagnosis of diabetes (Elliott et al, 1996; Kolb, Volker, 1999; PL/PL, 2000). Studies are also addressing whether nicotinamide may prevent the occurrence of diabetes (PL/PL, 2000).

Vitamin B6 is useful in women who have gestational diabetes, improving glucose tolerance. Vitamin B6 also appears involved in the production of neurotransmitters, the proper secretion of insulin and glucagon, and the metabolism of fat and protein. Poorer control of blood glucose levels, especially in children, is correlated with lower B6 levels (Wilson, David, 1977).

The ability of vitamin B12 to reduce nerve damage caused by diabetes has been countered in a variety of studies. No evidence exists that B12 deficiency (pernicious anemia) is causally associated with diabetes mellitus (Reed, Mooradian, 1990).

Vitamin C research shows reduced glycosylation and lower sorbitol formation (i.e., the polyol pathway) in people with diabetes (Davie et al, 1992). One study suggests that lack of vitamin C in the body may be associated with the development of microangiopathy (Jennings et al, 1987). Higher dietary requirements appear needed for people who have type 2 diabetes because of the higher turnover of ascorbic acid (Som et al, 1981). With vitamin C, evidence exists for decreased duration and severity of symptoms of upper respiratory infections and possibly decreased frequency under certain circumstances, such as stress (Hemila, 1997). Whether vitamin C elevates blood sugar remains controversial.

Vitamin D, usually associated with rickets and osteoporosis, now also appears to be associated with diabetes. Vitamin D is needed for adequate blood levels of insulin and, more recently, has been found to increase insulin secretion for some individuals with type 2 diabetes (Boucher, 1998).

Vitamin E has been shown to improve glucose tolerance in people with type 2 diabetes (Paolisso et al, 1993), and a high dietary intake of vitamin E has been associated with a reduced risk of type 1 diabetes (Knekt et al, 1999). In addition, vitamin E may play a part in improving nerve conduction and in endothelial function in type 1 diabetes (Andrew et al, 2000), as well as increasing retinal blood flow (PL/PL, 2000). In a preliminary study of 21 subjects with diabetic peripheral sensory motor polyneuropathy, people who took vitamin E for 6 months had improvement of nerve conduction when compared with a placebo group (Tutuncu, Bayraktar, Varli, 1998). Additionally, alpha-tocopherol therapy (RRR-AT supplementation of 1200 international units [IU]/day) "decreases markers of thrombosis in diabetic patients and control subjects and could be an adjunctive therapy in the prevention of atherosclerosis" (Devaraj et al, 2002, p. 524). High doses (greater than 2500 IU/day) can interfere with the production of vitamin K–dependent clotting factors (PL/PL, 2000); and because vitamin E is a fat-soluble vitamin, a potential for toxicity exists, thus doses need to be monitored.

The trace element trivalent chromium (Cr^{+3}) is needed for glucose metabolism and appears useful in people who have a deficiency. However, at this time, no accurate biochemical indicator of Cr^{+3} status exists (O'Connell, 2001). Cr^{+3} appears to improve the processing of glucose in people who have glucose intolerance and has been found useful in decreasing insulin resistance in patients with type 2 diabetes (Morris et al, 2000). Cr^{+3} research has shown mixed results ranging from nonsignificance in association with blood sugar improvement to improvements in blood sugar and increasing insulin sensitivity, as well as a decreased need for oral hypoglycemics and improvement in blood sugar control with the use of insulin (Anderson, 1997, 2001; Fox, 1998; O'Connell, 2001; PL/PL, 2000; Ravina et al, 1995; Trow et al, 2000).

Cr^{+3} has drug interactions and numerous adverse effects when too much is ingested. Cr^{+3} is likely safe in amounts of 50 to 200 micrograms per day (PL/PL, 2000), and the adequate intake (AI) is 25 micrograms for women and 35 micrograms for men (O'Connell, 2001). If their blood glucose levels have not improved within a few weeks to a few months, patients probably do not need a supplement.

Magnesium has been found to be lower in people with type 2 diabetes (deValk et al, 1998). Assessment of magnesium status is difficult because less than 0.3% is found in serum. "Serum magnesium is a specific, but not sensitive, indicator of magnesium deficiency; low serum magnesium levels indicate low magnesium stores, but a deficiency must be severe before serum levels decline" (O'Connell, 2001, p. 138). Low serum magnesium has been associated with a number of diabetic-related concerns, including retinopathy, neuropathy, cardiovascular disease, and possibly hypertension. According to an ADA panel, supplementation with magnesium is recommended for people who are at risk for complications or who are documented to have hypomagnesemia (McGrady, Horner, 1999). Because people with diabetes are at risk for numerous complications, testing for deficiencies or advising supplementation in all people with diabetes would perhaps be prudent. Deficiency state may be best diagnosed by administering a test load of magnesium and then measuring the percentage retained versus the amount excreted in the urine. Normal individuals have about 20% retention, but those with deficiency will retain more (Sacher, McPherson, 2000).

Vanadium is a trace element and exists in several forms, with vanadyl sulfate and sodium metavanadate being the common supplement forms. Accurate assays and established recommended daily allowance (RDA) for vanadium do not exist. In animal studies, vanadium has been shown to facilitate glucose uptake and to facilitate glucose, lipid, and amino acid metabolism; it also improved thyroid function and enhanced insulin sensitivity. In large doses, vanadium has a negative effect on bone and teeth development (O'Connell, 2001). In human research, vanadium does appear to improve glucose control in people with type 2 diabetes and possibly type 1 individuals. The usual diet provides approximately 10 to 60 micrograms a day, and more than 100 micrograms per day was thought to be unsafe and is considered as the upper limit of therapeutic treatment (Boden et al, 1996; Cam et al, 2000; O'Connell, 2001). The tolerable upper limit (UL) is set at 1.8 mg/day (*www.nap.edu*). In some cases, patients with diabetes have used very high doses (100mg/day) safely for up to 4 weeks. However, there is concern that prolonged use of high doses might cause serious side effects including kidney damage. Tell patients to avoid exceeding the UL (PL/PL, 2002, p. 1265).

Zinc is essential for the function of numerous enzymes and is involved in insulin metabolism; in addition, zinc has a protective effect against beta-cell destruction and has an effect on immune functioning (Godfrey et al, 2001; Murray, Pizzorno, 1999). Very high or very low concentrations appear to impair insulin secretion (Cunningham et al, 1994; Figlewicz et al, 1980). If high doses are taken, zinc may impair immune functioning, and a balance of copper, iron, and zinc is necessary.

Other Nutrients

Gamma linolenic acid (GLA), an omega-6 essential fatty acid, is known to affect nerve function. The body converts cis-linoleic acid, another omega-6 fatty acid, to GLA. However, in people with diabetes, conversion of linoleic acid to GLA is impaired (Benbow, Cossins, MacFarlane, 1999; Horrobin, 1997). Deficiencies have been associated with diabetic neuropathy. Administration of GLA corrects the impaired nerve function in animal models of diabetes (Cameron, Cotter, 1996). In humans, GLA in the form of evening primrose oil has been found to reduce symptoms and diabetic peripheral nerve damage (Jamal, 1994; Keen et al, 1993; Shane-McWhorter, 2001). Borage oil and black currant are less expensive forms of GLA.

In addition to omega-6 GLA, omega-3 oils have also been used in diabetes and seem to increase insulin sensitivity and improve glucose tolerance (PL/PL, 2000; Sheehan et al, 1997). Omega-3s are found in cold-water fish (salmon, tuna, trout, mackerel, sardines, herring, and anchovy), flaxseed oil, and pecans. This essential oil is often lacking in the American diet. Whether improvement in triglycerides and cholesterol exists in diabetes is not known. In addition, fish oil has a number of side effects, including bad taste, belching, and heartburn.

Alpha lipoic acid (ALA), or thioctic acid, is a vitaminlike substance and a disulfide compound synthesized in the liver (Shane-McWhorter, 2001). ALA research studies support its use in reducing pain in people with neuropathy (Reljanovic et al, 1999; Ziegler et al, 1999). A double-blind, multicenter study of 328 patients with type 2 diabetes and symptomatic peripheral neuropathy showed that ALA, an antioxidant and coenzyme, reduced symptoms of neuropathy, including pain, burning, paresthesia, and numbness (Ziegler, Gries, 1997; Ziegler et al, 1995). The subjects were given 100 mg, 600 mg, 1200 mg of intravenous ALA or placebo daily over a 3-week period. The 600-mg intravenous treatment with ALA was found to be safe and effective in reducing symptoms of diabetic peripheral neuropathy. Researchers also found a significant improvement in two out of the four heart rate variability parameters when giving oral ALA (800 mg/dl for 4 months) to people with diabetes who had cardiac autonomic neuropathy (Ziegler et al, 1997). Ziegler and Gries (1997) also critiqued previous studies of ALA citing research flaws in studies that indicated minimal response with ALA. Anecdotally, even after improved blood glucose levels, individuals have found an additional decrease in neuropathic symptoms with ALA use.

Coenzyme Q10 is a cofactor in many metabolic pathways and acts as a free-radical scavenger and membrane stabilizer. Coenzyme Q10 does not seem to be effective on its own, in either type 1 or type 2 diabetes, but ubiquinol (a form of coenzyme Q10) may potentiate vitamin E's antioxidant effects. In addition, coenzyme Q10 does have a use in maternally inherited diabetes and deafness (MIDD) because it seems to prevent progressive hearing loss and increase insulin secretion (Henricksen et al, 1999; PL/PL, 2000, 2002). Coenzyme Q10 is also used in heart disease.

Herbals

Herbals may help lower blood glucose or provide symptom relief. Only one glucose-lowering herb should be taken at a time to determine effectiveness. In addition, if kidney or liver complications from diabetes already exist, then herbs (and vitamins and minerals) can become toxic at lower doses. When starting on an herb (vitamin or mineral), patients are requested to be aware of any untoward responses in the following few days. The person may then add another, if it is appropriate, and again monitor blood glucose levels and any changes. Patients may ask about taking vitamins, minerals, or herbs, or they may only reveal such intake at assessment after being asked. Education as to safety, dose amount, and frequency of use are then given. Individuals are supported in this manner so that further questions or concerns may be comfortably discussed.

Topical botanical therapy   Other than topicals used to soften, cleanse, or protect the skin, capsaicin is the main topical therapy used in diabetes. Capsaicin is used for arthritis and neuralgias, including postherpetic and diabetic neuropathy. Capsaicin is the main component of the oil from capsicum or cayenne pepper and is a naturally occurring chemical derived from the Solanaceae family (Facts and Comparisons, 2001; Fetrow, Avila, 1999). Capsaicin (0.025%, 0.075%, or 0.25%) lasts approximately 4 to 6 hours and comes in cream, gel, or lotion. Capsaicin is a substance P depleter (pain transmitter substance) and, if used repeatedly (initially four to five times a day, subsequently two to three times a day), can limit pain transmission. However, the patient must be prepared for a 4- to 6-week trial and some initial burning with application (Belgrade, 1999).

Side effects include local burning, stinging, and erythema. These sensations resolve because of desensitization of the skin tissues (Benbow, Cossins, MacFarlane, 1999). Patients must remember to wear gloves with application and to wash their hands immediately after application and to avoid getting the substance into the eyes. Brand names include Capsin, Zostrix, Zostrix HP, Dolorac, No Pain HP, and Capzasin.

Testing a site with a small amount of capsaicin is recommended to determine if an allergic reaction results. Patients should be warned that the burning discomfort experienced in the first week or so is part of the counter-irritant therapy.

Oral herbals   Brinker (1998) lists 72 herbs that lower and nine that raise blood glucose levels. (See Table 10-2 for a list of some of these herbs.) Botanicals (herbs) may have a hypoglycemic effect because they act as bulk laxatives, increase insulin sensitivity, enhance insulin release, or mimic the effects of insulin (PL/PL, 2000; Tyler, 1993). Because of individual needs and type of diabetes, people may respond to herbs quite differently. Following are a few of the herbs that affect diabetes.

Bulk laxatives include psyllium, fenugreek, flaxseed, glucomannan, oat bran, and xanthan gum. Bulk laxatives increase the viscosity of the intestinal contents, slow gastric emptying, and act as a barrier to diffusion. This action appears to slow the absorption of carbohydrates, tending to reduce postprandial blood glucose levels. These herbs might be helpful at mealtimes for individuals who experience elevated postprandial blood sugars. An increased fluid intake must be taken with bulk laxatives; and they are not to be used by people who may choke easily. Additionally, some of these bulk herbs may have other benefits as well (Facts and Comparisons, 2001; PL/PL, 2000). For example, fenugreek's action may be from the high-fiber content or possibly the saponins or alkaloids in the seed. Fenugreek (*Trigonella foenum-graecum*) has been shown to lower both blood glucose levels and cholesterol levels in animal models, and this herb has a long history of use, even though few controlled studies have been conducted (Facts and Comparisons, 2001; Madar et al, 1988; PL/PL, 2000; Shane-McWhorter, 2001; Sharma et al, 1990, 1996).

Bilberry (*Vaccinium myrtillus*) was eaten as a jam by night-flying English pilots during World War II, purportedly to help their vision. Bilberry may improve circulation, decrease retinopathy, and reduce blood sugar. The mechanism of action in diabetes may be related to the high chromium content in the leaves, and the anthocyanoside (bioflavonoid) composition of the fruit may be responsible for its vascular effects. Side effects include gastrointestinal distress, drowsiness, and rash. This herb is probably not for long-term consumption, and human studies are few (Blumenthal et al, 2000; Cignarella et al, 1996; Fetrow, Avila, 1999; Muth et al, 2000; O'Connell, 1999; PL/PL, 2000; Shane-McWhorter, 2001).

Bitter melon (*Momordica charantia*) is a vegetable that has been found to have action similar to that of insulin. The fruit and seeds are thought to exert hypoglycemic effects (Ahmad et al, 1999; PL/PL, 2000; Shane-McWhorter, 2001). Animal studies found an effect on both normal and diabetic rat models, with a difference noted in the response to fruit pulp, the seeds, and the whole plant, with fruit pulp being most effective (Ali et al, 1993). Lack of standardization and purity are a problem with this product (Shane-McWhorter, 2001)

Ginseng is used to enhance physical and psychomotor performance and cognitive function, as well as being an immunomodulator.

Ginseng comes in numerous varieties. Commonly used varieties include Asian or Korean ginseng *(Panex ginseng)* and American ginseng *(Panax quiniquefolium L.)*. There is also "Siberian" ginseng *(Eleutherococcus senticosus)* that is eleuthero root and not a Panax. Eleuthera and Panax are in the same family *(Araliaceae)* however, and Eleutherococcus or Siberian ginseng is used for some of the same indications as are the Panax forms (Blumenthal et al, 2000; Facts and Comparisons, 2001; Fetrow, Avila, 1999; La Valle et al, 2000).

The mechanism of action for these energy-producing herbs is unknown, including whether it is the herb or the resultant increased activity and energy output that results in lowered blood glucose levels. Korean and American ginseng (Panax) have been studied:

> Panax and American ginseng might be beneficial in lowering blood glucose. Clinical evidence shows that Panax ginseng at 100 mg daily can lower blood glucose. At twice that dose, it can lower Hb A1c and improve mood. A new study shows that 3 grams of American ginseng before a glucose challenge can reduce postprandial glucose. Some researchers think ginseng acts by inhibiting cortisol, which opposes the effects of insulin. Others think ginseng's glycan constituents have direct hypoglycemic effects, but no mechanism has been proven with certainty. (PL/PL, 2000, p. 20)

If patients use both ginseng and hypoglycemic medications, additive effects may occur, thus close monitoring is necessary. In addition, ginseng abuse syndrome may be an adverse effect because it was reported in 14 of 133 long-term users who were taking high daily doses (PL/PL, 2000; Shane-McWhorter, 2001; Siegel, 1979; Sotaniemi et al, 1995). Ginseng abuse syndrome, although debated whether the syndrome exists:

> occurs when large doses of the herb are taken concomitantly with other psychomotor stimulants, such as tea and coffee; symptoms include diarrhea, hypertension, restlessness, insomnia, skin eruptions, depression, appetite suppression, euphoria, and edema. (Fetrow, Avila, 1999, p. 284)

Ginkgo biloba is used in Germany for cerebrovascular insufficiency and dementia, and it may help with peripheral circulatory problems and sexual dysfunction. Studies of ginkgo biloba indicate an increase in blood flow, which aides the eyes (Chung et al, 1999), decreases intermittent claudication (Pittler, Ernst, 2000), and improves erectile dysfunction (Shon, Sikora, 1991).

Milk thistle (Silybum marianum) may be helpful in people with hepatic damage, and it may diminish insulin resistance, although its use in diabetes is preliminary. People with diabetes may have preexisting liver damage, or hepatotoxicity can be a side effect of some of the antihyperglycemic medications. Milk thistle has been used in viral hepatitis, mushroom poisoning, and alcoholic cirrhosis (Blumenthal et al, 2000; Facts and Comparisons, 2001; Flora et al, 1998; Shane-McWhorter, 2001; Velussi et al, 1997).

Other nutrients and herbals are used for diabetes treatment. A credible herbal or nutrition source for indications should be consulted. Table 10-2 lists biologic-based therapies for diabetes.

MANIPULATIVE AND BODY-BASED METHODS FOR DIABETES

Pain can raise blood glucose, increase muscle tension, and cause psychologic and spiritual distress. Body-based methods may help lower blood glucose levels by decreasing pain, promoting relaxation, and relieving muscle tension. Included in body-based methods are chiropractic, osteopathy, and various massage methods.

Shekell and colleagues (1998) found that 25% of patients treated with chiropractic manipulations were treated for indications that were judged inappropriate, thus chiropractors need to be well informed about any patient with diabetes. A holistic chiropractic practitioner will ensure that a therapeutic intervention will enhance the diabetes regimen. Osteopathic manipulation has a more conventional assessment format very similar to allopathic practitioners. However, manipulation, alignment, and the ensuing possible comfort may help general function and decrease stressors that affect diabetes.

Rose (2001), a massage therapist who also has type 1 diabetes, writes of the beneficial effects of massage for diabetes. Effects include increasing circulation, promoting relaxation, and helping to increase mobility and tissue elasticity. Cautions for massage include the care that needs to be taken if the person with diabetes has complications, such as peripheral neuropathy or vascular problems.

Field (2000, 1998; Field et al, 1997) reports on the improvement of 24 children, ages 5 to 8 years, with insulin-dependent diabetes, who had massage administered by their parents. The parents were given massage training sessions. The children were given one daily 15-minute bedtime massage for a 4-week period; a standardized massage was taught and given to the children. Comparisons were made using The Family Environment Scale, The Parenting Stress Index, The Self Care Inventory, and glucose levels. Parent and child anxiety decreased, children's salivary cortisol decreased, and blood glucose levels decreased to the normal range (from 168 to 118 mg/dl) (9.3 to 6.5 mmol/L). In addition, food and insulin adherence scores improved.

Massage resulting in favorable outcomes was one of several options for treating 100 people with diabetes mellitus (Elson, Meredith, 1998). In addition, Ezzo and colleagues (2001) reviewed scientific literature regarding massage for people with diabetes. The authors found few studies or reports on massage and acupressure (Dillon, 1983; Field, 1995; Field et al, 1997; Valtonen, Lilius, 1973;

Table 10-2 Biologic-Based Therapies for Diabetes

A complete prescribing source should be consulted before using biologic therapies. Nutrient doses may be above the recommended daily allowance or tolerable upper limit. In illness or deficiency, such doses may be acceptable; however, long-term use may not be appropriate. Herbs may cause allergic reactions and interactions. Herbs are generally contraindicated or not recommended for women during pregnancy and lactation and for children unless research data or a long history of safe use has been established.

Intervention	Management	Treatment Regimen	Cautions, Precautions, Interactions	References
Diet and foods	For glucose control and thus helps prevent complications	Macrobiotic diet; Ornish diet; vegetarian diet	Blood glucose and medication use should be monitored	Kushi, 1979, 1996; Ornish, 1990; Snowdon, Phillips, 1985
Omega-3 fatty acids	Increases insulin sensitivity; may lower BP and decrease microvascular albumin leakage; may treat nephropathy	Omega-3 fatty acids best through consumption of coldwater fish or flaxseed; the supplement is fish oil, (but can have adverse effects if dosing too large)	Fish oil can cause belching, nausea, loose stools, nosebleeds; use lower doses of under 2.5 g of omega-3 fatty acid fish oil, otherwise can have adverse effects; can decrease pulmonary function in	Murray, Pizzorno, 1999; PL/PL, 2000

Continued

Omega-6 fatty acid	For diabetic neuropathy, hyperlipidemia	GLA (an omega-6 fatty acid); 360 mg/day has been used; found in black currant, borage oil, evening primrose	aspirin-sensitive individuals; interacts with antidiabetic agents and cyclosporin; increased bleeding with anticoagulants, antiplatelets, aspirin	PL/PL, 2002; Shane-McWhorter, 2001
			Headache, bloating, loose stools	
Bulk laxatives	As bulk laxatives, stimulates insulin synthesis or release from beta cells	Fenugreek, flaxseed, glucomannan, oat bran, psyllium (blond), xanthan gum; example dose: 1 tbsp of ground flaxseed with 150 ml water, bid-tid	Products must be without added sugar; must be taken with large amounts of fluid; not to be taken by people who choke easily; fenugreek has a bad taste and smell	PL/PL, 2000, 2002

Vitamins and minerals

B vitamins	Stimulates insulin synthesis or release from beta cells;	Niacinamide (or nicoti-namide) to slow disease progression of type 1	Vitamin B3 occurs in 2 forms (niacinamide and nicotinic acid);	O'Connell, 2001; NAP, 2002; PL/PL,

Table 10-2 Biologic-Based Therapies for Diabetes—cont'd

Intervention	Management	Treatment Regimen	Cautions, Precautions, Interactions	References
Vitamins and minerals—cont'd				
B vitamins, cont'd	may enhance "honeymoon" period in type 1 diabetes; possibly prevents type 1 diabetes. Decreases homocysteine levels and thus decreases risk of vascular disease; B vitamins may decrease neuropathy symptoms, especially if a B deficiency exists; thiamine needed for carbohydrate metabolism	diabetes; niacinamide 25 mg/kg of body weight daily has been used. Other B vitamins, including: B1 (thiamine), B6 (pyridoxine), folate, and B12. Many recommend a 25- or 50-mg B-complex formula: Adult RDA; folic acid 400 μg/day; adult UL: folate, 1000 μg/day. Adult RDA thiamine, 1.1-1.2 mg/day. Adult UL thiamine not determined. Niacin, 14-16 mg/day; adult UL:	both have similar effects as vitamins; however, in pharmacologic doses, nicotinic acid (although effective for dyslipidemia) has a negative effect on glycemic control. Metformin may reduce folate and vitamin B12 and thus increase homocysteine levels. See side effects for individual vitamins	2000, 2002; Abbas, Swai, 1997; NAP, 2002; O'Connell, 2001; PL/PL, 2000

Vitamin C	Lack of vitamin C may be associated with micro-angiopathy	niacin, 35 mg/day. Pyridoxine RDA, 1.3-1.7 mg/day; adult UL: pyridoxine, 100 mg/day. Riboflavin RDA, 1.1-1.3 mg/day; adult UL not determined. Vitamin B12 RDA, 2.4 µg/day; adult UL not determined. Vitamin C for slowing atherosclerosis; 250 mg bid taken with vitamin E. Adult RDA: 75-90 mg/day. Adult UL: 2000 mg/day. Higher requirements than for the general population are possibly needed for diabetics.	Jennings, 1987; PL/PL, 2002; Som et al, 1981
Vitamin D	Help ensure adequate blood levels of insulin; help increase insulin secretion	Vitamin D (calciferol); adult AI: 5-10 µg/day (200 to 400 IU); adult UL: 50 µg/day (2000 IU); sunshine also 15-20 min/day without sunscreen	A fat-soluble vitamin and thus stored in body and can be overdosed	Boucher, 1998; NAP, 2002

Continued

Table 10-2 Biologic-Based Therapies for Diabetes—cont'd

Intervention	Management	Treatment Regimen	Cautions, Precautions, Interactions	References
Vitamins and minerals—cont'd				
Vitamin E	Antioxidant may increase insulin sensitivity and glycemic control; may decrease complications such as retinopathy, nephropathy, neuropathy	Vitamin E (wheat germ, seeds, nuts, vegetable oils); natural d'alpha tocopherol more bioavailable; for peripheral neuropathy, 900 mg/day has been used. Adult RDA; 15 mg/day; Adult UL: 1000 mg/day	Increased risk of hemorrhagic stroke in smokers; vitamin E has anticoagulant properties, thus may interact with any herbs or medications that decrease blood clotting; interacts with bile acid sequestrants; amounts over 2500 IU/day can interfere with production of vitamin K–dependent clotting factors	NAP, 2002; O'Connell, 2001; PL/PL, 2000, 2002
Chromium	Required for maintenance of normal glucose metabolism; may	Chromium; for lowering blood glucose in type 2 diabetes: 200-1000 μg/day in divided	Likely safe in dose of 50-200 μg/day; blood sugars must be closely monitored; adverse	Anderson, 2001; NAP, 2002; O'Connell,

| | | doses. Adult AI: 20-30 μg/day. Adult UL not determined. | reduce Hgb A₁C and FBS and reduces need for oral hypoglycemics; increases insulin sensitivity; may improve blood sugar when insulin used; may be helpful in gestational diabetes | effects include cognitive, perceptual, and motor dysfunction at 200-400 μg/day; anemia, thrombocytopenia, hemolysis, hepatic dysfunction, and renal failure when given in doses of 1.2-2.4 mg/day; interacts with beta-blockers, corticosteroids; modest increase in serum HDL; has effects on serotonin, dopamine; caution with renal insufficiency | 2001; PL/PL, 2000, 2002 |
| Magnesium | Increases insulin sensitivity; magnesium is required for glucose metabolism; up to 25% of people with diabetes have | Magnesium to improve glycemic control in type 2 diabetes; 1000 mg elemental magnesium/day has been used. Adult RDA: 320-420 mg/day. Adult UL: | | Kidney regulates magnesium homeostasis (hypermagnesemia may occur with renal insufficiency); assessment of | NAP, 2002; O'Connell, 2001; PL/PL, 2000, 2002 |

Continued

Table 10-2 Biologic-Based Therapies for Diabetes—cont'd

Intervention	Management	Treatment Regimen	Cautions, Precautions, Interactions	References
Vitamins and minerals—cont'd				
Magnesium, cont'd	less than optimal levels of magnesium; helps lower BP	350 mg/day (UL is from a pharmacologic agent only; does not include food and water)	magnesium status difficult because less than 0.3% is found in serum; deficiency must be severe before serum levels decline	
Vanadium	Enhances action of insulin	Vanadium for type 2 diabetes, vanadyl sulfate, 50 mg bid for 4 wks was given but this is a very high dose and concern regarding kidney damage; vanadyl sulfate contains 31% elemental vanadium. Adult RDA not determined. Adult UL: 1.8 mg/day.	Small doses are potentially toxic; keep intake limited to less than 100 μg/day; green discoloration of tongue, nausea and vomiting, cramping, flatulence, diarrhea, anorexia, weight loss; long-term neurologic, hematologic, nephrotoxic, hepatotoxic,	NAP, 2002; O'Connell, 2001; PL/PL, 2000, 2002

Continued

| Zinc | For appropriate synthesis, secretion, and utilization of insulin; has protective effect against beta-cell destruction; involved in carbohydrate and protein digestion; people with diabetes excrete large amounts of zinc | Zinc; adult doses over 50 mg/day have increased HgbAic. RDA: 8 mg/day (women), 11 mg/day (men); adult UL: 40 mg/day; must have proper zinc/copper ratio; ratio of zinc to copper fed to humans of 2:1, 5:1, and 15:1 had limited effects on copper absorption, thus stay within that range | reproductive and developmental effects; may have additive effects with diabetes medications; may enhance digoxin and anticoagulants

SE: nausea, vomiting, diarrhea, dizziness, anemia; high doses impair immune response; increased zinc can lead to depletion of copper, iron, calcium, and magnesium; elevated copper, calcium, or iron can deplete zinc; can interfere with glucocorticoids and other immunosuppressants; doses over 50 mg/day can lower HDL levels; different salt forms contain | La Valle, 2000; Murray, Pizzorno, 1999; NAP, 2002; PL/PL, 2002 |

Table 10-2 Biologic-Based Therapies for Diabetes—cont'd

Intervention	Management	Treatment Regimen	Cautions, Precautions, Interactions	References
Vitamins and minerals—cont'd				
Zinc, cont'd			different amounts of zinc; vegetarians and people with diarrhea need more zinc	
Other nutrients	For improvement in diabetic neuropathy symptoms: ALA	ALA; 1200 mg/day or 600 mg tid	Can cause skin rash; high doses can cause thiamine deficiency; interacts with ETOH; ADA does not sanction use of ALA	Shane-McWhorter, 2001; Reljanovic et al, 1999; PL/PL, 2000, 2002
Herbs				
Basil	May help lower blood sugar	Basil (Ocimum basilicum); dose given is the one for flatulence since no diabetes dose given in PL/PL. Tea is made with 2-4 g basil leaf in	Safe when used at low levels as in food; however, possibly unsafe if used long term; contains estragole, which may	PL/PL, 2002

	Uses	Preparation/Dosage	Cautions	References
		150 ml boiling water, steeped 10-15 min, strained, bid-tid	produce liver tumors and mutagenic. Caution with long-term treatment.	Blumenthal et al, 2000; Facts and Comparisons, 2001; Fetrow, Avila, 1999; La Valle, 2000; PL/PL, 2000, 2002; Shane-McWhorter, 2001
Bilberry	Dried fruit is used for diabetic retinopathy, cataracts, night vision, visual acuity; decreases vascular permeability. Leaf used for lowering glucose levels.	Bilberry (Vaccinium myrtillus) leaf for diabetes, circulatory disorders, cataracts; steep 1 g or 1-2 tsp finely chopped dried leaf in 150 ml water for 5-10 min; strain; short-term use only; the bilberry fruit is used to improve night vision and visual acuity	Long-term use avoided; dosages exceeding 480 mg/day may be dangerous; long-term consumption of bilberry leaves can be poisonous; possible interaction with anticoagulants, ASA. Hypoglycemia effects need to be monitored.	
Bitter melon	For insulinlike effects	Bitter melon (Momordica charantia) 1-2 g/day of powdered leaf in tablets or capsules	Blood sugar should be closely monitored; insulin dose adjustments might be needed; interaction with other hypo-glycemics reported	PL/PL, 2000, 2002; Shane-McWhorter, 2001
Capsaicin	For neuropathy	Capsaicin (topical only); 0.025%-0.075% cream	Gloves should be worn; hands washed	PL/PL, 2000, 2002

Continued

Table 10-2 Biologic-Based Therapies for Diabetes—cont'd

Intervention	Management	Treatment Regimen	Cautions, Precautions, Interactions	References
Herbs—cont'd				
Capsaicin, cont'd		tid-qid; may take up to 3 days to feel effect	thoroughly; not to get in eyes; diluted vinegar solution used to remove; sometimes higher concentrations used with neuropathy	
Fenugreek	May lower blood glucose	Fenugreek (Trigonella foenum-graecum) 1-2 g of seeds tid	Can cause flatulence and diarrhea; subsides after a few days. Hypersensitivity reported; is member of the Leguminosae family, which includes peanuts. May potentially enhance anticoagulant activity; may interact with corticosteroid, hormone, MAOI. Is high mucilage, thus may cause decreased	PL/PL, 2000, 2002; Shane-McWhorter, 2001; Sharma et al, 1990, 1996

Ginko biloba	May help with peripheral circulatory problems (including microcirculation and intermittent claudication), sexual dysfunction, cerebrovascular insufficiency, dementia	_Ginkgo biloba_ leaf 120-240 mg/day in divided doses; begin with lower dose	absorption of other medications Can cause headache, dizziness, palpitations, GI upset, dermatologic reactions; has additive antiplatelet activity	Blumenthal, 2000; Facts and Comparisons; 2001; La Valle et al, 2000; PL/PL, 2000; Shane-McWhorter, 2001
Panax ginseng	May lower blood glucose in type 2 diabetes; action unknown; may possibly inhibit cortisol; two different ginsengs have study findings	Ginseng (_Panax ginseng_) 200 mg daily or (_Panax quinquefolius_) 3 g up to 2 hrs before a meal Note: the difference in the 2 ginsengs; time period is 3 wks to 3 mos Need a ginseng-free period of about 2 wks between consecutive courses.	Hypoglycemia a concern; can cause nervousness, headache, hypertension, insomnia, estrogenic effects (including mastalgia, vaginal bleeding); ginseng abuse syndrome; interacts with diuretics, MAOIs, diabetes agents, warfarin, stimulants;	PL/PL, 2000, 2002; Shane-McWhorter, 2001

Continued

Table 10-2 Biologic-Based Therapies for Diabetes—cont'd

Intervention	Management	Treatment Regimen	Cautions, Precautions, Interactions	References
Herbs—cont'd				
Panax ginseng, cont'd			close monitoring needed	PL/PL, 2002
Guar gum	Lowers postprandial blood sugars when taken with meals	Guar gum (*Cyamopsis tetragonolobus* or *psoralioides*) 5 g tid just before or with meals with at least 8 oz of water	Is a bulk laxative; must have plenty of water to avoid esophageal obstruction; SE: flatulence, nausea, diarrhea; can reduce nutrient absorption	
Gymnema sylvestre	Promotes or enhances insulin release	Gymnema sylvestre (GS4 extract) 400 mg/day	Blood glucose should be monitored	Baskaran et al, 1990; Shane-McWhorter, 2001; PL/PL, 2002; Shanmugasundaram et al, 1990
Milk thistle	May diminish insulin resistance,	Milk thistle (*Silybum marianum*) 70%-80%	Allergy to thistle, aster, or daisy; GI	PL/PL, 2002; Shane-

	especially in people with hepatic damage	silymarin 420 mg/day for cirrhosis; no dose given for decreasing insulin resistance	disturbance	McWhorter, 2001; Velussi et al, 1997
Nopal	For hypoglycemic effects with type 2 diabetes	Nopal or prickly pear cactus (Opuntia ficus indica) broiled stems 100-500 g/day in three divided doses	Increased stools, abdominal fullness, dermatitis; additive with chlorpropamide; most trials published in Spanish	PL/PL, 2002; Shane-McWhorter, 2001

ADA, American Diabetes Association; AI, adequate intake; ALA, alpha lipoic acid; ASA, acetylsalicylic acid; bid, twice daily; BP, blood pressure; ETOH, ethyl alcohol; FBS, fasting blood sugar; GI, gastrointestinal; GLA, gamma linolenic acid; HDL, high-density lipoprotein; Hgb, hemoglobin; IU, international units; MAOI, monamine oxidase inhibitor; NAC, National Academy Press; RDA, recommended daily allowance; tid, three times daily; UL, upper limits—the maximum level of daily nutrient that is likely to pose no risk of adverse effects. Includes intake from food, water, and supplements.Dietary recommended intake (DRI) values expands on the RDAs and contain four categories of recommendations (i.e., RDA, AI, UL, EAR [estimated average requirement]). Check for the latest data.

Both the AI and the RDA are goals for intakes, but are defined differently.

RDA is the intake at which risk of inadequacy is very small (2% to 3%); RDA is expected to meet the nutrient needs of 97% to 98% of the individuals in a life stage and gender group.

AI is the observed average or experimentally set intake by a defined population or subgroup that appears to sustain a defined nutritional status, such as growth rate, normal circulating nutrient values, or other functional indicators of health. An AI is used to derive an EAR. AN AI IS NOT AN RDA.

EAR is the intake that meets the estimated nutrient needs of one half of the individuals in a group.

From the Food and Nutrition Board, National Academy of Sciences, Institute of Medicine (www.nap.edu).

Vest, 2000). The authors found no studies pertaining to chiropractic. A study by Dillon (1983) showed improved absorption of insulin when patients massaged their insulin sites for 3 minutes with an electric vibrator. Serum glucose levels "fell 8.3% (P < 0.05) lower, 30 minutes after massage and 44 minutes post-injection, compared to the control day when participants did not massage their injection sites, and this was significant" (Ezzo et al, 2001, p. 220).

Vest (2000) reported on improved blood sugar levels, decreased physical symptoms, and an increased perception of well being in a study of 12 people. These subjects received 15-minute sessions of breath awareness, light touch, and acupressure weekly for 6 weeks. Details of when and how glucose was measured, length of follow-up, or definition of clinically significant glucose level change were not published.

Valtonen and Lilius (1973 in Ezzo, 2001) reported on improved subjective symptoms of neuropathy after using syncardial massage on 25 patients with symmetrical diabetic neuropathy of the lower limbs. The symptoms had averaged 14 months. Massage was administered every 2 days for a total number of treatments from 20 to 30 in participants who appeared to benefit. After 1 month, 14 people noted good results, 8 noted improvement, and 3 noted no effect. Syncardial massage is a mechanical leg massage technique that uses an inflatable cuff, and, in this study, the cuff was used around the thigh and leg. Ezzo and colleagues also reported on two of Field's publications, one of which has been previously discussed.

Reflexology is a type of massage. Carter and Weber (1994) anecdotally relate a situation in which the pancreas area had been massaged, and decreased medication (insulin) was needed. Reflexology areas are located on the abdomen, face, hands, and feet. Blood sugar lowering might also happen with other types of massage, such as shiatsu.

ENERGY THERAPIES FOR DIABETES

Healing touch, Therapeutic Touch, Reiki, polarity, or acupressure-acupuncture may be useful energy therapies. Reiki is being studied as part of a treatment regimen for neuropathy. Reiki has been found to have an empowering effect on individuals and appears to focus on the endocrine and lymph systems (Nield-Anderson, Ameling, 2001). Patient empowerment is an important approach to self-care (Feste, Anderson, 1995).

Therapeutic Touch (TT) promotes relaxation, helps decrease anxiety and pain, and accelerates wound healing (Egan, 1998; Gagne, Toye 1994; Keller, Bzdek, 1986; Kramer, 1990; Wirth et al, 1993) thus fostering lower blood sugars. In Delores Krieger's classic study (1974), TT increased hemoglobin; one wonders if such a therapy might theoretically affect glycosylated hemoglobin.

Anecdotally, Reiki combined with TT and other healing touch techniques may be useful in individuals who have peripheral neuropathy. A family member can be taught TT for daily treatments. This learning may provide a more comfortable adjustment period while awaiting the reversal of the neuropathy following normalization of blood glucose levels.

The transcutaneous electrical nerve stimulation (TENS) unit consists of a battery power source; controls for frequency, waveform, and amplitude; and electrodes. TENS consists of selective and repetitive stimulation of the large nonnociceptive alpha and beta fibers that inhibit nociceptive impulse transmission (Puntillo, Tesler, 1993). Researchers randomized 31 patients with type 2 diabetes and peripheral neuropathy to either a TENS or a sham treatment group (Kumar, Marshall, 1997). Subjects treated each of their lower extremities for 4 weeks with daily 30-minute sessions. Symptom relief was seen in 83% (15 out of the 18) of the electrotherapy cases versus 38% in the sham group.

By providing comfort, magnetic field therapy and electromagnetic currents may be indirectly useful for people with diabetes (Bassett, 1993; Weintraub, 2001). "The pulse of a magnetic field produces an electric current in tissue, which causes depolarization of a nerve membrane and the generation of an action potential" (Weintraub, 2001, p. 281). People have used this therapy for healing of fractures, for reduction of inflammation, for peripheral neuropathy and burning feet syndrome, and for the reduction of pain, such as in Charcot joint (neuroarthropathy) (Hanft et al, 1998; Weintraub, 2001). Anecdotally, people also use magnets in their shoes to treat residual peripheral neuropathy symptoms and have reported positive outcomes. Weintraub (1998 in Weintraub, 2001) reports on the use of permanent magnetic footpads (used 24 hours a day for 4 months of 475 G (Gauss, a measure of magnetic field strength) to treat people with diabetes and people with other diagnoses who had peripheral neuropathy and burning feet syndrome:

> Pilot data demonstrated that six out of eight subjects (75%) with diabetes experienced reduction or reversal of symptoms, whereas only 50% in the group with other etiologies improved. Burning dysesthesia was reversed in all four subjects who had diabetes and in one subject who did not. The entire cohort (9 out of 14 or 64%) experienced an unexpected clinical benefit. Visual analog scale (VAS) pain scores were considered significant only in the diabetic peripheral neuropathy group. (Weintraub, 2001, p. 284)

Eak and Tiszka (1998) describe the need for creative management approaches, especially for people who have diabetes. Box 10-3 represents a selection of potential program choices for people with peripheral neuropathy.

Box 10-3

NAC Therapies Suggested for Peripheral Neuropathy

Vitamins, Minerals, and Other Nutrients
Vitamins A, B complex, C, D, E
Alpha-lipoic acid
Chromium
Coenzyme Q10
Gamma linolenic acid
Magnesium
Omega-3 fatty acids
Vanadium (CAUTION)
Zinc

Topicals
Capsaicin

Body-Based and Energy Therapies
Acupuncture
Biofeedback
Magnetic, electromagnetic
Reiki
Swedish massage
Transcutaneous electrical nerve stimulation
Therapeutic touch

Adapted from Huebscher R: Peripheral neuropathy: alternative & complementary options, NP Forum 11(2):73, 2000.

NAC PRACTICES FOR THYROID CONDITIONS

Two of the most common functional disorders of the thyroid are hyperthyroidism and hypothyroidism. Hyperthyroidism occurs when thyroid hormone synthesis and release are increased. Several conditions can lead to hyperthyroidism, including Graves' disease, toxic multinodular goiter, toxic adenoma (Plummer's disease), coexistant Hashimoto's thyroiditis and Graves' disease, and pituitary adenoma release. Hyperthyroidism can also be induced by iodide from ingesting iodine or kelp (seaweed), from iodine-containing drugs, or contrast media (Rakel, 2000). All of these precursor conditions can lead to the same clinical picture of hyperthyroidism; however, diagnosis of the underlying cause is imperative so that the proper therapy can be selected. Signs and symptoms for hyperthyroidism can be highly variable. The "typical" patient expresses with one or more of the following complaints: weight loss, palpitations, hyperactivity, nervousness, irritability, heat intolerance, increased appetite, fatigue, weakness, frequent defecation, and (for women) menstrual abnormalities. Key signs include tachycardia, arrhythmia, systolic hypertension, hyperreflexia, tremor, eyelid retraction, stare, goiter, psychiatric manifestations, and warm, moist, smooth skin. The thyroid gland may be palpably enlarged, and a bruit may be auscultated over the enlarged lobes (Rakel, 2000).

Hypothyroidism is a metabolic state that occurs when the thyroid gland underproduces free thyroxin (T4) (Rakel, 2000). Even though hypothyroidism is the most common disorder of thyroid function, patients present with a broad spectrum of symptoms, and hypothyroidism may often be an unsuspected illness (Shames, Shames, 2001). The cause of hypothyroidism may be related to a primary thyroid disorder or a central pituitary disorder. Primary hypothyroidism can be caused by: (1) autoimmune thyroid disease (Hashimoto's thyroiditis, idiopathic hypothyroidism, Graves' disease remission, polyglandular failure); (2) postablative therapy for hyperthyroidism; (3) thyroiditis; (4) drug therapy (antithyroid drugs, iodine excess, lithium); (5) ingesting large amounts of kelp (seaweed); and rarely (6) from iodine deficiency, genetic biosynthetic defects, sporadic cretinism, or infiltrative disorders (scleroderma, amyloidosis, hemochromatosis, sarcoidosis, Riedel's thyroiditis). Central hypothyroidism is caused by either a deficiency of thyroid-stimulating hormone (secondary hypothyroidism) or thyrotropin-releasing hormone (tertiary hypothyroidism). Clinical manifestations of hypothyroidism are variable, often with an insidious onset. Therefore the following signs and symptoms associated with hypothyroidism may go unnoticed by the patient. Common symptoms include fatigue, lethargy, cold intolerance, muscle ache, constipation, mental impairment, menstrual abnormalities, weight gain, dry skin, hair loss, and paresthesias. Key signs associated with hypothyroidism are bradycardia, bradykinesia, hyporeflexia, muscle weakness, nonpitting edema (myxedema), delayed relaxation phase of reflexes, goiter; dry, coarse, thick skin; and low basal body temperature (Rakel, 2000, Shames, Shames, 2001). Laboratory tests often used to diagnose hypothyroidism include: T-4; thyroid panel (T-4, T-3 uptake, and free thyroxine index); thyroid-stimulating hormone (TSH); total T-3; free T-3; and free T-4. If all of these tests are normal, and if the patient still has clinically suspicious symptoms, another blood test to measure the amount of circulating thyroid antibodies produced by the immune system is imperative to determine if the body "thinks" the thyroid gland is a "foreign invader" (Shames, Shames, 2001, p. 65). The most common two antibody tests are the antimicrosomal antibody, or thyroid peroxidase test, and the antithyroglobulin antibody test (Shames, Shames, 2001).

Individuals who experience hypothyroidism or hyperthyroidism should examine their home and work environments for possible exposure to toxins. Radioactive iodine (Schmidt et al, 1997), polybrominated biphenyls (Bahn et al, 1980), organic hydrocarbons in drinking water (Gaitan et al, 1983), and pentachlorophenol (van Raaji et al, 1991) have all been identified as environmental substances that can directly or indirectly affect thyroid function. Certain foods such as rapeseed (canola oil), cabbage, Brussels sprouts, broccoli, turnips, cauliflower, lima beans, sweet potatoes, and pearl millet contain goitrogens (Paynter et al, 1988), a natural substance that can cause development of goiter (Lininger et al, 1999). Furthermore, foods such as walnuts, apples, almonds, sorghum, and cassava contain cyanogenic glycosides that can inhibit the thyroid gland's ability to concentrate iodine, thereby leading to a diseased glandular state (Rea, 1996). Therefore a thorough dietary evaluation is critical for patients with hypothyroidism or hyperthyroidism.

For patients with hypothyroidism, a biologic therapy that has been used instead of levothyroxine is desiccated thyroid (Bunevicius et al, 1999; Gaby, 1989; Lininger et al, 1999). Intact desiccated thyroid is available only by prescription. Glandular thyroid products purchased over the counter are ineffective and standardization of these products has been questioned.

Two supplements, selenium and zinc, have been used with some success for patients with an underactive thyroid. Selenium plays a role in the conversion of T4 to T3. If the patient does not have iodine deficiency–induced goiter and is selenium deficient, supplementing with selenium may improve hypothyroidism (Contempre et al, 1991; Diplock, 1992; Thilly et al, 1993). Zinc may also improve hypothyroidism by increasing thyroxine levels (Argiratos, Samman, 1994; Crofton et al, 1989; Sandstead, 1995; Spencer et al, 1994).

Patients with either an overactive or an underactive thyroid experience a variety of physical complaints that can be emotionally depleting. Treatment helps plus encouraging these individuals to use Swedish massage (Sunshine et al, 1996), relaxation techniques (Jacobs et al, 1986), visualization (Samuels, Samuels, 1988), guided imagery (McKinney et al, 1997), or prayer (Shuler et al, 1994; Wirth, Cram, 1994) can decrease fatigue and depression and relieve stress. Furthermore, practicing yoga (Ornish, 1990), Qi gong (Horstman, 1999), or Tai chi (Wolf et al, 1996; Wolfson et al, 1996) can further reduce stress and enhance relaxation if practiced regularly. Energy work such as healing touch, TT, or Reiki may also promote comfort and relaxation and help decrease pain and anxiety.

The practitioner should obtain a thorough knowledge of traditional therapies that the patient currently uses to ensure safe introduction of NAC regimens. Tables 10-3 through 10-6 present a selection of NAC therapies that are recommended for the treatment of hyperthyroidism and hypothyroidism.

Table 10-3 Alternative Health Care Systems for Thyroid Concerns

Intervention	Management	Treatment Regimen	Cautions, Precautions, Interactions	References
Ayurveda				
Yoga	Reduces stress; loosens chronically tense muscles; improves relaxation	Varies with individual; daily practice encouraged; breath work is part of yoga	Instructor needed at the beginning to ensure correct movements; often combined with meditation, prayer, and relaxation techniques	Ornish, 1990
Traditional Chinese Medicine				
Moxibustion	May improve thyroid function in Hashimoto's thyroiditis	Varies with individual	Skilled practitioner needed	Hu et al, 1993
Qi gong	Builds muscle strength; improves balance, relieves stress, improves depression	Daily practice	Instructor needed to ensure correct movements	Horstman, 1999
Tai chi	Builds muscle strength; improves balance; relieves stress; improves depression	Daily practice	Instructor needed to ensure correct movements	Wolf et al, 1996; Wolfson et al, 1996

Table 10-4 Mind Body Spirit Interventions for Thyroid Concerns

Intervention	Management	Treatment Regimen	Cautions, Precautions, Interactions	References
Guided imagery (with or without music)	Improves mood; relieves depression, fatigue; decreases cortisol levels	Recordings or trained provider	Instruction needed; must practice technique to sustain therapeutic effects	McKinney et al, 1997; Wynd, 1992
Personal and intercessory prayer	Reduces pain; promotes emotional, physical, spiritual healing; reduces stress, depressive symptoms, perceived worries; controls anger	Varies with individual	Health care providers are not expected to assume the role of spiritual advisor to patients; however, they can encourage patients to explore the potential benefits that prayer may have on their physical and mental well being	Byrd, 1988; Ornish, 1990; Shuler et al, 1994; Wirth et al, 1994
Relaxation techniques	May strengthen immune response; reduces stress; improves flexibility; reduces blood pressure; controls anger	Progressive muscle, autogenics, and breath work	Some relaxation techniques use various yoga techniques; often combined with prayer, meditation, visualization, yoga	Jacobs et al, 1986; Kiecolt-Glaser et al, 1984; Ornish, 1990
Visualization	Promotes healing; may strengthen immune system	Recordings	Often combined with prayer, meditation, visualization, yoga	Ornish, 1990; Samuels et al, 1988

Table 10-5   Biologic-Based Therapies for Thyroid Concerns

A complete prescribing source should be consulted before using biologic therapies. Nutrient doses may be above the recommended daily allowance or tolerable upper limit. In illness or deficiency, such doses may be acceptable; however, long-term use may not be appropriate. Herbs may cause allergic reactions and interactions. Herbs are generally contraindicated or not recommended for women during pregnancy and lactation and for children unless research data or a long history of safe use has been established.

Intervention	Management	Treatment Regimen	Cautions, Precautions, Interactions	References
Desiccated thyroid	Can be used as an alternative for synthetic thyroid hormones levothyropine	Dosage depends on the source of glandular tissue and severity of hypothyroidism	Intact desiccated thyroid is available only by prescription; glandular thyroid products sold in health food stores are basically ineffective because most of the thyroid hormone has been removed	Bunevicius et al, 1999; Gaby, 1989; Lininger et al, 1999
Dietary modifications: goitrogen-containing foods	1. Prevents or reduces goiter by patient avoiding foods containing	Goitrogen-containing foods: rapeseed (canola oil), cabbage, Brussels sprouts, broccoli, turnips,	Patient education should emphasize importance of balanced diet with the exclusion of the	Boyages, 1993; Paynter et al, 1988; Rea, 1996;

Continued

Table 10-5 Biologic-Based Therapies for Thyroid Concerns—cont'd

Intervention	Management	Treatment Regimen	Cautions, Precautions, Interactions	References
goitrogen-containing foods, cont'd	goitrogens, a natural substance that can cause goiter	cauliflower, lima beans, sweet potatoes, pearl millet, rutabaga	foods containing goitrogens and cyanogenic glycosides	Schmidt et al, 1997
Dietary: Cyanogenic glycoside foods	2. Promotes ability of thyroid gland to concentrate iodine by avoiding foods containing cyanogenic glycosides	Cyanogenic glycoside foods: walnuts, apples, sorghum, cassava are avoided		
Selenium	Plays a role in thyroid hormone metabolism (conversion of T4 to T3); replacement may relieve symptoms of hypothyroidism if	50-200 μg/day. Adult RDA: 55 μg/day; adult UL: 400 μg/day	Use of selenium avoided in the cases of iodine deficiency-induced goiter, because supplementation can exacerbate low thyroid function	Contempre et al, 1991; Diplock, 1992; Thilly et al, 1993

			patient is selenium deficient	
Zinc	May increase thyroxine levels, thereby relieving hypothyroidism	15-25 mg of zinc gluconate daily. Adult RDA: 8-11 mg/day; adult UL: 40 mg/day	Should also take a multimineral containing copper, iron, calcium, magnesium because zinc inhibits or competes with absorption of these minerals	Argiratos et al, 1994; Crofton et al, 1989; Sandstead, 1995; Spencer et al, 1994

Dietary recommended intake (DRI) values expand on the RDAs and contain four categories of recommendations (i.e., RDA, AI, UL, EAR [estimated average requirement]). Check for the latest data.

Both the AI and the RDA are goals for intakes, but are defined differently.

RDA is the intake at which risk of inadequacy is very small (2% to 3%); RDA is expected to meet the nutrient needs of 97% to 98% of the individuals in a life stage and gender group.

AI is the observed average or experimentally set intake by a defined population or subgroup that appears to sustain a defined nutritional status, such as growth rate, normal circulating nutrient values, or other functional indicators of health. An AI is used if sufficient scientific evidence is not available to derive an EAR. AN AI IS NOT AN RDA.

EAR is the intake that meets the estimated nutrient needs of one half of the individuals in a group.

From the Food and Nutrition Board, National Academy of Sciences, Institute of Medicine (www.nap.edu).

Table 10-6 Manipulative and Body-Based Methods and Energy Therapies for Thyroid Concerns

Intervention	Management	Treatment Regimen	Cautions, Precautions, Interactions	References
Identify harmful environmental and occupational hazards	For detoxification of environmental toxins; for early identification and treatment of individuals exposed to toxins	Exposure to radioactive iodine, polybrominated biphenyls, organic hydrocarbons (in drinking water), pentachlorophenol avoided	Early identification of toxic exposures can either prevent or initiate early treatment of resultant thyroid disease that can range from thyroid cancer to hypothyroidism	Bahn et al, 1980; Gaitan et al, 1983; Schmidt et al, 1997; van Raaij et al, 1991
Swedish massage	Decreases pain, fatigue, anxiety; improves sleep	Varies with massage; full-body Swedish very relaxing; takes about 1 hr	Trained and experienced massage therapist needed	Sunshine et al 1996
Therapeutic touch, healing touch, or Reiki	Provides comfort; decreases anxiety and pain	30-60-min sessions; first 3 Reiki sessions as close together as possible, such as daily for 3 days	Permission needed	

REFERENCES

Abbas ZG, Swai: Evaluation of the efficacy of thiamine and pyridoxine in the treatment of symptomatic diabetic peripheral neuropathy, *East African Med J* 74(12):803, 1997.

Abuaisha BB, Costanzi JB, Boulton AJ: Acupuncture for the treatment of chronic painful peripheral diabetic neuropathy: a long-term study, *Diabet Res Clin Pract* 39(2):141, 1998.

Ahmad N et al: Effect of Momordica charantia extracts on fasting and postprandial serum glucose levels in NIDDM patients, *Bangladesh Med Res Coun Bull* 25:11, 1999.

Ali L et al: Studies on hypoglycemic effects of fruit pulp, seed, and the whole plant of Momordica charantia on normal and diabetic model rats, *Planta Medica* 56:408, 1993.

American Diabetes Association: Report of the expert committee on the diagnosis and classification of diabetes mellitus, *Diabet Care* 26(suppl 1):S5, S12, 2003a.

American Diabetes Association: Gestational diabetes mellitus, *Diabet Care* 26(suppl 1):S103, 2003b.

American Diabetes Association: Standards of medical care for patients with diabetes mellitus, *Diabet Care* 26:(suppl 1):S33, S50, 2003c.

American Diabetes Association: Position statement on unproven therapies, *Diabet Care* 26(suppl 1):S142, 2003d.

American Diabetes Association: Stress management lowers blood glucose levels. ADA: In the News, 2002. Retrieved 01/06/02. URL: www.ada.yellobrix.com

Anderson J: Nutrition management of diabetes mellitus. In Goodhart R, Young VR, eds: *Modern nutrition in health and disease*, Philadelphia, 1988, Lea and Febiger.

Anderson R: *Clinician's guide to holistic medicine*, New York, 2001, McGraw-Hill.

Anderson R et al: Elevated intakes of supplemental chromium improve glucose and insulin variables in individuals with type II diabetes, *Diabet* 46(11):1786, 1997.

Andrew R et al: Vitamin E supplementation improved endothelium function in type 1 diabetes mellitus: a randomized, placebo-controlled study, *J Am Coll Cardiol* 36:94, 2000.

Argiratos V, Samman S: The effect of calcium carbonate and calcium citrate on the absorption of zinc in healthy female subjects, *Eur J Clin Nutr* 48:198, 1994.

Bahn AK et al: Hypothyroidism in workers exposed to polybrominated biphenyls, *N Engl J Med* 302:31, 1980.

Baskaran K et al: Antidiabetic effect of a leaf extract from Gymnema sylvestre in non-insulin dependent diabetes mellitus patients, *Ethnopharmacol* 30:295, 1990.

Bassett CA: Beneficial effects of electromagnetic fields, *J Cell Biochemistr* 51(4):387, 1993.

Belgrade MJ: Following the clues to neuropathic pain, *Postgrad Med* 106(6):127, 1999.

Benbow SJ, Cossins L, MacFarlane IA: Painful diabetic neuropathy, *Brit Diabet Assoc Diabet Med* 16:632, 1999.

Benson H, Stuart EM: *The wellness book: the comprehensive guide to maintaining health and treating stress-related illness*, New York, 1992, Simon and Schuster.

Blumenthal M, Goldberg A, Brinckmann J: *Herbal medicine*, Newton, Mass, 2000, Integrative Medicine Communications.

Boden G et al: Effects of vanadyl sulfate on carbohydrate and lipid metabolism in patients with non-insulin dependent diabetes mellitus, *Metabol* 45:1130, 1996.

Boucher BJ: Inadequate vitamin D status: does it contribute to the disorders comprising syndrome "X"? *Brit J Nutr* 79(4):315, 1998.

Boullata JI, Nace AM: Safety issues with herbal medicine, *Pharmacother* 20:257, 2000.

Boyages SC: Iodine deficiency disorders, *J Clin Endocrinol Metab* 77:587, 1993.

Brinker F: *Herb contraindications and drug interactions,* Sandy, Oreg, 1998, Eclectic Medical Publications.

Bunevicius R et al: Effects of thyroxine as compared with thyroxine plus triiodothyronine in patients with hypothyroidism, *N Engl J Med* 340:424, 1999.

Byrd RC: Positive therapeutic effects of intercessory prayer in a coronary care unit population, *South Med J* 81:826, 1988.

Cam MC et al: Mechanisms of vanadium action: insulin mimetic or insulin enhancing agent? *Am J Physiol Pharmacol* 78:829, 2000.

Cameron NE, Cotter MA: Comparison of the effects of ascorbyl gamma linolenic acid and gamma-linolenic acid in the correction of neurovascular deficits in diabetic rats, *Diabetologia* 39:1047, 1996.

Carter M, Weber T: *Body reflexology: healing at your fingertips,* New York, 1994, Parker Publishing.

Chang SL et al: An insulin dependent hypoglycemia induced electro acupuncture at the Zhongivan (CV 12) acupoint in diabetic rats, *Diabetologica* 42(2):250, 1999.

Chopra DP: *Journey into healing,* New York, 1999, Random House.

Chung HS et al: Ginkgo biloba extract increases ocular blood flow velocity, *J Ocul Pharmacol Ther* 15:276, 1999.

Cignarella A et al: Novel lipid-lowering properties of Vaccinium myrtillus L. leaves, a traditional antidiabetic treatment, in several models of rat dyslipidemia: a comparison with ciprofibrate, *Thromb Res* 84(5):311, 1996.

Contempre B et al: Effect of selenium supplementation in hypothyroid subjects of an iodine and selenium deficient area: the possible danger of indiscriminate supplementation of iodine-deficiency subjects with selenium, *J Clin Endocrinol Metab* 73:213, 1991.

Crofton RW et al: Inorganic zinc and the intestinal absorption of ferrous iron, *Am J Clin Nutr* 50:141, 1989.

Cunningham JJ et al: Hyperzincuria in individuals with insulin-dependent diabetes mellitus: concurrent zinc states and the effect of high dose zinc supplements, *Metabol* 43:1558, 1994.

Davie SJ et al: Effect of vitamin C on glycosylation of protein, *Diabet* 41:167, 1992.

deValk HW et al: Oral magnesium supplementation in insulin requiring type 2 patients, *Diabet Med* 15:503, 1998.

Devaraj S, Chan A, Jialal I: Alpha-tocopherol supplementation decreases plasminogen activator inhibitor-1 and P-selectin levels in type 2 diabetic patients, *Diabet Care* 25:524, 2002.

Diabetes Control and Complications Trial [DCCT] Research Group: The effect of intensive treatment of diabetes on the development and progress of long-term complications in insulin-dependent diabetes mellitus, *N Engl J Med* 329:977, 1993 (updated 1996).

Dillon R: Improved serum insulin profiles in diabetic individuals who massaged their insulin injection sites, *Diabet Care* 6:399, 1983.

Diplock A: Selenium, antioxidant nutrition and human diseases, *Biol Trace Elem Res* 33:155, 1992.

Duke JA: *Handbook of medicinal herbs,* ed 2, New York, 2002, CRC Press.

Eak GA, Tiszka R: Chronic complications of diabetes: a creative management approach, *NP Forum* 9(2):74, 1998.

Egan E: Therapeutic touch. In Snyder M, Lindquist R, editors: *Complementary/alternative therapies in nursing*, New York, 1998, Springer.

Elliott RB et al: A population-based strategy to prevent insulin-dependent diabetes mellitus using nicotinamide, *J Pediatr Endocrinol Metabol* 9:501, 1996.

Elson DF, Meredith M: Therapy for type 2 diabetes mellitus, *West Med J* 97(3):49, 1998.

Ernst E: *The desktop guide to complementary and alternative medicine: an evidence-based approach*, St Louis, 2001, Mosby.

Ezzo J et al: Is massage useful in the management of diabetes? A systematic review, *Diabet Spectr* 14(4):218, 2001.

Facts and Comparisons: *The review of natural products*, St Louis, 2001, Facts and Comparisons.

Feste C, Anderson RM: Empowerment: from philosophy to practice, *Pat Ed Coun* 26(103):139, 1995.

Fetrow C, Avila J: *Professional's handbook of complementary and alternative medicine*, Springhouse, Penn, 1999, Springhouse.

Field TM: *Touch therapy*, Edinburgh, 2000, Churchill Livingstone.

Field TM: Massage therapy effects, *Am Psychol* 53(12):1270, 1998.

Field TM: Massage therapy for infants and children, *J Dev Behav Pediatr* 16:105, 1995.

Field TM et al: Massage therapy lowers blood glucose levels in children with diabetes, *Diabet Spectr* 10(3):237, 1997.

Figlewicz DP et al: Effect of exogenous zinc on insulin secretion in vivo, *Endocrinol* 108:730, 1980.

Flora K et al: Milk thistle for therapy of liver disease, *Am J Gastroenterol* 93:139, 1998.

Fox GN et al: Chromium picolinate supplementation for DM, *J Fam Pract* 46(1):83, 1998.

Frawley D: *Ayurvedic healing: a comprehensive guide*, ed 2, Twin Lakes, Wisc, 2000, Lotus Press.

Gaby AR: Treatment with thyroid hormone [letter], *JAMA* 262:1974, 1989.

Gagne D, Toye L: The effect of therapeutic touch and relaxation therapy on reducing anxiety, *Arch Psychiatr Nurs* 8(3):184, 1994.

Gaitan E et al: In vitro measurement of antithyroid compounds and environmental goitrogens, *J Clin Endocrinol Metabol* 56:767, 1983.

Gill GV et al: Diabetes and alternative medicine: a cause for concern, *Diabet Med* 11(2):210, 1999.

Giugliano D: Cardiovascular health and the Mediterranean diet, *Cardiovas Dis Manag* 795:5, 2001.

Godfrey H et al: A randomized clinical trial on the treatment of oral herpes with topical zinc oxide/glycine, *Alt Ther Health Med* 7(3):49, 2001.

Good M: Biofeedback. In Snyder, M, Lindquist R, editors: *Complementary/alternative therapies in nursing*, New York, 1998, Springer.

Griffith V: Eastern and western paradigms: the holistic natures of traditional Chinese medicine, *Austral J Holistic Nurs* 6(2):35, 1999.

Guthrie D: The use of short term concentrated biofeedback of hospitalized patients with diabetes, *Clin Biofeedback Health* 8(1):1410, 1995.

Guthrie DW, Guthrie RA: *Nursing management of diabetes mellitus: a guide to the pattern approach*, ed 5, New York, 2002, Springer.

Guthrie DW, Moeller T, Guthrie RA: Biofeedback and its application to the stabilization and control of diabetes mellitus, *Am J Clinical Biofeedback* 6(2):82, 1983.

Guthrie DW et al: Effects of parental relaxation training on glycosylated hemoglobin of children with diabetes mellitus, *Pat Educ Counsel* 16(3):247, 1990.

Haines N: Diabetes: treatment by acupuncture, *J Chin Med* 43:5, 1993.

Hanft JR et al: The role of combined magnetic field bone growth stimulation as an adjunct in the treatment of neuroarthropathy/Charcot joint: an expanded pilot study, *J Foot Ankle Surg* 37(6):510, 1998.

Heidenry C: *An introduction to macrobiotics: a beginner's guide to the natural way of health*, Garden City Park, New York, 1991, Avery Publishing Group.

Hemila H: Vitamin C and infectious disease. In Packer L, Fuchs J, editors: *Vitamin C in health and disease*, New York, 1997, Marcel Dekker.

Henricksen JE et al: Impact of ubiquinone (coenzyme Q10) treatment on glycemic control, insulin requirement and well-being in patients with type 1 diabetes mellitus, *Diabet Med* 16(4):312, 1999.

Hernandez NE, Kolb KS: Effects of relaxation on anxiety in primary caregivers and chronically ill children, *Pediatr Nurs* 24(1):51, 1998.

Horrobin DF: Essential fatty acids in the management of impaired nerve function in diabetes, *Diabet* 46(suppl 2):S90, 1997.

Horstman J: *The arthritis foundation's guide to alternative therapies*, Atlanta, Ga, 1999, Arthritis Foundation.

Hu G et al: A study on the clinical effect and immunological mechanism in the treatment of Hashimoto's thyroiditis by moxibustion, *J Tradit Chin Med* 13:14, 1993.

Huebscher R: Peripheral neuropathy: alternative and complementary options, *NP Forum* 11(2):73, 2000.

Hunt LM, Arar NH, Akana LL: Herbs, prayer, and insulin: use of medicinal and alternative treatment by a group of Mexican American diabetes patients, *J Fam Pract* 49:216, 2000.

Jacobs RG et al: Relaxation therapy for hypertension, *Arch Intern Med* 146:233, 1986.

Jamal GA: The use of gamma linolenic acid (GLA) in the prevention and treatment of diabetic neuropathy, *Diabet Med* 11:145, 1994.

Jennings PE et al: Vitamin C metabolites and microangiopathy in diabetes mellitus, *Diabet Res* 6:151, 1987.

Jossa F et al: The Mediterranean diet in the prevention of arteriosclerosis, *Recent Progress Med* 87(4):175, 1996.

Kapoor LD: *Handbook of Ayuveda medicinal plants*, Boca Raton, Fla, 1990, CRC Press.

Keen H et al: Treatment of diabetic neuropathy with gamma linolenic acid, *Diabet Care* 16(1):8, 1993.

Keller E, Bzdek V: Effects of therapeutic touch on tension headache pain, *Nurs Res* 35(2):101, 1986.

Kiecolt-Glaser JK et al: Psychosocial modifiers of immunocompetence in medical students, *Psychosom Med* 46:7, 1984.

Knekt P et al: Low vitamin E status is a potential risk factor for insulin-dependent diabetes mellitus, *J Intern Med* 245(1):99, 1999.

Kolb H, Volker B: Nicotinamide in type 1 diabetes: mechanism of action revisited, *Diabet Care* 22(suppl 2):B16, 1999.

Kramer N: Comparison of therapeutic touch and casual touch in stress reduction of hospitalized children, *Pediatr Nurs* 16(5):483, 1990.

Krieger D: Healing by the laying-on of hands as a facilitator of bioenergetic change: the response of in-vivo human hemoglobin, *Psychoenerget Sys* 1:121, 1974.

Kuhn MA: *Complementary therapies for health care providers*, Philadelphia, 1999, Lippincott Williams & Wilkins.

Kumar D, Marshall H: Diabetic peripheral neuropathy: amelioration of pain with TENS, *Diabet Care* 20:1702, 1997.

Kushi M: *Natural health through macrobiotics*, New York, 1979, Japan Publications (Kushi's works now available through Becket, Mass, 1979, One Peaceful World Press).

Kushi M: *Standard macrobiotic diet*, Becket, Mass, 1996, One Peaceful World Press.

Lad V: *The complete book of Ayurvedic home remedies*, New York, 1998, Harmony.

La Valle J et al: *Natural therapeutics pocket guide*, Hudson, Ohio, 2000, LexiComp.

Leese GP et al: Prevalence of complementary medicine usage within a diabetes clinic, *Pract Diabet Int* 14(7):207, 1997.

Lerner M: *Choices in healing, integrating the best of conventional and complementary approaches to cancer*, Cambridge, Mass, 1994, MIT Press.

Lininger SW et al: *The natural pharmacy*, ed 2, Roseville, Calif, 1999, Prima Publishing.

Ma J, Peng A, Lin S: Mechanisms of the therapeutic effect of astragalus membranaceus on sodium and water retention in experimental heart failure, *Chin Med J* 111(1):17, 1998.

Madar KS et al: Glucose-lowering effect of fenugreek in non-insulin dependent diabetics, *Euro J Clin Nutr* 42:51, 1988.

Mao-liang Q: The treatment of diabetes by acupuncture, *J Chin Med* 15:3, 1984.

Maras MJL et al: Effects of meditation on insulin-dependent diabetes mellitus, *Diabet Educ* 10(1):22, 1984.

McGrady A, Bailey BK, Good M: Biofeedback-assisted relaxation in insulin dependent diabetes mellitus: a controlled study, *Diabet Care* 14:185, 1992.

McGrady A, Graham G, Bailey B: Biofeedback-assisted relaxation in insulin dependent diabetes mellitus: a replications and extension study, *Ann Behav Med* 18(3):47, 1996.

McGrady A, Horner J: Complementary/alternative therapies in general medicine: diabetes mellitus. In Spencer J, Jacobs J, editors: *Complementary/alternative medicine*, St Louis, 1999, Mosby.

McKinney T et al: Effects of guided imagery and music (GIM) therapy on mood and cortisol in healthy adults, *Health Psychol* 16:390, 1997.

Monahan P, Opichka P, Alseth B: MCN spotlight, *MCN* 17:323, 1992.

Morris BW et al: Chromium supplementation improves insulin resistance in patients with type 2 diabetes mellitus, *Diabet Med* 17(9):684, 2000.

Murray M, Pizzorno J: Diabetes mellitus. In Pizzorno J, Murray M, editors: *Textbook of natural medicine*, Philadelphia, 1999, Churchill Livingstone.

Muth ER, Laurent JM, Jasper P: The effect of bilberry nutritional supplementation on night visual acuity and contrast sensitivity, *Alt Med Rev* 5:164, 2000.

Naparstek B: *A meditation to help you control diabetes* [audiotape], Akron: Ohio, 1991, Image Paths and Health Journeys. Also Stress I and II, 1995.

National Academies Press: Vitamins (also elements), 2002. www.nap.edu. Accessed 1/03.

Nield-Anderson L, Ameling A: Reiki: a complementary therapy for nursing practice, *J Psychosoc Nurs Ment Serv* 39(6):42, 2001.

O'Connell B: Select vitamins and minerals in the management of diabetes, *Diabet Spect* 14(3):133, 2001.

O'Connell B: Herbal supplements in diabetes: one dietitian's perspective. On the cutting edge, *Diabet Care Educ* 20(6):11, 1999.

Ornish D et al: Can lifestyle changes reverse coronary heart disease? *Lancet* 336:129, 1990.

Ornish D: *Reversing heart disease,* New York, 1990, Ballentine Books.

Paolisso G et al: Pharmacologic doses of vitamin E improve insulin action in healthy subjects and non-insulin dependent diabetic patients, *Am J Clin Nutr* 57(5):650, 1993.

Paynter OE et al: Goitrogens and thyroid follicular cell neoplasia: evidence for a threshold proces, *Regul Toxicol Pharmacol* 8:102, 1988.

Persaud SJ et al: Gymnema sylvestre stimulates insulin release in vitro by increased membrane permeability, *J Endocrinol* 163:207, 1999.

Pharmacist's Letter/Prescriber's Letter [PL/PL]: *Natural medicine comprehensive database,* ed 4, Stockton, Calif, 2002, Therapeutic Research Faculty.

PL/PL, Continuing Education Booklet: Natural medicines in clinical management of diabetes, *Nat Med Clin Manag* 2:6, 2000.

Pittler MH, Ernest, E: Ginkgo biloba extract for the treatment of intermittent claudication: a meta-analysis of randomized trials, *Am J Med* 108:276, 2000.

Puntillo K, Tesler M: Pain. In Carrieri-Kohlman V, Lindsey A, West C, editors: *Pathophysiological phenomena in nursing,* Philadelphia, 1993, WB Saunders.

Rakel RE: *Saunders manual of medical practice,* ed 2, Philadelphia, 2000, WB Saunders.

Ravina A et al: Clinical use of the trace element chromium (III) in the treatment of DM, *J Trace Elem Exp Med* 8(3):183, 1995.

Rea W: *Chemical sensitivity,* Boca Raton, Fla, 1996, Lewis Publishers.

Reed RL, Mooradian AD: Nutritional status and dietary management of elderly diabetic patients, *Clin Geriatr Med* 6: 883, 1990.

Reljanovic M et al: Treatment of diabetic polyneuropathy with the antioxidant thioctic acid (ALA): a 2-year multi-center randomized double-blind placebo-controlled trial (ALADIN II), *Free Radical Biol Med* 31:171, 1999.

Rice BI, Schindler JV: Effects of thermal biofeedback-assisted relaxation training on blood circulation in the lower extremities of a population with diabetes, *Diabet Care* 15(7):853, 1992.

Rose M: Diabetes: a personal story, *Massage and Bodywork* Feb/March:84, 2001.

Rosensweig L: *New vegetarian cuisine,* Emmaus, Penn, 1994, Rodale.

Sabo CE, Michael SR, Temple LL: The use of alternative therapies by diabetes educators, *Diabet Educ* 25(6):945, 1999.

Sacher R, McPherson R: *Widmann's clinical interpretation of laboratory tests,* Philadelphia, 2000, FA Davis.

Samuels M, Samuels N: *The well adult,* New York, 1988, Summit Books.

Sandstead HH: Requirements and toxicity of essential trace elements, illustrated by zinc and copper, *Am J Clin Nutr* 61(suppl):621S, 1995.

Schmidt DC, Bland JS: Thyroid gland as sentinel: interface between internal and external environment, *Alt Ther Health Med* 3:78, 1997.

Sears B: *A week in the zone,* New York, 2000, Harper.

Sears B: *The zone: a dietary road map,* New York, 2001, Regan Books.

Sears B: *The zone,* New York, 1995, Regan Books.

Shames R, Shames K: *Thyroid power,* New York, 2001, Harper Collins.

Shane-McWhorter L: Biological complementary therapies: a focus on botanical products in diabetes, *Diabet Spectr* 14(4):199, 2001.

Shanmugasundaram E et al: Use of Gymnema sylvestre leaf extract in the control of blood glucose in insulin-dependent diabetes mellitus, *J Ethnopharmacol* 30:281, 1990.

Sharma RD et al: Use of fenugreek seed powder in the management of non-insulin dependent diabetes mellitus, *Nutr Res* 16:1331, 1996.

Sharma RD, Raghuram TC, Sudhaker R: Effect of fenugreek seeds on blood glucose and serum lipids in type I diabetes, *Eur J Clin Nutr* 44:301, 1990.

Sheehan JP et al: Effect of high fiber intake in fish oil-treated patients with non-insulin dependent diabetes mellitus, *J Clin Nutr* 66:1183, 1997.

Shekell PG et al: Congruence between decisions to initiate chiropractic spinal manipulation for low back pain and appropriateness criteria in North America, *Ann Intern Med* 129:9, 1998.

Shon M, Sikora R: Ginkgo biloba extract is the therapy of erectile dysfunction, *J Sex Educ Treatment* 17:53, 1991.

Shuler PA et al: The effects of spiritual/religious practices on psychological well-being among inner city homeless women, *NP Forum* 5:106, 1994.

Siegel RK: Ginseng abuse syndrome: problems with the panacea, *JAMA* 241:1614, 1979.

Sims J: The mechanism of acupuncture analgesia: a review, *Complemen Ther Med* 5(2):102, 1997.

Snowdon D, Phillips R: Does a vegetarian diet reduce the occurrence of diabetes? *Am J Publ Health* 75(5):507, 1985.

Som S et al: Ascorbic acid metabolism in diabetes mellitus, *Metabol* 30:572, 1981.

Sotaniemi EA et al: American ginseng reduces post prandial glycemia in non-diabetic subjects and subjects with type 2 diabetes mellitus, *Arch Intern Med* 160:1009, 1995.

Spencer H et al: Inhibitory effects of zinc on magnesium balance and magnesium absorption in man, *J Am Coll Nutr* 13:479, 1994.

Sunshine W et al: Fibromyalgia benefits from massage therapy and transcutaneous electrical stimulation, *J Clin Rheumatol* 2:18, 1996.

Surwit R et al: Stress management improves long-term glycemic control in type 2 diabetes, *Diabet Care* 25:30, 2002.

Surwit RS, Feinglos MN: The effects of relaxation on glucose tolerance in non-insulin dependent diabetes mellitus, *Diabet Care* 6:176, 1983.

Suzuki J et al: Fasting therapy for psychosomatic diseases with special reference to its indications of therapeutic mechanism, *Tohoku J Experiment Med* 118(suppl): 245, 1976.

Thilly CH et al: The epidemiology of iodine-deficiency disorders in relation to goitrogenic factors and thyroid-stimulating-hormone regulation, *Am J Clin Nutr* 57(suppl 2):267S, 1993.

Time/Life: *The Diet Advisor*, Alexandria, Va, 2000, Time/Life Books.

Tirtha S: *The Ayurvedic encyclopedia: natural secrets to healing, prevention and longevity*, ed 2, Bayville, New York, 1998, Ayurveda Holistic Center Press.

Trow LG et al: Lack of effect of dietary chromium supplementation on glucose tolerance, plasma insulin and lipoproteins levels in patients with type 2 diabetes, *Int J Vit Nutr Res* 11:149, 2000.

Trumbo P et al: Dietary reference intakes: vitamin A, vitamin K, arsenic, boron, chromium, copper, iodine, iron, manganese, molybdenum, nickel, silicon, vanadium, and zinc, *J Am Diebet Assoc* 101(3):294, 2001.

Tutuncu NB, Bayraktar M, Varli K: Reversal of defective nerve conduction with vitamin E supplementation in type 2 diabetes: a preliminary study, *Diabet Care* 21(11):1915, 1998.

Tyler VE: *The honest herbal: a sensible guide to the use of herbs and related remedies*, New York, 1993, Pharmaceutical Products Press.

Valtonen EJ, Lilius HG: Syncardial massage in diabetic and other neuropathies of lower extremities, *Dis Nerv Sys* 34:192, 1973.

van Raaji JA et al: Neurotoxic chlorinated hydrocarbons penetrate the blood-brain barrier possibly by binding to thyroid hormone transport proteins, *Neurotoxicology* 12:818, 1991.

Velussi M et al: Long-term (12 months) treatment with an anti-oxidant drug (silymarin) is effective on hyperinsulinemia, exogenous insulin need and malondialdehyde levels in cirrhotic diabetic patients, *J Hepatol* 26:871, 1997.

Vest G: Acupressure, breath awareness help diabetes patients, *Massage Magazine* 86:64, 2000.

Weintraub M: Magnetic biostimulation in neurologic illness. In Weintraub M, ed: *Alternative and complementary therapies in neurologic illness*, Edinburgh, 2001, Churchill Livingstone.

Wilson RG, David RE: Serum pyridoxal (B6) concentrations in children with diabetes mellitus, *Pathology* 9:95, 1977.

Wirth D, Cram J: The psychophysiology of nontraditional prayer, *Int J Psychsom* 41:68, 1994.

Wirth D et al: Full thickness dermal wounds treated with non-contact therapeutic touch: a replication and extension, *Complement Ther Med* 1:127, 1993.

Wolf SL et al: Reducing frailty and falls in older persons: an investigation of tai chi and computerized balance training, *J Am Geriatr Soc* 44:489, 1996.

Wolfson LR et al: Balance and strength training in older adults: intervention gains and tai chi maintenance, *J Am Geriatr Soc* 44:498, 1996.

Wynd CA: Relaxation imagery used for stress reduction in the prevention of smoking relapse, *J Adv Nurs* 17:294, 1992.

Zhizhou S et al: Blood sugar lowering action of "He Xiang Zuang Qi Gong" and its mechanism on diabetes mellitus, *Clin J Integrat Med* 7(131):146, 1987.

Ziegler D, Gries FA: Alpha-lipoic acid In the treatment of diabetic peripheral and cardiac autonomic neuropathy, *Diabet* 46(suppl 2):S62, 1997.

Ziegler D et al: The ALADIN III Study Group: treatment of symptoms of diabetic polyneuropathy with the anti-oxidant ALA: a 7-month multi-center randomized controlled trial, *Diabet Care* 22:1296, 1999.

Ziegler D et al: The ALADIN Study Group: the treatment of symptomatic diabetic peripheral neuropathy with the anti-oxidant a-lipoic acid: a 3-week multi-centre randomized controlled trial (ALADIN Study I), *Diabetologia* 38:1425, 1995.

Ziegler D et al: Cerebral glucose metabolism in type 1 diabetic patients, *Diabet Med* 11(2):205, 1994.

Ziegler D et al: Effects of treatment with the antioxidant alpha-lipoic acid on cardiac autonomic neuropathy in NIDDM patient: a 4-month randomized controlled multi-center trial (DEKAN Study), *Diabet Care* 20(3):369, 1997.

WEB SITES

http://medherb.com
www.aadenet.org
www.ahmaholistic.com
www.ahna.org
www.alnature.com
www.alternativediabetes.com
www.amtamassage.org
www.childrenwithdiabetes.com
www.diabetes.com

www.diabetes.org
www.diabetesworld.com
www.endocrine@medscape.com
www.feist.com/~dguthrie
www.healingtouch.net
www healthy.net
www.insulin.org/managing/discussion.html
www.jdf.cure
www.nccam.nih.gov
www.neuropathy.org
www.pns.ucsd.edu
www.webmaster@eatright.org

The following categorizations provide a framework for presenting natural-alternative-complementary (NAC) therapies and are a brief overview for understanding NAC modalities from an organized perspective. The categories are divided into chapters: Chapter 11 Alternative Health Care Systems; Chapter 12 Mind-Body-Spirit Interventions; Chapter 13 Biologic-Based Therapies; Chapter 14 Manipulative and Body-Based Methods; and Chapter 15 Energy Therapies. Obviously, NAC modalities often overlap. For example, having a massage, a body-based modality, often affects the mind and spirit. In addition, massages can include energy work, such as shiatsu or polarity. Overlap also occurs with most alternative health care systems because they employ modalities from several other categories. From a holistic perspective, a person cannot be separated into parts, and one modality cannot be identified as biologic and the other as mind-body-spirit. However, the presented framework is convenient and is modeled after (with a few word changes) the National Center for Complementary and Alternative Medicine (NCCAM) format. The reader is referred to references and web sites for details on modalities, including cautions, contraindications, side effects, and specific credentialing and regulation of practitioners. Chapter 11 is more detailed than are other chapters because alternative health care systems often are the most unfamiliar to conventional health care providers yet provide rich cultural information and create the basis for many of the other modalities.

ALTERNATIVE HEALTH CARE SYSTEMS

Asha K. Anumolu ▪ Helen Miller ▪ Mercy Mammah Popoola ▪ Brenda Talley ▪
Alison Rushing ▪ Roxana Huebscher ▪ Pamela Shuler

Alternative health care systems (called alternative medical systems by NCCAM) are health care systems that have their own theory, philosophy, and practice, often differing markedly from conventional Western medical philosophy. Traditional systems from other countries are in this category, including Traditional Chinese Medicine, Ayurveda (East Indian), and curanderismo. In addition, several well-entrenched health care systems in the United States include homeopathy, naturopathy, African practices, and Native-American health practices that have been in existence for thousands of years. Box 11-1 lists examples of alternative health care systems. Chapter 11 offers detail on a few of these alternative health care systems, as well as an overview of shamanism. In addition, an example of a traditional yet current United States health care system is offered, that of the Georgia Low Country. Several of these narratives are culturally rich, offering a first-person point of view.

Box 11-1

Examples of Alternative Health Care Systems

Aboriginal
African
Ayurveda
Mexican, Central and South American (including curanderismo)
Homeopathy
Middle-Eastern (including Unani)
Native American (including shamanism)
Naturopathy
Tibetan
Traditional Chinese Medicine
Traditional North American Health Care Practices

■ AYURVEDA: SCIENCE OF LIFE

Asha K. Anumolu

May all beings find happiness
May all be free of disease
May all see what is auspicious
May no one suffer
OM, peace, peace, peace (Frawley, 1999, p. 12)

Ayurveda is the knowledge of life. "Ayuh" means "life" and "veda" means "knowledge." Ayurveda connotes a combination of sharira (body), indriya (perceptory organs), satwa (mind), and atma (soul) (Frawley, 1999). Ayurveda proposes that the human is a microcosm, a universe within self. Ayurveda views health and "disease" in holistic terms with an inherent relationship among the individual, cosmic spirit, consciousness, energy, and matter. Ayurveda is often defined as medical-metaphysical healing life science (Frawley, 1998; Lad, 1984; Rhyner, 1998; Sharma, 1998). Ayurveda dates back to the Vedic period of India (Frawley, 1998; Lad, 1984; Sharma, 1998) and has been the health care system of India for 5000 years (Mishra et al, 2001a). Ayurveda is not only a science, but also a philosophy of pure existence (Frawley, 1999; Lad, 1984). The quest for a happy life and good health has been an incessant urge in human beings for thousands of years. To satisfy themselves, humans have endeavored to explore all possible avenues in search of good health. The uniqueness of this science is that it deals not only with the cure of the disease, but also with the maintenance of physical and psychosocial health of an individual and of society as a whole (Frawley, 1999; Lad, 1984). In this chapter, the major concepts surrounding Ayurveda are described, including a definition, five basic elements (pancha mahabutas), tridoshic concept, trigunas, and determination of constitution. As a drop in the ocean, the information presented here is only a small part of Ayurvedic science.

AYURVEDA *PANCHA MAHABHUTAS:* THE FIVE BASIC ELEMENTS

According to Ayurveda, all matter is composed of the following five elements:

Akasa: ether, the most subtle of the elements and the source of the other four

Vayu: air, the equivalent of the gaseous state of matter

Tejas: fire, the equivalent of the transformative power of matter

Ap: water, the equivalent to the liquid state of matter

Prithvi: earth, matter is solid state (Lad, 1998; Livingstone-Shealy, 1998)

A cell consists of all five elements. The earth element gives structure to the cell. Cytoplasm or liquid in the cell is the water element. The fire element governs the metabolism. The air element predominates in the gases in the cell, and the space occupied by cell represents the ether element (Lad, 1998; Livingstone-Shealy, 1998).

DISEASE CAUSES

People are made up of mind and body, the mind being *atma* (soul, spirit) and *nana* (mood, cognition). The body is made up of *dhatus* (body tissues), *malas* (waste products), and *doshas*. When these factors are balanced, good health results. When unbalanced state or imperfect functioning occurs, then disease results (Mishra et al, 2001a).

TRIDOSHIC CONCEPT

According to Ayurveda, the physiologic system has three basic constituents (bioenergies) called *doshas* (Livingstone-Shealy, 1998; Edward, 1998). The Tridoshic concept is a pivotal principle in Ayurveda. Biologic existence is considered to be a combination of the three doshas: *Vata, Pitta,* and *Kapha.* These doshas are the physical expressions of the five elements (Sharma, 1998).

Vata
Vata predominates at age 55 and up. Vata dosha is made up predominantly of ether and air elements and is a principle of movement. Vata is responsible for the functions of the central and sympathetic nervous system, respiration, movements, excretion, and normal processing of all body constituents such as blood, muscles, fats, and bones. The large intestine, bones, skin, pelvis, thighs, and ears are the seats of vata. Vata also governs feeling and emotions, such as nervousness, anxiety, fear, and pain (Lad, 1998; Livingstone-Shealy, 1998).

Pitta
Pitta predominates at puberty and lasts through middle age. Pitta dosha has a predominance of fire and water elements. Pitta deals with the functions of heat production and metabolism; the processes of vision, digestion, and secretion; hunger and thirst; and softness and luster of the body. Pitta influences intellect and cheerfulness. Pitta arouses anger, hate, and jealousy. The small intestine, stomach, eyes, sweat glands, blood, fat, and skin seat pitta (Lad, 1998; Livingstone-Shealy, 1998).

Kapha
Kapha predominates in childhood. Kapha dosha has a predominance of water and earth elements. Normal functions of kapha include firmness, binding, heaviness, potency, and strength. Kapha is responsible for reproduction and nourishment of cells and tissues in the body, and it provides biologic strength, vigor, stability, and supports memory retention. Psychologically, kapha is responsible for emotional attachment, greed, and envy. The chest is the seat of kapha (Lad, 1998; Livingstone-Shealy, 1998).

INDIVIDUAL CONSTITUTION

Each person is considered to have a preponderance of certain elements in the body when born. This preponderance of elements and a particular dosha that defines the qualities of a person is called the individual's constitution. Seven possible constitutions have been identified: (1) vata, (2) pitta, (3) kapha, (4) vata-pitta, (5) pitta-kapha, (6) vata-kapha, and (7) vata-pitta-kapha (Lad, 1998; Edward, 1998). The basic constitution of the individual is known to have been determined at the time of conception, based on the constitutions demonstrated by the parents' bodies, and it tends to remain unaltered throughout life because it is genetically determined.

However, changes in the environment can alter the combination of elements. Life is defined as a dynamic interaction between the external and internal environments. The external environment comprises the cosmic forces (macrocosm), and the internal forces (microcosm) are governed by the basic principles of vata-pitta-kapha. A balance among the three doshas is necessary for health (Lad, 1998; Sharma, 1998; Svoboda, 1999).

DETERMINING THE INDIVIDUAL CONSTITUTION

The descriptions in Table 11-1 reflect the pure aspect of each constitutional element. However, no individual constitution is made up solely of any one element. Rather, each person is a combination of all three elements, with a predominant tendency toward one or two.

TRIGUNAS CONCEPT

Trigunas, called the gunas of mind, are a concept referring to the three basic constituents of the individual's psychosocial system. *Satwa, Rajas,* and *Tamas* are the trigunas of the mind (Baidynath, 1990). *Satwa* is the consciousness or knowledge; it is the neutral or balancing force. *Satwa* imparts virtues such as faith, honesty, self-control, truthfulness, and modesty (Baidynath, 1990). *Rajas* is the motion or action that initiates change; it is the quality of passion and agitation. *Rajas* gives rise to emotional fluctuations of attraction and repulsion, fear and desire, and love and hate (Baidynath, 1990). *Tamas* is the inertia and quality of darkness and is responsible for ignorance and attachment. *Tamas* causes dullness, heaviness, emotional clinging, and stagnation (Baidynath, 1990). These trigunas are demonstrated in temperament, constitution, and behavior and are therefore responsible for personality development.

DIAGNOSIS *(NIDAN)* AND TREATMENT *(CHIKITSA)*

Diagnosis is made by observation, touch, questioning, pulse diagnosis, and the examination of urine and stool, tongue, bodily sounds, eye, and skin, as well as total body appearance. Digestive capacity, personal habits, and a patient's resilience are also obtained (Mishra et al, 2001b).

Table 11-1	Ayurveda: Determining the Constitution		
Constitutional Element, Aspect	**Vata**	**Pitta**	**Kapha**
Frame	Thin	Moderate	Large
Weight	Under	Moderate	Over
Skin	Dry, cool, rough	Oily, warm, soft	Oily, thick, cool
Hair	Dry, kinky	Oily, soft, early graying, hair loss	Oily, thick, wavy
Teeth	Crooked	Moderate in size	Strong, white, well formed
Eyes	Small, active	Sharp, penetrating	Big, attractive, thick lashes
Appetite	Variable	Strong, excessive	Slow but steady
Faith	Wavering, changeable	Determined, fanatic	Steady, loyal
Memory	Recent: good; Remote: poor	Sharp	Slow but excellent
Dreams	Fearful, flying, jumping	Anger, war, passionate	Watery, swimming, romantic, ocean
Sleep	Scanty, interrupted	Little but sound	Heavy, prolonged
Thirst	Variable	Excessive	Slight
Elimination	Hard, dry, constipated	Soft, oily, loose	Thick, oil
Physical activity	Very active	Moderate	Lethargic
Mental activity	Restless, active, curious	Aggressive, intelligent	Calm, slow

Baidynath, 1990; Frawley, 1998; Lad, 1984, 1998; Sharma, 1998; Tiwari, 1995.

Ayurvedic treatment consists of cleansing (shodan), palliation or reduction in the intensity of the disease (shaman), rejuvenation (rasayan), and mental nurturing and spiritual healing (satwajaya) (Mishra et al, 2001b). Cleansing includes five processes called panchakarma: cleansing the intestines, cleansing the stomach and duodenum, medicated enemas, medicated nasal oils, and bloodletting (seldom used). These actions are not all done simultaneously. These cleansings rid the body of ama or "undigested, unabsorbed, or unassimilated food products that look like sticky substances" (Mishra et al, 2001b, p. 45).

Palliation involves kindling the digestive fire, burning toxic waste, fasting, observing thirst, practicing yoga, lying in the sun, breathing exercise, and meditation. Herbs may be used in some of these processes. Rasayanas are herbal and dietary supplements and are taken daily with food (Mishra et al, 2001b). Removing serious worry (chinta) and spiritual nurturing are also a part of treatment.

Some other terminology used in this text that is related to treatment includes herb combinations and a reference to ghee. Ghee is made by two methods, either from butter or from unhomogenized milk that is turned into yogurt (dahi), then mixed with water and churned; when the cream comes out on top, it is heated until the milk solids precipitate out (Sharma, Clark, 2000). For the first method, butter is melted until the water evaporates; for a pound of unsalted butter this process takes about 30 to 40 minutes with the heat low. The milk solids are strained off and discarded; what is left is the ghee. The ghee is cooled, covered, and stored at room temperature. The whole process takes about 1½ hours. Ghee is made in glass, enameled, or stainless steel cookware and never left unattended while making (Sharma, 2000).

Ayurveda, the traditional healthcare system of India, offers many therapies and a unique perspective when compared with conventional Western medicine. Ayurvedic therapies could be used for many conditions.

REFERENCES

Baidynath: Book of Ayurvedic knowledge, Nagpur, 1990, Swati Enterprise.

Edward T: Ayurveda revolutionized: integrating ancient and modern Ayurveda, Delhi, 1998, Motilal Banarsidass Publishers Private Limited.

Frawley D: Ayurvedic healing: a comprehensive guide, Salt Lake City, Utah, 1998, Passage Press.

Frawley D: Yoga and Ayurveda: self-healing and self-realization, Twin Lakes, Wisc, 1999, Lotus Press.

Lad V: Ayurveda: the science of self-healing, Santa Fe, NM, 1984, Lotus Press.

Lad V: The complete book of Ayurvedic home remedies, New York, 1998, Harmony.

Livingstone-Shealy CN: The illustrated encyclopedia of healing remedies, Boston, 1998, Element Books.

Mishra L, Singh B, Dagenais S: Ayurveda: a historical perspective and principles of the traditional health care system in India, *Alt Ther Health Med* 7(2):36, 2001a.

Mishra L, Singh B, Dagenais S: Healthcare and disease management in Ayurveda, *Alt Ther Health Med* 7(2):44, 2001b.

Rhyner H: *Ayurveda: the gentle health system*, Delhi, 1998, Motilal Banarsidass Publishers Private Limited.

Sharma H, Clark C: *Contemporary Ayurveda*, Edinburgh, 2000, Churchill.

Sharma P: *Essentials of Ayurveda: sodasangahrdayam*, ed 2, Delhi, 1998, Motilal Banarsidass Publishers Private Limited.

Svoboda R: *Ayurveda for women: a guide to vitality and health*, Newport Devon, Italy, 1999, LEGO SpA.

■ TRADITIONAL CHINESE HEALTH CARE PRACTICES

Helen Miller

Chinese medicine is a system of logical theory and thought developed over more than 2000 years. Traditional modalities of treatment have included herbs, acupuncture and moxibustion, Tai chi, Qi gong, Tui na (Chinese massage), feng shui, and astrology. A Consensus Panel of the National Institutes of Health (NIH Consensus, 1998) has approved acupuncture for postoperative nausea; chemotherapy and pregnancy nausea; and postoperative dental pain. In addition, the Panel found that acupuncture might be "useful as an adjunct treatment or an acceptable alternative or be included in a comprehensive management program" (NIH Consensus, 1998, p. 1518) for addiction, stroke rehabilitation, headache, menstrual cramps, epicondylitis, fibromyalgia, myofascial pain, osteoarthritis, low back pain, carpal tunnel syndrome, and asthma (NIH Consensus, 1998; Villaire, 1998). Chinese health care principles include yin-yang balance, energy flow along channels, and the concept of Qi (pronounced "chee"), as well as the other basic substances of the body in the presence of assessing, describing, and treating problems (Kaptchuk, 1983).

VITAL SUBSTANCES

Qi is the body's vital energy and is considered most important in the harmonious working of the body. The functions of Qi are numerous: transports nutrients through the digestive system; warms the entire body, including the extremities; holds fluids in their normal place; protects the body from outside invasion through the skin and immune system; transforms fluids and nutrients into both useable and waste products; and rises along the mid-line of the body to keep the organs in their proper place (Maciocia, 1989). When Qi becomes *deficient*, general symptoms such as fatigue, cold hands and feet, or edema may occur. *Stagnant* Qi feels like pain, bloating, or congestion. *Counterflow* Qi produces symptoms such as vomiting or coughing. *Sinking* Qi may demonstrate as a prolapsed organ or hernia.

Blood as a substance is fairly similar to the Western medical concept of Blood; it moistens and nourishes our bodies. In Chinese medicine, Blood also stabilizes the mind. If Blood becomes *deficient*, fatigue and dizziness (as in anemia) may occur; the person may also feel restless and sleep poorly as part of that pattern of imbalance. If Blood becomes *stagnant*, sharp stabbing pains may occur, as with an acute injury or menstrual cramps with clot formation (Maciocia, 1989).

Jing, or "essence," is a specific kind of energy housed in the Kidney. (See expanded description in section on menopause.) Jing encompasses a hereditary energy that helps determine constitution and is also involved in growth, development, and reproduction (Maciocia, 1989). If Jing is *deficient*, children may grow poorly, or adults may have problems with sexual function or brain activity.

Body fluids include saliva, mucus, and sweat, as well as urine and excretory fluids. *Deficiency* of body fluids produces dryness in the body; and *stagnant* fluid may appear as edema or thickened secretions.

Shen includes the mental, emotional, and spiritual aspects of a person. (See expanded description in section on anxiety.) Shen also involves the memory and consciousness. A *deficiency* of Shen presents as a loss of interest in life; thus Shen is one of the most crucial indicators of prognosis in a patient. *Disturbed* Shen appears as inappropriate behavior or reactions.

Qi is considered the basis of all other substances of the body. Qi has many functions in the working of the body and mind: without Qi, the Blood cannot be formed and flow through the vessels; the persons would be unable to use the Jing to grow, develop, and reproduce; the body fluids would not be distributed through the tissues and organs; and the person would not have mental and emotional stability (Maciocia, 1989). Thus all of these substances work together to produce a healthy state. When an imbalance in the flow or supply of substances to the organs and limbs of the body occurs, pain or other symptoms result.

MERIDIAN SYSTEM

Qi flows through the meridian system of the body. Each of the 12 principal meridians relates to an internal organ and connects the interior of the body with the exterior (Beinfield, Korngold, 1991). The 12 principal meridians are Lung, Large Intestine, Stomach, Spleen, Heart, Small Intestine, Urinary Bladder, Kidney, Pericardium, Triple Burner, Gallbladder, and Liver. (The Triple Burner is the only meridian related to a concept rather than a solid organ, referring to a threefold division of the body trunk into sections that function to distribute Qi and fluids throughout the body [Maciocia, 1989].) Appendix B contains diagrams. The meridian's acupuncture points are needled to influence the circulation of Qi and Blood in the local area and to the related organ. For instance, Lung disorders may be treated by puncturing points along the Lung meridian, treating points over the lung area, or both.

YIN AND YANG

Another basic premise of Chinese medicine is the importance of the balance of Yin and Yang. Yin represents the moist, cooling, substantial aspects of nature—the water element. Yang represents the warm, dry, insubstantial aspects of nature—the fire element. Yin and Yang are interactive, dynamic, interdependent symbols of nature itself. The human body is seen as a microcosm of the world around us, using language of Yin and Yang to describe problems of imbalance relating to the specific organs (Gerber, 1988). The supply and orderly flow of the substances of the body help maintain the Yin-Yang balance of the body.

CHINESE DIAGNOSIS

Two methods of diagnosis are specific to Chinese medicine: pulse diagnosis and observation of the tongue. The pulse is palpated at the radial artery on both wrists in three positions. The right wrist yields information about the lung, stomach, and kidney yang energy; the left wrist yields information about the heart, liver, and kidney yin energy. Several complementary pulse positions are listed for the gallbladder, esophagus, and diaphragm. The depth and quality of the pulse in each position give an indication of the amount of energy available in that organ system and the condition of that energy, whether it is stagnant, disturbed, or hot. A normal range for the rate of the pulse depends on the age of the patient (Maciocia, 1989).

The tongue is observed for its color, shape, coating, and moisture. A normal color is pink, and the coating should be very light or absent. The shape should be not too large or too small, no creases or cracks, and no teeth imprints. A normal tongue should be slightly moist (Maciocia, 1989).

EXAMPLE OF CHINESE DIAGNOSIS

The case of a menopausal woman with hot flashes and low back pain is an example of the way in which the concepts of Chinese medicine are used in practice. The diagnosis is a deficiency of Yin, the moistening and cooling element, which causes the woman to feel abnormally warm. The Yin and Yang elements are not balancing each other. This imbalance is comparable to a machine running with too little lubrication and becoming overheated. The moisture is essential for cooling the body and regulating the Yang or fire energy. The deep quality of the Kidney position on pulse palpation indicates a deficiency of Kidney Qi. This deficiency is contributing to the woman's low back pain and her Yin deficiency, because the Kidney is the main regulator of Yin and Yang balance. Treatment consists of an herbal formula (to help cool and moisten the system and support the Kidney) and acupuncture (to open stagnation in the meridians and relieve the back pain). Acupuncture in the kidney area and on the Kidney meridian helps restore Yin-Yang balance in the body and stabilize the kidney energy.

TREATMENT WITH ACUPUNCTURE

In a typical treatment, 10 to 14 points may be chosen to address a painful area or to balance organ energies. Needles are presterilized and disposable. A typical treatment lasts 20 to 30 minutes with the patient lying in a comfortable position. Certain points are not used on pregnant women to ensure stability of the pregnancy. Adverse effects are rare, with bruising seen occasionally (Ehling, 2001).

Sham Acupuncture in Research

One of the commonly used methods of study comparison is to do real acupuncture on one group of research participants and to do sham acupuncture on a comparison group. Improvement is sometimes seen in both groups, and so the conclusion is made that real acupuncture is a placebo effect. In fact, acupuncture, even sham points, can be very regulating to the entire system, and in some conditions the acupuncture points do not need to be as specific as in other cases.

> Placement of a needle in any position elicits a biological response that complicates the interpretation of studies involving sham acupuncture. Thus, there is substantial controversy over the use of sham acupuncture in control groups. (NIH Consensus, 1998, p. 1520)

An example involves acupuncture in the knee area for arthritis pain. The sham acupuncture points were in fact very close to the "real" points and might be considered "ashi" or "ouch" points that may be needled in a clinical situation to help the circulation in the painful area. Both the "real" and the "sham" groups improved (Takeda, Wessel, 1994). This finding illustrates some of the difficulties with the scientific methods of research in looking at an energetic modality.

Another type of example involves two asthma studies. Results indicated that lung function did not significantly improve, but the patient's feeling of well being did improve (Biernacki, Peake, 1998; Yu, Lee, 1976). This finding may be an indication that the overall system was functioning better, and the subjects felt a change in their anxiety involving their breathing processes. The subjects, in turn, would be able to rally their own resources more effectively to deal with stimuli affecting breathing, as was shown by a decrease in the use of bronchodilators.

QI GONG

Qi gong is mentioned several times in the text as an alternative modality. "Qi gong is an ancient Chinese meditative moving exercise that is similar to, but more profound, than T'ai Chi Ch'uan. Qi gong has been practiced in China for thousands of years to improve health and longevity" (Sancier, Hole 2001, p. 197). "The practice of qi gong is divided into three main applications: medical, spiritual, and martial" (p. 197). "The benefits of qi gong can be achieved by self-practice, but for serious illness a qi gong therapist may be required to diagnose the illness and recommend suitable exercises. In diagnosing, the qi gong therapist senses the patient's body field for blocks to the flow of qi. The therapist may also diagnose according to traditional Chinese medicine by examining the tongue, eyes, and pulses at the radial artery of the wrist" (p. 197-198). The principles of qi gong are mediation, awareness, breathing and movement.

RESOURCES AND REGULATION

For more information or to find a qualified practitioner who uses acupuncture, contact the American Association of Oriental Medicine at 610-266-1433. Additionally, the NCCAM at the NIH can be accessed at http://www.nih.gov. To view the acupuncture position paper, see http:// odp.od.nih.gov/consensus/statements/cdc/107/107 stmt.html.

States vary regarding regulation of acupuncture and oriental medicine. The National Commission for the Certification of Acupuncturists and Oriental Medicine (NCCAOM) has established standards. States may use the NCCAOM examination as part of meeting licensing and registration requirements.

REFERENCES

Beinfield H, Korngold E: *Between heaven and earth*, New York, 1991, Ballantine Books.

Biernacki W, Peake M: Acupuncture in treatment of stable asthma, *Res Med* 92:9, 1998.

Ehling D: Oriental medicine: an introduction, *Alt Ther Health Med* 7(4):71, 2001.

Gerber R: *Vibrational medicine*, Santa Fe, NM, 1988, Bear and Company.

Kaptchuk T: *The web that has no weaver*, New York, 1983, Congdon and Weed.

Maciocia G: *The foundations of Chinese medicine*, New York, 1989, Churchill Livingstone.

National Institutes of Health [NIH] Consensus Development Panel on Acupuncture: Acupuncture, *JAMA* 280(17):1518, 1998.

Sancier K, Hole L: Qigong and neurologic disease. In Weintraub M, ed: *Alternative and complementary treatment in neurologic illness*, Edinburgh, 2001, Churchill Livingstone.

Takeda W, Wessel J: Acupuncture for the treatment of pain of osteoarthritic knee, *Arthr Care Res* 7(3):11, 1994.

Villaire M: NIH consensus confirms acupuncture's efficacy, *Alt Ther Health Med* 4(1):21, 1998.

Yu D, Lee S: Effect of acupuncture on bronchial asthma, *Clin Sci Mol Sci* 51:503, 1976.

■ TRADITIONAL AFRICAN HEALING PRACTICES

Mercy Mammah Popoola

AFRICA: A HUGE CONTINENT

As of 2001, there were 44 African countries. Africa is rooted in the center of human civilization and is composed of many cultures and a rich history of vast and diverse traditions. Countries include Niger, located in North Africa and predominantly a desert nation; Somalia, located in East Africa, unique for its homogenous language, culture, and severe famine; Kenya, located on the equator on the east coast, known for the wildlife environment and safaris; Morocco, located on the northwestern coast, popular for its close proximity to Spain; Ghana, located on the Gulf of Guinea in West Africa (formally known as the Gold Coast), known for its Kente cloth; Namibia (formerly southwest Africa), bound in part by South Africa; Mozambique, which stretches along the southeast coast where civil war, drought, and famine have made the country among the world's poorest; South Africa, located in the southern tip of Africa and famous for its place in history with apartheid and Nelson Mandela; and finally, Nigeria, Africa's most populous black country, situated on the southern border along the Gulf of Guinea in West Africa and famous for its oil production and overpopulation. One similarity among the diversity of the countries is that NAC modalities have been and still are a major aspect of health care practices in Africa. For example, Egypt, a country that occupies the northeast corner of Africa, has documented traditional health care and healing practices since the beginning of civilization and is currently known for its NAC practice of aromatherapy (Buckle, 2001; Mentgen, 2001; Kozier et al, 2000). The author of this portion of the text, although now a citizen of the United States, is originally from Nigeria.

SUPERNATURAL POWER AND BELIEF

What follows is the author's perspective on traditional African healing beginning with a case history of a patient. A well-known traditional healer, whom the author interviewed several years ago, introduced the patient, Mr. Ojo. The following is Mr. Ojo's story:

> Twenty years ago I was taken to a native doctor who chained me and gave me some herbs and tea to drink, which helped me with some of my anxiety and behavior problems. Prior to this treatment, I used to be very noisy and thought that everyone was going to kill or harm me.

I had many frightful dreams and could not go to work or to church. Some of my family members left me, but some of them took me to the Aladura Church (Celestial Church). I had never been to a celestial church before, but no sooner had I started going to this church than I began to feel normal again. I made new friends in church and continued to take my herb and tea. We always danced in the church and that tends to help to alleviate some of my fears and anxieties. After five months in this church, I left because I was able to go to work again. Three weeks after I left the church, all my initial problems started again, and my family had to take me back to that church. I have now been here six years with no problems, and I even helped others who came here for similar or different problems get well and return to work.

A similar story is reported in Erinosho's (1981) book. Erinosho noted that, in Africa, churches such as the celestial church are well known not only for helping with the healing of physical illnesses, but more so for treating mental illnesses. Herbs, dance therapy, prayers, holy water, and imagery are some of the NAC health care therapies used throughout Africa (Kelly, 1995; Morrison, Thornton, 1999; Hilderbrandt, 1997; Wilkinson, Gcabashe, Lurie, 1999).

Traditional African health care practices are ancient and have evolved in the last 2 centuries. Traditions have been passed down from generation to generation or are learned or acquired as a spiritual encounter or calling. With the recent interest in NAC modalities, the need to revisit the origin and root of some of these NAC practices has increased (Kelly, 1995; Morrison, Thornton, 1999; Hodes, 1997; Stone, 2001). These interests have led to study of native doctors and traditional healers (Cocks, Dold, 2000; Homsy et al, 1999; Chipfakacha, 1997; Ntuli, 1997; Courtright, 1995; Alexander, 1985). In this part of the text, traditional African health care practices are presented from the perspective of a holistic African nurse trained in the African and Western worldview who has traveled and lived in several African countries. Information is provided from interviews with several African traditional and spiritual experts, healers, health care providers, and citizens about their experiences and understanding of the traditional African health care and healing practices within their countries. Subjects from 10 African countries participated in the interviews. A total of 45 Africans were interviewed. Common health care practices include herbs, Christian and Islamic treatments of religious prayers and verses, and the appeal to different spirits. The research is part of an ongoing data-collection process to continue the second edition of the book, *Where in Africa? A Cultural Saga From Denver* [Colorado, USA] *to Lagos* [Lagos, Nigeria] (Popoola, 2000).

The story of Joan of Arc is similar to the way in which traditional African healers operate. At the age of 13, Joan of Arc began hearing what she believed to be "celestial voices." As the voices, and sometimes visions, continued to appear to Joan, she eventually became certain that the voices she heard were those of St. Michael, St. Catherine, and St. Margaret, all angels. The voices told Joan that she needed to save her people and reunite France. The young woman led her army to a defeat over the English at Compiegne, near Paris. Joan was tried by the church for heresy, and, because of her strong will and beliefs, she was put to death for not admitting that she was wrong about her claim of hearing celestial voices.

Similarly traditional healers of any culture are often a strong and powerful male or female with strong celestial, syncretic, spiritual, and magical powers (Jarret, 1981; Erinosho, 1981; Coppo, 1985; Tsey, 1997). These healers are unwilling to deny their power no matter the circumstances. Many traditional healers claim to have the ability to communicate with a higher being such as God, Allah, other gods, some space, or objects. Such powers may be used to save an entire community, as in the case of "town criers"; or powers are used to treat simple or complex physical or mental illnesses, stresses, and injuries.

Most African societies are still male-dominated, polygamous, and have many different languages with diverse ethnic and cultural beliefs. African countries are still developing, and the majority of the citizens are very poor. Even with the presence of modern health care systems, many African citizens cannot afford modern health care. In addition, many of the countries, after building hospital and clinic infrastructures, found that they were unable to afford medical equipment and supplies or even pay their health care providers. Today, traditional healers and therapies coexist in conjunction with modern medicine (biomedical), and traditional health practices are closely linked with religious and cultural traditions.

The predominant traditional African health care practices of most Africans are native doctors, as well as cultural, magical, and religious ethnic healers. The concept of supernatural forces, spiritual power, and the notion of "hot-cold" energy balances are the roots of traditional practices. The biomedical or modern practices, though present in every African country, have not replaced traditional practices (Ataudo, 1995).

A belief in supernatural power or being is strong. Traditional healers may have consultation with a priest and with God to seek luck and to avoid evil and illness. Some illnesses are perceived to originate from supernatural, magical, religious beliefs and must therefore be cured by traditional and ethnic treatments or magical spells. Traditionally, people still may believe in the practice of sorcery, and take daily precautions or make periodic sacrifices, to protect self and family against harm, jealousy, or evil spirits.

Christian, Islamic, and pagan treatments, such as prayers, verses, amulets, and the art of appealing to different icons, or spirit or God, are among the beliefs central to African health care practice. In addition, some of the general beliefs underlying traditional African health care practices as a whole include the following:

1. Human beings have two parts: body (mass) and spirit.
2. The mind is a part of the spirit that makes the whole (holistic) person.
3. Spiritual and cultural beliefs are important for healing the body, mind, spirit, and for the whole well being [holistic healing].
4. Health care is a mix of biomedical, magical, spiritual, traditional, holistic, and supernatural beliefs and practices.
5. The origin of modern medicine has its roots in the practice of traditional and herbal healers.
6. Most medicines come from roots, trees, herbs, plants, flowers, and seeds that are the tools of traditional healers.
7. Traditional healers act as facilitators who assist the person to rebalance energy from illness to wellness.

TRADITIONAL HEALING PRACTICES

African traditional healers use many healing therapies. In areas with limited biomedical practices, some very rural areas still favor traditional practices such as healing by cauterization and bloodletting that claim to "burn out" or "let out" evil spirits. Additionally, traditional healing practices include many respected and skilled bonesetters who are located throughout the rural and urban parts of different African countries and are famous for their orthopedic and wound healing skills. Traditional healers or native doctors treat sprains, swellings, and other selected problems, as well as other physical and mental illnesses. These healers are also counselors who give advice and use healing cultural artifacts and icons such as stones, beads, and roots. These healers are generally known as the shaman (Rankin-Box, 2001). Some specific NAC therapeutic practices include ancient healing practices or native doctors, herbal healing practices, folk remedies (acupuncture, massage, and chiropractor), dermabrasive techniques (cupping, pinching, rubbing, and burning), amulets, prayers, holy water, ashes, rituals (birth and death practices), healing dance, town criers, magic hand or touch practices, and a combination of home remedies.

ROLE OF THE HERBALIST AND HOMEOPATHY

Herbalists are people who are skilled in the use of herbs, roots, and plants. Homeopaths, as local chemists or pharmacists, have the ability to mix extracts from roots, food, tea, and plants that are used to treat specific illnesses. However, herbs are not the only healing tools that herbalists use. For example, herbalists treat common disorders and specialize in the treatment of the "evil eye." The evil eye is supposed to cast spells or curses that can lead to illness and death. This belief cuts across many African countries.

Herbalists and homeopaths often boil ingredients and roots into tea or steam inhalants, and they frequently promote self-care and self-medications. Such steam inhalants are frequently used as bronchodilators.

SPIRITUAL AND IMAGINARY HEALERS

Spiritual and imaginary healing involves the mind, the spirit, and the relationship to the body. Prophets of various celestial or syncretic churches are classified as traditional healers or shamans. Today, some of these NAC practices are known as relaxation exercises, biofeedback, massages, healing touch, imagery, yoga, meditation, prayer, music therapy, humor, laughter, and hypnosis (Dossey et al, 1988; Campbell, 2000; Saeki, 2000; Mentgen, 2001).

Spiritual healers and imaginative healers have their roots in ancient spiritual practices, as well as in Christian churches. Prayers and the healing power of God are used for protection against misfortune, and holy water is used as a symbol of communion with the healer. Christian healing churches, such as the celestial, or Aladura and/or faith-healing churches, are common. In some religious practices, such as Islam, that dictate health-promotion practices, the citizens take a passive role in the healing process.

FOLK HEALERS AND AMULETS

Folk healers have special areas of expertise and therapeutics. Folk remedies include a variation of massage, herbal remedies, and dermabrasive practices such as cupping, pinching, rubbing, and burning. These dermabrasive therapies and practices are believed to release the bad energy or evil spirits, thereby restoring health. Amulets on a bracelet, necklace, or pinned to clothing provide some protection against evil and certain illnesses. Wrist strings, also worn around the neck, ankles, and waist, are worn to prevent harm. Amulets inscribed with verses of the Koran or the Bible, turquoise stones, or a charm of a hand with five fingers enhance protection powers against the evil spirit or "evil eye."

BIRTH PRACTICES AND RITUALS

Many babies are still delivered at home with the mother in a squatting position or being tied to some object (as in some African countries). Traditionalists will use bellybands after the delivery to assist with the expulsion of the placenta and to decrease the size of the abdomen. Traditionally, the newborn is believed to be susceptible to evil influences during the first week of life, and caution is taken as to the number and type of visitors. For male infants, the natives usually perform circumcision in the first 2 weeks following birth. Immediately after the birth, bowls of clear water soup, prepared during the delivery process, are offered if the birth is successful to give thanks to the spirit; and the baby may then be taken away for a brief time (a few hours) if the baby is a son. Mothers are usually instructed not to drink iced drinks but to have only warm foods and liquids (Odebiyi, 1989; Ogaga, 1999). Traditional practices include numerous birth taboos, which, if broken, are thought to affect the pregnancy and the newborn baby. Traditional birth attendants are often used for deliveries outside the hospital.

PREVENTIVE AND HOLISTIC PRACTICES

Other health care practices include touch therapy, such as therapeutic body massage, foot massage, and reflexology; acupuncture; food therapy, such as garlic and onions hung in the home or on the body and used for cooking to prevent illnesses; "magic hand" for healing and pain management; and traditional healing dance. Traditional healers frequently use a combination of therapies or holistic practices, such as the one used for and by Mr. Ojo (as described previously). Parts of preventative and holistic therapy are self-medication, self-care, herbal medicines, religious arts, and traditional dance treatment and praxis. Although some people regard African healing and health care practices as inflexible, unchanging, voodoo, mystical, and magical, their role and impact cannot be underestimated.

REFERENCES

Alexander GA: A survey of traditional medical practices used for the treatment of malignant tumors in an East African population, Soc Sci Med 20(1):53, 1985.

Ataudo ES: Traditional medicine and biopsychosocial fulfillment in African health, Soc Sci Med 21(12):1345, 1995.

Buckle J: The role of aromatherapy in nursing care, Nurs Clin North Am 36(1):47, 2001.

Campbell A: Acupuncture, touch, and the placebo response, Complem Ther Med 8:43, 2000.

Chipfakacha VG: STD/HIV/AIDS knowledge, beliefs and practice of traditional healers in Botswana, Aids Care 9(4):417, 1997.

Cocks M, Dold A: The role of African chemists in health care system of the Eastern Cape Province of South Africa. Amayeza stores, Soc Sci Med 51(10):1505, 2000.

Coppo P: Ethnopsychiatric observations apropos of the ritualization of deviation, Med Tropics 45(1):67, 1985.

Courtright P: Eye care knowledge and practice among Malawian traditional healers and the development of collaborative blindness prevention programs, Soc Sci Med 41(11):1569, 1995.

Dossey B et al: Holistic nursing: a handbook for practice, Rockville, Md, 1988, Aspen.

Erinosho OA: Behavioral science for nursing and medical students in Nigeria, London, 1981, George Allen and Unwin.

Hilderbrandt E: Have I angered my ancestors? Influences of culture on health care elderly black South Africans as an example, J Multicult Nurs Health 3(1):40, 1997.

Hodes RM: Cross-cultural medicine and diverse health beliefs: Ethiopians abroad, West J Med 166(1)29, 1997.

Homsy J et al: Evaluating herbal medicine for the management of herpes zoster in human immunodeficiency virus-infected patients in Kampala, Uganda, *J Alt Complem Med* 5 (6):553, 1999.

Jarret R: Caring power, or the restoring myth, *Med Tropics* 41(3):327, 1981.

Kelly L: What occupational therapists can learn from traditional healers, *Br J Occup Ther* 58(3):111, 1995.

Kozier B et al: *Fundamentals of nursing: concepts, process, and practice*, Upper Saddle River, NJ, 2000, Prentice Hall Health.

Mentgen JL: Healing touch, *Nurs Clin North Am* 36(1):143, 2001.

Morrison EF, Thornton KA: Influence of southern spiritual beliefs on perceptions of mental illness, *Iss Ment Health Nurs* 20(5):443, 1999.

Ntuli PB: Study to discover the influence and effects of non-medical practitioners on black terminally ill patients in Edendale, Pietermaritzburg, *S African J Nurs* 20(1):60, 1997.

Odebiyi AI: Food taboos in maternal and child health: the views of traditional healers in Ile-Ife, Nigeria, *Soc Sci Med* 28(9):985, 1989.

Ogaga A: Special herbal complex for women, *Healthcare* 14(6):13, 1999.

Popoola MM: *Where in Africa? A cultural saga from Denver to Lagos*, Lagos, Nigeria, 2000, Mace.

Rankin-Box D, ed: *The nurse's handbook of complementary therapies*, Edinburgh, London, 2001, Bailliere Tindall.

Saeki Y: The effect of foot-bath with or without the essential oil of lavender on the autonomic nervous system: a randomized trial, *Complem Ther Med* 8:2, 2000.

Stone J: How might traditional remedies be incorporated into discussion of integrated medicine? *Complem Ther Nurs Midwif* 7:55, 2001.

Tsey K: Traditional medicine in contemporary Ghana: a public policy analysis, *Soc Sci Med* 45(7):1065, 1997.

Wilkinson D, Gcabashe L, Lurie M: Traditional healers as tuberculosis treatment supervisors: precedent and potential, *Int J Tuberc Lung Dis* 3(9):838, 1999.

■ NATIVE-AMERICAN HEALING

Pamela Shuler[*]

"Native American medicine is based on widely held beliefs about healthy living, the repercussions of disease-causing activity or behavior, and the spiritual principles that restore balance" (Cohen, 1998, p. 45). In addition to balance, "Bear Hawk" Cohen (1998), who practices Native-American healing, identifies wholeness as a basic underlying principle of Native-American health culture. Bear Hawk relates the perspective of wholeness to healing. He reiterates what Native-American spiritual leaders, who gathered at the University of Lethbridge, Alberta, in 1982, said:

> All things are inter-related. This connectedness derives from the reality that everything is part of a single whole that is greater than the sum of its parts. Hence any given phenomenon can only be under-

---

[*]Excerpts from Ken "Bear Hawk" Cohen: Native American medicine, *Alt Ther Health Med* 4:45, 1998.

stood in terms of the wholeness out of which it comes" (The Four Worlds Development Project, 1982). The ultimate source of this wholeness is known by many names: *Kitchi Manitou* ("the Great Mystery," Ojibway), *Wakan Tanka* ("the Great Sacred" or "Great Spirit," Lakota), *Achadadea* ("Maker of All Things Above," Crow), *Shongwàyadíhs:on* ("the Creator," Iroquois), or simply God. (Cohen, 1998, p. 47)

Bear Hawk goes on to quote the spiritual leaders when defining health in terms of balance and wholeness:

...health "can be understood in terms of the wholeness out of which it comes" (The Four Worlds Development Project, 1982). Thus, health and disease always have both physical and spiritual components. Speaking of Iroquois concepts of disease etiology, Herrick and Snow (1995) write: "Because each causal agent is thought to be influencing the balanced, yet constantly fluctuating life force of the individual, there is necessarily the element of spirituality involved in the treatment and diagnosis of all illness." Health means restoring the body, mind, and spirit to balance and wholeness: the balance of life energy in the body; the balance of ethical, reasonable, and just behavior; balanced relations within family and community; and harmonious relationships with nature. (Cohen, 1998, p. 47)

When looking at the cause of disease, Bear Hawk relates that:

Native American medicine, unlike Western medicine, tends to consider disease in terms of morality, balance, and the action of spiritual power rather than specific, measurable causes. Native American medicine is based on a spiritual rather than a materialistic or Cartesian view of life. (Cohen, 1998, p. 47)

Diseases can be categorized into two broad and interrelated categories: internal and external causes. In Box 11-2, the internal and external causes as described by Bear Hawk are listed.

However, Native Americans believe that some illnesses are untreatable or are not easily treated. Bear Hawk (p. 47) explains:

...inherited conditions, such as birth deformities or retardation (including fetal alcohol syndrome), may be caused by the parents' unhealthy or immoral behavior and are not easily treatable. Native healers believe that, among adults, some diseases are the patient's responsibility and the natural consequence of his or her behavior; to treat these conditions may be to interfere with important life lessons...Some illnesses are not treated because they are considered "callings" or diseases of initiation: physical and spiritual crises engendered by the breakdown of previous ways of being or by the acquisition of guardian-spirit power..." The 'calling' comes in the form of a dream,

---

Box 11-2

Causes of Disease

Internal Causes:
Negative thinking (e.g., low self-esteem, anger, jealousy, greed, self-centeredness)
Disturbances in flow of life energy and healing power within the individual or to and from the environment

External Causes:
Pathogenic forces, objects (including microbes), people (sorcerers), and/or spirits
Environmental poisons, pollution, and contaminants, including alcoholic drinks and unhealthy food
Traumatic events: physical, emotional, spiritual, or any combination
Breach of taboo: imbalanced living and inconsiderate behavior; not demonstrating proper respect toward an animal, person, place, object, event, or spirit; improper performance of ritual or care of ritual objects

---

(*Cohen K: Native American medicine*, Alt Ther Health Med 4:48, 1998.)

accident, sickness, injury, disease, near-death experience, or even actual death. (Lake, 1991)

With respect to methods of diagnosing, Bear Hawk relates that:

...there are numerous methods of diagnosing disease. Diagnostic ability depends more on the intuition, sensitivity, and spiritual power of the healer than on the precision of a particular diagnostic technique. Therefore, diagnostic methods may vary not only from tribe to tribe, but also from healer to healer. Healers may create new diagnostic methods or find creative adaptations of practiced techniques in any particular healing session. As in Western medicine, the Native healer observes presenting symptoms and frequently asks the patient to describe them. The healer pays attention to the age and gender of the patient, the history and duration of the problem, and nonverbal cues, such as posture, breathing, tone of voice, and general deportment. (Cohen, 1998, p. 50)

Healers also use divination to determine the underlying cause of illness or to make a diagnosis:

Medical divination is the attempt to elicit medical information from divine or spiritual forces. It is commonly practiced by interpreting dreams, waking visions, or omens seen in such apparently random events as a toss of coins, a pattern in flowing water, or the crackling of a fire...Native Americans employ water, fire, smoke, stones, crystals, or other objects as projective fields in which they can "see" the reason and course of a disease. Sometimes the patient is asked to read the markings on a stone in a type of free association to help both the patient and the healer discover relevant information from the *realm of Spirit*—what we might call the *unconscious*, both personal and collective...It must be emphasized, again, that the essence of Native American diagnostics is not the technique, but the ability of the healer to see the patient with the inner eye of spirit, to sense disturbances of energy with the hands and heart, and to commune with higher sources of knowledge. For this reason, the diagnostic procedures are ineffective if merely imitated and cannot be easily taught to those who do not participate in Native tradition. (Cohen, 1998, p. 50)

Treatment methods vary from healer to healer and from tribe to tribe; however, the most common methods include prayer, chanting, music, smudging-purification with the smoke of sacred herbs, herbalism, laying on of hands, counseling, and ceremony. Table 11-2 lists the therapeutic methods along with the purpose of the treatment.

In addition to the power given to healers, within the Native-American culture is the recognition of the power of healing in nature and spirit (Cohen, 1998).

For example, natural elements, such as earth, water, mountain, and sun, are considered *elder healers;* by harmonizing with them, patients may experience spontaneous healing or find intuitive solutions to their problems. Native Americans also recognize the healing power of fasting and inner silence as ways to become more receptive to any healing influence. Family and community are also important facets of many healing sessions. (Cohen, 1998, p. 54)

The length of time that a person will experience symptoms of the illness after treatment varies from person to person:

...even in serious or chronic disease, long-term therapy may not be required. The intensity of the therapy is generally considered more important than the duration, (Duran, Duran, 1995)...The healing ritual shocks the patient into a new awareness of self and Creation. Healing may not be a gradual process but rather a quantum leap. However, Native healers recognize that patients must make lifestyle and behavioral changes that reinforce and maintain the improved

Table 11-2	Native American: Common Therapeutic Methods*
Method	**Purpose**
Prayer and chant	Prepare and focus the mind; induce altered state of consciousness; commune with, invoke, empower, and express gratitude to sacred healing forces; attend gathering and administration of herbs or other medicines
Music: voice, drum rattle	Same as prayer and chant; entrain consciousness of healer, patient, and helpers; accompaniment to dance and ceremony
Smudge: sage, cedar, sweetgrass	Cleanse space, healer, patient, helpers, and ritual objects; induce altered state of consciousness and increased sensitivity.
Herbs	Establish physical, mental, and spiritual balance; combat specific physical or spiritual pathogens
Laying on of hands: massage noncontact treatment	Aid healing of body, mind, and spirit; relieve pain; transmit healing energy and spiritual power
Counseling: talking things out; advice of elder/advisor; dream and vision interpretation; "Native-American Rorschach": stones, fire, water, and other projective fields; healing imagery; humor	Discover emotional or psychologic correlate of problem; help patient find new sources of inner strength and understanding; strengthen family and community relations
Ceremony	Support and context for any methods above; commune with natural and spiritual forces, the Great Spirit, and the spirit of the disease; induce altered consciousness; affirm cultural identity and values

See Footnote on next page.

Nature, social support, and sacrifice are common elements that may increase the efficacy of therapy. The patient may expose himself or herself to the healing power of nature, or the healer may invoke their presence. Family and community are frequently asked to join healer and patient in administering any of the therapeutic methods. Patient and healer may practice fasting or other forms of personal sacrifice as purging or purification and to demonstrate courage, commitment, and dedication to Spirit.
From Cohen K: Native American medicine, Alt Ther Health Med 4(6):52, 2001.

---

condition. Although healing may occur quickly, way of life makes healing last. (Cohen, 1998, p. 54)

In the Native-American culture, the belief holds that:

healing power can be inherited from ancestors, transmitted from another healer, or developed through training and initiation (Johnny Moses, oral communication to Bear Hawk, 1988). However, the best way to develop, strengthen, and maintain healing power is through rigorous personal training. Among the Snohomish, "individuals sometimes inherit a power from a grandmother, grandfather, aunt or uncle... If they want that power to be strong, they have to fast and go through a lot of sacrifice" (White, 1991). The only prerequisite is patience. (Cohen, 1998, p. 54)

With respect to payment for "healing services," Bear Hawk explains the Native-American perspective:

The exorbitant fees charged by Western medical practitioners are, from the Native American point of view, a sign of contemptible professional ethics. Because healing is a gift from the Great Spirit, it is beyond price and should never be equated with a specified bundle of "frog skins." Although many healers accept monetary or material offerings, most do not charge a set fee. Illness is a time for generosity by a caring community. One should not take advantage of someone when he or she is down. (Cohen, 1998, p. 55)

REFERENCES

Cohen K: Native American medicine, *Alt Ther Health Med* 4:45, 1998.
Duran E, Duran B: *Native American postcolonial psychology,* Albany, NY, 1995, State University of New York Press.
The Four Worlds Development Project: *Overview: the Four Worlds development project,* Lethbridge, Alberta, Canada, 1982, University of Lethbridge.
Herrick JW, Snow DR, eds: *Iroquois medical botany,* Syracuse, NY, 1995, Syracuse University Press.
Lake MG: *Native healer,* Wheaton, Ill, 1991, Quest Books.
White T: *Northwest coast medicine teachings: an interview with Johnny Moses,* Shaman's Drum, 1991, p. 23.

■ A TRADITIONAL UNITED STATES HEALING PRACTICE EXAMPLE: TRADITIONAL HEALTH BELIEFS AND PRACTICES OF THE GEORGIA LOW COUNTRY

Brenda Talley

The following story exemplifies the numerous traditional healing practices and cultural heritages in the United States. Speaking in the first person, the author describes a nurse's perspective in the Georgia Low Country.

CULTURAL HERITAGE OF THE GEORGIA LOW COUNTRY

The Low Country of Georgia includes approximately 30 miles of wide flat coastal plain and a string of small barrier islands separated from the mainland by the narrows of the intercoastal waterways. It reaches from gentle ocean waves on sugar sand beaches to slow deep rivers stained dark from the tannin of thousands of trees. It is a land of grackles and gulls, of sea grasses, tall cypress, ancient live oak trees, and flowing Spanish moss. It is long-needled pines that sing in gentle breezes and it is the dramatic palmetto that can both nourish and injure. It is a lush land, jungle-like, temperate and fertile. I was born here and it is my home still. Although storms may chase the waves to wildness and the rush of waters from the inland rains may suddenly reshape the sandbars and so the rivers, it is a land that appears calm and serene, a land that seems to change only slowly. It is a land of many secrets, and a land that shows only glimmers of its truths, as secretive as the Blue Heron who disappears into the deepness of the cypress groves, leaving us only a flash of color and an echoing cry. The cities and towns of the Georgia Low Country are small. Farming and belief in God are important, although perhaps not as much as in years past. The largest city is Savannah, a city born around formal squares. Savannah was planned carefully and with a mind toward elegance and grace, and history is honored here. Many of the formerly safe caches of culture, long preserved on the formerly "bridge-less" barrier islands and rural "pocket" communities, are disappearing.

I grew up thinking that I did not have a culture. I was of small-town, white-bread America and *ordinary*. My parents didn't have a foreign accent. Nobody danced at family weddings in great circles with their arms linked. Exotic spices never made their way into *our* kitchen. When I did realize that indeed I was a member of a unique cultural group, I found that things southern and rural rarely seemed valued by others. Sometimes southernness and ruralness were even scorned and became sources for poor comedy and cheap novels. It took my first year as a registered nurse to understand the importance of culture to well-being. It took me longer to honor and value this culture myself.

My first job in nursing was in an Intensive Care Unit in Savannah. One day I had a patient—we'll call him Mr. Greene—who was from one of the small barrier islands that, to this day, does not have a bridge (although it does have condos, a golf course, and a heliport). He was a quiet, dignified man, an oysterman, who went out to the oyster banks every day during season in his bateau. I enjoyed talking with him. During my growing up years, we had a four by four fishing cabin on the next island that was built on tall palm tree pilings high over a salt water creek. We spent much of our summers there, fishing, crabbing and walking on the beach. Mr. Greene and I decided that my father had likely bought oysters from him on many occasions. When lunchtime came, I reported Mr. Greene's condition to my colleague and left the unit. When I returned, my colleague and an orderly were in Mr. Greene's room attempting to restrain him. "He's become combative and his speech is unintelligible. Maybe he's had a CVA," they said. What was "wrong" was that Mr. Greene spoke only Gullah; I had not thought to mention his language, and he desperately needed to go to the bathroom. The nurses could not understand what he was saying. Gullah is a patois spoken by the African-Americans living on the barrier islands. The language is mostly English with some other European influence, and full of African words. The cadence and accents on words are very different than "standard" English. Closer inland a similar dialect is called Geechee, after the Ogeechee River.

THE HISTORY OF THE GEORGIA LOW COUNTRY

Native Americans, including the Yamasee, the Yamacraw, and others had been present since ancient times. The first Europeans were the Spanish who left some fortifications and churches on the barrier islands but minimal impact on the culture. Georgia became an English colony in 1732, and alliances were quickly formed with the coastal tribes. Later in the 1730s the colony granted safe haven for Austrian Lutherans ousted from their homes. They established thriving towns along the inland rivers. Jewish refugees from Spain and Portugal were welcomed into the young colony. After the Revolution, Scotch-Irish and others having served in the Continental Army, were given land grants in Georgia. Early in the nineteenth century, a number of Irish settled in the area. All the while, African slaves were being brought to the large plantations that developed along the coast and on some of the islands.

I experienced this as a constellation of beliefs, as an integrated set of knowledge. Perhaps some healing magic arises from African Shamanism. The notion of spirituality in all things surely has Celtic origins as well. Spiritual healing has arisen from Christianity, Judaism, and other religions and involves the use of scriptures and evoking the assistance of God. Often this is linked with very ancient healing rituals such as the "pulling out" and "talking out" healing, originating in Western Europe.

Immigrants to this land were often without physicians; and European medications were very scarce. Some of the arrivals had knowledge about natural healing, but found the botanicals in this world different from those they knew. Probably, some of the native tribes shared knowledge with their new friends. There was (and still is) a wealth of biologics with which to experiment. One must honor those who first experimented with new forms of plant life for healing. With a few, the logic of choice is apparent. For example, the dog fennel plant is used to enhance general vitality. This tough tenacious plant, though delicate in appearance, has a strong root that will survive the winter and expand with new shoots each year. It also re-seeds itself, paying attention to the environment and blooming just 6 weeks before the first frost of the season for optimal seeding. That this plant might gift us with vitality is not, perhaps, a far reach. But the one who first had the notion of the tiny blue mushroom growing around barns helping epilepsy should be commended for courage. (Or perhaps the one partaking of it should be.)

THREE ASPECTS OF HEALING

The traditional healing of the Georgia Low Country has three aspects: medicinal, magical, and religious/spiritual. Medicinals involve the use of herbs, chemicals, poultices, feathers, etc. Magical healing calls for transference, exorcism, and talismans. Religious healing includes prayer, the recitation of scripture, and the use of consecrated ground.

Medicinals
Medicinals, products ingested or used on the body, are a familiar form of healing. Included are herbs, roots, and (because of the heavy pine forests) naval products such as rosin and terpentine. Some plants, such as sweet bay and wax myrtle, are used for both medicinal and magical purposes.

Transference, Exorcism, and Talismans
Transference means placing the illness or affliction elsewhere, such as in an object, animal, or another person. Many of the cures for warts involve the use of transference. In exorcism, the practitioner removes the problem (a curse or a spirit that is within the person) and ensures that it will not return. Talismans are objects or colors that have the power to protect. A talisman may be a single object or a group of objects. Some objects, such as a button from a dead man's coat, have inherent power. Others are "created" by instilling protective qualities. Sometimes, a collection of charms (gris gris) are worn around the neck and should not be removed.

Table 11-3	Three Aspects of Healing
Medicinals	Herbs and roots; chemicals such as rosins, kerosene; poultices; smoke
Magical	Transference; exorcism; talismans
Religious-spiritual	Prayer; quoting scripture; use of consecrated ground

Religious/Spiritual Healing

The restorative and protective power of God is clearly a part of the Low Country healing traditions. The use of religion in healing often has a mystic quality. Scriptures may be recited in languages understood only by God. Healing rituals may need to be conducted in sacred places, in the darkness of night. Many times a patient will wear a cloth, pinned to clothing, that has been blessed. These also should not be removed. If they are removed, in order to change clothes, they should be treated with reverence and transferred to the clean garment quickly. [Table 11-3 provides an overview of these aspects of healing.]

THE PRESCRIPTION

Rarely does a practitioner use only one modality. Often all three of the healing aspects are used, or at least two are called upon. It may seem paradoxical or strange to combine the magical or superstitious with the religious, but this seems to distress few. I remember hearing stories of how my great-great uncle, known as a warlock, consecrated ground deep in the woods for his healing rituals. He was a tall Irishman, with long red hair that he never cut, and he was a blacksmith by trade. These wonderful stories were passed on to me by my grandfather. His first teachings to me were the secrets of how to remove warts. Grandpa was an elder in the Primitive Baptist Church, which disdains secretiveness but honors the knowledge of healing, and recognizes that this precious knowledge warrants protecting.

Much of the responsibility of healing rests with the patient. Almost always, the patient is given a prescription of behaviors, and noncompliance results in failure of the intervention. Often objects must be buried in a certain place at a certain time. One must go to the crossroads and turn around three times at midnight. Worse yet, something might have to be buried in a graveyard at midnight. Graveyards and grave dirt are very important to healing and protection against harm. However, the intervention does not always work; one cannot alter the laws of nature or the will of God.

THE HEALERS

Healers are those born with gifts, chosen because of special characteristics, and/or have been "called" to healing. Traditionally there are several layers of healers. Persons who provide basic care for family members, friends and neighbors, usually don't undergo special training but are willing to use the everyday kinds of knowledge to render aid to loved ones in a lay manner. Others, including root doctors, faith healers, conjure women, granny women, and talkers/pullers, study with other practitioners, often for several years. Their knowledge was carefully guarded and those with whom it was shared were carefully selected.

Lay Healers

Family members used many healing and protective techniques, although most were medicinal in nature. Most everyone knew that rubbing a cut green walnut over a ringworm infection would cure it. Blackberry root was known to be good for diarrhea. Turpentine was used as an antiseptic and even taken internally. A few drops on a teaspoon of sugar will help a chest cold (although it *tastes awful!*). Some practices and beliefs were aimed at preventing illness and bad fortune. A pregnant woman must not attend a funeral for fear of harming the baby. Girls should not whistle, lest they risk a misfortune (*A whistling girl and a crowing hen will always come to the same bad end*). Homes could be protected with talismans and techniques to inhibit bad spirits. Wearing dimes made in one's birth year or leap year brought good fortune.

Root Doctors, Warlocks, Spiritual Healers, and Conjure Women

Root doctors, warlocks, and spiritual healers are all terms used to describe those who have devoted their lives to learning and practicing the traditional work. Usually they are male. The female counterpart is called a conjure woman although the term root doctor can also refer to women. I recently was told by the local root doctor that the preferred term by root doctors now is spiritual healer. Although practice clearly does include "rooting," many other modalities, such as herbs and other medicinals, incense, and counseling are used. The term root doctor, he believes, gives an imprecise and limited view of their work. The "root" in root doctor is not referring to a medicinal use, or the simple ingestion of a botanical root. The root is both the organic material and the spell, or conjuring that is cast. To "put a root on someone" is to have a conjure against or to protect a person and that involves evoking spirits.

Several years ago, I received a phone call from an MD with an urgent request to have a root doctor come to see a patient in the hospital. A man was dying, saying that he had an evil eye cast upon him and no one except a root doctor could help him. His vital signs were crashing. The physician could not find an explanation for his condition but it was clear that he WAS dying. The root doctor came to the hospital immediately and the man lived. Root doctors/spiritual healers and conjure women receive their knowledge in an apprenticeship with an experienced practitioner. The knowledge base of the spiritual healers is secretive, as is often their identities, at least to the general public. Sometimes they will take the names of animals— Dr. Buzzard is the root doctor mentioned in the movie "Midnight in the Garden of Good and Evil." Of course, the garden of good and evil is the cemetery, a powerful and sacred place, and midnight is the time when spirits are about.

Firetalkers and Pullers

When I was 17, my hands and arms were badly burned in an accident. It looked as though I would be badly scarred. Though my mother was not usually given to folk medicine, she took me to a firetalker. Firetalkers and pullers "remove" the fire from a person. The aim is to reduce the pain and inhibit scarring. The practitioner whom I visited chanted (I was told later that the chant was verses from the Bible, although I could not understand her words) and simultaneously moved her hands near the surface of the burns. Her hand movements looked very much like therapeutic touch. She refused payment, saying that her skill was a gift from God. My burns healed well and the scars are almost invisible. I no longer know a firetalker, although one of my former students knows one.

Granny Women

Granny women are women who use medicinals and knowledge of healing. Granny women include the midwives and, although they may involve superstitions and taboos, they generally do not use conjuring. After the turn of the century, many of the granny women in our region were incorporated into the public health department as midwives. In order to deliver babies in rural areas where physicians were in short supply, they were enrolled in a training program and were provided with supplies and support. Years ago when I was a home health nurse, one of my patients was a granny woman. She was nearing 100 but still able to talk about her practice. As we talked, we discovered that she had delivered at least two of my uncles, in 1910 and 1912. My uncle said that Grandpa had brought her on horseback to their home.

BEING A HOME HEALTH NURSE IN THE LOW COUNTRY OF GEORGIA

My years as a home health nurse taught me much about traditional healing. I learned to begin my assessment before I entered the home.

Although traditional beliefs are not important to everyone, they are critically important to many. Before I entered a home where the traditions were important, I could see that those within were protected from harm. Evil spirits (hags) and malevolent ghosts (haints) were being kept at bay with the bright blue painted window frames and by sprigs of evergreen placed on the window sills. Additional protection was sought by scrubbing the porch and steps with Red Devil lye. If I dared to look under the steps, likely I would find talismans buried.

One 90-year-old patient confided in me that her leg ulcers would not heal because evil spirits were in her legs. She took both my hands in hers. "You have the power in your hands to make them leave, I can feel it. Please make them leave." I do not consider myself a practitioner of the traditional arts, but since she asked, I commanded the spirits to leave in the manner that my grandfather had taught me. Interestingly, as with the firetalker, these hand movements look very much like therapeutic touch. I then found some wax myrtle growing nearby and placed sprigs on her windows and above the doors so the evil spirits could not return. Perhaps her ulcers would have healed anyway, but this "nursing intervention" was more important to her than just for the purposes of healing the leg ulcers; this was important to her total well-being.

It took me many years to understand and appreciate my own culture. It took many more years to realize the importance of culture and of healing beliefs on well-being. The story above is based on a presentation I did in Huntsville, Alabama at the 2001 annual Conference of the American Holistic Nurses Association. I kept noticing that one member of the audience frequently nodded her head and smiled broadly. She came to me after the presentation and said, "Thank you for taking me home again. My family is from Hilton Head Island." We spoke for a while on our common heritage and I felt that, if one from the area could feel it so intensely, then indeed I had provided a "snapshot" of the Low Country.

Resources

Only one book accurately describes the aspects of magic in the Low Country. It was actually written about the Beaufort, South Carolina area, just over the river. (The state line is more a political than a sociocultural boundary in this regard.) Someone born and raised in the region wrote this book, which is: Pickney R: *Blue roots: African-American folk magic of the Gullah people,* St Paul, Minn, 2000, Llewellyn Publications. Also, the "Foxfire" series of books, although written about the culture of the North Georgia mountains, provides insight to healing and other traditions, primarily of the Scotch-Irish.

■ SHAMANISM

Alison Rushing

WHAT IS SHAMANISM?

Historically, shamanism is a religious phenomenon of Siberia and central Asia that has been used for centuries. Shamans are found in numerous cultures, and shamanism is one of the oldest healing traditions found among indigenous peoples all over the world. A shaman is one possessed by "magico-religious" powers and may act as a magician and medicine man who is believed to cure and perform miracles; beyond this, he is a "psychopomp, priest, mystic and poet" (Eliade, 1964, p. 4) and a master of ecstasy (the ability to create the healing imagery he uses in an altered state of reality). Eliade equates shamanism with techniques of ecstasy.

> The shaman is an individual endowed with supernatural power to heal, or one who by calling his spirit(s) can find out what is beyond time and space" (Rogers, 1982). Rogers' description represents the essence of shamanism as perceived by the patients served. It embodies the major focus of the shaman and his/her capability to deal with issues in ordinary as well as non-ordinary realms of consciousness. The empirically-based Western allopathic medical model explains sickness within an internalizing system where physiological and psychological symptomatology is essential for treatment. Shamanism, by contrast, is based on an externalizing system in which the problems of illness originate from the activities of spiritual forces or deities. (Rogers, 1982, p. 107)

A distinction must be made between illness and disease. Disease refers to the pathologic condition that afflicts the person; illness refers to the total personal impact of the disease on the person who is afflicted. McClenon (1993) states that, "most Western physicians limit their help to the cure of a *disease*—a biological disorder. They are generally unprepared to heal *illness*—(that is) the way a person experiences his/her disorder in a social or personal context. Shamanism, by contrast, appears to address illness more than disease" (p.117). Imaginative techniques employed by the shaman to achieve health are most likely to be regarded to affect the illness and not the pathologic condition (Achterberg, 1985). In the realm of imaginative healing however, "the various psychic powers attributed to (the shaman) must not be too readily dismissed as mere primitive magic and 'make-believe' for many of them have specialized in the working of the human mind and in the influence of mind on body and mind on mind" (Elkin, 1998, p. xiv).

A shaman is a "constructor of worlds" (Overing, 1990, p. 602), endowed with special power, by birth, training, or inspirational experience, to intervene with supernatural beings or forces on behalf of patients (Wallace, 1966: in Overing, 1990, p. 602). A shaman has the "ability to contact the supernatural—with or without the benefit of ritual" (Malefijit, 1968: in Overing, 1990, p. 602). Shamans "order the gods or spirits for the securing of good and averting evil" (Mathews, Smith, 1921: in Overing, 1990, p. 602). One characteristic of shamans is "their familiarity with realities other than those of three dimensional space and linear time known to our usual waking consciousness" (Nicholson, 1987, p. 1) and their ability to mediate between this ordinary world and that alternate, nonordinary reality. Through the use of various techniques, the shaman moves at will between an ordinary reality, called the ordinary state of consciousness (OSC) and a nonordinary reality or the shamanic state of consciousness (SSC).

BECOMING A SHAMAN

A person can become a shaman in several ways. Some cultures believe that the shaman is preordained from birth to his or her profession; others believe that the shaman receives a "call" that must be accepted, or he or she might incur great bodily harm or suffering from the "spirits." Other cultures believe that a person is destined to become a shaman evidenced through suffering physical or mental afflictions or experiencing a high frequency of anomalous experiences that include seeing apparitions, having precognitive dreams, experiencing extrasensory perception (ESP) or night paralysis, or having out-of-body or near-death experiences that support the belief in spirits, souls, or life after death (McClenon, 1993). These experiences or afflictions mark the person and must be attended to so as not to incur the ire of their ancestors. These people, once healed of their affliction, are then obligated to pass the healing on to others. In this sense, shamans fall into the realm of the "wounded healer" archetype.

ROLE OF THE SHAMAN

Shamanic practice emanates from both religious and healing tradition. Shamans are the keepers of tribal wisdom and healing secrets. Additionally they have been assigned the roles of artist, dancer, musician, singer, dramatist, intellectual, poet, psychopomp, ambassador, advisor, weatherman, artisan, and culture hero (Achterberg, 1985, p.3). Numerous sources (Walsh, 1994; Achterberg, 1985; Harner, 1990; Rogers, 1982) attest to the universal role of a shaman as being one of both practice and intent. The practice of shamanism is marked by several commonalities that are consistent worldwide and over time. One commonality is the shaman's ability to voluntarily enter a shamanic state of consciousness (SSC) that is different from that observed in psychopathology or religious practice. Another belief asserts that the shaman's soul or spirit leaves his or her body to travel to other worlds or realms to acquire knowledge or power, to engage spirit helpers, and to assist people in the community. A third commonality is the ability to command, control, interact, and intercede with spirits on behalf of their patients, to whom they then interpret their intercessions (Walsh, 1994). One of the most distinguishing commonalities is "that shamans have been recognized throughout recorded history as having the ability to heal with the imagination par excellence" (Achterberg, 1985, p. 13). In addition to the role as an imaginative healer are numerous functions and techniques used to bring about healing.

CREATING THE IMAGE

Shamans communicate with their patients on an emotional and symbolic level rather than intellectually. Shamans manipulate symbols that resonate with the needs of people in their society. Because shamans perform wondrous events, observers accept (or increase their faith in) a particular therapeutic ideology. Belief is not based so much on a body of orderly knowledge (as in allopathic medicine, although the shaman is the keeper for a vast amount of knowledge) but rather on the experiential "proofs" the patient gains from observing the ceremony. This belief contributes to changes in attitudinal and physiologic states that coincide with healing (McClenon, 1993). The shaman creates and maintains this image and mystique in several ways.

First are the peculiar circumstances under which shamans receive their "call" or the occurrence of the initiation crisis. Many times, the call occurs in the late teens or early adulthood and is marked by observable changes in behavior. The shamans-to-be become withdrawn, demonstrate erratic behavior and mood swings, sleep more, have visions, or are subject to seizures; they appear ill, either physically or mentally. These people often emerge from their illness as exceptionally functional community members who demonstrate remarkable energy and stamina; unusual levels of concentration; high intelligence and leadership skills; a grasp of complex knowledge, myths, and rituals; and control of altered states of consciousness (Walsh, 1994).

Second, the shaman creates the image of "apartness" by maintaining boundaries between himself or herself and the community so that the sacred domain is delineated as a special domain. Through the procedures and rituals used, the means by which the shaman enters his or her world and engages and channels its powers are kept "separate." Additionally, the shaman remains physically removed from the community through the maintenance of special living quarters that are separated from the rest of the community, even though he or she is highly involved in community life (Chernela, Leed , 1996).

A third aspect of the image created by the shaman is the healing rituals. As someone who is able to manipulate spiritual powers, the shaman helps patients "transcend their ordinary definition of reality, including the definition of themselves as ill" (Harner, 1990, p. xvii). The shaman demonstrates to patients that he or she is self-sacrificing through (1) sharing self to show patients that they are not emotionally or spiritually alone in their struggle with illness and death and (2) sharing his or her special powers to convince the patient that another person is willing to offer personal skills to come to his or her aid.

Two approaches that a shaman uses to guide the healing rituals are to restore beneficial or personal power to a patient and to remove harmful or blocking powers from the patient's body. A shaman may be needed to return a personal guardian spirit or even the patient's soul to one who is "dis-spirited." At other times, the shaman may be called on to remove magical darts that may cause disease ("dis-ease") or the loss of soul or spirit. The shaman is considered an expert seer whose work is carried out in darkness or with the eyes covered so that he or she can "see" clearly. For this reason, the shaman usually performs the functions at night because in the darkness, things or events that are perceived in ordinary reality are not a distraction. This measure allows him or her to focus on the aspects of nonordinary reality necessary for him or her to carry out healing (Harner, 1990).

The aspect of shamanism that contributes most to the creation of healing in an imaginative realm is the use of altered states of consciousness or SSC. Harner (1990) says that the use of some amount of ecstasy or altered consciousness, the SSC, is absolutely necessary to shamanic practice. Additionally, the shaman must be able to use what he or she has learned while in this state to heal the patient.

The shaman enters the SSC through the use of sacred plants that are natural hallucinogens or through the use of sound vibration using drumming or rattles. A shaman may use natural hallucinogenics. However, for healing to occur, the shaman must remain in control to carry out tasks, as well as to maintain control of the spirits with which he or she is dealing; therefore the shaman is never "out of control" or "out of touch" with this altered reality.

Another method for achieving the SSC involves a drum, a rattle, or both. Harner (1990) cites studies revealing that the energy from the rhythm and the sound (both of which become monotonous) affect sensory and motor areas of the brain and produce an altered state of awareness. The resonance that the sound of the drum produces causes vibrations that are within a certain frequency range and, if continuous, can produce a trancelike state. Andrews (1992) discusses the use of the drum and the rattle in achieving a meditative resonance within the body.

The shaman, with or without the help of an assistant, beats a drum at a certain tempo that may or may not change during the ritual. The beating drum may be accompanied by chants or "power songs" sung by either the shaman or the assistant (if one is used) both of which increase in tempo and intensity as the SSC is approached. Many times, the audience joins in singing or chanting. This combination may act as a catalyst to extend the trancelike state to members of the audience and the patient, and may aid in creating the image of healing sought by the shaman. The shaman is such an expert that he or she is able to enter the SSC at will, aided by the sound and rhythm of the instruments.

The purpose of attaining a SSC is to journey to other worlds to reclaim spirits that may have been lost by the patient, to gain wisdom and knowledge, and to acquire power spirits in the form of animals (to assist the shaman while journeying). Usually, the more power animals and spirits a shaman can command, the more powerful he or she is considered to be. A shaman typically journeys to the "Lower World" (the realm where the spirit lives and works) to accomplish his or her tasks. Entrances to this world are to be found in or around hollow tree stumps, in caves, holes that have been made by animals, and special holes in the dirt floors of houses. Additionally, as the SSC is entered, the shaman may sink to the floor symbolizing the beginning of the journey. Some cultures envision the shaman entering the Lower World through the bottom of the sea or a body of water. Whichever way the shaman exits, the journey is the most important task the shaman undertakes. The entrance into the Lower World usually leads into a tunnel that winds downward until the shaman exits the tunnel into a bright and beautiful world in which he or she communicates with all living things as they or the shaman wishes or finds necessary. The power animals or guardian spirits that are encountered on the journey display the ability to speak to humans or to take on a human form as an indicator of their power. When the shaman possesses one of these power animals, it acts as his or her alter ego imparting to the shaman the power to transform from human to animal and back again. This action, in turn, enhances the power of the shaman and his or her ability to recover a patient's lost spirit (Harner 1990). The "limitations of time and space are transcended...rocks and stones speak...men are turned into animals and animals into men. It is a world replete with archaic symbolism in which the shaman travels the breadth of the universe on missions of utmost importance to his people" (Achterberg, 1985, p. 11).

When the shaman has returned with the power animal, he or she blows it back into the patient usually through the chest or fontanel on the top of the head. Once the spirit or power animal has been returned to its owner, the person who has received the spirit is encouraged to dance the animal form to demonstrate association with the spirit and to keep the spirit happy so that it will remain with the person for its appointed duration. Dancing enhances the power of the protective spirit and the person who is its symbiont. Many times, the shaman dances these symbols of power during his or her entrance into the SSC.

The other function the shaman uses during his or her healing rituals involves removing magical darts (instruments that spirits use to cause disease or illness) or the spirits themselves, accomplished mostly by sucking out the darts or spirits. Usually taking the form of some kind of animal, these darts or spirits have both a material and a nonmaterial form and are seen by the shaman only during an altered state of consciousness, visualized by the shaman in an SSC before being sucked out of the patient's body during a healing ritual. When the shaman is ready to remove the darts, he or she keeps two spirits of the type visualized in the patient's body in his mouth, one in the front and one at the back of his or her mouth. The purpose of the spirit in the front of the mouth is to trap the essence of the offending spirit once the shaman has sucked it out. The spirit in the back of the mouth guards the shaman's throat so that if the invading spirit gets by the first, the second will trap it and keep it from invading and harming the shaman. The shaman then "vomits" out the trapped essence and removes it as soon as the healing ritual is concluded. The shaman has been accused of concealing objects in his mouth to produce as "evidence" to substantiate the claim that the offending dart or spirit has indeed been removed. Whether or not this claim is true is immaterial. The shaman focuses only on capturing and removing the nonmaterial essence of the invading dart or spirit and the illness with it.

STATE OF THE PRACTICE

A resurgence of interest in the practice of shamanism has taken place. Reasons include dissatisfaction with the way health care is currently practiced with its emphasis on curing diseases of the body and ignoring the totality of the patient. Second, a growing body of knowledge exists concerning holistic treatment of people. This holistic trend embodies an array of NAC therapies that may be less expensive, readily accessible, and easy to use. Shamanic practice and treatment appeals to an increasing number of people. The power of the image to heal is strongly recognized, and an expert shaman is a master at weaving the image that contributes to health and well being.

REFERENCES

Achterberg J: *Imagery in healing: shamanism and modern medicine*, Boston, London, 1985, Shambala.

Andrews T: *Sacred sounds, Transformation through music and words*, St Paul, Minn, 1999, Llewellyn Publications.

Chernela J, Leed E: Shamanistic journeys and anthropological travels, *Anthropol Q* 69(3):129, 1996.

Eliade M: *Shamanism: archaic techniques of ecstasy*, Princeton, NJ, 1964, Bollingen Series, Princeton University Press. Translated 1974.

Elkin AP: Aboriginal men of high degree. In Harner M, ed: *The way of the shaman*, San Francisco, 1998, Harper Collins.

Harner M: *The way of the shaman*, San Francisco, 1990, Harper Collins.

McClenon J: The experiential foundations of shamanic healing, *J Med Philos* 18:107, 1993.

Nicholson S, ed: *Shamanism*, Wheaton, Ill, 1987, Quest Books.

Overing J: The shaman as a maker of worlds: Nelson Goodman in the amazon, *Man* 25(4):602, 1990.

Rogers S: *The shaman: his symbols and his healing power*, Springfield, Ill, 1982, Charles C. Thomas.

Walsh R: The making of a shaman: calling, training, and culmination, *J Humanis Psychol* 34(3):7, 1994.

■ HOMEOPATHY

Roxana Huebscher

Homeopathy is a system of treatment whereby extremely small doses of a substance are administered. Such a substance, given in a stronger dose, might cause a *healthy* person to have symptoms of the concern that is being treated in the ill person. "The best therapy for any given patient is a single medicine whose adverse effects most closely mimic the symptoms of the illness" (Skinner, 2001, p. 9). Using the *Law of Similars*, homeopathy conveys this concept with: "Let likes be cured by likes." An example:

> An onion may cause the eyes to burn and water when being chopped, yet an onion prepared homeopathically may be given orally in small doses to treat eye burning and watering caused by allergies or the common cold. (Chapman, Wilson, 1999, p. 705)

Homeopathy uses many other terms and, in a sense, has its own language. Box 11-3 lists some homeopathic terminology. Important to remember is that homeopathic treatment is not the same as taking herbs. Homeopathy has its own philosophy and practice parameters that are quite different from those of both allopathic and herbal therapies.

HISTORY OF HOMEOPATHY

Homeopathy is used by approximately 3.4% of the American population (Eisenberg et al, 1998). The practice of homeopathy began with Samuel Hahnemann (1755-1843), a German physician, translator, chemist, and author who developed homeopathy after leaving his conventional medical practice. Conventional medical practice in Hahnemann's time consisted of bloodletting, blistering, leeching, purging, and doses of mercury, arsenic, and other toxic substances (Kaufman, 1971; Huebscher, 2000). After leaving his medical practice,

---

Box 11-3

Homeopathy Terminology

Case-taking
Law of Similars; *similia similibus curantur;* "Let likes be cured by
  likes."
Law of Simplex
Law of Infinitesimals
Law of Minimum
Hering's Laws of Cures
Homeopathic Materia Medica; Organon of Medicine; Repertory
  Homeopathy Pharmacopoeia of the United States
Potencies, potentization—X, C, M
Provings
Remedy
Succussion
Totality of Symptoms
Aggravation

Hahnemann began experimenting to find out why cinchona (which
contains quinine) cured malaria:

> In 1790, while experimenting with cinchona (Peruvian bark),
> Hahnemann decided to ingest a therapeutic dose. He soon felt cold,
> numb, drowsy, thirsty, and anxious, and experienced palpitations,
> prostration, and aching bones; he recognized these symptoms as those
> of *ague,* or intermittent fever, the syndrome that was being treated
> with cinchona (Bradford, 1895). He allowed the dose to wear off
> before taking a second and a third dose that confirmed his original
> results. Stunned by the implications of this finding, Hahnemann
> devoted the rest of his life to ascertaining the therapeutic properties
> of medicinal substances by administering them to healthy people—
> himself, his colleagues, and his students. His *Materia Medica Pura*
> records the detailed symptomatology of over 90 medicines, a truly
> monumental achievement that represents 20 years of painstaking
> labor. In these *provings,* as he called them, Hahnemann administered
> the substance in question to a group of reasonably healthy people in
> doses sufficient to elicit symptoms without provoking irreversible tox-
> icity, anatomical changes, or organic damage. A unique composite
> portrait, or symptom-picture, was assembled for each substance, dif-
> ferentiating it from every other. Therefore homeopathic remedy is a
> shorthand for the sum of observable responses of all people who have
> taken that remedy, a distinctive totality that must be studied as a

whole and for its own sake rather than simply as a weapon against a particular disease or a group of symptoms. (Jacobs, Moskowitz, 2001, pp. 88-89; Hahnemann, 1880; Hahnemann, 1833)

Brought to the United States by Constantine Hering in the early 1800s, homeopathy became a popular form of health care. "By the early 1900s there were 111 homeopathic hospitals, 22 homeopathic medical schools, and over 1000 pharmacies who sold homeopathic medicines, and 20-25% of all urban physicians practiced homeopathy" (Migodow, 1986, p. 164). However, following the Flexnor Report in 1914 calling for the standardization of medical education, homeopathy lost favor. By 1935, no more totally homeopathic hospitals were operating (Migodow, 1986). The practice of homeopathy did survive, however, and is once again becoming increasingly popular in the United States. Homeopathy has remained a mainstay of health care in Germany, France, and India, to name a few countries.

PROCESS OF CARE AND REMEDIES

The homeopathic process of care includes the homeopathic interview (case-taking), case evaluation, and prescribing (Lange, 2000). In this process, all symptoms are important, and the totality of symptoms must "take into account the living experience of the patient, including the full range of thoughts and feelings" (Jacobs, Moskowitz, 2001, p. 90). The case history includes that:

> ...an entire review of symptoms is recorded in descriptive detail, taking into consideration all modalities which affect a symptom. Hahnemann emphasized the general symptoms (i.e., those affecting the entire organism, as the leading indications for the remedy). These key symptoms include mental and emotional affects, the metabolism and its reactions to environmental stimuli, sleep positions, food cravings and aversions, thirst, body type, and all manifestations of unconscious and autonomic regulation. Unique characteristic symptoms, particularly those regarded as "strange, rare, and peculiar," are important considerations in the selection of the remedy. These might be the expression of a paradoxical or unusual relationship, such as pain ameliorated by pressure or the sensation of the legs being made of wood or glass. The association of the start of a disease or symptom complex with an environmental or emotional event can be very important and emphasizes the importance of an accurate and extensive interview. (Lange, 2000, p. 338)

The homeopath's job is to reconcile the patient's grouping of signs and symptoms (physical, mental, emotional, and spiritual) with the remedies. Homeopathic resources include the Materia Medica and repertories. The Materia Medica is a text listing remedies followed by the symptoms for which the remedies are used. A repertory lists symptoms and signs followed by remedies that work for these signs and symptoms (Boericke, 1999).

Homeopathic remedies include plant, mineral, and animal sources. More than 2000 remedies can be found in the homeopathic pharmacopeia (Jacobs, Moskowitz, 2001). Table 11-4 lists a few of the substances used in remedies. These remedies are highly dilute substances. Homeopathic remedies are regulated by the U.S. Food and Drug Administration, including regulation of manufacturing, labeling, and dispensing of remedies. Latin names are used for purposes of worldwide identification. The various dilutions of the remedies are termed *potencies*. Homeopathic remedies are created through a process called "potentization" and are serially diluted and shaken (called succussion). The more dilute the remedy is, the higher the potency is considered:

> The preparation of homeopathic medicines follows a rigorous process. For soluble substances one part of the original plant, mineral, or animal substance is diluted in water or lactose on a decimal (X; 1 part:9 parts) or centesimal (C; 1:99) scale, or the 50-millesimal scale (LM; $\frac{1}{50,000}$); each dilution then is agitated vigorously. For insoluble substances the material is serially diluted in lactose and ground in a mortar and pestle at each dilution, a process referred to as trituration.

Table 11-4	Examples of Homeopathic Remedy Substances	
Plant	**Mineral**	**Animal**
Aconite	Antimony	Venoms of: bee,
Arnica	Arsenic	jellyfish, crustaceans,
Belladonna	Carbon	fish, Spanish fly,
Cayenne	Copper	tarantula pit viper,
Chamomilla	Gold	bushmaster
Comfrey	Hydrochloric acid	Secretions: ambergris,
Digitalis	Hydrogen	cuttlefish ink, musk
Eyebright	Iodine	Nosodes (disease
Garlic	Lead	products): gonorrhea,
Ipecacuanha	Platinum	tuberculosis,
Marigold	Potassium chloride	syphilis, vaccines,
Mulmein	Silica	abscesses
Nux vomica	Silver	Sarcodes (glandular
Pulsatilla	Sodium chloride	and tissue extracts)
St John's wort	Sulfur	
Wild rosemary		
Yellow dock		

Eventually the lactose triturate is dissolved in water, and the process of potentization is continued using the liquid medium. Homeopaths refer to these dilutions as "potencies" or "remedies." Potency actually refers to the extent of dilution—low potency remedies range from 2X (0.01 molar) to 30C, and high potencies range from 200X (10 to the minus 200 molar) to 100,000C (10 to the minus 200,000 molar). (Chapman, Wilson, 1999, p. 706)

The Law of Simplex refers to using one remedy at a time as treatment, the single remedy (Jacobs, Moskowitz, 2001). This area is somewhat controversial, and some practitioners use several remedies. In addition, homeopaths use the smallest possible dose, the minimum dose, or infinitesimal doses (Jacobs, Moskowitz, 2001). If remedies are given in too large a dose, they can cause an aggravation or a temporary increase of symptoms (McCabe, 1997). Box 11-4 provides information according to Hering's Laws of Cure on how healing occurs in the body.

USES OF HOMEOPATHY

Jacobs and Moskowitz (2001) outline conditions for which homeopathic remedies are best used. Box 11-5 lists these conditions. In the area of research, the *provings* were the first study into the area of homeopathy. More recently, a meta-analysis was done of studies. Skinner (2001) discusses research on influenza, child birth, otitis media, allergy, vertigo, childhood diarrhea, and chronic illness, including traumatic brain injury, rheumatoid arthritis, and aphasia. Carlston (2003) reviews published studies from 1980 to 2001. In addition, Chapman and Wilson (1998) report on research specific to physical

---

Box 11-4

Hering's Laws of Cure—Symptom Movement in Healing

1. Healing progresses from upper to lower parts of the body (from head to foot).
2. Healing progresses from inside to the external parts, interior to peripheral (for example, from heart and lungs, or mental and emotional to the skin and extremities)
3. Healing progresses from more vital to less vital organs
4. Symptoms appear and disappear in the reverse of their original order of appearance (first to occur in life history of the patient are last to disappear).

(Cummings, Ullman, 1997; McCabe, 1997; Jacobs, Moskowitz, 2001.)

Box 11-5

Uses of Homeopathic Remedies

Functional complaints with little or no tissue damage, such as headache, insomnia, chronic fatigue, and premenstrual syndrome

Conditions for which no effective conventional treatment is available, such as viral illnesses, traumatic injuries, surgical wounds, multiple sclerosis, and acquired immunodeficiency syndrome

Conditions that require chronic use of conventional drugs, such as allergies, recurring infections, arthritis, skin conditions, and digestive problems

Conditions for which elective surgery has been proposed, but immediate attention is unnecessary, such as fibroid tumors, gallstones, and hemorrhoids

Conditions that have not been cured by conventional treatments because of the inappropriateness of the medications, the determined nature of the disease, or patient's noncompliance

(Jacobs, Moskowitz, 2001, p. 97.)

rehabilitation, including for migraine headache, aphasia, fibromyalgia, head injury, vertigo, sprains, and soft tissue injury.

EDUCATION AND REGULATION

The National Center for Homeopathy (www.homeopathic. org/edudir) lists educational programs. Each of the programs listed is either approved or under review for approval by the Council on Homeopathic Education. Arizona, Nevada, and Connecticut have licensing boards for homeopathic practitioners. Other states vary. The Homeopathic Pharmacopoeia of the United States (www. hpus.com) also "is the official standard for the preparation of homeopathic medicines" (Jacobs, Maskowitz, 2001; Chapman, Wilson, 1999). Homeopathic practitioners include nurses, physicians, osteopaths, chiropractors, naturopaths, acupuncturists, and dentists, as well as homeopaths with no other professional affiliation.

REFERENCES

Boericke W: *Pocket manual of homoeopathic materia medica and repertory*, New Delhi, 1999, B Jain Publishers.

Bradford T: *The life and letters of Samuel Hahnemann*, Philadelphia, 1895, Boericke and Tafel.

Carlston M: *Classical homeopathy*, New York, 2003, Churchill Livingstone.

Chapman E, Wilson J: Homeopathy in rehabilitation medicine. In Schulman R et al, eds: *Physical Med Rehab Clin North Am* 10(3):705, 1999.

Cummings S, Ullman D: *Everybody's guide to homeopathic medicines*, New York, 1997, Tarcher Putnam.

Eisenberg D et al: Trends in alternative medicine use in the United States, *JAMA* 280:1569, 1998.

Hahnemann S: *Materia medica pura*, Dudgeon E [translator], Liverpool, UK, 1880, Hahnemann Publishing Society.

Hahnemann S: *Organon of medicine*, ed 5, Boericke W, Dudgeon E [translators], Calcutta, India, 1833, Roy.

Huebscher R: Homeopathy: let likes be cured by likes, *NP Forum* 11(3):155, 2000.

Jacobs J, Moskowitz R: Homeopathy. In Micozzi M, ed: *Fundamentals of complementary and alternative medicine*, Edinburgh, 2001, Churchill Livingstone.

Kaufman M: *Homeopathy in America*, Baltimore, 1971, The Johns Hopkins Press.

Lange A: Homeopathy. In Pizzorno J, Murray M, eds: *Textbook of natural medicine*, vol 1, Edinburgh, 2000, Churchill Livingstone.

McCabe V: *Let like cure like: the definitive guide to the healing power of homeopathy*, New York, 1997, Martin's Press.

Migodow JA: An introduction to homeopathic medicine and the utilization of bioenergies for healing, *Alt Med* 1(2):163, 1986.

Skinner S: *An introduction to homeopathic medicine in primary care*, Gaithersburg, Md, 2001, Aspen.

■ NATUROPATHY

Roxana Huebscher

WHAT IS NATUROPATHY?

Naturopathy is a distinct system of health care that "stresses promotion of health, prevention of disease, patient education, and self-

---

Box 11-6

Principles of Naturopathic Medicine

The healing power of nature — *Vis medicatrix naturae*
The healing power of nature is an inherent property of the living organism.
First do no harm.
Find the cause.
Treat the whole person.
Preventive medicine
Wellness
Physician as teacher

(Bradley, 1999; Pizzorno, Snider, 2001)

responsibility" (Pizzorno, Snider, 2001, p. 173). Naturopathic medicine is based on vitalism rather than mechanism. Mechanism maintains that life can be explained as the "product of a complex series of chemical and physical reactions" (Bradley, 1999, p. 42), whereas with vitalism, "life is more than just the sum of biochemical processes" (Pizzorno, Snider, 2001, p. 173). "Vitalism is the proposition that more is needed to explain life than just physical or mechanical laws" (Micozzi, 2001, p. 44). With naturopathy, a strong belief holds that the body has the ability to heal itself. The principles of naturopathic medicine are outlined in Box 11-6.

HISTORY OF NATUROPATHY

Naturopathy began with the teachings and therapy of Benedict Lust. Lust came to the United States in 1892 to promote hydrotherapy, having himself been "cured" by Father Kneipp's water therapy. Lust purchased the term "naturopathy" in 1902 from John Sheel (who had coined the term in 1895 to describe his method of health care). Lust eventually became an osteopathic physician, acquired a chiropractic and homeopathic education, and became a conventional physician because of his homeopathic education (which was possible at that time in the United States). Lust opened the first health food store and began both the American School of Chiropractic and the New York School of Massage (Cody, 1999). Nutrition was also important; Kellogg, a physician who maintained a sanatorium in Battle Creek, Mich., defended vegetarianism and believed that humans during the meat digestion process produced "self-poisons that contributed to 'auto-intoxication'" (Cody, 1999, p. 32). Kellogg wrote *The New Dietetics* in 1921, which, resulting from Lust's influence, became a popular naturopathic reference. In addition, exercise was important; Bernarr MacFadden, a friend of Lust's, opened a physical culture school of health and healing, leading to the opening of gymnasiums across the country. Lust also helped publicize "zone therapy," popularized by a chiropractor named Riley. Zone therapy is similar to acupressure (Cody, 1999). In the early 1920s, some of the established medical profession began to malign Lust and colleagues. With the advent of more drugs, and the death of Lust in 1945, naturopathy declined. However, a resurgence has occurred since the late 1960s, and naturopathy is once again becoming popular.

PROCESS OF CARE AND THERAPIES

A history and physical examination are done. Applying the principles of naturopathic medicine, the naturopathic practitioner does a case analysis that includes asking a set of questions. Briefly, the questions include the following areas:

What is the first cause; what is contributing now?

How is the body trying to heal itself?

What is the minimum level of intervention needed to facilitate the self-healing process?

What are the patient's underlying functional weaknesses?

What education does the patient need to understand why they are sick and how to become healthier?

How does the patient's physical disease relate to their psychological and spiritual health? (Pizzorno, Murray, 1999, p. 1)

Some states allow standard diagnostic privileges such as venipuncture or ordering radiologic procedures. Some states allow assistance with natural childbirth and limited prescriptive privileges. Minor or superficial surgery may also be done (Downey, 2000).

Therapies include nutrition, botanicals, fasting, detoxification, homeopathy, standard medications, acupuncture, biofeedback, hydrotherapy, physical medicine (touch, heat, cold, electricity, and sound), exercise, counseling, spirituality, health psychology, and lifestyle modification (Downey, 2000; Pizzorno, Snider, 2001).

USES OF NATUROPATHY

Naturopathy is used for both acute and chronic care. Examples are as diverse as are those in any primary care practice, from hypertension, rosacea, arthritis, menopause, and migraine (Pizzorno, Murray, 1999) to human immunodeficiency virus (HIV) and acquired immunodeficiency syndrome (AIDS) (Standish et al, 1999). A naturopathic physician (ND) who is an associate dean at a naturopathic college of medicine writes:

> Naturopathic medicine is a primary care form of practice that is applicable to acute as well as chronic disease. It is this author's opinion that the first physician a patient should see is a naturopathic doctor. Drugs and surgery would then become the "alternative" medicine. All too frequently, people come to naturopathic medicine as a last resort. They are hoping for a way to avoid surgery or they have exhausted all that allopathic medicine has to offer them and are told to seek the aid of a psychiatrist. They still do not believe it is all in their heads if no disease can be named. Often people with cancer are seeking ways to ease the side effects of chemotherapy, or those who are HIV-positive want help strengthening their immune system. Patients seek out NDs when they are tired all the time or have insomnia. They want natural therapies to treat their children's chronic otitis media, asthma, or allergies. Patients want alternatives to antibiotics or cortisone. Women find that plant-based hormones, vitamins, minerals, and herbs address their menopause symptoms more effectively than prescription synthetic estrogen and progesterone preparations. Young mothers want advice on nutrition for their children and older men are helped with benign prostate hypertrophy without drugs and surgery. Arthritis responds well to our natural therapies as do migraines and other types of chronic

pain. As with all alternative therapies, use of naturopathic medicine does not preclude the use of mainstream medical therapies in addition. Naturopathic doctors do not perform heroic medicine. They do not compete with medical physicians in the emergency room or in major surgery. Sometimes surgery is best for the patient and NDs refer to their colleagues in the hospital. (Downey, 2000, pp. 278-279)

EDUCATION AND REGULATION

The American Association of Naturopathic Physicians (AANP) describes an ND as a person who:

> Attends a four-year graduate level naturopathic medical school and is educated in all of the same basic sciences as an MD but also studies holistic and nontoxic approaches to therapy with a strong emphasis on disease prevention and optimizing wellness. In addition to a standard medical curriculum, the naturopathic physician is required to complete four years of training in clinical nutrition, acupuncture, homeopathic medicine, botanical medicine, psychology, and counseling (to encourage people to make lifestyle changes in support of their personal health). A naturopathic physician takes rigorous professional board exams so that he or she may be licensed by a state or jurisdiction as a primary care general practice physician. (AANP@ www.naturopathic.org, Accessed 2/1/2003.)

Naturopaths are licensed in a limited number of states. In addition, Canada has licensing in several provinces (Ernst, 2001). In states without licensing, the consumer needs to be aware of credentials that the provider has to be sure that the practitioner graduated from a 4-year accredited college. AANP supports licensing requirements. Examples of schools in North America include the National College of Naturopathic Medicine in Portland, Oregon (www.ncnm.edu); Bastyr University in Kenmore, Washington (www.bastyr.edu); Southwest College of Naturopathic Medicine and Health Sciences in Tempe, Arizona (www.scnm.edu); and the Canadian College of Naturopathic Medicine in Ontario, Toronto. In addition, the University of Bridgeport College of Naturopathic Medicine has candidacy status granted by the Council on Naturopathic Medical Education (AANP@ www.naturopathic.org, accessed 2/1/2003).

REFERENCES

American Association of Naturopathic Physicians [AANP]: Education and licensing; and Accredited Schools, www.naturopathic.org, accessed 2/1/2003.

Bradley R: Philosophy of naturopathic medicine. In Pizzorno J, Murray M, eds: *Textbook of natural medicine*, ed 2, Edinburgh, 1999, Churchill Livingstone.

Cody G: History of naturopathic medicine. In Pizzorno J, Murray M, eds: *Textbook of natural medicine*, ed 2, Edinburgh, 1999, Churchill Livingstone.

Downey C: Naturopathic medicine. In Novey D, ed: *Clinician's complete reference to complementary and alternative medicine*, St Louis, 2000, Mosby.

Ernst E: *The desktop guide to complementary and alternative medicine: an evidence-based approach*, St Louis, 2001, Mosby.

Micozzi M: History of vitalism. In Micozzi M, ed: *Fundamentals of complementary and alternative medicine*, ed 2, New York, 2001, Churchill Livingstone.

Pizzorno J, Murray M: *Textbook of natural medicine*, ed 2, Edinburgh, 1999, Churchill Livingstone.

Pizzorno J, Snider P: Naturopathic medicine. In Micozzi M, ed: *Fundamentals of complementary and alternative medicine*, ed 2, New York, 2001, Churchill Livingstone.

Standish L, Wines R, Reeves C: Complementary/alternative therapies in select populations: women with HIV and AIDS. In Spencer J, Jacobs J, eds: *Complementary and alternative medicine: an evidence-based approach*, St Louis, 1999, Mosby.

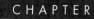
MIND-BODY-SPIRIT INTERVENTIONS

Roxana Huebscher ▮ Pamela Shuler

The National Center for Complementary and Alternative Medicine (NCCAM, 2002) defines mind-body interventions as:

> A variety of techniques designed to enhance the mind's capacity to affect bodily function and symptoms. Some techniques that were considered CAM [complementary and alternative medicine] in the past have become mainstream (for example, patient support groups and cognitive-behavioral therapy). Other mind-body techniques are still considered CAM, including meditation, prayer, mental healing, and therapies that use creative outlets such as art, music, or dance. (NCCAM, 2002)

In this text, the NCCAM definition of mind-body interventions is modified by adding the spiritual dimension to the title, recognizing that something beyond the "mind" exists. Mind-body-spirit (MBS) interventions refer to the variety of ways of being and doing that affect and enhance mind, body, and spirit function, symptoms, and processes.

Many MBS interventions are used within alternative health care systems (see Chapter 11), and some overlap with each other. For example, meditation is a part of Ayurveda; movement is important in naturopathy, Ayurveda, and Traditional Chinese Medicine; and shamanism certainly involves altered states of consciousness. Box 12-1 lists examples of MBS interventions. Interventions are circumspectly divided into three categories: the creative and expressive; altered states of consciousness; and social support and personal interaction. This method of categorization is for reading ease and grouping the numerous modalities. However, individual modalities may fit into another categorization. For example, when an individual is engrossed in a hobby (creative and expressive), the relaxation response may be elicited (altered state of consciousness); any creative endeavor may produce an altered state of consciousness. Examples are discussed for each category.

CREATIVE AND EXPRESSIVE INTERVENTIONS

The creative and expressive refers to various modalities that bring forth or create. "Creative work comes out of an intense and passionate

Box 12-1

Examples of Mind-Body-Spirit Interventions

The creative and expressive, including creating, performing, viewing, listening, sensing
Acting
Bibliotherapy
Drawing
Hobbies
Journaling
Literature
Movement
Meditative movement, such as Baguan, circle walking, labyrinth walking, Tai chi, yoga, aikido, sufi
Exercise movement, such as dance, aerobics
Music
Painting
Photography
Poetry
Pottery
Sculpting
Storytelling
Writing

Altered states of consciousness
Affirmation
Assertiveness
Biofeedback
Breathing techniques
Centering/presence
Humor/laughter
Hypnosis
Imagery/visualization
Meditation
Mental healing
Neurolinguistic programming
Prayer
Relaxation techniqies such as autogenics, progressive muscle relaxation
Spiritual healing
Values clarification

Social support and personal interaction
Family and friends
Hobby groups
Pet therapy
Support groups
Therapy with another person
Volunteerism

involvement...as one (the artist) interacts with the 'other' to bring something new into being. This 'other' may be a painting, a dance form, a musical composition, a sculpture, a poem or a manuscript, a new theory or invention, that for a time is all-absorbing and fascinating. Creativity is also a 'sensual' process for many people; it is an in-the-moment sensory experience involving touch, sound, imagery, movement, and sometimes even smell and taste" (Bolen, 1984, p. 241).

Drawing, painting, sculpting, dancing, making music, acting, writing, and other creative endeavors can be healing interventions. In addition, viewing-listening, or sensing such works in other ways, may provide a healing intervention. Samuels (1995) writes that:

> ...healing, art, and prayer all come from the same source, the soul. And when we travel deeply into the inner realms, we reach the insights, emotions, and transformation that are our birthright.... I see healing and art as one. They are the two sides of the split between rational and the intuitive; their separation historically is as profound as that between mind and body. And just as it is our task to bring mind and body together to heal the whole person, it is our task to unite healing and art to heal our bodies and the world. (p. 38)

Cameron (1992) outlines a 12-week program for discovering and recovering the creative self. The topics are in the area of recovering a sense of safety, identity, power, integrity, possibility, abundance, connection, strength, compassion, self-protection, autonomy, and faith. The following are a few examples of modalities included in the creative and expressive. Health care providers (HCPs) can help patients recover their creative spirit by offering suggestions and resources. In addition, art therapy may prove useful for some patients.

Art and Art Therapy

According to The American Art Therapy Association (AATA, 1998), art therapy is:

> A human service profession which utilizes art media, images, the creative art process, and patient/client responses to the created art productions as reflections of an individual's development, abilities, personality, interests, concerns, and conflicts. Art therapy practice is based on knowledge of human developmental and psychological theories which are implemented in the full spectrum of models of assessment and treatment including educational, psychodynamic, cognitive, transpersonal, and other therapeutic means of reconciling emotional conflicts, fostering self-awareness, developing social skills, managing behavior, solving problems, reducing anxiety, aiding reality orientation, and increasing self-esteem. Art therapy is an effective treatment for the developmentally, medically, educationally, socially,

or psychologically impaired; and is practiced in mental health, reha-bilitation, medical, educational, and forensic institutions. Populations of all ages, races, and ethnic backgrounds are served by art therapists in individual, couples, family and group therapy formats. (p. 1)

Horovitz (2000) lists a diagnostic guide to help an HCP know who would be an appropriate patient to refer:

Adjustment disorder; antisocial behavior; agoraphobia; Alzheimer's disease; anxiety disorders; autistic disorders; bipolar disorders; border-line personality disorder; body dysmorphic disorder; cognitive disor-ders; depressive personality disorder; attention deficit and disruptive behavior disorders; eating disorders; elective mutism; impulse control disorders; learning disorders (specifically dyslexia); mood disorders; schizoaffective disorders; sexual abuse; sexual dysfunction; trichotillo-mania; and obsessive-compulsive disorders. (p. 23)

Numerous graduate schools in the United States provide art ther-apy training and education, and there is also an Art Therapy Credentialing Board (www.atcb.org) (Horovitz, 2000). In addition to formal art therapy, individuals may view artistic works, have a hobby or gain personal gratification from their own artistic practices.

Bibliotherapy, Journaling, Storytelling, and Writing

"Word" therapies, whether reading, writing, or telling, can promote health. Sources of reading can be literature, poetry, fiction or non-fiction, or self-help. Rojcewicz (2000) explains bibliotherapy or poetry therapy as the "intentional use of poetry and other forms of literature for healing and personal growth" (p. 105). Allende (1996) believes that a "story is a living creature, with its own destiny, and my job is to listen to its voice and write it down" (p. 2). The author describes writing as "a silent introspection, a journey to the dark caverns of the memory and the soul" (p. 2):

Writing has been very healing for me, because it has allowed me to exorcise some of my bad spirits and to transform most of my defeats into strengths. After my daughter's death, writing was the only thing that kept me relatively sane, when Prozac, therapy and vacations in Hawaii couldn't help. I was paralyzed with pain until my mother came up with the idea that grief was a long and dark tunnel that one has to go through...Trust the life force, she said...A year later I was at the end of the tunnel, and I could see the light, and I discovered, amazed, that I did not pray to die anymore. I wanted to live. By that time there were four hundred pages on my desk. It looked like a book. (p. 2)

Writing can be a way to express oneself when talking will not work. "Journaling provides an opportunity for catharsis about highly emotional events" (Pennebaker, 1997 in Snyder, 2002, p. 136).

Self-discovery and self-reflection are possible, as well as positive coping. Writing or journaling need not be done every day, nor is any special equipment required; whatever the person wants to work with is possible. Writing can be narrative or poetry, and it can be free flowing, or structured. Day (2001) describes several forms of journaling with various topics. An interesting format is the "AlphaPoem." Writing an AlphaPoem consists of copying the alphabet, one letter per line, down the left side of a page and then simply writing a poem using the letters consecutively. Each line can have a word or a line, whichever works best, before coming to the next letter. The writing is done quickly and then edited as needed.

In addition, Day (2001) suggests writings within the categories of: captured moments, character sketch, clustering (free association around a central word), dialogue, inner wisdom, list of 100 (such as 100 ways to nurture the self), different points of view, and unsent letter. Snyder and colleagues (2002) discuss writing techniques in terms of free flowing, topical, and intensive journaling. Progoff's (1975) intensive journaling workshops teach a structured method of writing. Topics include areas such as a life history log; stepping stones; intersections, roads taken and not taken; dialogues with people, work, society, events, the body, inner wisdom; and dream logs and imagery extensions (Snyder et al, 2002). Journaling is a private and confidential thing. HCPs can give patients encouragement or even start them with a small journal. Advise clients to mark the journal as personal and private and keep the journal safe from anyone else's reading. Whether patients want to discuss the journal with the HCP is an individual matter.

Several chapters in this text cover journaling as therapy (general well being, respiratory, and neuropsychology, for example). In addition, the HCP can lend out helpful literature or reference citation lists to patients.

Movement Therapies

Movement therapy can be categorized as meditative such as Tai chi, yoga, or labyrinth walking, or more active movement such as aerobic exercise and dancing. Physical activity is vital for physical and mental health; "our bodies were designed to move, stretch and run" (Northrup, 1998, p. 740). Movement helps maintain or restore the "rhythm" or synchronized connection between our bodies and emotional selves (Hoban, 2000). As the body moves repetitively and rhythmically, as in swimming, walking, or dancing, the mind can be stimulated for general well being and healing, as well as for creative and intuitive thinking (Northrup, 1998). Therefore exercise can kindle the mind, as well as the body.

The benefits of being physically active are many (Anderson, 1987), and these benefits have been well documented (U.S. Preventive

Services Task Force [USPSTF], 1996). "Evidence exists that physical activity and fitness reduce morbidity and mortality for at least six chronic conditions: coronary heart disease, hypertension, obesity, diabetes, osteoporosis, and mental health disorders" (USPSTF, 1996, p. 611). In the area of mental health, exercise can be an effective component of psychotherapy. Studies have shown that regular, supervised aerobic exercise improves symptoms associated with panic disorders and agoraphobia and reduced depression, agitation, and hallucinations in patients with schizophrenia (Tkachuk et al, 1999). Furthermore, physical activity has been successfully used in the behavioral treatment of chronic pain, while dance can be used as a form of psychotherapy for emotional, cognitive, social, and physical integration (American Dance Therapy Association [ADTA], 2001).

Regular exercise has been linked with improved immune system function in patients with cancer (Anderson, 1987), decreased risk for breast cancer (Thune et al, 1997), increased restful sleep (Griffin et al, 1978), increased insulin sensitivity (Helmrich et al, 1991), and improved symptoms associated with premenstrual syndrome (Prior, 1987). Yoga and Tai chi are other options for physical activity that can improve flexibility, muscle tone, mental clarity, and reduce stress (American Yoga Association, 2002; Jones, 1998; Iyengar, 1979; Frawley, 1999; Wolf et al, 1996; Wolfson et al, 1996). These more gentle forms of activity are beneficial throughout the life span but may be particularly important for the elderly population.

For some individuals, physical activity becomes addictive and therefore destructive (Northrup, 1998). To avoid using exercise as a "drug," using physical activity to "run away from stress or disconnect from our deepest selves" must be avoided (Northup, 1998, p. 749). Exercise can be an important component of stress management, but it should not prevent the honest examining and dealing with stressful events in people's lives.

When discussing exercise with patients, the primary focus should be on determining what activity the patient will actually do on a regular basis. Several activities may be alternated throughout the week. Patients should be encouraged to "make a commitment to move their bodies" at least three times a week for 20 to 30 minutes at a moderate pace, or most days of the week doing some activity (National Heart, Lung and Blood Institute [NHLBI], 2001; Northrup, 1998, p. 754). The HCP can help people select an "enjoyable" activity and one that can be started simply. The patients should be taught to monitor their body's physical and emotional response over a month. During this brief period, patients may experience an improved sense of well being and may commit to making regular physical activity a gratifying and healthy part of their lives. Healthfinder, a government-based information source, has physical activity guidelines from many organizations that may be helpful for use with patients (Healthfinder, 2003).

Music and Music Therapy

Music is sound, or vibration, that a person can hear between 20 and 25,000 cycles per second. Music may be performed or listened to. Music therapy is the application of pleasant sounds to produce desired changes in behaviors, emotions, or physiologic responses (Dossey et al, 1995). "The playing of appropriate music produces alpha and theta brain waves, which are known to stimulate creativity" (Guzzetta, 1995, p. 677). In addition, music aids relaxation, improves learning, and is used to enhance audio and video recordings that reprogram thought patterns (including subliminal recordings). Music is used for suggestion and in thanatology as a way of addressing the needs of people who are dying (Guzzetta, 1995). Music affects heart rate, skin conductivity, respiration, blood pressure, muscular tension, motor-postural response, peripheral skin temperature, blood volume, and biochemical response (Hunter, 2000).

Numerous schools are available to train music therapists at bachelor's, masters', and doctoral levels; approximately 5000 music therapists are registered in the United States. The American Music Therapy Association lists information (www.musictherapy.org). Credentialing consists of: music therapist-board certified (MT-BC), certified music therapist (CMT), advanced certified music therapist (ACMT), and registered music therapist (RMT) (Hunter, 2000).

ALTERED STATES OF CONSCIOUSNESS

Altered states of consciousness refer to a focus that is different from that which occurs during a person's alert awake times. Altered states can be of several degrees, from the deeply altered states of some healers and spiritual practitioners to the person deeply engrossed in an enjoyable hobby. Relaxation response, imagery, and hypnosis are examples of altered states, as well as the everyday times when a person is "daydreaming" in an altered state. Naparstek (1994) defines an altered state as:

> ...a state of relaxed focus, a kind of calm but energized alertness, a focused reverie. Attention is concentrated on one thing, or on a very narrow band of things. As this happens, we find we have a heightened sensitivity to what we are focused on, and a decreased awareness of the other things going on around us, things we would ordinarily notice...In practical terms, this kind of altered-state experience allows us to reach peak performance levels in many areas of endeavor. There is a kind of self-forgetfulness and disregard for outcome that characterizes this state, allowing us to outreach what we thought we could do. This state is sometimes called "flow" or being "in the zone." In it,

artists and athletes can extend their normal range of achievement. Proposal writers can propose better; rescuers can rescue better, charmers can charm better. (p. 23)

Example descriptions of a few of these altered states of consciousness follow. In addition, the chapter on general well being covers assertiveness, attitude, and thought stopping.

Affirmations

Affirmations are positive, personal, present-tense statements that express a desirable outcome as if it has already occurred. No negative words are used in an affirmation. (The reader should note the two negative words used in the previous sentence, "no" and "negative.") Additionally, no future tense or "trying to" words are used. A person immerses the consciousness in the affirmation to produce a positive outcome. Repeating the affirmation many times is a way of accomplishing this task. The premise is that people are what they say they are; and if a person continually repeats affirmations, he or she achieves what is said. "Life experiences mirror our beliefs" (Hay, 1988, p. 4). Box 12-2 gives examples of affirmations, and the general well being Chapter 2 of this text has more details on affirmation.

Biofeedback

Biofeedback is "a training technique in which people are taught to improve their health and performance by using signals from their own bodies" (Association for Applied Psychophysiology and Biofeedback [AAPB], 1998). Equipment is used for learning biofeedback. The equipment has a sensor that monitors the physiologic

---

Box 12-2

Sample Affirmations

- am healthy and happy.
- am strong and confident.
- am stress-free (or fill in the condition).
- have excellent grades.
- am a loving sister, brother, mother, father, husband, wife, friend.
- am a competent and caring health care provider.
- do what I need to do effectively and with care.
- say what I need to say in a gentle way.
- exercise three times a week for 20 minutes each time.
- am smoke-free.
- have a wonderful relationship with...

function and a transducer that converts what is measured into some visual or audio signal.

The Biofeedback Certification Institute of America (BCIA) recognizes two different types of biofeedback procedures: general biofeedback and electroencephalogram (EEG) biofeedback, called neurotherapy or neurofeedback (BCIA, 2001; AAPB, 1998). EEG is used for conditions such as attention deficit disorder (ADD), attention deficit and hyperactivity disorder (ADHD), and anxiety. General biofeedback usually uses readings from muscle tension, skin temperature, or both to treat disorders such as anxiety, chronic pain, headaches, hypertension, and urinary incontinence (BCIA, 2001).

> The electromyogram (EMG) has been the workhorse of biofeedback...EMG biofeedback procedures are based on the fact that muscles produce an instantaneous electric discharge when they are activated. Typically, two electrodes and one reference electrode are attached to the skin in close proximity to the muscular activity, [usually] pasted or held with straps. The level of activity is usually read in microvolts (mv) of electrical output within a range of 100 Hz to 200 Hz. A measurement of 5 mv or higher is defined as a stressed or spastic muscle; 2 Hz to 4 Hz defines an active muscle; and 0.5 Hz to 1.5 Hz defines a relaxed or flaccid muscle. (Freeman et al, 2001, p. 200)

Biofeedback training is available through several programs in the United States. The BCIA can help locate a trained practitioner (www.bcia.org).

Hypnosis

Hypnosis is "an induced, sleeplike state involving motivation, relaxation, concentration and application. In this state, the person is relaxed and the mind is directed inward" (Halo Shames, 1996, p. 38). Hypnosis is a combination of imagery and suggestive techniques. With hypnosis, the inductee (person being hypnotized) has a focus, some work to do.

Generally, there are two schools of thought about hypnosis: the "paternal-authoritarian" or traditional school, and the "maternal or Ericksonian," a popular form of hypnosis introduced by Milton Erickson (Saichek, 2000). "There has been a movement away from more traditional authoritarian techniques (telling the patient what they are going to do) because this tends to threaten some patients with fear for the loss of control" (Hrezo, 1998, p. 218); suggestion is used instead. Hypnosis is used in psychotherapy, surgery, childbirth, medical outpatient processes (e.g., smoking cessation programs), and as self-hypnosis or autosuggestion.

Hrezo (1998) includes a basic induction script, chronic pain management script, and trance termination in his article on pain management. The American Society of Clinical Hypnosis has a variety of materials available for people who are interested in hypnosis (www.asch.net). Backgrounds of hypnosis practitioners are numerous and varied, and some people believe hypnosis is not an acceptable form of patient care.

The National Board for Certified Clinical Hypnotherapists (NBCCH) (www.natboard.com) is responsible for certifying hypnotherapists. The NBCCH is an "educational, scientific, and professional organization dedicated to professionalizing the mental health specialty/subspecialty of hypnotherapy" (NBCCH brochure). To be certified, a hypnosis practitioner needs a degree, a minimum of 60 hours of classroom instruction, a minimum of 1 year of clinical hypnosis experience, including 100 to 250 hours of face-to-face hypnotherapy; and also needs to be licensed as a mental health professional in the state of practice, or have other certification.

Imagery

Imagery may be done with any of the senses and refers to imagining. Gawain (1978, 1997) refers to imagery as creative visualization or "using your imagination to create what you want in your life" (p. 13). Zahourek (1988) calls imagery a mental process. Naparstek (1994) says guided imagery is:

> ...a process of deliberately using your imagination to help your mind and body heal, stay well, or perform well. It's a kind of directed, deliberate daydream, a purposeful creation of positive sensory images—sights, sounds, smells, tastes, and feel—in your imagination. (p. 198)

Imagery can be used for numerous problems, including physical, mental, and spiritual. For example, Naparstek has imagery recordings for asthma, cancer, chemotherapy, depression, diabetes, grief, headache, healing trauma, healthy heart, help for infertility, multiple sclerosis, pain, rheumatoid arthritis, smoking cessation, stress, stroke, and weight loss (www.healthjourneys.com).

See scripts for allergy in this text's respiratory chapter and for pain, headache, and general relaxation in the neuropsychology chapter.

Meditation

"Meditation is a self-directed practice for relaxing the body and calming the mind that has been used by people in many cultures since ancient times" (Kreitzer, 2002, p. 101); it is the "art of inner listening" (Kornfield, 1996, p. 1). Meditation can be practiced in several ways. Three basic ways of meditating are with a mantra, breath counting, and gazing meditations (Davis, Eshelman, McKay, 1998). Two popular types of meditation are mindfulness meditation and Transcendental meditation. *Vipassana* meditation emphasizes:

...mindful attention or immediate awareness of one's experience in all spheres of activity. Even the most mundane, repetitive experiences—such as eating, walking, or answering the phone—are drawn into the field of meditative awareness through practice of *vipassana*. (Kornfield, 1996, p. 1)

Four basic exercises in *vipassana* (to see things as they really are) practice include a breathing meditation, a body awareness–naming of sensation meditation, a thoughts-feelings-moods meditation, and a forgiveness and loving kindness mediation (Kornfield, 1994, 1996b). Mindfulness means paying attention "on purpose, in the present moment, and nonjudgmentally" (Kabat-Zinn, 1994, p. 4):

People think of meditation as some kind of special activity, but this is not exactly correct. Meditation is simplicity itself. As a joke, we sometimes say: "Don't just do something, sit there." But meditation is not just about sitting, either. It is about stopping and being present, that is all. Mostly we run around doing. Are you able to come to a stop in your life, even for one moment? What would happen if you did? (Kabat-Zinn, 1994, p. 11)

Transcendental meditation (TM) was popularized in the West by Maharishi Mahesh Yogi (Sharma, Clark, 2000). The term "transcendental" refers to the mind transcending subtleties, including the mantra (or sound) that the meditator may be using. Practicing TM requires approximately 20 minutes twice a day. The person is in a comfortable seated position. TM produces not only relaxation, but also a state of mental alertness (Sharma, Clark, 2000).

Follow-up investigations in the landmark study by Ornish and colleagues (1990), showed that patients with coronary atherosclerosis, using lifestyle modifications, were able to reverse coronary artery disease. Modifications included meditation (along with dietary measures, exercise programs, smoking cessation, and group support):

The ancient swamis, and yogis, rabbis, and priests, nuns and monks didn't develop mind-body techniques to get cholesterol down, or unclog arteries, or help people lose weight, or perform better at board meetings. Their techniques are tools for transformation and transcendence that can help us quiet the mind and body, and experience an inner sense of peace and joy and well-being...People who meditate on a regular basis may ultimately find it leads to a direct experience of transcendence. (Ornish, 1993, p. 8)

Snyder (1998, 2002) and Freeman and Lawlis (2001) summarize the conditions and research in which meditation has been used. These conditions include anxiety, asthma, pain, heart conditions, drug abuse, epilepsy, hypertension, headache, health promotion, insomnia, menstrual discomfort, posttraumatic stress disorder, and psychotherapy.

In a retrospective study in Canada, the use of TM by patients appeared to reduce healthcare costs (government payments). "After beginning TM practice, subjects' adjusted expenses declined significantly. The several methods used to assess the rate of decline showed estimates ranging from 5% to 7%" (Herron et al, 1996, p. 208). In an older study, male students between the ages of 21 and 30 who were heavy social drinkers (at least 45 drinks each month) were placed in an exercise, meditation, or control group (Murphy et al, 1986). The meditators were to sit comfortably for 20 minutes a day and repeat a mantra. The subjects in the running group decreased their alcohol consumption, but the total decrease for the meditators was not significant. However, subjects who were high compliers with the meditation schedule decreased consumption by 60% compared with the low compliers who decreased by only 24%. Because this study was small and the researchers were working with a complicated issue, future research in this area may help shed light on interventions.

Several popular meditation learning resources include Jack Kornfield's materials (1996a,b). Kornfield has both audio and video recordings and discusses "insight" meditation, emphasizing "mindful attention, or immediate awareness of one's experience in all spheres of activity" (p. 1). *The Inner Art of Meditation* (1996b), a videotape, is especially good for beginners. Jon Kabat-Zinn (1994) has recording and texts. Thich Nhat Hanh (1997) has writings and recordings on the practice of mindfulness; these media present Buddhist principles for daily life.

Neurolinguistic Programming

Neurolinguistic programming (NLP) is a therapy model:

> ...that focuses on resolving problems by identifying the way that individuals create and also maintain their problems through the way they think and what they believe. The problem then can be resolved by changing the patients' thought patterns and mental strategies in order to give the patients more—and better—choices. (Brookhouse, 2000, p. 96)

All senses are used and are discussed in terms of being *representational systems*. People are thought to demonstrate the way they think by their "words, body language and eye movements" (Brookhouse, 2000, p. 97). For example, visual people will talk using visual terms such as, "I see"; a feeling person would use words such as "feel," "grasp," and "let's touch on that"; and an auditory person would use terms such as, "I hear you" or "that rings a bell."

When a person makes initial contact with another person, he or she will probably be thinking in one of these three main *representational systems*. Internally he or she will be generating visual images, having feelings, or talking to himself or herself and hearing sounds.

One of the ways this activity can be acknowledged is by listening to the kinds of process words (the predicates: verbs, adverbs, and adjectives) that the person uses to describe his or her experience. If the listener is attentive to that information, he or she can adjust behavior to get the response that is wanted. If good rapport is the aim, the person can speak using the same kind of predicates that the other person is using. If the aim is to alienate the other person, deliberately *mis*matching predicates will work (Bandler, Grinder, 1979).

NLP has been used with phobias, feelings of inadequacy, smoking cessation, stress management, assertiveness, neurosis, weight control, performance enhancement, gender dysphoria, and schizophrenia (Brookhouse, 2000).

Prayer

Prayer is a universal form of communication with a higher power. In most cultures, a desire exists to connect with the higher power for direction in life, for healing purposes, or both. Various names are given to this source of power, depending on the underlying religious or spiritual beliefs that the community or individual embraces. For the purposes of this book, the higher power is not defined by a particular religion and will be referred to as God, Great Spirit, or higher power. Most cultures believe that power associated with God exists that can heal the mind, body, and spirit (Davis, 1990). Prayer is often the mechanism used to connect with this power. "They (prayers) are like the lightening rod, they pierce the clouds and bring down the mighty and mysterious power from on high" (Carter, 1988, p. 153).

During times of plenty or good health, people often forget to pray and communicate with God, "but when sickness comes, God is remembered" (White, 1942, p. 225). This provision implies an underlying belief that a higher power not only listens to prayers, but also answers them, often in the form of healing. Most cultures embrace some form of personal and intercessory or distant prayer; however, a realization exists that prayers are not always answered according to our wishes. According to Mother Teresa, "prayer is not asking. Prayer is putting oneself in the hands of God, at His disposition, and listening to His voice in the depths of our hearts" (Gonzalez-Balado, 1996, p. 9). Catherine Marshall (1975) says that most people try to tell God how to "fix" things in life through prayer, but realize at some point that trusting in the higher power's wisdom and will is the better path to take, because this omnipotent being knows the person's past, present, and future. Praying in terms of "God's will be done" can enable individuals to pray for others more readily and with less risk of imposing their personal religious-spiritual beliefs inappropriately or offensively. Dossey (1999), a spiritually-focused physician, seems to support this premise in a commentary on prayer and health, stating, "if a physician simply prays, 'may Thy will be done' or 'may the best outcome prevail for my patient,' he or she is not attempting to manipulate or control a patient, but is asking for a greater wisdom to prevail" (p. 18). Dossey (1999) encourages HCPs to embrace the opportunity to explore the relationship between spirituality and health with their patients. Through the simple act of prayer, the HCP and patient can benefit. First, wisdom can be sought regarding patient evaluation or care; and second, healing within the patient can be promoted. Although this premise may be "new" news in the United States, it is "old" news in most other cultures. In his writings on Native-American medicine and healing, Ken "Bear Hawk" Cohen (1998) points out that, "healing always begins with prayer" (p. 50). Cohen goes on to say, "the healer prays each day to prepare himself or herself for the work ahead. The healer may also pray with and for the patient" (p. 50). Davis (1990) similarly points out that traditional healers often use various healing remedies and strategies, including herbal baths, massage, and the ingestion of medicinal plants when treating ailments. However, healers believe that intervention on the spiritual plane ultimately determines the patient's fate. "For early humanity and for most societies around the world today, priest and physician are one, for the condition of the spirit determines the physical state of the body. Health is a state of balance, of harmony, and for most societies it is something holy" (Davis, 1990, pp. 11-12).

Today's society offers many instances in which prayer in health care is beneficial, However, one area of particular importance is when a HCP must tell a patient, family members, or both that the patient has a very serious or even fatal health problem (Holland et al, 1999). Prayer can be a source of strength for the bearer of bad news, as well as for the recipient. Most patients welcome spiritual support and have improved health outcomes when personal or intercessory prayer is implemented (Anderson et al, 1993; Creagan, 1997; Harris et al, 1999; Helm et al, 2000; King et al, 1994; Maugans et al, 1991). Furthermore, research indicates that spiritual activities, including prayer, have a positive impact on quality of life, recovery, and survival among patients with cancer and patients during rehabilitation (Anderson et al, 1993; Maugans et al, 1991). Platt (2001) has developed a helpful tool that directs the HCP systematically through the process of presenting "bad news" to patients. Other resources for HCPs who strive to develop or improve the skill of relating "bad news" to patients includes Dahlin (1999), Holland (1999), Maynard (1997), Vaidya (1999), and Vetto (1999).

Even though the concept of prayer and healing is ancient, this relationship has not been given serious scientific consideration until recently (Dossey, 1999). The effects of personal and intercessory prayer on health outcomes have been a topic of great discussion over the last few years. The effect of prayer is a difficult topic to study, because "extraneous prayer" can be easily introduced into the control group (Dossey, 1997). Nevertheless, the results of several studies have strongly indicated that prayer apparently "works" (Dossey, 1997). "An impressive body of evidence (Larson et al, 1995) suggests that prayer and religious devotion are associated with positive health outcomes" (Dossey, 1997, p. 10). One of the most well-known studies regarding intercessory prayer was conducted by Byrd (1988) at the University of California at San Francisco School of Medicine. In this experimental group, Christians anonymously prayed for patients in the coronary care unit. Patients in the control group who did not receive the assigned intercessory prayer had poorer health outcomes; they required ventilatory assistance, antibiotics, and diuretics more frequently than did patients who received prayer. A recent study by Harris and colleagues (1999) replicated the Byrd (1988) study with a few methodologic improvements. Study findings similarly showed improved health outcomes for patients who received intercessory prayer.

Meisenhelder and colleagues (2000) examined the effects of personal prayer on health status, with results supporting the relationship between frequent prayer and positive mental health status. Personal prayer has also been identified as a strategy for improving feelings of connectedness to self, others, and a larger purpose (Bellington et al, 1989). Shuler and colleagues (1994) in their work with inner-city homeless women found that prayer had a soothing effect for these impoverished women and somewhat restored their feelings of being connected to self. Psychologic well being was also enhanced for the homeless women who perceived personal prayer as an effective coping strategy. The women who coped with prayer reported fewer concerns, worries, and depressive symptoms, which improved their psychologic well being. Furthermore, prayer served as a deterrent for self-destructive, addictive behavior by strengthening the women's ability to refrain from alcohol and cocaine use.

As the evidence mounts for improved patient outcomes as a result of spiritual interventions, possibly some HCPs and patients will be more willing to delve into this ubiquitous domain of healing. Fox (1940), in his book, *Power Through Constructive Thinking,* explains that, "what you think about any situation is your treatment of that condition" (p. vii). The author goes on to explain that people's "considered attitude" regarding such questions as, "Do you think that prayer really makes any difference?" determines, among other things, the "state of their bodies" (Fox, 1940, pp. viii-ix). Fox is implying that prayer can affect health status, if the person believes in prayer. According to this premise, research findings may encourage people to believe in the healing power of prayer, thereby making their bodies more receptive to the properties of spiritual healing.

Second, scientific inquiry may increase awareness of how the mind, body, and spirit interact and what impact these interactions can have on healing. Learning better ways to connect with the power of spiritual healing might revolutionize modern medicine. However, in spite of the importance of evidence-based practice, Dossey (1997) asserts that "people test prayer in their individual lives and one's life is the most important laboratory of all" (p. 118). Therefore, regardless of what findings are statistically significant, if a patient has found prayer to be "significant" in his or her healing experience, what else really matters?

Prayer appears to be a powerful resource for many people. As HCPs who treat the "whole" person, inclusion of spiritual matters that can have health consequences is a professional responsibility (Dossey, 1999). Some HCPs may feel the need to become more skilled in making spiritual inquiries with patients and seek resources and training, while others may prefer to include spiritual or religious professionals as members of the multidisciplinary health care team (Dossey, 1999; Shuler et al, 1994). Either route of "wholistic" patient care is acceptable and demonstrates a true desire to respect, preserve, protect, and heal the MBS connection. Information and teaching materials for HCPs regarding learning how to make spiritual inquiries with patients is available through the National Institute for Healthcare Research, 6110 Executive Blvd., Suite 908, Rockville, MD 20852.

In addition, Shuler developed a wholistic (whole person) clinical practice model that directs the HCP in providing wholistic health care, including identification of spiritual strengths and needs in relation to health (Shuler, 1991; Shuler et al, 1993a). Shuler developed two model-based wholistic assessment forms for use with either comprehensive or episodic patient visits (Shuler et al, 1993b). Each form contains a brief spiritual assessment. (See Appendix A.)

Relaxation Techniques

Relaxation techniques are defined as:

> ...a group of behavioral therapeutic approaches that differ widely in their philosophical bases as well as in their methodologies and techniques. Their primary objective is the achievement of nondirected relaxation, rather than direct achievement of a specific therapeutic goal. They all share 2 basic components: (1) repetitive focus on a word, sound, prayer, phrase, body sensation, or muscular activity, and (2) the adoption of a passive attitude toward intruding thoughts and a return to the focus. (NIH [National Institutes of Health] Technology Assessment Panel [TAP] on Integration of Behavioral and Relaxation Approaches into the Treatment of Chronic Pain and Insomnia, 1996, p. 313.)

Relaxation techniques generally alter sympathetic activity. Thus respiratory rate, heart rate, and oxygen consumption decrease, and electroencephalographic slow wave activity increases. Relaxation is practiced in several ways, including Benson's relaxation response, progressive muscle relaxation, autogenics, and some brief methods of deep breathing. Meditation is also considered a form of relaxation (NIH TAP, 1996).

Although Herbert Benson developed the formal term "relaxation response" and process (1975), the philosophy is based in ancient meditative principles. The relaxation response is defined as:

> ...a set of integrated physiologic changes that may be elicited when a subject assumes a relaxed position, often with closed eyes, within a quiet environment, engages in a repetitive mental action and passively ignores distracting thoughts. (Benson, 1977, p. 1152)

The four elements—relaxed position, quiet environment, repetitive mental action, and passive attitude (e.g., ignoring distractions by saying, "Oh, well" or some other soothing sound)—are key to the response. The relaxation response can be elicited in many ways, including walking, breathing, concentration, repetitive exercise, meditation, or complete absorption in a pleasant experience such as a hobby.

Progressive Muscle Relaxation

In the 1930s and 1940s, 40 years before the development of Benson's relaxation response, Jacobsen developed progressive muscle relaxation (PMR). This technique consists of:

> ...progressive tensing and relaxing of successive muscle groups. A person's attention is drawn to discriminating between the feelings experienced when the muscle group is relaxed and when it is tensed. With continued use of PMR, an individual can sense muscle tension without having to progress through the tensing and relaxing of specific muscle groups. (Snyder, 1998, p. 1)

Several forms of PMR are now practiced, including active, passive, self-control, and rapid forms. The active form is one of the most widely used (Snyder, 1998).

Lichstein (1988) details an induction procedure for 16 muscle groups. Participants tense muscles for about 7 seconds and relax them for 45 seconds while concentrating attention on the muscle sensations. The therapist provides the "tension patter" in a crisp voice and the "relaxation patter" in a soothing tone. Each tension phase is ended with the term "relax." Induction starts with the participant comfortably seated, eyes closed. For example, "Tense the muscles of your right hand and forearm by clenching your fist" would be the first:

When I say "now", go ahead and tense the muscles of your right hand and forearm by clenching your fist. Now. Keep it tight, feel the strain, the tension, the muscles are working so hard, and relax (7 seconds). Relax completely, relax immediately. Just give up control of the muscles and let them lie there quietly. Compare in your mind the feelings of tension you were feeling just a few seconds ago in your right hand and forearm to the restful relaxation that is gradually emerging now. The more carefully you focus your attention on the feelings of serenity and tranquility, the greater the relaxation effect you will enjoy. Feel the peaceful, calm sensations growing more and more (45 seconds). (Lichstein, 1988, pp. 120-121)

The rest of the muscle groups that follow are left arm and forearm, right then left biceps, forehead, middle portion of face, lower face, neck, upper back, chest and abdomen, right upper leg, then calf, then ankle, followed by the left. Variation to the patter and comment can be made, such as, "Try to tense only the intended muscle" or "Your face was relaxed" or "That was done well." Variations are made also depending on participant's condition (Lichstein, 1988).

Autogenic Training

Autogenic training (AT) is an imaginal relaxation method in which participants develop a relaxed, passive, and casual attitude, imaging themselves in a comforting, peaceful place. The subjects then follow a set of six standard exercises with the themes of heaviness, warmth, cardiac regulation, respiration, abdominal warmth, and cooling of the forehead. First, the heaviness and warmth are used with arms and legs. The sequence is right arm, left arm (or left first if the person is left-handed), both arms, right leg, left leg, both legs, then arms and legs together. The statement that is continued by the provider in a soothing voice, for approximately 30 seconds, is:

I am at peace...My right (or left) arm (or leg) is heavy...My right arm is heavy...I am at peace. My right arm is heavy...My right arm is heavy...I am at peace. (Lichstein, p. 110)

A brief period of silence for about 30 seconds is given as the participants continue on their own with each limb and imagining themselves in their peaceful place. This period is followed by the warmth exercises in similar fashion, then adding both warmth and heavy as a statement. Then, each of the other exercises ("My heartbeat is calm and regular." "My breathing is calm." "My abdomen is warm." "My forehead is cool.") are individually stated, combining each of the previous exercises until the final exercise:

I am at peace...My arms and legs are heavy and warm, heartbeat calm and regular...I am at peace...My breathing is calm...My abdomen is warm...My forehead is cool...My forehead is cool...I am at peace...My breathing is calm...My abdomen is warm...My forehead is cool...My forehead is cool...I am at peace...My forehead is cool....My forehead is cool...My forehead is cool. (Lichstein, 1988, p. 111)

Freeman and Lawlis (2001) give an example with explanatory mechanism:

My arm is very heavy (muscular relaxation)
My arm is very warm (vascular dilation)
My heartbeat is very regular (stabilization of heart function)
It breathes me (regulation of breath)
Warmth is radiating over my stomach (regulation of visceral organs)
There is a cool breeze across my forehead (regulation of blood flow in the head) (p. 253)

Benefits and Uses of Relaxation Techniques

Research evidence suggests a correlation between relaxation therapy and reducing chronic pain (NIH TAP, 1996), including research for other diseases and symptoms. Box 12-3 lists relaxation uses and

---

Box 12-3

Relaxation Techniques Uses and Research

Acute pain (Cole, Brunk, 1999)
Anxiety (Kanji, Ernst, 2000; Crocker, Grozelle, 1991)
Asthma (Freedberg et al, 1987; Henry et al, 1993)
Cancer (Bridge et al, 1988; Cotanch, 1983; Sloman et al, 1994)
Chronic obstructive pulmonary disease (Gift et al, 1992)
Chronic pain (Freeman, 2001; NIH TAP, 1996)
Dysmenorrhea (Freeman, 2001)
Eczema (Ehlers et al, 1995)
Glaucoma (Ernst, 2001)
Headache pain (Blanchard et al, 1991; Freeman, 2001 ; Ernst, 2001; Rolicki, 1997; Freeman, 2001)
Hypertension (Freeman, 2001; Hahn et al, 1993; Kanji et al, 1999)
Insomnia (NIH TAP, 1996)
Irritable bowel (Guthrie, 1991)
Myocardial infarction rehabilitation and angina (Linden et al, 1994)
Nausea and vomiting relief (Ernst, 2001; Freeman, 2001)
Panic disorder (Beck et al, 1994; Ost et al, 1993)
Seizure reduction (Ernst, 2001; Freeman, 2001; Whitman et al, 1990)

references. Ernst (2001) and Freeman and Lawlis (2001) review some relaxation research.

SOCIAL SUPPORT AND PERSONAL INTERACTION

Last, but far from least, social support and personal interaction adds the dimension of compassion, sharing, and caring to any situation. Interactive events help form social structure and give meaning, depth, and learning experiences to life. These social and interactive aspects include family; friends; pets; work, social, and religious groups; and support groups. Social support can include even therapists, HCPs, and people encountered on a casual but regular basis who do not fit any of the aforementioned roles.

Social and personal interaction provides companionship and support. This aspect of life has numerous implications for well being and health status. Chapter 2 on well being in this text covers information on the importance of social support and lists social and interactive factors that promote health, including the importance of helping others, forming relationships based on trust, and having the capacity to confide in others (Dreher, 1995). In addition, several studies are mentioned regarding social support.

Pet Therapy

Pet therapy and service animal programs are two structured ways that pets help humans. In addition, animals are involved in human lives in many other ways. Pet therapy programs, in which pets are brought to patients, provide companionship, "affection, attention, diversion, and relaxation" (McCloskey, Bulechek, 1992, p. 68). Moreover, pet ownership itself has health benefits. Jennings (1997) says that "a pet may become a stimulus for exercise, reduce anxiety, and provide an external focus of attention. Pets are also a source of physical contact and comfort and may decrease loneliness and depression while promoting an interesting lifestyle" (p. 358). Research has shown that pets help buffer physiologic responses to stress, decrease blood pressure, increase survival following critical care discharge and following myocardial infarction, and help promote relaxation. In addition, people with pets have lower systolic blood pressure and triglycerides and have improved health than do those without pets (Jennings, 1997). Furthermore, most pets offer unconditional love.

Service animal programs provide a valuable health benefit and independence to people who use such animals. These organizations help with people who are sight or hearing impaired or have other physical, developmental, mental, or emotional concerns. Resources include: Guide Dog Foundation for the Blind (www.guidedog.org);

Canine Companions for Independence (www.caninecompanions. org); Paws with a Cause (www.pawscause.org); The Delta Society National Service Dog Center (www.deltasociety.org); and Helping Hands: Simian Aides for the Disabled (www.helpinghandsmonkeys.org).

In addition, we have therapy with dolphins and hobbies with animals, such as horseback riding, bird watching, and fishing, and also dog and horse races. On a more somber note, there are dogs that search for humans in cases of lost or escaped persons. These are mice, rats, sheep, guinea pigs, and dogs, among other animals, used in health care experimentation so that humans may have safer medicines, products, and cosmetics. There are some animals that work as beasts of burden to ensure a food supply; and, of course, animals that we slaughter for food. These examples may seem a bit remote, but they exemplify how animals impact heavily on our lives and our health. (Huebscher, 2000, p. 1)

RESOURCES

Academy for Guided Imagery (www.interactiveimagery.com)
Nurse's Certificate Program in Interactive Imagery (email: ncpii@aol.com; web site: www.imageryrn.com)
The American Art Therapy Association (www.arttherapy.org)
American Dance Therapy Association (www.adta.org)
American Music Therapy Association (infor@musictherapy.org; www.musictherapy. org)
American Society of Clinical Hypnosis (www.asch.net)
American Yoga Association (www.americanyogaassociation.org)
Association for Applied Psychophysiology and Biofeedback Information Area (www.aapb.org/public)
Biofeedback Certification Institute of America (www.bcia.org)
International Association of Interactive Imagery (www.iaii.org)
National Association for Poetry Therapy (202-966-2536)
The Transcendental Meditation Program (www.tm.org)

REFERENCES

Allende I: Dreams and stories: the spirit in everyday life, *Noetic Sciences Bulletin*, Summer, 1996.
American Art Therapy Association [AATA]: Frequently asked questions, 1998. www.arttherapy.org Accessed 2/1/2003.
American Dance Therapy Association [ADTA]: What is dance/movement therapy? 2001. URL: http://www.adta.org Accessed 7/31/2001.
American Yoga Association [AYA]: yoga and wellness, 2001. Accessed 4/3/2003. URL: http://www. americanyogaassociation.org
Anderson JM et al: Pastoral needs and support within an inpatient rehabilitation unit, *Arch Phys Med Rehab* 74:574, 1993.

Anderson RA: *Wellness medicine*, Emmaus, Penn, 1987, Rodale Press.

Association for Applied Psychophysiology and Biofeedback [AAPB]: AAPB Website Public Information Area, 1998. URL: www.aapb.org/public. Accessed 6/4/2001.

Bandler R, Grinder J: *Frogs into princes: neuro linguistic programming*, Moab, Utah, 1979, Real People Press.

Beck et al: comparison of cognitive therapy and relaxation training for panic disorder, *J Consult Clin Psychol* 62:818, 1994.

Bellington R et al: Connectedness: some skills for spiritual health, *Am J Health Promo* 4:18, 1989.

Benson H: *The relaxation response*, New York, 1975, Avon.

Benson H: Systemic hypertension and the relaxation response, *N Engl J Med* 296(20):1152, 1977.

Biofeedback Certification Institute of America [BCIA]: How to search for a practitioner, 2001. URL: www.bcia.org/generalinfo. Accessed 6/5/2001.

Blanchard EB et al: The role of regular home practice of relaxation treatment for tension headache, *J Consult Clin Psychol* 59:467, 1991.

Bolen J: *Goddesses in every woman*, New York, 1984, Harper and Row.

Bridge et al: Relaxation and imagery in the treatment of breast cancer, *Br Med J* 297:1169, 1988.

Brookhouse S: Neuro linguistic programming. In Novey D, ed: *Clinician's complete reference to complementary and alternative medicine*, St Louis, 2000, Mosby.

Byrd RC: Positive therapeutic effects of intercessory prayer in a coronary care unit population, *South Med J* 81:826, 1988.

Cameron J: *The artist's way*, New York, 1992, Tarcher Putnam.

Carter T: *Spurgeon at his best*, Grand Rapids, Mich, 1988, Baker Book House Company.

Cohen K "Bear Hawk": Native American medicine, *Alt Ther Health Med* 4:45, 1998.

Cole B, Brunk Q: Holistic interventions for acute pain episodes: an integrative review, *J Holistic Nurs* 17(4):384, 1999.

Cotanch P: Relaxation training for control of nausea and vomiting in patients receiving chemotherapy, *Cancer Nurs* 6:272, 1983.

Creagan ET: Attitude and disposition: do they make a difference in cancer survival? *Mayo Clin Proc* 72:160, 1997.

Crocker PR, Grozell C: Reducing induced state anxiety: effects of acute aerobic exercise and autogenic relaxation, *J Sports Med Phys Fitness* 31:277, 1991.

Dahlin CM: Care and compassion in conveying bad news, *Clin J Oncol Nurs* 3:73, 1999.

Davis M, Eshelman E, McKay M: *The relaxation and stress reduction workbook*, Oakland, Calif, 1998, New Harbinger.

Davis W: The many paths of a healer. In Smolan R, Moffitt P, Naythons M, eds: *The power to heal: ancient arts and modern medicine*, New York, 1990, Prentice Hall Press.

Day A: The journal as a guide for the healing journey, *Nurs Clin North Am* 36(1):131, 2001.

Dossey B et al: *Holistic nursing: a handbook of practice*, Gaithersburg, Md, 1995, Aspen.

Dossey L: Do religion and spirituality matter in health? A response to the recent article in the Lancet, *Alt Ther Health Med* 5:16, 1999.

Dossey L: The return of prayer, *Alt Ther Health Med* 3:10, 113, 1997.

Dreher H: *The immune power personality*, New York, 1995, Dutton.

Ehlers A, Stangier U, Gieler U: Treatment of atopic dermatitis: a comparison of psychological and dermatological approaches to relapse prevention, *J Consult Clin Psychol* 63:624, 1995.

Ernst E: *The desktop guide to complementary and alternative medicine*, St Louis, 2001, Mosby.

Fox R: *Power through constructive thinking*, New York, 1940, Harper and Row.

Frawley D: *Yoga and Ayurveda*, Twin Lakes, Wisc., 1999, Lotus Press.

Freedberg PD et al: Effect of progressive muscle relaxation on the objective symptoms and subjective responses associated with asthma, *Heart Lung* 16:24, 1987.

Freeman L: Relaxation. In Freeman L, Lawlis F, eds: *Mosby's complementary and alternative medicine*, St Louis, 2001, Mosby.

Freeman L, Lawlis F: *Mosby's complementary and alternative medicine*, St Louis, 2001, Mosby.

Gawain S: *Creative visualization*, New York, 1978, (updated 1997), Bantam Books.

Gift AG, Moore T, Soeken K: Relaxation to reduce dyspnea and anxiety in COPD patients, *Nurs Res* 41:242, 1992.

Gonzalez-Balado JL: *Mother Teresa: in my own words*, Liguori, Mo, 1996, Liguori Publications.

Griffin SJ, Trinder J: Physical fitness, exercise and human sleep, *Psychophysiol* 15:447, 1978.

Guthrie E et al: A controlled trial of psychological treatment for the irritable bowel syndrome, *Gastroenterol* 100:450, 1991.

Guzzetta C: Music therapy: hearing the melody of the soul. In Dossey B et al, eds: *Holistic nursing: a handbook of practice*, Gaithersburg, Md, 1995, Aspen.

Hahn YB: The effect of thermal biofeedback and progressive muscle relaxation training in reducing blood pressure of patients with essential hypertension, *Image* 25:204, 1993.

Halo Shames K: *Creative imagery in nursing*, Albany, New York, 1996, Delmar.

Harris WS et al: A randomized, controlled trial of the effects of remote, intercessory prayer on outcomes in patients admitted to the coronary care unit, *Arch Intern Med* 159:2273, 1999.

Hay L: *Heal your body*, Carlsbad, Calif, 1988, Hay House.

Healthfinder: Prevention and wellness: exercise, 2003. URL: www.healthfinder.gov/scripts/searchcontext.asp?topic=297&super=112&branch=5. Accessed 2/1/2003.

Helm HM et al: Does private religious activity prolong survival? A six-year follow-up study of 3,851 older adults, *J Gerontol Biol Sci Med Sci* 55:M400, 2000.

Helmrich SP et al: Physical activity and reduced occurrence of non-insulin-dependent diabetes mellitus, *N Eng J Med* 325:3, 1991.

Henry M et al: Improvement of respiratory function in chronic asthmatic patients with autogenic therapy, *J Psycho Res* 17:265, 1993.

Herron R et al: The impact of the transcendental meditation program on government payments to physicians in Quebec, *Am J Health Promot* 10(3):208, 1996.

Hoban S: Motion and emotion: the dance/movement therapy experience, *Nurs Homes Long Term Care Manag* 49:2, 2000.

Holland JC, Almanza J: Giving bad news: is there a kinder, gentler way? *Cancer* 86:738, 1999.

Horovitz E: Art therapy. In Novey D, ed: *Clinician's complete reference to complementary and alternative medicine*, St Louis, 2000, Mosby.

Hrezo R: Hypnosis and pain management, *NP Forum* 9(4):217, 1998.

Huebscher R: Pets and animal-assisted therapy, *NP Forum* 11(1):1, 2000.

Hunter B: Music therapy. In Novey D, ed: *Clinician's complete reference to complementary and alternative medicine*, St Louis, 2000, Mosby.

Iyengar BKS: *Light on yoga*, New York, 1979, Schocken Books.

Jennings L: Potential benefits of pet ownership in health promotion, *J Holistic Nurs* 15(4):358, 1997.

Jones A: *Yoga: a step-by-step guide*, Boston, 1998, Element Books.

Kabat-Zinn J: *Wherever you go there you are*, New York, 1994, Hyperion.

Kanji N, Ernst E: Autogenic training for stress and anxiety: a systematic review, *Compl Ther Med* 8:106, 2000.

Kanji N, White AR, Ernst E: Anti-hypertensive effects of autogenic training: a systematic review, *Perfusion* 12:279, 1999.

King DE et al: Beliefs and attitudes of hospital inpatients about faith, healing and prayer, *J Fam Pract* 39:349, 1994.

Kornfield J: *Meditations of the heart* [audiotape], Boulder, Colo, 1994, Sounds True.

Kornfield J: *The inner art of meditation* [videotape], Boulder, Colo, 1996, Sounds True.

Kornfield J: *The inner art of meditation. Program guide to the inner art of meditation* [videotape], Boulder, Colo, 1996a, Sounds True.

Kornfield J: *The inner art of meditation* [videotape], Boulder, Colo, 1996b, Sounds True.

Kreitzer M: Meditation. In Snyder M, Lindquist R, eds: *Complementary and alternative therapies in nursing*, ed 4, New York, 2002, Springer.

Larson DB et al: Are religion and spirituality clinically relevant in health care? *Mind/Body Med* 1:147, 1995.

Lichstein K: *Clinical relaxation strategies*, New York, 1988, Wiley Interscience.

Marshall C: *Adventures in prayer*, New York, 1975, Ballantine Books.

Maugans TA, Wadland WC: Religion and family medicine: a survey of physicians and patients, *J Fam Pract* 32:210, 1991.

Maynard DW: How to tell patients bad news: the strategy of forecasting, *Clev Clin J Med* 64:181, 1997.

McCloskey J, Bulechek G: *Nursing interventions classification* [NIC], St Louis, 1992, Mosby.

Meisenhelder JB, Chandler EN: Prayer and health outcomes in church members, *Alt Ther Health Med* 6:56, 2000.

Murphy T, Pagano R, Marlatt GA: Lifestyle modification with heavy alcohol drinkers: effects of aerobic exercise and meditation, *Addictive Behav* 11:175, 1986.

Naparstek B: *Staying well with guided imagery*, New York, 1994, Time Warner.

National Center for Complementary and Alternative Medicine (NACCAM): What is complementary and alternative medicine, 2002. URL: http://nccam.nih.gove/health/whatiscom. Accessed 2/1/2003.

National Heart, Lung and Blood Institute [NHLBI]: Guide to physical activity, 2001. URL: http://www.nhlbi.org. Accessed 7/17/2001.

National Institutes of Health [NIH], Technology Assessment Panel [TAP] on Integration of Behavioral and Relaxation Approaches into the Treatment of Chronic Pain and Insomnia: Integration of behavioral and relaxation approaches into the treatment of chronic pain and insomnia, *JAMA* 276(4):313, 1996.

Northrup C: *Women's bodies, women's wisdom*, New York, 1998, Bantam Books.

Ornish D: Opening your heart: anatomically, emotionally and spiritually, *Noetic Sci Rev* Winter, 4, 1993.

Ornish D et al: Can lifestyle changes reverse coronary heart disease? *Lancet* 336:129, 1990.

Ost LG, Westling BE, Hellstrom K: applied relaxation, exposure in vivo and cognitive methods in the treatment of panic disorder with agoraphobia, *Behav Res Ther* 31:383, 1993.

Pennebaker J: *Opening up: the healing power of expressing emotions*, New York, 1997, Guilford Press.

Platt A: A systematic approach to presenting bad news, *Clin News* July/August 20:22, 2001.

Prior J: Conditioning exercise decreases premenstrual symptoms: a prospective, controlled 6-month trial, *Fertility Sterility* 47:402, 1987.

Progoff I: *At a journal workshop*, New York, 1975, Dialogue House Library.

Rojcewicz S: Poetry therapy. In Novey D, ed: *Clinician's complete reference to complementary and alternative medicine*, Philadelphia, 2000, Mosby.

Rolicki LA et al: Change mechanisms associated with combined relaxation/EMG biofeedback training and chronic tension-type headache, *Appl Psychophysiol Biofeedback* 22:187, 1997.

Saichek K: Hypnotherapy. In Novey D, ed: *Clinician's complete reference to complementary and alternative medicine*, St Louis, 2000, Mosby.

Samuels M: Art as a healing force, *Alt Ther* 1(4):38, 1995.

Sharma H, Clark C: *Contemporary Ayurveda*, Edinburgh, 2000, Churchill Livingstone.

Shuler PA: Homeless women's wholistic and family planning needs: an exposition and test of the Shuler nurse practitioner practice model (Doctoral dissertation, University of California, Los Angeles, 1991). Ann Arbor: University Microfilms International/Dissertation Information Service (Order number 9126912).

Shuler PA et al: The effects of spiritual/religious practices on psychological well-being among inner city homeless women, *NP Forum* 5:106, 1994.

Shuler PA, Davis J: The Shuler nurse practitioner practice model: a theoretical framework for nurse practitioner clinicians, educators and researchers, part 1, *J Am Acad Nurs Pract* 5(1):11, 1993a.

Shuler PA, Davis J: The Shuler nurse practitioner practice model: clinical application, part 2, *J Am Acad Nurs Pract* 5(2):73, 1993b.

Sloman R et al: The use of relaxation for the promotion of comfort and pain relief in persons with advanced cancer, *Contemp Nurs* 3(1):6, 1994.

Snyder M: Journaling. In Snyder M, Lindquist R, eds: *Complementary and alternative therapies in nursing*, ed 4, New York, 2002, Springer.

Snyder M: Progressive muscle relaxation. In Snyder M, Lindquist R, eds: *Complementary and alternative therapies in nursing*, ed 3, New York, 1998, Springer.

Thich Nhat Hanh: *The blooming of a lotus: guided meditation exercises for healing and transformation*, Boston, 1997, Beacon. (Also others from 1976.)

Thune I et al: Physical activity and the risk of breast cancer, *N Engl J Med* 336:1269, 1997.

Tkachuk, GA, Martin, GL: Exercise therapy for patients with psychiatric disorders: research and clinical implications, *Prof Psychol: Res Pract* 33:275, 1999.

U.S. Preventive Services Task Force: *Guide to clinical preventive services*, Baltimore, 1996, Williams and Wilkins.

Vaidya DU et al: Teaching physicians how to break bad news: a 1-day workshop using standardized parents, *Arch Pediatr Adolesc Med* 153:419, 1999.

Vetto JT et al: Teaching medical students to give bad news: does formal instruction help? *J Cancer Educ* 14:13, 1999.

White E: *The ministry of healing*, Mountain View, Calif, 1942, Pacific Press Publishing.

Whitman S: Progressive relaxation for seizure reduction, *J Epilepsy* 3:17, 1990.

Wolf SL et al: Reducing frailty and falls in older persons: an investigation of tai chi and computerized balance training, *J Am Geriatr Soc* 44:489, 1996.

Wolfson LR et al: Balance and strength training in older adults: intervention gains and tai chi maintenance, *J Am Geriatr Soc* 44:498, 1996.

Zahourek R: *Relaxation and imagery: tools for therapeutic communication and intervention*, Philadelphia, 1988, Saunders.

CHAPTER 13

BIOLOGIC-BASED THERAPIES*

Roxana Huebscher

Biologic-based therapies refer to "substances found in nature, such as herbs, foods, and vitamins" (NCCAM, 2002, p. 2). Within this category are nutritional supplements that include vitamins, minerals, and herbs; dietary therapy; and other biologic therapies such as shark cartilage, bee pollen, melatonin, antineoplastins, chelation therapies, and flower essences, as well as additional practices and products (Novey, 2000). The biologic-based therapies are prevalent within the Alternative Health Care Systems category. For example, Ayurveda, Traditional Chinese Medicine, and Native-American Medicine have many herbal preparations. Box 13-1 lists some examples of biologic-based products and substances.

DIET

Dietary variations are numerous. Most specialty diets have both good and caution points. The reader should refer to individual chapters of the text for dietary recommendations for diseases and symptoms and then to nutritional resources and references for particular diets.

NUTRITIONAL SUPPLEMENTS

Before 1994, only substances such as vitamins, minerals, and proteins were considered dietary supplements. However, in 1994 the Dietary Supplement Health and Education Act (DSHEA) broadened the definition. The DSHEA provides minimal U.S. Food and Drug Administration (FDA) regulation of dietary supplements and gives manufacturers the freedom to market more products as dietary supplements. Currently, a dietary supplement is considered:

> ...a product taken by mouth that contains a "dietary ingredient" intended to supplement the diet. The "dietary ingredients" in these products may include: vitamins, minerals, herbs or other botanicals,

---

*Note: This chapter is not a prescribing source. Readers are cautioned to use a complete prescribing text for biologic-based therapies.

Box 13-1

Examples of Biologic-Based Products and Substances

Algae (chlorella, spirulena)
Amino acids and enzymes
Antineoplastins
Antioxidants (alpha lipoic acid; vitamins C, E; beta carotene; selenium; copper; zinc; bioflavenoids; cysteine)
Aromatherapy
Bacteria such as *Lactobacillus*
Bee by-products (pollen, propolis, honey-royal jelly)
Chelation therapy
Coley's toxins
Diet: Atkins, Diamond, Elimination, Fasting, Gerson, Juice Therapy, Macrobiotics, Mediterranean, Ornish, Pritikin, Vegetarian, Whole Foods, Zone
Dimethylsulfoxide (DMSO)
Essential fatty acids and lecithin
Fiber (bran, cellulose, gum, hemicellulose, lignin, mucilage, pectin)
Flower essences (such as Bach flower remedies)
Glandulars and organ tissues (bovine cartilage, shark cartilage)
Herbs
Hormones (such as melatonin and dehydroepiandrosterone [DHEA])
Hyperbaric oxygen
Minerals and elements
Mushrooms (maitake, reishi, shitake, etc.)
Spices (allspice, cinnamon, cloves, ginger, etc.)
Vinegar
Vitamins
Yeast

Sources: Balch J, Balch P: Prescription for nutritional healing, *Garden City Park, New York, 1997, Avery; DerMarderosian A, ed:* Facts and comparisons, *St Louis, 2000, Facts and Comparisons; Novey D:* Clinician's complete reference to complementary and alternative medicine, *St Louis, 2000, Mosby.*

amino acids, and substances such as enzymes, organ tissues, glandulars, and metabolites. Dietary supplements can also be extracts or concentrates, and may be found in many forms such as tablets, capsules, soft-gels, gel-caps, liquids, or powders. They can also be in other forms, such as a bar, but if they are, information on their label must not represent the product as a conventional food or a sole item of a

meal or diet. Whatever their form may be, DSHEA places dietary supplements in a special category under the general umbrella of "foods,"
not drugs, and requires that every supplement be labeled a dietary supplement. (FDA, Center for Food Safety and Applied Nutrition
[CFSAN], 2001, p. 1)

Thus the FDA considers an herb, vitamin, and mineral to be neither a drug nor a substitute for a conventional diet. Drugs are
intended to "diagnose, treat, cure, or prevent disease" and effectiveness, safety, possible interactions, and dosages must be FDA-
reviewed before the drug is marketed (FDA/CFSAN, 2001a, p. 1).
In contrast, the FDA does not authorize or test dietary supplements.
Thus consumers need to be wary because the FDA premarket review
for dietary supplements is less than it is for regulated products (such
as drugs or food additives). Consumers therefore have the responsibility to determine if a product is safe, that labels are truthful, and
the product is what it says it is. This task is time-consuming and
requires either an extensive knowledge base or access to reputable
nutritional and supplement experts who are up-to-date and knowl-
edgeable themselves.

The FDA has published regulations defining the type of statements that can be made about the effects of dietary supplements on
the structure or function of the body. The FDA 2000 regulations
help differentiate claims of treat/cure/diagnose from those of
structure/function (FDA, 2000, 2001a,b). For example, unless a
dietary supplement has FDA approval, the label cannot make a *disease* claim such as "prevents osteoporosis" or "prevents bone
fragility." Dietary supplement labels can, however, make health
maintenance statements such as "maintains a healthy circulatory system," for "muscle enhancement," or "helps you relax"; and they can
make claims for alleviating common minor symptoms such as: "for
hot flashes." Obviously, confusion exists in the subtleties of these
regulations (FDA, 2001b, p. 1).

Vitamins, Minerals, and Elements

Recently, new vitamin and element recommendations have been
released (Food and Nutrition Board, 2001). (See Appendix D.)
Included are several new dietary reference intakes (DRIs) other than
recommended dietary allowances (RDAs). These values are the estimated average intake (EAR), adequate intake (AI), and tolerable
upper limit (UL). Important to note is that many alternative recommendations exceed the AI and RDA. Care should be taken when a
natural-alternative-complementary (NAC) recommendation exceeds
the UL, because this is the amount beyond which the supplement
may produce adverse effects.

Herbs

Phytomedicine refers to ingested and topical use of medicinal herbs, including plants or plant parts (Fetrow, Avila, 1999). Herbs are rooted in, steeped, and infused throughout ancient cultures, with evidence dating to Neanderthal times, 60,000 BCE. Herbal use is reported for Ayurvedic, Unanic (Middle Eastern), Mesopotamian, Egyptian, and Greek cultures. The Chinese have texts dating back 5000 years (including mention of the opium poppy and ephedra), and early European settlers exchanged herbal information with Native Americans (Chavez, Chavez, 2000). In the early twentieth century, United States physicians used many herbs, and herbal medicine was a part of routine medical practice. However, herbal use waned for many years. Recently, interest has increased and several herbal resources have been published, including a frequently updated Natural Medicines Comprehensive Database that has information about herbs, vitamins, minerals, and other supplements (PL/PL, 2003).

Germany, certain Asian countries, Italy, Spain, Netherlands, and Belgium have used herbs more consistently than the United States (Fetrow, Avila, 1999). In Germany, as in other European countries, the use of herbals has a long history and monograph documentation. The German Commission E (GCE) was formed in 1978 using a group of experts who worked together to approve herbals. Approval was based on evidence from a long history of human use combined with a moderate amount of scientific data, called the "Doctrine of Reasonable Certainty." The GCE monographs have been translated into English and are currently available (Blumenthal et al, 1998, 2000).

Phytomedicinal medications are made by extracting herbs with various solvents to make teas, infusions, extracts, tinctures, decoctions, powders, capsules, tablets, and topicals. Various plant parts are used, and different species may have differing amounts of active principles. For example, the ginkgo leaf, ginseng root, and flaxseed are the plant parts that carry the active constituents for common use of ginkgo, ginseng, and flax (DerMarderosian, 2001). Additionally, accurate plant identification is extremely important because some toxic plants resemble medicinal herbs (and some medicinal herbs can be toxic at incorrect dosages). Thus clear and extensive knowledge of herbs is necessary for correct use and identification, and to avoid possible poisoning. Box 13-2 describes types of herbal preparations.

Active ingredients in herbs include alkaloids, bitters, enzymes, essential oils, gums, glycosides, mucilage, saponins, tannins, vitamins, and minerals (Bremness, 1994). Furthermore, each of these ingredients is complex. For example, several thousand alkaloids have been identified. Alkaloids are alkaline compounds that generally

Box 13-2

Types of Herbal Preparations

Teas: dried herbs steeped in water that was boiling; steeped for a short (5 minutes) period of time

Infusions: made from flowers, leaves, and stems; infusions are stronger than teas; a standard infusion recipe is ½ to 1 rounded teaspoon of dried herb per cup of boiling water, steeped for 10 to 20 minutes; to use fresh herb, rather than dried, double the amount. Often, infusion-type preparations are referred to as teas.

Decoctions: similar to infusions, except made from roots, bark, or seed. Active ingredients are more difficult to extract, so rather than steeping, the ingredients are boiled in water, then allowed to simmer for 10 to 20 minutes.

Extracts: substance is treated with water, alcohol, or ether; extracts thicker than tincture; also are dry extracts that are evaporated liquid extracts, almost like a powder

Tinctures: extracts made with alcohol rather than water; are highly concentrated and have longer shelf lives

Powders: crushed and ground dried herbs; used on their own or in mixtures

Pills, tablets, syrups, lozenges: herb may be mixed with other substances and compressed or put into syrup

Capsules: a dose of herb (oil or dried) in a soluble case, usually made of gelatin

Topical: lotions, oils, salves and ointments, liniments, compresses, poultices, herbal baths; for example, add ½ to 1 teaspoon of tincture per ounce of commercial skin lotion; for cuts and burns, a clean cloth can be dipped into a cool infusion or decoction and draped over affected area (a compress)

Sources: Bascom A: Incorporating herbal medicine into clinical practice, *Philadelphia, 2002, FA Davis; Bremness L: Herbs, London, 1994, Dorling Kindersley; Bunney S, ed: The illustrated encyclopedia of herbs: their medicinal and culinary uses, New York, 1992, Dorset; Hoffman D: The complete illustrated holistic herbal, Rockport, Mass, 1997, Element Books.*

have an effect on the nervous and circulatory system. Such substances include atropine, caffeine, codeine, morphine, nicotine, and strychnine (Bunney, 1992). In addition, herbal products may contain a variety of compounds from various classes:

> Often, therapeutic action is due to the combined action of several constituents. Some, like the primary metabolites (cellulose, starches, sugars,

fixed oils), are not particularly active pharmacologically. Others, like the secondary metabolites (alkaloids, cardiac glycosides, and steroids), are quite active pharmacologically. Content varies depending on genetics, environment (sunlight and rainfall), and fertilization. In fact, it is possible to see mixed activity depending on which compounds predominate. Selection at different times of the year also affects herb quality and clinical efficacy. (DerMarderosian, 2001, p. ix)

Thus quality control is extremely important. Attention is needed regarding the plant, how it is grown and harvested, the processing, the manufacturer's standards and qualifications, and the storage of products. Additionally, after extraction occurs, concentration of active ingredients is often higher than it is in the crude herb; thus risk with crude herb is often less than with the concentrated product. Thus in order to ensure safety and quality, health care providers (HCPs) must seek out reliable manufacturers with good manufacturing practices (GMP) (DerMarderosian, 2001).

Standardized Extracts

A standardized extract refers to extracting the specific plant properties that are theorized to have the healing substances. Using a standardized extract means someone, optimally an expert, has identified the correct plant species and that a consistency in the strength of the finished botanical product has been found. Thus a resulting reliability in dosing should exist. Standardized extracts are most often based on a "marker" substance, usually the active principle or principles that has been shown by appropriate trials to reflect the activity of the product. Standards can vary among manufacturers. Standardized preparations are good if the standardized ingredient is the one doing the healing work. However, if the active substance is not known, or a different plant part is needed, or the whole plant in combination is needed to produce the effect, then standardized substances may not be the best. Herein lies the problem with standardized extracts or parts of whole plants. If just part of the garlic is used or just part of the carrot, and no beneficial effects are found, should the phytomedicinal be called ineffective and therefore abandoned; or are we oversimplifying the process to satisfy an experimental procedure?

Box 13-3 outlines several considerations when using herbals. Table 13-1 lists commonly used herbs and Box 13-4 lists some of the herbs that have safety concerns.

AROMATHERAPY

Most of the development of modern aromatherapy began around the mid-twentieth century in France; however, the origins are from thousands of years ago in herbal medicine. Findings date back 60,000

Box 13-3

Herbal Considerations

FDA regulations are less stringent for herbs than they are with drugs.

Adulterations can occur especially with expensive herbs such as Echinacea, ginseng, goldenseal, and saffron.

Beware of products that do not indicate quantity or permit calculation of herb dose.

Natural does not automatically mean safe; herbs can have side effects and interactions.

Do not exceed recommended dose; check for interactions before starting.

Stop herb immediately if adverse effects occur.

Crude herbs often have lower concentrations of active ingredient than extracted or concentrated products.

In general, herbs are not used in pregnant or nursing mothers or in children under 2 years of age; exceptions do exist.

In elderly patients, start with one half the usual dose.

Standardized extracts may be best, or not—the evidence must be known.

Herbs take longer than conventional medications to work, sometimes weeks.

Different plant formulations may be used, thus dosages vary.

Plants or plant parts may be unsafe; an expert must be consulted.

Misuse of a product does not mean the product should be discarded.

Unproven or inadequate research does not mean an herb is ineffective.

Herbal medicine must not be confused with homeopathy.

All people must be encouraged to inform their health care provider or pharmacist of all medications and herbs consumed.

Herbs can cause allergies and drug-herb interactions.

Other ingredients in addition to the herb must be determined.

years to a Neanderthal skeleton that was found (in Iraq) near concentrated extracts of yarrow, knapweed, grape hyacinth, mallow, and other plants. In addition, history of use in Mesopotamia, Egypt, China, India, Tibet, Greece, Arabia, Europe (France and Germany), and England has been discovered (Buckle, 1997).

Buckle (2001), a nurse, defines aromatherapy as:

Table 13-1   Commonly Used Herbs

Current herbal references should be consulted for appropriate part of herb to be used, doses, other uses, side effects, interactions, contraindications, and new information. In general, herbs are not used in women during pregnancy and lactation or in children unless information and evidence exists for safety and benefits. Any herb is contraindicated when allergy to the plant exists. Several of these herbs are considered unsafe.

Herb (Latin Name)	Common Use	Herb (Latin Name)	Common Use
Aloe (Aloe barbendenis)	Constipation (oral); burns (external use)	Garlic (Allium sativum)	To lower cholesterol, lipids, blood sugar; for mild hypertension; antibacterial
Angelica root (Angelica archangelica); family: Apiaceae umbelliferae	GI concerns, respiratory complaints, arthritis	Ginger (Zingeber officinale)	GI concerns, motion sickness
Arnica (Arnica Montana or chamissonis)	External use; injuries (hematomas, dislocations, contusions, etc.)	Ginkgo biloba (Ginkgo biloba)	Organic brain syndrome, memory problems, peripheral arterial occlusive disease, tinnitus
Artichoke (Cynara scolymus)	GI concerns, dyspepsia associated with biliary disease, reduce cholesterol (LDL)	Ginseng root (Panax ginseng or P. quinquefolium); also called true ginseng, Asian, Chinese, or Korean ginseng	Fatigue, for invigoration, antistress

Continued

Table 13-1 Commonly Used Herbs—cont'd

Herb (Latin Name)	Common Use	Herb (Latin Name)	Common Use
Astragalus (Astragalus membranaceus)	Immune function, HIV, diabetes, cancer	Goldenseal (Hydrastis canadensis)	Respiratory, GI, GU infections
Bilberry (Vaccinium myrtillus)	Visual problems, diarrhea	Hawthorn (Crataegus monogyna)	Heart failure, cardiovascular conditions
Black cohosh (Cimicifuga racemosa)	Menopause	Horse chestnut (Aesculus hippocastanum); also called buckeye; FDA classified as unsafe herb	Venous insufficiency
Calendula (Calendula officinalis)	Wounds (external use), fever, dysmenorrhea	Kava kava (Piper methysticum) (currently there are serious concerns regarding liver toxicity with kava use)	Anxiety, for sedation
Cayenne pepper (Capsicum species)	Arthritic pain, neuromuscular pain	Lemon balm (Melissa officinalis)	Sedative; cold sores (external use)
Chamomile (German) (Chamomilla recutita)	GI concerns, sleep disorders	Milk thistle (Silybum marianum)	Reduces liver damage; amanita mushroom poisoning
Chaste tree fruit (Vitex agnus castus)	Menstrual concerns	Mint (Mentha arvensis)	GI and gallbladder disorders, upper respiratory disorders; myalgias (topical)

Cinnamon (Cinnamomum verum or aromaticum)	Loss of appetite, GI concerns	
Cranberry (Vaccinium macrocarpon)	Urinary tract infection and prevention	
Dandelion (Teraxacum officinale)	GI concerns, diuresis, disturbances of bile flow (not for use with obstruction)	
Devil's claw (Harpagophytum procumbens)	Disorders of musculoskeletal system, GI concerns	
Dong quai (Angelica sinensis); family: Apiaceae umbelliferae	Gynecologic concerns	
Echinacea (Echinacea augustifolia, pallida, or purpurea)	Stimulation of immune response; colds and infections	
Eleuthero root (leutherococus senticosus); Siberian ginseng	Fatigue	
Mistletoe (Phoradendron serotinum) (very toxic)		Cancer
Myrtle (Myrti communis) (likely unsafe because of cineol content)		Bronchitis, TB, whooping cough, worm infestation, bladder conditions, diarrhea
Peppermint (Mentha piperita)		Irritable bowel, GI symptoms, abdominal pain, gallbladder symptoms such as spasm
Saw palmetto (Serenoa repens)		BPH, prostate cancer
St. John's wort (Hypericum perforatum)		Depression, anxiety; contusions and burns (topical)
Stinging nettle (Urtica dioica)		Urinary disorders including BPH, diuretic, allergic rhinitis; rheumatic ailments (topical)
Teatree (Melaleuca alternifolia)		External use for skin conditions; antimicrobial effects

Continued

Table 13-1 Commonly Used Herbs—cont'd

Herb (Latin Name)	Common Use	Herb (Latin Name)	Common Use
Evening primrose (Oenothera biennis)	Gynecologic, skin, and cardiovascular concerns, rheumatoid arthritis, multiple sclerosis	Valerian (Valeriana officinalis)	Sleep disorders, restlessness
Feverfew (Tanacetum parthenium)	Headache, arthritis, fever	Witch hazel (Hamamelis virginiana)	Minor skin injuries, local inflammation of skin and mucous membranes, hemorrhoids, varicose veins (topical)

BPH, Benign prostatic hypertrophy; FDA, U.S. Food and Drug Administration; GI, gastrointestinal; GU, genitourinary; HIV, human immunodeficiency virus; TB, tuberculosis.

Sources: Blumenthal M, Goldberg A, Brinckmann J, eds: Herbal medicine: expanded commission E monographs, *Newton, Mass, 2000, Integrative Medicine Communications; Bunney S, ed: The illustrated encyclopedia of herbs: their medicinal and culinary uses, New York, 1992, Dorset; DerMarderosian A, ed: Facts and comparisons, St Louis, 2000, Facts and Comparisons; Fetrow C, Avila J: Professional's handbook of complementary and alternative medicine, Springhouse, Penn, 1999, Springhouse; Novey D: Clinician's complete reference to complementary and alternative medicine, St Louis, 2000, Mosby; Pharmacist's Letter/Prescriber's Letter [PL/PL]: Natural medicine's comprehensive database, Stockton, Calif, 2002, Therapeutic Research Faculty; PDR for herbal medicines, Montvale, NJ, 1998, Medical Economics.*

Box 13-4

Herbs with Safety Concerns

Many herbs, including some of those in Table 13-1, have risks. The herbs listed below have documented health risks. Remember that risks with any herb may be from the herb itself, misuse of the herb, adulteration, or improper identification or processing. The list is not all-inclusive.

Aconite (monkshood)
Aloe (internal use)
Arnica (internal use)
Betel nut
Blue cohosh
Boneset
Broom
Buckthorn
Chamomile
Chaparral
Coltsfoot
Comfrey
Corkwood tree
Dong quai
Ephedra (ma huang)
Germander
Ginseng
Horse chestnut
Kava kava
Licorice
Mistletoe
Myrtle
Pennyroyal
Sassafras
Yew
Yohimbe

Sources: Blumenthal M, Goldberg A, Brinckmann J, eds: Herbal medicine: expanded commission E monographs, Newton, Mass, 2000, Integrative Medicine Communications; DerMarderosian A, ed: Facts and comparisons, St Louis, 2000, Facts and Comparisons; Novey D: Clinician's complete reference to complementary and alternative medicine, St Louis, 2000, Mosby; Pharmacist's Letter/Prescriber's Letter [PL/PL]: Natural medicine's comprehensive database, Stockton, Calif, 2002, Therapeutic Research Faculty.

...the controlled, therapeutic use of essential oils. Essential oils are the "volatile, organic constituents of fragrant plant matter" that are extracted by steam distillation or expression. No other methods of extraction produce an essential oil. When essential oils are used to target specific conditions and the outcomes are measured, aromatherapy becomes clinical. (p. 57)

Clarke (2002), however, describes three types of materials used in aromatherapy. These are essential oils, absolute oils, and aromatherapy oils:

...an essential oil is an aromatic, volatile substance extracted by distillation or expression from a single botanical species. The resulting oil should have nothing added or removed...An absolute oil is an aromatic, volatile substance obtained by solvent extraction from a single botanical species (e.g. rose absolute, jasmine absolute). The resulting oil should have nothing added or removed during the process...An aromatherapy oil is not an essential oil. It is a product that meets the requirements of the profession of aromatherapy. It contains blends of undefined percentages, consisting of vegetable oils and essential oils and sometimes absolutes. (p. 116)

Blended with essential oils are other oils such as carrier oils and herbal oils. Essential oils are diluted before skin application often in a carrier oil. Carrier oils are vegetable-based or seed oils. A few examples are sweet almond, grape seed, apricot kernel, and avocado oil. Herbal oils are "infused oils," in a base of olive or sunflower oil. "A selected herb is macerated in the oil over a period of time" (Buckle, 1997, p. 69). Many aromatherapists, including Buckle, prefer that only pure essential oils (not absolutes or blends) be used in aromatherapy and that carrier oils should be cold-pressed.

Essential oils come from various plant parts, and correct species identification is important. For example, several varieties of lavender and chamomile have been identified. Essential oils are inhaled or used topically, including vaginally. The most common use is inhalation. Inhalation diffusers, nebulizers, and vaporizers are available. Another option is to place one to five drops of essential oil on a cloth, cotton ball, or tissue or in a steaming bowl of water. Common inhalation indications include depression, insomnia, sinusitis, upper respiratory infection (URI), and relaxation. Before topical use, essential oils are diluted with a carrier oil, such as almond oil. Topical uses include contusions, skin complaints, muscle strain, aches and pains, on scar tissue, and vaginally for yeast infections or cystitis. Topical techniques include aromatherapy massage, compresses, bathing, or douching. For vaginal use, essential oils diluted in carrier oil are used, and only oils high in alcohols, such as Teatree, are recommended (Buckle, 2001).

There are numerous essential oils. Four essential oils that Buckle (2001) considers safe in nursing practice include lavender (*Lavandula augustifolia*), teatree (*Melaleuca alternifolia*), Blue gum (*Eucalyptus globulus*), and rose (*Rosa damascena*). Each of these four oils has several uses. (In addition, some safe essential oils have analgesic properties; these are listed in the neuropsychology chapter of this text.) *Lavandula augustifolia* (lavender) has sedative, relaxant, antispasmodic, and hypotensive properties. Lavender is skin regenerative and "useful for burns, abscesses, acne, mild eczema, insect bites, lice, psoriasis and ringworm" (Buckle, 2001, p. 62). Lavender has antimicrobial action, is an analgesic, and can be used for arthritis and earache. Lavender is also used to enhance sleep (Buckle, 1997, 2001).

Teatree is used for infection. Buckle (2001) recommends the terpineol chemotype of teatree because of its alcohol content; this is gentler on mucous membranes than is the cineol (oxide) content. Teatree is used for fungal infections, impetigo and other bacterial infections, herpes, acne, insect bites, and poison ivy. Carrier oil is not used with poison ivy, but rather Buckle suggests aloe vera gel (as carrier) for providing relief of poison ivy.

Eucalyptus is used for respiratory complaints, including asthma, and is in many conventional medications. Buckle discusses its use for tuberculosis and states that eucalyptus may enhance the action of the conventional antibiotics used for tuberculosis. Eucalyptus is also a muscle relaxant, an antiparasitic (it helps kill house mites) and mosquito repellant, and it may help with virus such as shingles and herpes (Buckle, 2001).

Rose is an antispasmodic, mild sedative, antidepressant, is used to sooth radiodermatitis, is thought to lower blood pressure and has antibacterial properties. Rose is soothing to the skin, and the pure rose otto oil should be used and not the rose absolute (Buckle, 2001).

Contraindications to essential oils include allergy to the substance; contact dermatitis has been reported (Robins, 1999). In addition, spike lavender (*Lavandula latifolia*) and rosemary should be avoided in people with hypertension or seizures (Buckle, 1999). Additionally, some odors may be offensive to some people. The steam-distillate essential oils should be 100% pure. Inexpensive oils may not be pure essential oils; pure essential oils tend to be expensive, and adulteration has been known to occur.

Training in clinical aromatherapy is available through RJ Buckle Associates, LLC at rjbinfo@aol.com. This program is endorsed by the American Holistic Nurses Association. In addition, the M-technique is offered, a very gentle touch method that can enhance aromatherapy and is useful for patients who are critically ill or dying.

HERB AND NUTRITION RESOURCES

American Botanical Council (www.herbalgram.org)

American Herbal Products Association (www.ahpa.org)

American Herbalist Guild (www.americanherbalistguild.com)

American Society of Pharmacognosy (www.phcog.org)

Botanical Society of America (www.botany.org)

HerbalGram—Journal of the American Botanical Council and Herb Research Foundation (www.herbalgram.org)

Herb Research Foundation (www.herbs.org)

National Academy of Science (www.nap.edu and www4.nationalacadamies.org)

U.S. Food and Drug Administration for nutrition information (www.cfsan.fda.gov)

REFERENCES

Balch J, Balch P: *Prescription for nutritional healing,* Garden City Park, New York, 1997, Avery.

Bascom A: *Incorporating herbal medicine into clinical practice,* Philadelphia, 2002, FA Davis.

Blumenthal M, Goldberg A, Brinckmann J, eds: *Herbal medicine: Expanded commission E monographs,* Newton, Mass, 2000, Integrative Medicine Communications.

Blumenthal M, et al, eds: *The complete German commission E monographs,* Boston, 1998, Integrative Medicine Communications.

Bremness L: *Herbs,* London, 1994, Dorling Kindersley.

Buckle J: The role of aromatherapy in nursing care. In Colbath J, Prawlucki P, eds: *Nurs Clin North Am* 36(1):57, 2001.

Buckle J: Use of aromatherapy as a complementary treatment for chronic pain, *Alt Ther Health Med* 5(5):42, 1999.

Buckle J: *Clinical aromatherapy in nursing,* San Diego, 1997, Singular.

Bunney S, ed: *The illustrated encyclopedia of herbs: their medicinal and culinary uses,* New York, 1992, Dorset.

Chavez M, Chavez P: Herbal medicine. In Novey D, ed: *Clinician's complete reference to complementary and alternative medicine,* St Louis, 2000, Mosby.

Clarke S: *Essential chemistry for safe aromatherapy,* Edinburgh, 2002, Churchill Livingstone.

DerMarderosian A, ed: *Facts and comparisons,* St Louis, 2000, Facts and Comparisons.

Fetrow C, Avila J: *Professional's handbook of complementary and alternative medicine,* Springhouse, Penn, 1999, Springhouse.

Food and Drug Administration (FDA): Regulations on statements made for dietary supplements concerning the effect of the product on the structure or function of the body, 2000. URL: www.cfsan.fda.gov. Accessed 4/3/2003.

FDA: Overview of dietary supplements, 2001a. URL: www.cfsan.fda.gov. Accessed 2/5/2003.

FDA: Claims that can be made for conventional foods and dietary supplements, 2001b. URL: www.cfsan.fda.gov. Accessed 2/5/2003.

Food Nutrition Board: Dietary reference intakes: Elements and vitamins, 2001. URL: www4.nationalacademies.org. Accessed 2/5/2003.

Hoffman D: *The complete illustrated holistic herbal,* Rockport, Mass, 1997, Element Books.

National Center for Complementary and Alternative Medicine [NCCAM]: *What is complementary and alternative medicine [CAM]*, 2002. URL: nccam.nih.gov Accessed 2/1/2003.

Novey D: *Clinician's complete reference to complementary and alternative medicine*, St Louis, 2000, Mosby.

Pharmacist's Letter/Prescriber's Letter [PL/PL]: *Natural medicine's comprehensive database*, Stockton, Calif, 2002, Therapeutic Research Faculty.

PDR for herbal medicines, Montvale, NJ, 1998, Medical Economics.

Robins J: The science and art of aromatherapy, *J Holist Nurs* 17(1):5, 1999.

U.S. Food and Drug Administration, Center for Food Safety and Applied Nutrition [CFSAN]: *Overview of dietary supplements*, 2001. Accessed 3/13/02. URL: www.cfsan.fda.gov

CHAPTER *14*

MANIPULATIVE AND BODY-BASED METHODS

Roxana Huebscher ▮ Pamela Shuler

Manipulative and body-based methods are practices that are "based on manipulation and/or movement of one or more parts of the body (NCCAM, 2002, p. 2). These methods include chiropractic, osteopathy, and massage. Massage has many forms and techniques.

CHIROPRACTIC MEDICINE

Chiropractic is a system of health care based on the premise that a significant relationship exists in the human body between structure and function and that the relationship between the spinal column and the nervous system that innervates the entire body positively or negatively affects health status.

Three theories for chiropractic include:
1. Disturbances of the nervous system influence pathologic disease processes.
2. Disturbances of the nervous system may be the result of derangements of the musculoskeletal structure.
3. Disturbances of the nervous system may aggravate pathologic processes in various parts or with various functions of the body. Vertebral and pelvis subluxations may be involved in common functional disorders of a visceral and vasomotor nature and at times may produce phenomena that relate to the special organs. (Chiropractic First Source, 2003a)

The focus of chiropractic treatment has been to correct vertebral subluxations. Subluxations are defined as misalignments of spinal vertebrae (Haldeman, Hooper, 2001) leading to joint, nerve, tissue, and muscle damage, as well as overall health degeneration and pain (Haldeman, Hooper, 2001; Koren, 1997). In addition to the theory of subluxation:

> Chiropractic theories have since evolved and today focus on the restoration of joint mobility, relaxation of muscle spasm, modulation of spinal reflexes, and the soothing or psychosocial effects of manual therapy. It is now widely believed that immobility of spinal joints is one factor that can lead to joint inflammation, formation of adhesions, and degenerative joint disease. Spinal manipulation is thought to improve joint mobility and restore normal joint function, especially when

associated with an exercise and rehabilitation program. (Haldeman, Hooper, 2001, p. 97)

Chiropractors use mobilization, manipulation, and massage. Mobilization is "rhythmic repetitive movements that are performed within the client's range of motion" (Haldeman, Hooper, 2001, p. 96). Mobilization does not have rapid movements; however, manipulation does. The manipulation that doctors of chiropractic (DC) use is "a treatment using the doctor's hands to apply body leverage and a physical thrust to one joint or a group of related joints to restore joint and related tissue function" (Chiropractic First Source, 2003b, p. 1). Chiropractic treatment is thought to improve a vast array of health problems ranging from low back pain to migraine headaches. In addition, chiropractic care is promoted as a preventative therapy that can enhance the immune system and general overall function of internal organs and bodily processes (Koren, 1997). Four levels of chiropractic care have been identified: level 1—intensive spinal correction; level 2—reconstructive-corrective or spinal healing; level 3—health enhancement; and level 4—health optimization (Koren, 1997).

Founded by D. D. Palmer, chiropractic originated in the late 1800s in Iowa. Chiropractic is the third largest independent health profession in the United States (after allopathic medicine and dentistry). Some research shows that spinal manipulation is "of short-term benefit in some patients, particularly those with uncomplicated, acute low-back pain" (Shekelle et al, 1992, p. 590). In addition, chiropractic may relieve headache (ACA, 2003; Chiropractic First Source, 2003b).

Chiropractic education requires at least 2 years of prerequisite undergraduate work with credits in the biologic and basic sciences. Chiropractic colleges require a minimum of 4 years of undergraduate academic study and 4 to 5 years of professional study in an accredited chiropractic college (ACA, 2001). Study areas include anatomy, physiology, neurology, embryology, pathology, microbiology, biochemistry, radiology, diagnostics, dermatology, toxicology, psychiatry, dietetics, physical therapy, spinal analysis, and orthopedics. Additional offerings include manipulation, mobilization, manual therapy, and adjustive techniques and clinical practice in a teaching clinic (ACA, 2003; Chiropractic First Source, 2003b; Koren, 1997).

The Council on Chiropractic Education (CCE) is a national organization that sets curricular standards and accredits eligible colleges (Chiropractic First Source, 2003b). The CCE has a Commission on Accreditation that is recognized by the U.S. Department of Education. After graduating from chiropractic college, the chiropractor must pass a state licensing examination before working as a DC. Chiropractors are licensed in all 50 states (ACA, 2003). Each state has established licensing laws with corresponding licensing examinations. In addition, the Federation of Chiropractic Licensing Boards recommends regulatory nomenclature stating graduation from an accredited chiropractic college is necessary (Chiropractic First Source, 2003b; Koren, 1997).

OSTEOPATHIC MEDICINE

Osteopathic medicine (OM) or osteopathy combines manual manipulation of the body with conventional forms of allopathic medicine (www.naturalhealers, 2001). In the United States, a doctor of osteopathic medicine (DO) is fully licensed as a physician and can work in any type of health care setting. The goals of OM are to alleviate pain, restore freedom of movement, and enhance the body's healing power. Andrew Still developed osteopathy in the late 1800s out of a desire to reduce the need for harmful drugs and invasive treatment procedures. Still believed that methods or techniques can be established for stimulating the body's ability to fight disease (American Osteopathic Association, 2002; www.naturalhealers, 2001). "Some of the most commonly used osteopathic medical techniques (OMTs) include articulatory techniques, counterstrain, cranial treatment, myofascial release treatment, lymphatic techniques, soft tissue techniques and thrust techniques" (www.naturalhealers, 2001, p. 2). These techniques are combined with traditional medical practices.

The educational preparation for DOs is similar to that for general physicians; however, "the osteopathy curricula emphasizes family medicine, preventive health and ways in which the musculoskeletal and nervous systems influence the functioning of the entire body" (www.naturalhealers, 2001, p. 2). Thus DOs receive extra training in the musculoskeletal system and learn osteopathic manipulative treatment (American Osteopathic Association, 2002). DOs are licensed in all 50 states within the United States. To qualify for licensure, the DO must graduate from an accredited U.S. college of osteopathic medicine, successfully complete internship and residency requirements, and pass state medical board examinations.

MASSAGE THERAPY

Massage, bodywork, and somatic therapy refer to:

> ...the application of various techniques to the muscular structure and soft tissues of the human body. The application of massage, bodywork and somatic therapy techniques may include, but is not limited to stroking, kneading, tapping, compression, vibration, rocking, friction, pressure, and techniques based on manipulation or the application of pressure to the muscular structure or soft tissues of the human body. This may also include non-forceful passive or active movement and/or application of techniques intended to affect the energetic

systems of the body. The use of oils, lotions, powders, or other lubricants may also be included. (Associated Bodywork and Massage Professionals [ABMP], 2000, p. 1)

Massage is based in the ancient practice of laying-on-of-hands. In the past, massage was a technique that all nurses learned in their training (the back rub). Massage satisfied the patient need for touch, allowed time with the patient, and provided attention. Unfortunately, massage is no longer a standard routine treatment for inpatients.

Swedish massage, probably one well-known form of massage, originated in the early 1800s. Per Henrik Ling, a fencing master and gymnastic instructor, established the Central Royal Institute of Gymnastics in Stockholm in 1813 and practiced and taught Swedish massage following his travels to China, where he was cured of his gouty elbow and where he studied with Taoist priests. Massage then spread throughout Europe. The French added manipulation of the head, neck, face, and arms; the English added physiotherapy; and the Germans added hydrotherapy. Approximately 100 forms of massage are practiced; most of these are less than 20 to 30 years old, however (Greene, 2000). Box 14-1 gives examples of types of massage therapy. A brief explanation of types of massage is given in Kuhn (1999), Lawrence (1986), and in Tappan (1988). Several texts explain the fundamentals, techniques, and sequences of basic massage (Beck, 1994; Domenico, Wood, 1997; Fritz, 1995; Lawrence, 1986; Tappan, 1988). Beck (1994) has a specific chapter on massage for nursing and health care. Box 14-2 reviews the basic steps of Swedish massage, which is the usual initial massage taught to therapists learning massage, and is a good therapy for those wishing to have a general relaxing massage. Massage therapy sessions generally last approximately an hour. The participant removes jewelry and clothing in privacy (but may choose to wear whatever pieces of clothing he or she wants); the person is covered except for the body part being massaged; and legitimate massage therapists never massage genitalia. A form of breast massage, however, is available for breast problems. Contraindications to massage are listed in Box 14-3. Massage therapists may use heat sources or packs such as castor oil packs.

Special Situations

Massage is given in pregnancy, but appropriate support is used (pillows, bolsters, and cushions). The woman receiving the massage is usually on her left side from the second trimester onward. In addition, differences exist between a regular massage and a pregnancy massage, including the gentleness needed. Contraindications include increased blood pressure, severe edema, or bleeding (Beck, 1994; Fritz, 1995).

Box 14-1

Types of Massage Therapy/Bodywork

Some of these therapies also include energy therapy.

Acupressure	Myofascial Release
Alexander	Neuromuscular Therapy
Amma	Polarity Therapy
Aromatherapy	Prenatal Massage
Aston Patterning	Qigong
Ayurvedic	Reflexology
Bindegewebmassage	Rolfing
Bonnie Pruden Myotherapy	Rosen Method
Bowen	Rubenfeld Synergy
Chair-seated Massage	Russian Medical Massage
Cranial Sacral Therapy	Shiatsu
Deep-tissue Massage	Sports Massage
Esalen Massage	St. John's Method
Eucapnic Breath Retaining	Strain/Counterstrain
Feldenkrais	Structural Integration
Functional Integration	Swedish Massage
Hellerwork	Thai Massage
Infant Massage	Trager Work
Kripalu Bodywork	Tui Na
Lomi Lomi	Vodder's Manual Lymph
Lymphatic	Drainage
'M' Technique	Zero Balancing
Mariel	

Infant massage is another special situation. McClure's small book (1989) describes the basics and has photographs of techniques and sequencing. In addition, a chapter is written for fathers and for massage on infants with special needs.

Older adults and those with other special needs require gentler touch, special positioning, and help getting on and off the massage table; sometimes the person may not be able to get on the table. This situation is also true of people with mobility problems; then special settings or equipment are needed.

Face cradle (contains a cushion with a face hole) may be used for some people. The massage therapist needs to set up special areas for the home-based massage participant, including for terminally ill patients (Smith, 2001). In addition, chair massage, often done at work sites, is available. The therapist brings the chair to the site and during a work break or lunch hour the participant can sit, fully clothed for a short session of massage.

Box 14-2

Basic Swedish Massage Movements

Effleurage—stroking
Pétrissage—kneading
Friction—quick, short movements; hands or fingertips moving
    quickly over superficial tissue so that it moves over or against
    deeper tissues
Tapotement—percussion
    Tapping
    Slapping
    Hacking
    Cupping
    Beating
Shaking
Vibration
Range of motion

Box 14-3

Contraindications to Massage

Acute illness, fever, and recent surgery
No massage over varicosities, suspected phlebitis, open wounds,
    lesions, skin eruptions, or acute injuries, bruises, or fractures
Allergy to massage substances
Some psychological conditions

Regulation

Licensure varies from state to state. In addition, the National Certification Board for Therapeutic Massage and Bodywork (NCBTMB) administers a national certification examination. Before taking the exam, a number of practice hours are needed, including didactic and hands-on practice. Massage schools are located throughout the United States and generally offer approximately 600 hours of education, the minimum required to take the certification examination.

RESOURCES: JOURNALS

Journal of the American Chiropractic Association (www.amerchiro.org)
Massage and Bodywork, published by Associated Bodywork and Massage Professionals
    (www.abmp.com)

Massage Magazine, published by Massage Magazine, Inc., an independent publication (www.massagemag.com)

Massage Therapy Journal, the official publication of the American Massage Therapy Association (www.amtamassage.org)

RESOURCES: PROFESSIONAL ORGANIZATIONS

American Chiropractic Association
American Craniosacral Therapy Association
American Massage Therapy Association (AMTA)
American Osteopathic Association
Associated Bodywork and Massage Professionals (ABMP)
International Myomasethics Foundation (IMF)
National Association of Nurse Massage Therapist (NANMT)
National Association of Pregnancy Massage Therapy

REFERENCES

American Chiropractic Association [ACA]: What is chiropractic? 2003. URL: http://www.amerchiro.org. Accessed 2/7/2003.

American Osteopathic Association: Osteopathic medicine, 2002. URL: www.aoanet.org. Accessed 3/18/02.

Associated Bodywork and Massage Professionals [ABMP]: About massage, bodywork and somatic therapies, 2000. URL: www.abmp.com. Accessed 2/7/2003.

Beck M: *Milady's theory and practice of therapeutic massage*, Albany, New York, 1994, Delmar.

Chiropractic First Source: Scientific theories of chiropractic, 2003a. URL: www.Kansaschiro.com. Accessed 2/7/2003.

Chiropractic First Source: Answers to your questions, 2003b. URL: www.Kansaschiro.com. Accessed 2/7/2003.

Domenico G, Wood E: *Beard's massage*, Philadelphia, 1997, Saunders.

Fritz S: *Mosby's fundamentals of therapeutic massage*, St Louis, 1995, Mosby.

Greene E: Massage therapy. In Novey D, ed: *Clinician's complete reference to complementary and alternative medicine*, St Louis, 2000, Mosby.

Haldeman S, Hooper P: Chiropractic approach to neurologic illness. In Weintraub M, ed: *Alternative and complementary treatments in neurologic illness*, Edinburgh, 2001, Churchill Livingstone.

Koren T: *Chiropractic: bringing out the best in you*, ed 4, Philadelphia, 1997, Koren Publications.

Kuhn M: *Complementary therapies for health care providers*, Philadelphia, 1999, Lippincott.

Lawrence DB: *Massage techniques*, New York, 1986, Perigee.

McClure VS: *Infant massage: a handbook for loving parents*, New York, 1989, Bantam.

National Center for Complementary and Alternative Medicine[NCCAM]: What is complementary and alternative medicine [CAM], 2002. URL: www.nccam.nih.gov. Accessed 2/1/2003.

NaturalVillage.com, Inc: Natural Healers Osteopathic Medical Schools, Q and A, 2001. URL: http://www.naturalhealers.com/qa/osteopathic.html. Accessed 8/22/2001.

Shekelle P et al: spinal manipulation for low-back pain, *Ann Intern Med* 117(7):590, 1992.

Smith I: Massage for the ill in a home setting, *Massage Bodywork* 16(1):24, 2001.

Snyder M, Cheng WY: Massage. In Snyder M, Lindquist R, eds: *Complementary and alternative therapies in nursing,* New York, 1998, Springer.

Tappan F: *Healing massage techniques*, Norwalk, Conn, 1988, Appleton and Lange.

CHAPTER 15

ENERGY THERAPIES

Roxana Huebscher ■ Pamela Shuler

Energy therapies refer to either energy fields surrounding and penetrating the human body (biofields) or those from other sources (bioelectromagnetic based) (National Center for Complementary and Alternative Medicine [NCCAM], 2002). Such therapies include diverse forms of treatment ranging from the laying-on-of-hands and healing touch to electrical current, magnets, crystals, light, and sound. Box 15-1 gives examples of energy therapies.

BIOFIELD THERAPY

The biofield refers to the complex energy that surrounds or permeates an entity. The Chinese call the person's life force energy "Qi" (pronounced "chee") and also describe a system of energy channels in the body called meridians; the Japanese say "Ki" (pronounced "kee"); the Ayurvedic practitioner speaks of prana. The Therapeutic Touch or healing touch practitioner talks about the energy field, auric fields, chakras, and etheric levels (Brennan, 1993; Bruyere, 1990; Karagulla, Kunz, 1989; Krieger, 1993; Mentgen, 2001). Other terms: the Algonquin say "manitou"; the Huron, "oki"; the Iroquois,

---

Box 15-1

Examples of Energy Therapies

Acupressure (jin shin do and jin shin jyutsu)	Light therapy
	Magnetic fields
Alternating-current or direct-current fields	Pulsed fields
	Qi gong
Bioelectromagnetic	Reiki
Biofield	Sound therapy
Color therapy	Therapeutic touch
Crystal and gemstone therapy	
Healing touch	

"orenda"; the Inuit, "sila"; the Dakota, "ton"; and the Lakota say "wakan" (Hurwitz, 2001). This, as yet experimentally unproven, biofield is thought to be affected by a healer's hands. In biofield therapies, the assumption is that energy can be worked with and repatterned. Healing touch, Therapeutic Touch, and Reiki are examples of biofield therapy.

Healing Touch

Healing touch is a program of therapies and is defined as:

> ...an energy (biofield) therapy that encompasses a group of noninvasive techniques that utilize the hands to clear, energize, and balance the human and environmental energy fields....The North American Nursing Diagnosis Association (NANDA) identifies an Energy Field Disturbance as a disruption in the flow of energy surrounding a person's being that results in a disharmony of the body, mind, and/or spirit. Healing Touch interventions may be used to restore, energize, and balance an energy field disturbance. (Healing Touch International, 1998)

Healing touch energy principles assert that:

Energy permeates all animate and inanimate matter.
All healing is self-healing but it can by assisted by others.
Human beings are composed of interpenetrating layers or fields of energy and each layer vibrates to a different frequency.
The world and everything in it is interdependent.
A person can influence the energy system without being able to feel or see it.
All life experiences are recorded and stored within the energy system.
Potential illness appears in the energy system before signs of illness appear.
A person's health and quality of life are affected by the health and quality of the energy system and vice versa.
The energy system is influenced by the environment, thoughts, emotions, actions, and intentionality.
Energy can be experienced as movement, temperature, or density. (Mentgen, 2001, p. 146)

The healing touch program was developed by Janet Mentgen, an RN, who has practiced energy-based care for many years. Healing Touch International is a nonprofit membership and educational corporation that administers the healing touch certification process (Healing Touch International brochure) and provides standards, a code of ethics, and standards of practice. The program emphasizes energy-based therapy, and instructors teach various strategies of healing touch that combine conventional nursing and:

...complementary healing techniques derived from native cultures and Eastern and Western medicine and packages it into a therapeutic approach for application in the modern health care system. The program uses a collection of healing works developed by the author [Mentgen] and other healers (Mentgen, 2001, p.153). Dolores Krieger (1979), Dora Kunz (Karagulla, Kunz, 1989), W. Brugh Joy (1979), Rosalyn Bruyere (1990), Barbara Brennan (1987), and Alice Bailey (1953) also offer energy-based readings. Some of their works are included in the Healing Touch program.

The Healing Touch program has four levels, including an instructor level for those who wish to teach Healing Touch. Three levels of the program are needed for Healing Touch certification (Healing Touch International, 2000).

Therapeutic Touch

Therapeutic touch (TT) is a process and procedure defined as an "intentionally directed process of energy exchange during which the practitioner uses the hands as a focus to facilitate the healing process. It is the contemporary interpretation of several ancient healing practices" (Nurse Healers—Professional Associates International, 2000, p. 1). TT has several assumptions:

1. People are energy fields.
2. People are open systems.
3. Illness is an imbalance in energy or a shift in pattern of energy field.
4. Energy can be transferred from one person to another with intent to heal.

TT was developed by Delores Krieger (1979), an RN and professor at New York University, and Dora Kunz, a natural healer who had been working with touch for years. Both women had worked with another extraordinary healer, Oscar Estebani, a retired Hungarian cavalry officer who had immigrated to Canada. Kunz and Krieger began teaching nurses in 1972 (Horrigan, 1998). The Nurse Healers-Professional Associates International (NH-PAI) is the official organization of TT that provides standards, educational recommendations, and guidelines for the scope of practice (NH-PAI, 2000).

Krieger (1987) states that three characteristics of the person who successfully practices TT are "intentionality, motivation in the interests of the healee [the person to whom TT is focused], and an ability and willingness to confront oneself with the question: Why do I want to be a healer?" (p. 125). The process of TT is outlined in Box 15-2. A session lasts about 30 minutes, and receiving permission from the participant or family is essential before treatment.

Box 15-2

Process of Therapeutic Touch

Centering is the healer bringing his or her own body, mind, and emotions to a quiet focused state of consciousness. Centering involves being comfortable; taking quiet, full, slow breaths; and exploring the thoughts that come into consciousness while becoming aware of one's own subtle energies and finding an inner sense of equilibrium to connect with the inner core of wholeness and stillness. Kunz and Krieger have said that centering "brings energies to a focal point in the heart and a sense of peace throughout."

Assessing-scanning is the healer holding his or her hands 2 to 6 inches away from the "healee's" body. This position provides clues and cues to the healee's problems. The healee is seated or lying in a comfortable position. The healer's hands are moved from head to feet in a rhythmical and symmetrical manner. The healer does not stay in any one place for an extended length of time. If a particular area is of concern, the healer scans the entire energy field or body first, then rescans areas of concern, if necessary. Sensory cues may become apparent, such as warmth, heat, coolness, static, fullness, blockage, congestion, pressure, pulling, pulsations, change in rhythm, tingling, and vacuum. The healer may also get insights or intuition about a healee's condition.

Unruffling and clearing is the healer assisting the energy field flow. The healer uses hand movements from midline outward while moving the hands rhythmically and symmetrically from head to feet. This is a process of smoothing or freeing the energy from disturbances.

Intervention, treatment, balancing, rebalancing is the healer using the hands for projecting, directing, or modulating energy in the areas that need attention. This effect is dampening, toning down, sedating, vitalizing, quickening, strengthening, or stimulating energy flow. The aim is to establish rhythm or patterning. Treatment assists in reestablishing order in the system. Energy may be transferred if a deficit is present, or energy may be mobilized away from areas of congestion.

Evaluation or closure is finishing the treatment and knowing when to end. The healer reassesses the energy field and obtains feedback from the healee, using this input as well as professional judgment to know when to end the treatment.

From: *Krieger D*: Accepting the power to heal: the personal practice of therapeutic touch. *Santa Fe, NM, 1993, Bear and Co; www.therapeutic-touch.org, The Therapeutic Touch Process, 2000.*

Reiki Therapy

Reiki (pronounced "ray-kee") means universal life-force energy and has Tibetan origins from thousands of years ago. Reiki rediscovery is attributed to Mikao Usui, a Japanese minister and university president, who, in the mid-nineteenth century, went in search of answers as to why Jesus Christ and Buddha were able to heal the sick (Fairbass, 2001; Hurwitz, 2001; Wetzel, 1989). Mikao Usui journeyed to the United States, the Far East, India, and also Tibet where he read the ancient sutras:

> the doctrines of life revered by the Tibetan Buddhists. Within the sutras, he found the "keys" to healing, which claimed to activate and direct a universal life energy. The keys when applied, would enable one to channel this energy. Usui called this process "Reiki" a combination of the Japanese words *Rei* (meaning "free passage"), and *Ki* (meaning "universal life energy"). (Wetzel, 1989, p. 47)

With Reiki, the therapist acts as a conduit for the energy. Reiki therapy has hands-on placement in 12 to 16 specific areas of the body, both front and back. Hands are left on the body in each set position for approximately 2 to 5 minutes. The patient remains clothed, and the breasts and genitals are not touched. A treatment lasts from 1 to 1½ hours (Fairbass, 2001; Stein, 1995; Wetzel, 1989).

Practitioners go though several levels of training called degrees, with first-degree Reiki being the basic level and second-degree Reiki being more advanced. Attunements or rituals are also involved with each training. The third-degree designation is that of Reiki master or a teacher of Reiki; the master category is sometimes in two levels (Wetzel, 1989).

Uses of Biofield Therapy

Healing touch and TT have been studied and used for numerous conditions. Indications for use include enhancing well-being and reducing anxiety and stress, including agitation in dementia and for chemotherapy symptoms and soothing children (Gagne, Toye 1994; Giasson, Bouchard 1998; Heidt, 1981; Kramer, 1990; Olson et al, 1997; Olson, Sneed, 1995; Quinn, 1984; Simington, Laing, 1993; Snyder, 1995). Healing Touch and TT are also used for decreasing pain (including arthritis, headache, and postoperative pain) (Boguslawski, 1980; Gordon et al, 1998; Keller, Bzdek, 1986; Meehan, 1993; Peck, 1997), and relieving sleep problems (Braun et al, 1986; Heidt, 1991). Several studies have shown resulting relaxation, decreased anxiety, and decreased pain following treatment. In addition, Krieger, with an early TT study (1973), showed an increase in hemoglobin level. Wirth (1990, 1995) had contradictory results on differing studies with wound healing. Most studies have used TT as intervention. Other published works on healing touch and TT include Engle and Graney (2000), Horrigan (1998), Krieger (1979, 1987, 1993), Macrae (1987), Mentgen (2001), Mulloney and Wells-Federman (1996), Spence and Olson (1997), Quinn (1988, 1992), Starn (1998), and Wytias (1994).

Mentgen (2001) describes a 2-year medical center study using Healing Touch modalities as part of therapy for employees with back injuries. "Because of a positive financial impact, the hospital has chosen to analyze in depth the medical costs, work time loss, pain levels, and functional levels of the employees" (p. 156). Mentgen discusses other anecdotal organizational uses of Healing Touch.

Krieger (1993) anecdotally reports on good results with a person who had Parkinson's symptoms and of her assessment of a second patient who presented to her with the diagnosis of Parkinson's disease, whom she thought did *not* have the disease. Further testing proved that the woman did not have the disease. Krieger reports other intuitive information.

Literature regarding the TT controversy, how and if TT works, and criticism of the TT research has been published (Courcey, 2001; O'Mathuna, 2000; Pearson, 2001; Rosa et al, 1998). Some writings imply that TT is harmful (O'Mathuna, 1998).

Although Reiki has little research, several texts and articles give more depth (Arnold, 1982; Baginski, 1988; Fairbrass, 2000; Halcón, 2002; Hurwitz, 2001; Stein, 1995). One study was that of Olson and Hanson (1997) using Reiki to manage pain, including cancer pain, on 20 volunteers. Reiki was used as an adjunct to opioid therapy, and the intervention showed significance using both a Likert Scale and a visual analog scale.

Although several theories explain how biofield therapies work, no instrument or tool is available at this time to measure what is happening with TT, Healing Touch therapies, or Reiki. However, many health care providers (HCPs) believe that if these therapies provide comfort, reduce anxiety and pain, and promote relaxation and sleep, then they should be considered, and they should be used as treatment for, or as an adjunct to, whatever other comfort measures are needed. These treatment measures are provided with permission from the patient or family and are not to be provided if patients have religious, moral, or ethical objections, just as with any other therapy. Thus the HCP needs to read the information available and possibly experience a session of TT, a Healing Touch therapy, Reiki, or other biofield therapy, such as Qi gong, from an experienced practitioner so as to make an informed decision.

ELECTROMAGNETIC THERAPIES

Bioelectromagnetic-based therapies involve the use of "electromagnetic fields, such as pulsed fields, magnetic fields, or alternating current or direct current fields," (NCCAM, 2002, p. 3) to, for example, treat asthma or cancer, or manage pain and migraine headaches. Other electromagnetic energy therapies include microcurrent electrical therapy, light therapy, and color therapy.

Microcurrent Electrical Therapy

Microcurrent electrical therapy (MET) is thought to improve circulation and promote lymphatic drainage, waste product removal, and cellular metabolism, thereby promoting healing of soft tissue, ligaments, tendons, and muscles (Kirsch, 1995; www.neilprimack.com/neilprimack/whattoexpect.html, 2002). "MicroCurrents are weak electrical impulses, one-millionth the strength of household current," (www.neilprimack.com/neilprimack/whattoexpect.html, 2002, p. 1). Therapy is administered through an instrument called the Acuscope and Myopulse System. The system simultaneously measures and treats electrical imbalances in injured tissues, (www.neilprimack.com/neilprimack/whattoexpect.html, 2002). A growing body of research supports using MET for treating conditions such as bursitis, degenerative joint disease, ligament strain, neuralgia, tendinitis, dysmenorrhea, torn muscles and ligaments, fibromyalgia, decubitus and venous stasis ulcers, headache (tension, sinus, migraine), and degenerative or herniated disc (Lichtbroun et al, 2001; Matteson, Eberhardt, 1985; Meyer, Nebrensky, 1983; Noto, Grant, 1985; Radler, 1984; Tyers, Smith, 2001).

An HCP uses various types of probes to massage the injured area while current is flowing into the tissues. The patient feels little or no sensation as the microcurrent stimulates underlying tissues. Length of treatment ranges from 20 to 60 minutes, depending on the area of the body being treated. Multiple sessions are usually necessary because a cumulative effect is noted; however, most patients notice some improvement after the first treatment. No true side effects occur, although as a result of the action of therapy at the cellular level, some patients may experience some temporary discomfort such as headache, nausea, or even increased pain after the first few treatments (www.neilprimack.com/neilprimack/whattoexpect.html, 2002). Rarely, mild bruising can occur. U.S. Food and Drug Administration (FDA) regulations list two contraindications for MET treatment: patients wearing demand-type pacemakers and pregnant women (www.neilprimack.com/neilprimack/whattoexpect.html, 2002).

Light Therapy

Light therapy is the therapeutic application of electromagnetic energy in the visible spectrum to treat a wide range of health disorders. Phototherapies use ultraviolet, bright white, colored, monochrome, and laser light to treat health conditions. The treatment usually involves using instrumentation to produce specific frequencies of light energy that activate biochemical and energetic reactions. Therapy may require shining light on a person's body, into acupuncture points, into the eyes, or on the body using fiberoptics to balance and restore health (Wallace, 2000).

Light therapy has had research in the areas of seasonal affective disorder (Rosenthal, 1984; Terman et al, 1998) and sleep problems (Guilleminault et al, 1995) and is used for other concerns, including "cataracts, conjunctivitis, headaches, head trauma, hyperactivity, lazy eye, macular degeneration, migraine, night blindness, poor eyesight, stroke, and vision disorders" (Wallace, 2000, p. 158). Wallace, an optometrist, says that these disorders are responsive to light therapy but that it does not preclude mainstream medical therapies. The author lists other applications as well.

Light therapy varies. A person may sit in front of a colored light, white light, or a highly illuminated light box. The light may shine on the body or in the eyes, depending on type of therapy. Although light therapy practitioners are generally in the field of optometry or medicine, light is also used in homeopathy, chiropractic, osteopathy, physical and occupational therapy, psychology, Chinese medicine, naturopathy, and massage therapy. There is an Annual Conference of Light and Vision sponsored by the College of Syntonic Optometry, and training is available through attendance at continuing education programs and seminars (Wallace, 2000).

Color Therapy

Color therapy refers to "wavelengths of the energy of light to assist the body in self-healing" (Donnelly, 2000, p. 691). Therapy can be psychologic, Eastern influenced, or physical.

With psychologic color therapy:

> Color is used to identify states of mind and negative stress. When a patient prefers or detests a certain shade or tone, it has to do with both the properties inherent in that color plus the patient's energy status at that moment. When a patient is drawn towards a color, its energy is needed for psychologic balance and healing. (Donnelly, 2000, p. 691)

Color imagery, visualization, or self-hypnosis can be used with patients using psychologic color therapy. Eastern influence refers to Hindu, Tibetan, and Chinese teachings. Hinduism, for example, discusses the chakras and colors involved with the health state of the individual. Physical light therapy directs colored light to a diseased area of the body or the eyes. Physical light therapy is also used in conventional care (ultraviolet light for psoriasis and blue light for hyperbilirubinemia, as well as light to help establish circadian rhythms) (Donnelly, 2000).

Magnet Therapy

Magnet therapy is an age-old technique that healers in ancient Greece, Persia, China, Egypt, and India used (Epp, 1998; Livingston,

1996). Russia and Japan revitalized the therapy after World War II by using magnets to reduce amputation pain and for treating injuries. Recently, researchers in the United States have examined the benefits of using magnets to treat pain. The American public spurred this renewed interest. With over $200 million in magnet sales during 1999, American consumers showed great interest in magnet therapy (Consumers Union, 2000).

> Magnetic fields fall into two broad groups: static and time-varied. *Static* fields are either permanent or direct current (DC) (electromagnetic). *Time-varied* fields are either pulsed or sinusoidal (radio-frequency). Most therapeutic time-varied fields (either pulsed or sinusoidal) are modulated at slower "biologic" speeds or frequencies (1 to 100 cycles per second Hz) and can have various pulse and on-off cycle patterns. Permanent magnets only produce static fields, unless they are spun, during which they can act as sinusoidal fields. Electromagnets can be made to produce static, pulsed/sinusoidal, or radio-frequency (RF) fields, which are in megahertz or greater range. Magnetic field strength is measured in gauss or Tesla. One Tesla equals 10,000 gauss. Ten milliTesla (mT) is equal to 100 gauss (Pawluk, 2000, p. 164).

The exact mechanism of action for magnet therapy is unknown; however, several theories have been proposed. One theory focuses on the magnet's ability to increase circulation to the treatment area, thereby promoting oxygenation and nutrition to the injured tissues. A second explanation promotes the ability of magnets to cause changes in ions, the electrically charged particles that are responsible for nerve impulses and muscle contractions. Altering the electron state may affect transmission of nerve signals for pain (Livingston, 1996). Lawrence (2000) suggests purchasing magnets from companies that offer a 30-day money-back guarantee because magnets do not work for everyone.

Magnets come in all sizes, shapes, and strengths. Flat pads, rotating magnets, shoe inserts, and button or bar magnets are available (Pawluk, 2000). The strength of magnetism for medical magnets ranges from 450 to 10,000 gauss (as a comparison, the typical refrigerator magnet is approximately 10 gauss). Magnets range in price from about $10 to $900 (Lawrence, 2000). Magnets are usually placed locally on the painful area, close to the body, with no more than a layer of clothing. "If a systemic condition is being treated, then placement on one or more acupuncture points, spinal segments, or whole body exposure (using a mattress pad) would be considered" (Pawluk, 2000, p. 167). Other application techniques are also used.

The research base for magnet therapy is growing as more patients report benefits from the often self-prescribed therapies. One double-blind, placebo-controlled randomized study at Baylor University on patients with postpolio chronic pain used magnet therapy for a 45-minute treatment period (Vallbonna et al, 1997). Seventy six percent of the magnet-treated patients reported pain relief as compared with 19% of the control group who used sham magnets. Jacobson and colleagues (2001), in a double-blind study, used magnet therapy to treat osteoarthritis of the knee with significant reduction of pain. In addition, patients with Parkinson' disease (Sandyk, 1992a), multiple sclerosis (Sandyk, 1992b), and Alzheimer's disease (Anninos et al, 1991) have been treated with magnets. Pawluk (2000) suggests magnets for fractures, carpal tunnel syndrome, chronic bronchitis, corneal trauma, endometriosis, hypertension, skin wounds, and skin grafts. Magnets are FDA-approved only for fracture, nerve-conduction testing, and skin and soft-tissue ulcer treatment.

Acute and chronic pain has been treated with magnet therapy. Athletes with repetitive joint stress and muscle strain, such as baseball pitchers, football players, golf professionals, and baseball umpires, have reported relief from muscle pain and joint stiffness as a result of magnet therapy (Epp, 1998; Schindler, 1999). Patients with fibromyalgia may have reduced pain after sleeping on a mattress embedded with active magnets (Colbert et al, 1999); and people with both diabetes and peripheral neuropathy may have reduction of pain, numbness, and tingling sensation after wearing magnetized insoles (Weintraub, 1999). In addition, Lawrence (1998, 2000) suggests magnets for tennis elbow, aching feet, headache, and back pain.

Therapy should begin as soon as possible after onset of symptoms and can be used in conjunction with other treatments. If magnets do not work within the first 20 exposures, they may not be of much value (except for fractures that take approximately 30 days for the first signs of healing). Minimal exposure time is 10 minutes and the minimal number of exposures is 10; exposures should be "long and repeated" (Pawluk, 2000, p. 168).

Absolute contraindications to magnet use include pregnancy; pacemakers, defibrillators, and other implanted devices (because they may be turned off by magnets); myasthenia gravis; conditions with active bleeding; and hyperthyroidism, adrenal, hypothalamic, and pituitary dysfunction. In addition, decreased blood pressure and accompanying symptoms may occur (Pawluk, 2000).

The North American Academy of Magnetic Therapy (800-457-1853) offers an information package, product recommendations, and a referral service to HCPs who have an interest in magnet therapy. No formal training is required at this time, thus consumers need to investigate practitioners and magnet sources for credibility.

RESOURCES

Healing Touch International, Inc.
12477 West Cedar Drive, Ste 202
Lakewood, CO 80228
FAX: 303-980-8683
E-mail: htiheal@aol.com
Web site: www.healingtouch.net

Nurse Healers-Professional Associates International
Official Organization of Therapeutic Touch
E-mail: nhpai@therapeutictouch.org
Web site: www.therapeutic-touch.org

The Reiki Alliance
E-mail: reikialliance@compuserve.com

North American Academy of Magnetic Therapy
Phone: 800-457-1853

Society for Light Treatment and Biological Rhythms
Phone: 303-424-3694

REFERENCES

Baginski BJ, Sharamon S: *Reiki universal life energy*, Mendocino, Calif, 1988, Life Rhythm.

Bailey A: *Esoteric healing*, New York, 1953, Lucis.

Boguslawski M: Therapeutic touch: a facilitator or pain relief, *Topics Clin Nurs* 2(1):27, 1980.

Braun C, Layton J, Braun J: Therapeutic touch improves residents' sleep, *Am Health Care Assoc J* 12(1):48, 1986.

Brennan B: *Light emerging: the journal of personal healing*, New York, 1993, Bantam Books.

Brennan B: *Hands of light*, New York, 1987, Pleiades Books.

Bruyere R: *Wheels of light*, Arcadia, Calif, 1990, Bon Productions.

Colbert AP et al: Magnetic mattress pad use in patients with fibromyalgia: a randomized double-blind pilot study, *J Back Musculoskeletal Rehab* 13:19, 1999.

Consumers Union: Magnets: strong draw, weak evidence, *Consumer Reports on Health* 12:10, 2000.

Courcey K: Investigating therapeutic touch, *NP Forum* 26(11):12, 2001.

Donnelly T: Color therapy. In Novey D, ed: *Clinician's complete reference to complementary and alternative medicine*, St Louis, 2000, Mosby.

Engle V, Graney M: Biobehavioral effects of therapeutic touch, *J Nurs Scholar* 32(3):287, 2000.

Epp T: Stuck on magnets, *Vegetarian Times* 256:40, 1998.

Fairbass J: Reiki. In Novey D, ed: *Clinician's complete reference to complementary and alternative medicine*, St Louis, 2001, Mosby.

Gagne D, Toye RC: The effects of therapeutic touch and relaxation therapy in reducing anxiety, *Arch Psychiatr Nurs* 8(3):184, 1994.

Giasson M, Bouchard L: Effect of therapeutic touch on the well-being of persons with terminal cancer, *J Holistic Nurs* 16(3):383, 1998.

Gordon A et al: The effects of therapeutic touch on patients with osteoarthritis of the knee, *J Fam Pract* 47:271, 1998.

Guilleminault C et al: Nondrug treatment trials in psychophysiologic insomnia, *Arch Intern Med* 155:838, 1995.

Halcón L: Reiki. In Snyder M, Lindquist R: *Complementary/alternative therapies in nursing*, New York, 2002, Springer, pp. 197-203.

Healing Touch International: Home page: What is Healing Touch, 1998. URL: www.healingtouch.net. Accessed 3/18/2002.

Heidt P: Helping patients to rest: clinical studies in therapeutic touch, *Holistic Nurs Pract* 5(4):57, 1991.

Heidt P: Effect of therapeutic touch on anxiety level of hospitalized patients, *Nurs Res* 30(1):32, 1981.

Horrigan B: Dolores Krieger, RN, PhD: Healing with therapeutic touch [interview], *Alt Ther* 4:86, 1998.

Hurwitz W: Energy medicine. In Micozzi M, ed: *Fundamentals of complementary and alternative medicine*, New York, 2001, Churchill Livingstone.

Jacobson J et al: Low-amplitude, extremely low frequency magnetic fields for the treatment of osteoarthritic knees: a double-blind clinical study, *Alt Ther Health Med* 7(5):5, 2001.

Joy WB: *Joy's way*, Los Angeles, 1979, JB Tarcher.

Karagulla S, Kunz D: *The chakras and the human energy fields*, Wheaton, Ill, 1989, Quest.

Keller E, Bzdek V: Effects of therapeutic touch on tension headache pain, *Nurs Res* 35(2):101, 1986.

Kirsch D: *Alpha-Stim CES postmarketing survey*, Mineral Wells, Tex, 1995. Prepared for the U.S. Food and Drug Administration (PMA #950036).

Kramer N: Comparison of therapeutic touch and casual touch in stress reduction of hospitalized children, *Pediatr Nurs* 16(5):483, 1990.

Krieger D: *Accepting your power to heal: the personal practice of therapeutic touch*, Santa Fe, NM, 1993, Bear and Co.

Krieger D: *Living the therapeutic touch: healing as a lifestyle*, New York, 1987, Dodd Mead.

Krieger D: *The therapeutic touch: how to use your hands to help or to heal*, Englewood Cliffs, NJ, 1979, Prentice-Hall.

Krieger D: *The relationship of touch, with intent to help or heal to subjects' in-vivo hemoglobin values: a study in personalized interaction*, 1973. In Proceedings of ninth ANA Nursing Research Conference, San Antonio, Tex, March 21-23, 1973.

Lawrence R: Controlling chronic pain with magnet therapy, 2000. URL: http://www.kick-n-stuff.com/controling_chronic_pain_with_magnetic_therapy.htm. Accessed 3/21/02.

Lawrence R, Plowden J, Rosch P: *Magnet therapy: the pain cure alternative*, Rocklin, Calif, 1998, Prima Publishing.

Lichtbroun AS, Raicer MC, Smith R: The treatment of fibromyalgia with cranial electrotherapy stimulation, *J Clin Rheumatol* 7(2):72, 2001.

Livingston JD: *Driving force: the natural magic of magnets*, Boston, 1996, Harvard University Press.

Macrae J: *Therapeutic touch: a practical guide*, New York, 1987, Knopf.

Matteson JH, Eberhardt T: Pain management and the new generation of "intelligent" TENS, *Am J Acupuncture* 13(2):149, 1985.

Meehan T: Therapeutic touch and postoperative pian: a Rogerian research study, *Nurs Sci Q* 6(2):69, 1993.

Mentgen J: Healing touch. In Colbath J, Prawlucki P, eds: *Nurs Clin North Am: Holistic Nurs Care* 36(1):143, 2001.

Meyer FP, Nebrensky A: A double-blind comparative study of micro stimulation and placebo effect, *Calif Health Rev* 2(1):19, 1983.

Mulloney S, Wells-Federman C: Therapeutic touch: a healing modality, *J Cardiovasc Nurs* 10(3):27, 1996.

National Center for Complementary and Alternative Medicine [NCCAM]: What is complementary and alternative medicine [CAM]? 2002. URL: www.nccam.nih.gov. Accessed 2/1/2003.

Noto K, Grant P: Comparative study of electro-Acuscope neural stimulation and conventional physical therapy modalities, *Physical Ther Forum* 4(11):1, 1985.

Nurse Healer's Professional Associates International [NH-PAI]: Therapeutic Touch, 2000. URL: www.therapeutic-touch.org. Accessed 2/7/2003.

Olson K, Hanson J: Using Reiki to manage pain: a preliminary report, *Cancer Prevent Control* 1(2):108, 1997.

Olson M, Sneed N: Anxiety and therapeutic touch, *Iss Ment Health Nurs* 16(2):97, 1995.

Olson M et al: Stress-induced immunosuppression and therapeutic touch, *Alt Ther* 3(2):68, 1997.

O'Mathuna D: Evidence-based practice and reviews of therapeutic touch, *J Nurs Scholar* 32(3):279, 2000.

O'Mathuna D: The subtle allure of therapeutic touch, *J Christian Nurs* 15(1):5, 1998.

Pawluk L: Magnetic field therapy. In Novey D, ed: *Clinician's complete reference to complementary and alternative medicine*, St Louis, 2000, Mosby.

Pearson L: "Unruffling" the mystique of therapeutic touch, *NP Forum* 26(11):10, 2001. (See also Letters to the Editor 2002, *NP Forum* 27(2):7, 2002.)

Peck S: The effectiveness of therapeutic touch for decreasing pain in elders with degenerative arthritis, *J Holistic Nurs* 15(2):176, 1997.

Primack N: Accelerated healing with microcurrent: A brief overview, 2000. URL: www.neilprimack.com/neilprimack/whattoexpect.html. Accessed 4/25/2000.

Quinn J: Holding sacred space: the nurse as healing environment, *Holistic Nurs Pract* 6(4):26, 1992.

Quinn J: Building a body of knowledge: research on therapeutic touch 1974-1986, *J Holistic Nurs* 6(1):37, 1988.

Quinn J: Therapeutic touch as energy exchange: testing the theory, *Adv Nurs Sci* 6(2):42, 1984.

Radler M: Dysmenorrhea, *Am Chiropract* March/April:29, 1984.

Rosa L et al: A close look at therapeutic touch, *JAMA* 279(13):1005, 1998. (See also the Letters to the Editor 1998, *JAMA* 280(22):1905, 1998.)

Rosenthal N: Seasonal affective disorder: a description of the syndrome and preliminary findings of light therapy, *Arch Gen Psychiatr* 41:72, 1984.

Sandyk R: Magnetic fields in the therapy of Parkinsonism, *Int J Neurosci* 66:209, 1992a.

Sandyk R: Successful treatment of multiple sclerosis with magnetic fields, *Int J Neurosci* 66:237, 1992b.

Schindler M: Boost your pain-fighting power with magnets, *Prevention* 51:111, 1999.

Simington JA, Laing GP: Effects of therapeutic touch on anxiety in the institutionalized elderly, *Clin Nurs Res* 2(4):438, 1993.

Snyder M, Egan E, Burns K: Interventions for decreasing agitation behaviors in persons with dementia, *J Gerontological Nurs* 21(7):34, 1995.

Spence J, Olson M: Quantitative research on therapeutic touch, *Scand J Caring Sci* 11:183, 1997.

Starn J: The path to becoming an energy healer, *NP Forum* 9(4):209, 1998.

Stein D: *Essential Reiki*, Freedom, Calif, 1995, Crossing Press.

Terman M, Terman J, Williams D: Seasonal affective disorder and its treatments, *J Pract Psychiatr Behav Health* 5:287, 1998.

Tyers S, Smith RB: A comparison of cranial electrotherapy stimulation alone or with chiropractic therapies in the treatment of fibromyalgia, *Am Chiropractor* 23(2):39, 2001.

Vallbonna C et al: Response of pain to static magnetic fields in postpolio patients: a double-blind pilot study, *Arch Phys Med Rehab* 78:1200, 1997.

Wallace L: Light therapy. In Novey D, ed: *Clinician's complete reference to complementary and alternative medicine*, St Louis, 2000, Mosby.

Weintraub MI: Alternative medicine; magnetic bio-stimulation in painful diabetic peripheral neuropathy: a novel intervention-a randomized, double-placebo crossover study, *Am J Pain Manage* 9:8, 1999.

Wetzel W: Reiki healing: a physiologic perspective, *J Holistic Nurs* 7(1):47, 1989.

Wirth D: Complementary healing intervention and dermal wound re-epithelization: an overview, *Int J Psychosom* 42(1):48, 1995.

Wirth D: The effect of non-contact therapeutic touch on the healing rate of full thickness dermal wounds, *Subtle Energies* 1(1):1, 1990

Wytias C: Therapeutic touch in primary care, *NP Forum* 5(2):91, 1994.

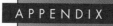

APPENDIX A

SHULER (WHOLISTIC PRACTICE) MODEL

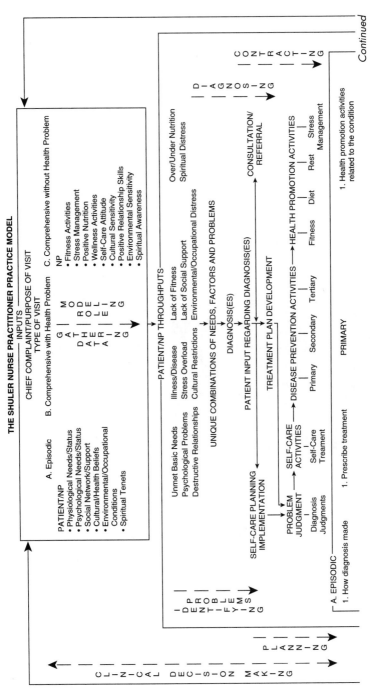

THE SHULER NURSE PRACTITIONER PRACTICE MODEL

Continued

THE SHULER NURSE PRACTITIONER PRACTICE MODEL

A. EPISODIC

1. How diagnosis made
2. Signs & symptoms of condition
3. How to know when to consult health care professional
4. How patient can make the diagnosis in future

1. Prescribe treatment
2. Pharmacological tx component
3. Non-pharmacological tx component
4. How to follow treatment regimen
5. Possible reactions to treatment components
6. Preconsult home treatment

PRIMARY
1. Prevent spread of contagious condition
2. 1° preventive measures specific to condition

SECONDARY
1. How to detect recurrent problem in future
2. 2° preventive measures specific to condition

TERTIARY
1. Rehabilitative measures specific to condition

1. Health promotion activities related to the condition

B. COMPREHENSIVE EXAM WITH AN EXISTING ACUTE PROBLEM

1. How diagnosis made
2. Signs & symptoms of condition
3. How to know when to consult health care professional
4. How patient can make the diagnosis in future

1. Prescribe treatment
2. Pharmacological tx component
3. Non-pharmacological tx component
4. How to follow treatment regimen
5. Possible reactions to treatment components
6. Preconsult home treatment

Primary
1. 1° preventive measures related to condition
2. General 1° preventive measures

SECONDARY
1. How to detect recurrent problem in future
2. 2° preventive measures related to condition
3. General 2° preventive measures

TERTIARY
1. Rehabilitative measures specific to condition

1. Health promotion activities related to the condition
2. Incorporate remainder of health promotion activities to strive for attainment of a higher health status

B. COMPREHENSIVE EXAM WITH AN EXISTING CHRONIC PROBLEM

1. Prescribe treatment
2. Pharmacological tx component
3. Non-pharmacological tx component
4. How to follow treatment regimen
5. Possible reactions to treatment components
6. Preconsult home treatment

PRIMARY
1. 1° preventive measures related to condition
2. General 1° preventive measures

SECONDARY
1. 2° Preventive measures related to condition
2. General 2° preventive measures

TERTIARY
1. Rehabilitative measures specific to condition

1. Health promotion activities related to the condition
2. Incorporate remainder of health promotion activities to strive for attainment of a higher health status

IMPLEMENTING

C. COMPREHENSIVE EXAM WITHOUT AN EXISTING HEALTH PROBLEM

PRIMARY
1. General 1 preventive measures

SECONDARY
1. General 2 preventive measures

1. All health promotion activities that can assist in attainment of a higher health status

EVALUATING

PATIENT OUTPUTS

Movement toward improved health status and wellness, including:

- attainment of basic needs;
- increasing ability to utilize self-care activities;
- setting nutritional goals & actions to meet goals;
- setting fitness goals & actions to meet goals
- setting stress management goals & actions to meet goals;
- increasing ability to function in social and work roles;
- increasing cognizance of spiritual & cultural belief system;
- assessing environmental occupational conditions;
- increasing confidence regarding health care needs, treatments & wellness activities;
- improving compliance to the mutually agreed upon treatment plan;
- decreasing complications & exacerbations of acute/chronic health conditions;
- improving quality of life.

NP OUTPUTS

Movement toward personal wellness, including:

- setting & moving toward own nutritional, fitness, spiritual, cultural, stress management, social, environmental & self-care goals.

Movement toward a professional wellness orientation including:

- role-modeling wellness behaviors;
- facilitating wellness behaviors & self-care activities within plan of care for patient.

Identification of professional learning needs including:

- patient education updates;
- new diagnostic testing options;
- new treatment modalities;
- alternative health care update;
- community resource update.

PROBLEM-FOCUSED WHOLISTIC ASSESSMENT FORM*
(Supplement to Episodic Health History)

Patient Name_____   **Date**_____

Interviewer signature/title_____

Health Problem
1. Type of problem_____
2. Date of onset_____ Duration of symptoms_____
3. Current conventional treatments_____
4. Current alternative treatments_____

Physiological Needs/Status
1. Effects on eating_____
2. Effects on sleeping_____
3. Effects on movement/exercise_____
4. Effects on sexual activities_____

Psychological Needs/Status
1. Psychological response to problem and/or limitations_____
   (depressed, anxious, angry, accepting)
2. Coping strategies_____
3. Perceived effectiveness of coping strategies_____
_____

Social Support/Networks
1. Family/friend responses to problem and/or limitation_____
2. Perceived adequacy of emotional support_____
3. Deficits in tangible support_____
   (self-care activities, housekeeping, cooking, transportation, childcare)

Cultural/Health Beliefs
1. Cultural beliefs regarding problem, treatments, prognosis_____
_____
2. Perceived effectiveness of conventional therapies_____
3. Perceived effectiveness of alternative therapies_____

Environmental/Occupational Conditions
1. Effects on ability to do usual work_____
_____
2. Presence of environmental impeding factors_____
   (air pollution; lack of heat; toxin exposure, refrigeration; unsanitary housing)

Spiritual Tenets
1. Usual spiritual practices_____
2. Perceived benefits of spiritual practices_____
3. Spiritual beliefs regarding problem, treatments, prognosis_____

*Based on the Shuler Nurse Practitioner Practice Model (Shuler, 1991)

WHOLISTIC HEALTH ASSESSMENT FORM*
(Supplement to Comprehensive Health History)

Patient Name_____   Date_____

Interviewer signature/title_____

Biographical Information
1. Age___ DOB_____
2. Country of origin_____
3. 1st language_____ 2nd_____
4. Ethnicity_____
5. Marital status_____
6. No. of children_____
7. Highest year of school_____
8. No. of years in USA_____
9. Recent international travel_____

Environmental/Occupational Conditions
1. Occupation_____
2. Occupational health risk_____
3. Type of housing_____
4. No. of people in home_____
5. Home water source_____
6. Environmental health risks_____
_____

Social Support/Network
(y = yes, n = no, explain)
_____ Has positive emotional support:
_____
_____ Has needed tangible support:
_____
_____ Has family support:
_____

Psychological Needs/Status
1. Depressive sx_____
2. Worries/concerns_____
_____
3. Coping strategies_____
_____

Spiritual Tenets
1. Religious preference_____
2. Spiritual activities (prayer, meditation, church or fasting)_____
3. Perceived benefits_____
4. Spiritual concerns about health___
_____
5. Spiritual beliefs that direct health care practices_____

Cultural/Health Beliefs
1. Alternative/cultural health care practices_____
2. Type of diet_____
3. Cultural health beliefs that direct health care practices_____

Nutrition/Eating Patterns
1. No. of meals per day_____
2. Concerns about eating or getting food:_____

Exercise Patterns
1. Type of exercise_____
2. Frequency of exercise_____
3. Duration of exercise_____

Sleep Patterns
1. Sleep during ____night ____day ____both
2. Usual amount of sleep in 24 hours
_____
3. Concerns about sleep_____

Substance Use (y = yes, n = no)
____Tobacco use: type____ amt____
____Alcohol use: type_____ amt____
____Drug use: type_____ amt____
____Caffeine use: type____ amt____

Referral Needs_____

* Based on the Shuler Nurse Practitioner Practice Model (Shuler, 1991)

MERIDIANS, ACUPUNCTURE, AND AURICULAR POINTS

LEGEND OF ACUPUNCTURE CHANNELS AND POINTS

Ear Points
Kidney
Liver
Upper Lung
Lower Lung
Relaxation
Shenmen
Spleen
Stomach
Sympathetic

Extra
Ding chuan

Diabetes (UB)
17.5

Conception Vessel (Ren mo)
4, 6, 8, 12, 14, 17, 22, 23

Gallbladder (GB)
3, 12, 13, 14, 19, 20, 21, 29, 30, 31, 34, 39, 41

Governing Vessel (Du mo)
3, 4, 8, 14, 16, 18, 19, 20, 21, 24.5 (3rd eye)

Heart (H)
5, 7

Kidney (K)
1, 3, 6, 10

Large Intestine (LI)
4, 10, 11, 15, 16, 20

Liver (Liv)
3, 8, 13, 14

Lung (L)
1, 5, 6, 7

Percardium (PC)
6, 7

Small Intestine (SI)
3, 17

Spleen (Sp)
3, 6, 9, 10

Stomach (ST)
2, 3, 8, 9, 17, 25, 32, 36, 37, 40, 41, 43

Triple Warmer or Burner (San Jiao)
3, 5, 6, 14, 17

Urinary Bladder (UB)
10, 12, 13, 14, 15, 17, 18, 20, 21, 22, 23, 25, 27, 38, 40, 43, 44, 47, 57, 60, 62

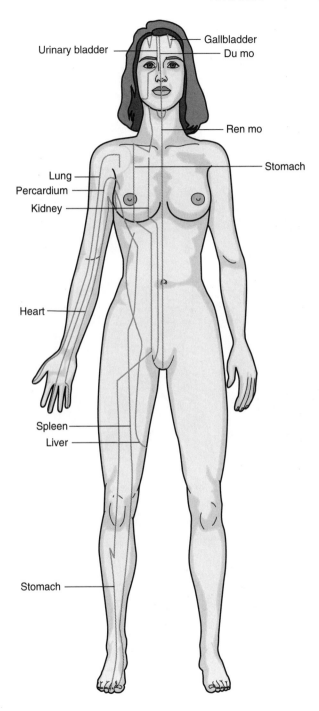

Urinary bladder

Gallbladder

Du mo

Ren mo

Lung

Percardium

Kidney

Stomach

Heart

Spleen

Liver

Stomach

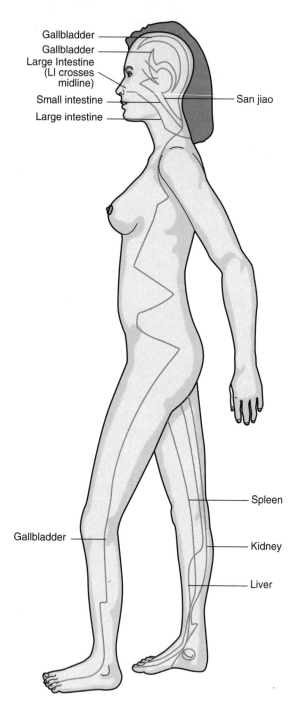

Gallbladder

Gallbladder

Large Intestine (LI crosses midline)

Small intestine

Large intestine

San jiao

Spleen

Kidney

Liver

Gallbladder

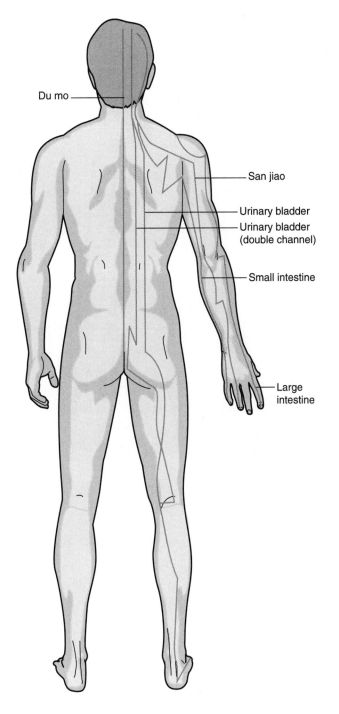

Du mo

San jiao

Urinary bladder

Urinary bladder
(double channel)

Small intestine

Large
intestine

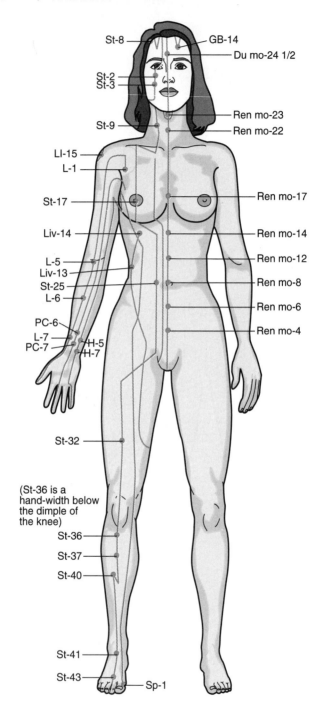

St-8

GB-14

Du mo-24 1/2

St-2
St-3

Ren mo-23

St-9

Ren mo-22

LI-15

L-1

St-17

Ren mo-17

Liv-14

Ren mo-14

L-5
Liv-13

Ren mo-12

St-25

Ren mo-8

L-6

Ren mo-6

PC-6

Ren mo-4

L-7
PC-7

H-5
H-7

St-32

(St-36 is a
hand-width below
the dimple of
the knee)

St-36

St-37

St-40

St-41

St-43

Sp-1

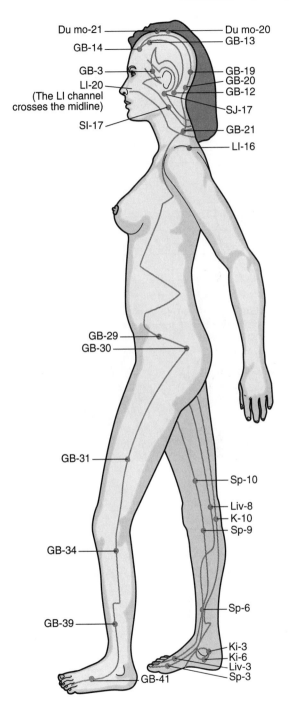

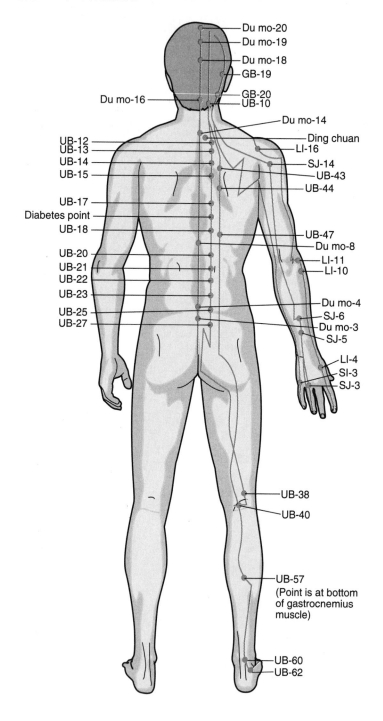

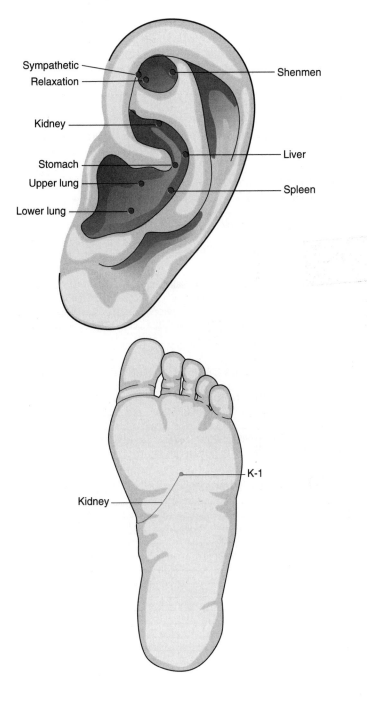

NAC Menopausal Treatment Plan

DATE: _____ **Initial or Follow-up Visit** **MD/FNP** _____
NAME: _____ **DOB** _____ **Age** _____

LABORATORY/DIAGNOSTIC RESULTS: **Date**: _____
Mammogram _____;
Pap Smear _____; Thyroid Profile _____;
TSH _____; CMP _____;
CBC _____; Lipid Profile _____;
Insulin_____; Other_____

HORMONE TESTING (Serum or Salivary) RESULTS: **Date**: _____
Estradiol _____; Estrone _____: Estriol _____:
Progesterone _____; Testosterone _____; DHEA _____;
Cortisol _____; Melatonin _____; Other _____
FSH _____; LSH _____

SELF-CARE TREATMENT PLAN

DIET RECOMMENDATIONS:
Water Intake (½ of Weight = # ounces) _____
Type of Diet _____
Caffeine, Sugar, Alcohol Restrictions _____
Flax Oil _____ Fish Oil _____

VITAMIN & MINERAL THERAPY:
Multiple Vitamin _____
Vitamin C (Rose Hips) _____
Vitamin E (d'alpha tocopheral) _____
B Complex (Contains B6)_____
Vitamin B5 (Pantothenic Acid) _____
Vitamin B8 (Inositol) _____
Vitamin B12 _____
Vitamin D _____
Calcium _____
Magnesium _____
Selenium _____
Chromium Picolinate _____
Boron _____
Other _____

HORMONE THERAPY:
Transdermal/Sublingual Therapies

Tri-Est Creme 2.5 mg or 1.25 mg (Estriol 80%, Estradiol 10%, Estrone 10%)
_____

   Plus: 20-100 mg Progesterone _____, 5-25 mg DHEA _____,
   2 mg Testosterone _____
Bi-Est Creme 2.5 mg or 1.25 mg (Estriol -80%, Estradiol -20%) _____
__ _____

   Plus: 20-100 mg Progesterone _____, 5-25 mg DHEA _____,
   1-2 mg Testosterone _____
Progesterone: _____
Testosterone: _____
DHEA Creme: _____

HORMONE THERAPY:

Oral Therapies

Isoflavones (Soy Protein): _____
Estradiol: _____
Progesterone: _____
Testosterone: _____
DHEA: _____
Pregnenolone: _____
Melatonin: _____
Other: _____

ADRENAL GLAND THERAPY:
   Adrenal Complex (Glandular) _____
   Adrenal Comp (Herbal) _____
   Adrenal Homeopathy _____

HERBAL THERAPY:
   Ashwagandha _____
   Black Cohosh _____
   Borage Oil _____
   Chasteberry _____
   Dong Quai _____
   Evening Primrose _____
   Flaxseed _____
   Korean Ginseng _____
   Ginkgo Biloba _____
   Licorice _____
   Red Clover _____
   Saw Palmetto _____
   Siberian Ginseng _____
   St. John's Wort _____
   Other _____

EXERCISE RECOMMENDATIONS: _____

_____

SPIRITUAL ACTIVITIES: _____

JOURNALING _____

STRESS MANAGEMENT _____

EVALUATION PLANS

FOLLOW-UP EXAM DATE(S) _____
Review-Treatment Adverse Rxns, Sx Improvement, Pt Education Needs,
Patient ?s, Revise Plan as Needed, Physical Exam as Indicated

FOLLOW-UP LAB/DIAGNOSTIC TESTS & DATES _____

_____
_____
_____

REFERRALS _____

_____

_____

*Form developed by Pamela A. Shuler, DNSc, CFNP, RN -Nurse Practitioner Consultant,
4503 Skyland Drive, Sylva, NC 28779, (828) 586-6058 -01/01, Revised 4/03*

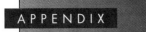

DIETARY REFERENCE INTAKES: VITAMINS AND ELEMENTS

Table D-1 Vitamins

Nutrient	Function	Life Stage Group	RDA/AI*	UL^a	Selected Food Sources	Adverse Effects of Excessive Consumption	Special Considerations
Biotin	Coenzyme in synthesis of fat, glycogen, and amino acids	Infants	(µg/d)		Liver and smaller amounts in fruits and meats	No adverse effects of biotin in humans or animals were found. This does not mean that there is no potential for adverse effects resulting from high intakes. Because data on the adverse effects of biotin are limited, caution may be warranted.	None
		0-6 mo	5*	ND b			
		7-12 mo	6*	ND			
		Children					
		1-3	8*	ND			
		4-8 y	12*	ND			
		Males					
		9-13 y	20*	ND			
		14-18 y	25*	ND			
		19-30 y	30*	ND			
		31-50 y	30*	ND			
		51-70 y	30*	ND			
		> 70 y	30*	ND			
		Females					
		9-13 y	20*	ND			
		14-18 y	25*	ND			
		19-30 y	30*	ND			
		31-50 y	30*	ND			
		51-70 y	30*	ND			
		> 70 y	30*	ND			
		Pregnancy					
		≤18 y	30*	ND			
		19-30y	30*	ND			
		31-50 y	30*	ND			
		Lactation					
		≤18 y	35*	ND			
		19-30y	35*	ND			
		31-50 y	35*	ND			

844

Choline		(mg/d)	(mg/d)	Milk, liver, eggs, peanuts	Fishy body odor, sweating, salivation, hypotension, hepatotoxicity	Individuals with trimethylaminuria, renal disease, liver disease, depression and Parkinson's disease, may be at risk of adverse effects with choline intakes at the UL. Although AIs have been set for choline, there are few data to assess whether a dietary supply of choline is needed at all stages of the life cycle, and it may be that the choline requirement can be met by endogenous synthesis at some of these stages.
Precursor for acetylcholine, phospholipids and betaine	Infants		ND			
	0-6 mo	125*	ND			
	7-12 mo	150*				
	Children					
	1-3 y	200*	1000			
	4-8 y	250*	1000			
	Males					
	9-13 y	375*	2000			
	14-18 y	550*	3000			
	19-30 y	550*	3500			
	31-50 y	550*	3500			
	51-70 y	550*	3500			
	> 70 y	550*	3500			
	Females					
	9-13 y	375*	2000			
	14-18 y	400*	3000			
	19-30 y	425*	3500			
	31-50 y	425*	3500			
	51-70 y	425*	3500			
	> 70 y	425*	3500			
	Pregnancy					
	≤18 y	450*	3000			
	19-30y	450*	3500			
	31-50 y	450*	3500			
	Lactation					
	≤18 y	550*	3000			
	19-30y	550*	3500			
	31-50 y	550*	3500			

Continued

Table D-1 Vitamins—cont'd

Nutrient	Function	Life Stage Group	RDA/AI*	UL^a	Selected Food Sources	Adverse Effects of Excessive Consumption	Special Considerations
Folate Also known as: Folic acid Folacin Pteroyl- polyglutamates Note: Given as dietary folate equivalents (DFE). 1 DFE = 1 µg food folate= 0.6 µg of folate from fortified food or as a supplement consumed with food = 0.5 µg of a supplement taken on an empty stomach.	Coenzyme in the metabolism of nucleic and amino acids; prevents megaloblastic anemia		(µg/d)	(mcg/d)	Enriched cereal grains, dark leafy veggies, enriched and whole-grain breads and bread products, fortified ready-to-eat cereals	Masks neurological complication in people with vitamin B12 deficiency. No adverse effects associated with folate from food or supplements have been reported. This does not mean that there is no potential for adverse effects resulting from high intakes. Because data on the adverse effects of folate are limited, caution may be warranted. The UL for folate applies to synthetic forms obtained from supplements and/or fortified foods.	In view of evidence linking folate intake with neural tube defects in the fetus, it is recommended that all women capable of becoming pregnant consume 400 µg from supplements or fortified foods in addition to intake of food folate from a varied diet. It is assumed that women will continue consuming 400 µg from supplements or fortified food until their pregnancy is confirmed and they enter prenatal care, which ordinarily occurs after the end of the peri-conceptional period—the critical time for formation of the neural tube.
		Infants					
		0-6 mo	65*	ND^b			
		7-12 mo	80*	ND			
		Children					
		1-3	**150**	300			
		4-8 y	**200**	400			
		Males					
		9-13 y	**300**	600			
		14-18 y	**400**	800			
		19-30 y	**400**	1,000			
		31-50 y	**400**	1,000			
		51-70 y	**400**	1,000			
		>70 y	**400**	1,000			
		Females					
		9-13 y	**300**	600			
		14-18 y	**400**	800			
		19-30 y	**400**	1,000			
		31-50 y	**400**	1,000			
		51-70 y	**400**	1,000			
		>70 y	**400**	1,000			
		Pregnancy					
		≤18 y	**600**	800			
		19-30y	**600**	1,000			
		31-50 y	**600**	1,000			
		Lactation					
		≤18 y	**500**	800			
		19-30y	**500**	1,000			
		31-50 y	**500**	1,000			

Niacin Includes nicotinic acid amide, nicotinic acid (pyridine-3-carboxylic acid), and derivatives that exhibit the biological activity of nicotinamide. Note: Niacin requirements are met by nicotinic acid (niacin) and nicotinamide (niacinamide) in the diet; also by conversion from protein containing tryptophan. 60 mg tryptopah = 1 mg; niacin = 1 mg of niacin equivalents (NE)	Coenzyme or cosubstrate in many biological reduction and oxidation reactions—thus required for energy metabolism	Life stage group	(mg/d)	(mg/d)	Meat, fish, poultry, enriched and whole-grain breads and bread products, fortified ready-to-eat cereals	There is no evidence of adverse effects from the consumption of naturally occurring niacin in foods. Adverse effects from niacin containing supplements may include flushing and gastrointestinal distress hepatotoxicity. The UL for niacin applies to synthetic forms obtained from supplements, fortified foods, or a combination of the two. Niacin should be discontinued if liver function tests rise to 3 times the upper limit of normal.	Extra niacin may be required by persons treated with hemodialysis or peritoneal dialysis, or those with malabsorption syndrome.
		Infants					
		0-6 mo	2*	ND			
		7-12 mo	4*	ND			
		Children					
		1-3	6	10			
		4-8 y	8	15			
		Males					
		9-13 y	12	20			
		14-18 y	16	30			
		19-30 y	16	35			
		31-50 y	16	35			
		51-70 y	16	35			
		> 70 y	16	35			
		Females					
		9-13 y	12	20			
		14-18 y	14	30			
		19-30 y	14	35			
		31-50 y	14	35			
		51-70 y	14	35			
		> 70 y	14	35			
		Pregnancy					
		≤18 y	18	30			
		19-30y	18	35			
		31-50 y	18	35			
		Lactation					
		≤18 y	17	30			
		19-30y	17	35			
		31-50 y	17	35			

Continued

Nutrient	Function	Life Stage Group	RDA/AI*	UL^a	Selected Food Sources	Adverse Effects of Excessive Consumption	Special Considerations
Pantothenic Acid	Coenzyme in fatty acid metabolism	Infants	(mg/d)	(mg/d)	Chicken, beef, potatoes, oats, cereals, tomato products, liver, kidney, yeast, egg yolk, broccoli, whole grains	No adverse effects associated with pantothenic acid from food or supplements have been reported. This does not mean that there is no potential for adverse effects resulting from high intakes. Because data on the adverse effects of pantothenic acid are limited, caution may be warranted.	None.
		0-6 mo	1.7*	ND ^b			
		7-12 mo	1.8*	ND			
		Children					
		1-3	2*	ND			
		4-8 y	3*	ND			
		Males					
		9-13 y	4*	ND			
		14-18 y	5*	ND			
		19-30 y	5*	ND			
		31-50 y	5*	ND			
		51-70 y	5*	ND			
		> 70 y	5*	ND			
		Females					
		9-13 y	4*	ND			
		14-18 y	5*	ND			
		19-30 y	5*	ND			
		31-50 y	5*	ND			
		51-70 y	5*	ND			
		> 70 y	5*	ND			
		Pregnancy					
		≤18 y	6*	ND			
		19-30y	6*	ND			
		31-50 y	6*	ND			
		Lactation					
		≤18 y	7*	ND			
		19-30y	7*	ND			
		31-50 y	7*	ND			

Riboflavin Also known as: Vitamin B2

Coenzyme in numerous redox reactions

Life Stage Group	(mg/d)	(mg/d)	Selected Food Sources	Adverse Effects	Special Considerations
Infants			Organ meats, milk, bread products and fortified cereals	No adverse effects associated with riboflavin consumption from food or supplements have been reported. This does not mean that there is no potential for adverse effects resulting from high intakes. Because data on the adverse effects of riboflavin are limited, caution may be warranted.	None
0-6 mo	0.3*	ND			
7-12 mo	0.4*	ND			
Children					
1-3	**0.5**	ND			
4-8 y	**0.6**	ND			
Males					
9-13 y	**0.9**	ND			
14-18 y	**1.3**	ND			
19-30 y	**1.3**	ND			
31-50 y	**1.3**	ND			
51-70 y	**1.3**	ND			
> 70 y	**1.3**	ND			
Females					
9-13 y	**0.9**	ND			
14-18 y	**1.0**	ND			
19-30 y	**1.1**	ND			
31-50 y	**1.1**	ND			
51-70 y	**1.1**	ND			
> 70 y	**1.1**	ND			
Pregnancy					
≤18 y	**1.4**	ND			
19-30y	**1.4**	ND			
31-50 y	**1.4**	ND			
Lactation					
≤18 y	**1.6**	ND			
19-30y	**1.6**	ND			
31-50 y	**1.6**	ND			

Continued

849

Table D-1   Vitamins—cont'd

Nutrient	Function	Life Stage Group	RDA/AI*	UL[a]	Selected Food Sources	Adverse Effects of Excessive Consumption	Special Considerations
Thiamin Also known as: Vitamin B1 Aneurin	Coenzyme in the metabolism of carbohydrates and branched-chain amino acids	**Infants**	(mg/d)		Enriched, fortified, or whole-grain products; bread and bread products, mixed foods whose main ingredient is grain, and ready-to-eat cereals	No adverse effects associated with thiamin from food or supplements have been reported. This does not mean that there is no potential for adverse effects resulting from high intakes. Because data on the adverse effects of thiamin are limited, caution may be warranted.	Persons who may have increased needs for thiamin include those being treated with hemodialysis or peritoneal dialysis, or individuals with malabsorption syndrome.
		0-6 mo	0.2*	ND [b]			
		7-12 mo	0.3*	ND			
		Children					
		1-3	**0.5**	ND			
		4-8 y	**0.6**	ND			
		Males					
		9-13 y	**0.9**	ND			
		14-18 y	**1.2**	ND			
		19-30 y	**1.2**	ND			
		31-50 y	**1.2**	ND			
		51-70 y	**1.2**	ND			
		> 70 y	**1.2**	ND			
		Females					
		9-13 y	**0.9**	ND			
		14-18 y	**1.0**	ND			
		19-30 y	**1.1**	ND			
		31-50 y	**1.1**	ND			
		51-70 y	**1.1**	ND			
		> 70 y	**1.1**	ND			
		Pregnancy					
		≤18 y	**1.4**	ND			
		19-30y	**1.4**	ND			
		31-50 y	**1.4**	ND			
		Lactation					
		≤18 y	**1.4**	ND			
		19-30y	**1.4**	ND			
		31-50 y	**1.4**	ND			

Vitamin A Includes provitamin A carotenoids that are dietary precursors of retinol. Note: Given as retinol activity equivalents (RAEs). 1 RAE = 1 mcg retinol, 12 mcg beta carotene, 24 mcg alpha -carotene, or 24 mcg beta cryptoxanthin. To calculate RAEs from REs of provitamin A carotenoids in foods, divide the REs by 2. For preformed vitamin A in foods or supplements and for provitamin A carotenoids in supplements, 1 RE = 1 RAE.	Required for normal vision, gene expression, repro-duction, embryonic development and immune function		(µg/d) 400* 500*	(µg/d) 600 600	Teratological effects, liver toxicity Note: From preformed Vitamin A only.	Liver, dairy products, fish	Individuals with high alcohol intake, pre-existing liver disease, hyperlipidemia or severe protein malnutrition may be distinctly susceptible to the adverse effects of excess preformed vitamin A intake. Beta-carotene supplements are advised only to serve as a provitamin A source for individuals at risk of vitamin A deficiency.
		Infants					
		0-6 mo	400*	600			
		7-12 mo	500*	600			
		Children					
		1-3	300	600			
		4-8 y	400	900			
		Males					
		9-13 y	600	1,700			
		14-18 y	900	2,800			
		19-30 y	900	3,000			
		31-50 y	900	3,000			
		51-70 y	900	3,000			
		>70 y	900	3,000			
		Females					
		9-13 y	600	1,700			
		14-18 y	700	2,800			
		19-30 y	700	3,000			
		31-50 y	700	3,000			
		51-70 y	700	3,000			
		>70 y	700	3,000			
		Pregnancy					
		≤18 y	750	2,800			
		19-30y	770	3,000			
		31-50 y	770	3,000			
		Lactation					
		≤18 y	1,200	2,800			
		19-30y	1,300	3,000			
		31-50 y	1,300	3,000			

3000 mcg = 10,000 units

Continued

Table D-1 Vitamins—cont'd

Nutrient	Function	Life Stage Group	RDA/AI*	UL[a]	Selected Food Sources	Adverse Effects of Excessive Consumption	Special Considerations
Vitamin B6 Vitamin B6 comprises a group of six related compounds: pyridoxal, pyridoxine, pyridoxamine, and 5'-phosphates (PLP, PNP, PMP)	Coenzyme in the metabolism of amino acids, glycogen and sphingoid bases		(mg/d)	(mg/d)	Fortified cereals, organ meats, fortified soy-based meat substitutes	No adverse effects associated with Vitamin B6 from food have been reported. This does not mean that there is no potential for adverse effects resulting from high intakes. Because data on the adverse effects of Vitamin B6 are limited, caution may be warranted. Sensory neuropathy has occurred from high intakes of supplemental forms.	None
		Infants					
		0-6 mo	0.1*	ND b			
		7-12 mo	0.3*	ND			
		Children					
		1-3	**0.5**	30			
		4-8 y	**0.6**	40			
		Males					
		9-13 y	**1.0**	60			
		14-18 y	**1.3**	80			
		19-30 y	**1.3**	100			
		31-50 y	**1.3**	100			
		51-70 y	**1.7**	100			
		> 70 y	**1.7**	100			
		Females					
		9-13 y	**1.0**	60			
		14-18 y	**1.2**	80			
		19-30 y	**1.3**	100			
		31-50 y	**1.3**	100			
		51-70 y	**1.5**	100			
		> 70 y	**1.5**	100			
		Pregnancy					
		≤18 y	**1.9**	80			
		19-30y	**1.9**	100			
		31-50 y	**1.9**	100			
		Lactation					
		≤18 y	**2.0**	80			
		19-30y	**2.0**	100			
		31-50 y	**2.0**	100			

Vitamin B12 Also known as: Cobalamin	Coenzyme in nucleic acid metabolism; prevents mega-loblastic anemia		(µg/d)	Fortified cereals, meat, fish, poultry	No adverse effects have been asso-ciated with the consumption of the amounts of vitamin B12 normally found in foods or supple-ments. This does not mean that there is no potential for adverse effects resulting from high intakes. Because data on the adverse effects of vitamin B12 are limited, caution may be warranted.	Because 10 to 30 percent of older people may malabsorb food-bound vitamin B12, it is advisable for those older than 50 years to meet their RDA mainly by consuming foods fortified with vitamin B12 or a supplement containing vitamin B12.
		Infants				
		0-6 mo	0.4*	ND		
		7-12 mo	0.5*	ND		
		Children				
		1-3	**0.9**	ND		
		4-8 y	**1.2**	ND		
		Males				
		9-13 y	**1.8**	ND		
		14-18 y	**2.4**	ND		
		19-30 y	**2.4**	ND		
		31-50 y	**2.4**	ND		
		51-70 y	**2.4**	ND		
		> 70 y	**2.4**	ND		
		Females				
		9-13 y	**1.8**	ND		
		14-18 y	**2.4**	ND		
		19-30 y	**2.4**	ND		
		31-50 y	**2.4**	ND		
		51-70 y	**2.4**	ND		
		> 70 y	**2.4**	ND		
		Pregnancy				
		≤18 y	**2.6**	ND		
		19-30 y	**2.6**	ND		
		31-50 y	**2.6**	ND		
		Lactation				
		≤18 y	**2.8**	ND		
		19-30 y	**2.8**	ND		
		31-50 y	**2.8**	ND		

Continued

853

Table D-1   Vitamins—cont'd

Nutrient	Function	Life Stage Group	RDA/AI*	ULᵃ	Selected Food Sources	Adverse Effects of Excessive Consumption	Special Considerations
Vitamin C Also known as: Ascorbic acid Dehydroascorbic acid (DHA)	Cofactor for reactions requiring reduced copper or iron metalloenzyme and as a protective antioxidant		(mg/d)	(mg/d)	Citrus fruits, tomatoes, tomato juice, potatoes, brussel sprouts, cauliflower, straw- berries, cabbage and spinach	Gastrointestinal distur- bances, kidney stones, excess iron absorption	Individuals who smoke require an additional 35mg/d of vitamin C over that needed by nonsmokers. Nonsmokers regularly exposed to tobacco smoke are encouraged to ensure they meet the RDA for vitamin C.
		Infants					
		0-6 mo	40*	ND b			
		7-12 mo	50*	ND			
		Children					
		1-3	**15**	400			
		4-8 y	**25**	650			
		Males					
		9-13 y	**45**	1,200			
		14-18 y	**75**	1,800			
		19-30 y	**90**	2,000			
		31-50 y	**90**	2,000			
		51-70 y	**90**	2,000			
		> 70 y	**90**	2,000			
		Females					
		9-13 y	**45**	1,200			
		14-18 y	**65**	1,800			
		19-30 y	**75**	2,000			
		31-50 y	**75**	2,000			
		51-70 y	**75**	2,000			
		> 70 y	**75**	2,000			
		Pregnancy					
		≤18 y	**80**	1,800			
		19-30 y	**85**	2,000			
		31-50 y	**85**	2,000			
		Lactation					
		≤18 y	**115**	1,800			
		19-30 y	**120**	2,000			
		31-50 y	**120**	2,000			

Vitamin D Also known as: Calciferol Note: 1 µg calciferol = 40 IU vitamin D The DRI values are based on the absence of adequate exposure to sunlight.	Maintain serum calcium and phosphorus concentrations.		(µg/d)	(µg/d)	Fish liver oils, flesh of fatty fish, liver and fat from seals and polar bears, eggs from hens that have been fed vitamin D, fortified milk products and fortified cereals	Elevated plasma 25 (OH) D concentration causing hyper-calcemia	Patients on glucocorticoid therapy may require additional vitamin D.
		Infants					
		0-6 mo	5*	25			
		7-12 mo	5*	25			
		Children					
		1-3	5*	50			
		4-8 y	5*	50			
		Males					
		9-13 y	5*	50			
		14-18 y	5*	50			
		19-30 y	5*	50			
		31-50 y	5*	50			
		51-70 y	10*	50			
		>70 y	15*	50			
		Females					
		9-13 y	5*	50			
		14-18 y	5*	50			
		19-30 y	5*	50			
		31-50 y	5*	50			
		51-70 y	10*	50			
		>70 y	15*	50			
		Pregnancy					
		≤18 y	5*	50			
		19-30 y	5*	50			
		31-50 y	5*	50			
		Lactation					
		≤18 y	5*	50			
		19-30 y	5*	50			
		31-50 y	5*	50			

Continued

Table D-1 Vitamins—cont'd

Nutrient	Function	Life Stage Group	RDA/AI*	UL^a	Selected Food Sources	Adverse Effects of Excessive Consumption	Special Considerations
Vitamin E Also known as: alpha-tocopherol. Note: As α-tocopherol α-tocopherol includes *RRR*-α-tocopherol, the only form of α-tocopherol that occurs naturally in foods, and the 2R-stereoisomeric forms of α-tocopherol (*RRR*-, *RSR*-, *RRS*-, and *RSS*-α-tocopherol) that occur in fortified foods and supplements. It does not include the 2S-stereoisomeric forms of α-tocopherol (*SRR*-, *SSR*-, *SRS*-, and *SSS*-α-tocopherol), also found in fortified foods and supplements.	A metabolic function has not yet been identified. Vitamin E's major function appears to be as a non-specific chain-breaking antioxidant.	Infants	(mg/d)	(mg/d)	Vegetable oils, unprocessed cereal grains, nuts, fruits, vegetables, meats	There is no evidence of adverse effects from the consumption of vitamin E naturally occurring in foods. Adverse effects from vitamin E containing supplements may include hemorrhagic toxicity. The UL for vitamin E applies to any form of alpha-tocopherol obtained from supplements, fortified foods, or a combination of the two.	Patients on anticoagulant therapy should be monitored when taking vitamin E supplements.
		0-6 mo	4*	ND^b			
		7-12 mo	5*	ND			
		Children					
		1-3	**6**	200			
		4-8 y	**7**	300			
		Males					
		9-13 y	**11**	600			
		14-18 y	**15**	800			
		19-30 y	**15**	1,000			
		31-50 y	**15**	1,000			
		51-70 y	**15**	1,000			
		> 70 y	**15**	1,000			
		Females					
		9-13 y	**11**	600			
		14-18 y	**15**	800			
		19-30 y	**15**	1,000			
		31-50 y	**15**	1,000			
		51-70 y	**15**	1,000			
		> 70 y	**15**	1,000			
		Pregnancy					
		≤18 y	**15**	800			
		19-30 y	**15**	1,000			
		31-50 y	**15**	1,000			
		Lactation					
		≤18 y	**19**	800			
		19-30 y	**19**	1,000			
		31-50 y	**19**	1,000			

Vitamin K						
Coenzyme during the synthesis of many proteins involved in blood clotting and bone metabolism			(mcg/d)		Green vegetables (collards, spinach, salad greens, broccoli), brussel sprouts, cabbage, plant oils and margarine	No adverse effects associated with vitamin K consumption from food or supplements have been reported in humans or animals. This does not mean that there is no potential for adverse effects resulting from high intakes. Because data on the adverse effects of vitamin K are limited, caution may be warranted.	Patients on anticoagulant therapy should monitor vitamin K intake.
	Infants					
	0-6 mo	2.0*	ND			
	7-12 mo	2.5*	ND			
	Children					
	1-3	30*	ND			
	4-8 y	55*	ND			
	Males					
	9-13 y	60*	ND			
	14-18 y	75*	ND			
	19-30 y	120*	ND			
	31-50 y	120*	ND			
	51-70 y	120*	ND			
	>70 y	120*	ND			
	Females					
	9-13 y	60*	ND			
	14-18 y	75*	ND			
	19-30 y	90*	ND			
	31-50 y	90*	ND			
	51-70 y	90*	ND			
	>70 y	90*	ND			
	Pregnancy					
	≤18 y	75*	ND			
	19-30 y	90*	ND			
	31-50 y	90*	ND			

Continued

Table D-1   Vitamins—cont'd

Nutrient	Function	Life Stage Group	RDA/AI*	UL[a]	Selected Food Sources	Adverse Effects of Excessive Consumption	Special Considerations
Vitamin K, cont'd		Lactation					
		≤18 y	75*	ND			
		19-30 y	90*	ND			
		31-50 y	90*	ND			

AI, Adequate intake; DFE, dietary folate equivalents; DHA, dehydroascorbic acid; DRI, dietary reference intake; IU, international units; ND b, not determinable resulting from lack of data of adverse effects in this age group and concern with regard to lack of ability to handle excess amounts. Source of intake should be from food only to prevent high levels of intake; NE, niacin equivalents; PLP, pyridoxal phosphate; PMP, pyridoxamine phosphate; PNP, pyridoxine phosphate; RAEs, retinol activity equivalents; RDA, recommended daily allowance; REs, retinol equivalents; UL a, the maximum level of daily nutrient intake that is likely to pose no risk of adverse effects. Unless otherwise specified, the UL represents total intake from food, water, and supplements. Because of the lack of suitable data, ULs could not be established for vitamin K, thiamin, riboflavin, vitamin B12, pantothenic acid, biotin, or carotenoids. In the absence of ULs, extra caution may be warranted in consuming levels above recommended intakes.

Note: The table is adapted from the DRI reports (see www.nap.edu); it represents Recommended Dietary Allowances (RDAs) in **bold type**, Adequate Intakes (AIs) in ordinary type followed by an asterisk (*), and Upper Limits (UL)[a]. RDAs and AIs may both be used as goals for individual intake. RDAs are set to meet the needs of almost all (97% to 98%) individuals in a group. For healthy breast-fed infants, the AI is the mean intake. The AI for other life stage and gender groups is believed to cover the needs of all individuals in the group, but lack of data prevent being able to specify with confidence the percentage of individuals covered by this intake.

Sources: Dietary Reference Intakes for Calcium, Phosphorous, Magnesium, Vitamin D, and Fluoride (1997); Dietary Reference Intakes for Thiamin, Riboflavin, Niacin, Vitamin B6, Folate, Vitamin B12, Pantothenic Acid, Biotin, and Choline (1998); Dietary Reference Intakes for Vitamin C, Vitamin E, Selenium, and Carotenoids (2000); and Dietary Reference Intakes for Vitamin A, Vitamin K, Arsenic, Boron, Chromium, Copper, Iodine, Iron, Manganese, Molybdenum, Nickel, Silicon, Vanadium, and Zinc (2002). These reports may be accessed via www.nap.edu and www4.nationalacademies.org.

Table D-2	Elements						
Nutrient	Function	Life Stage Group	RDA/AI*	UL[a]	Selected Food Sources	Adverse Effects of Excessive Consumption	Special Considerations
Arsenic	No biologic function in humans although animal data indicate a requirement	Infants			Dairy products, meat, poultry, fish, grains and cereal	No data on the possible adverse effects of organic arsenic compounds in food were found. Inorganic arsenic is a known toxic substance. Although the UL was not determined for arsenic, there is no justification for adding arsenic to food or supplements.	None
		0-6 mo	ND b	ND			
		7-12 mo	ND	ND			
		Children					
		1-3 y	ND	ND			
		4-8 y	ND	ND			
		Males					
		9-13 y	ND	ND			
		14-18 y	ND	ND			
		19-30 y	ND	ND			
		31-50 y	ND	ND			
		51-70 y	ND	ND			
		> 70 y	ND	ND			
		Females					
		9-13 y	ND	ND			
		14-18 y	ND	ND			
		19-30 y	ND	ND			
		31-50 y	ND	ND			
		51-70 y	ND	ND			
		> 70 y	ND	ND			
		Pregnancy					
		≤18 y	ND	ND			
		19-30 y	ND	ND			
		31-50 y	ND	ND			
		Lactation					
		≤18 y	ND	ND			
		19-30 y	ND	ND			
		31-50 y	ND	ND			

Continued

Nutrient	Function	Life Stage Group	RDA/AI*	UL^a	Selected Food Sources	Adverse Effects of Excessive Consumption	Special Considerations
Boron	No clear biologic function in humans although animal data indicate a functional role			(mg/d)	Fruit-based beverages and products, potatoes, legumes, milk, avocado, peanut butter, peanuts	Reproductive and developmental effects as observed in animal studies	None. Because of potential estrogen effects, use caution.
		Infants					
		0-6 mo	ND	ND			
		7-12 mo	ND	ND			
		Children					
		1-3 y	ND	3			
		4-8 y	ND	6			
		Males					
		9-13 y	ND	11			
		14-18 y	ND	17			
		19-30 y	ND	20			
		31-50 y	ND	20			
		51-70 y	ND	20			
		>70 y	ND	20			
		Females					
		9-13 y	ND	11			
		14-18 y	ND	17			
		19-30 y	ND	20			
		31-50 y	ND	20			
		51-70 y	ND	20			
		>70 y	ND	20			
		Pregnancy					
		≤18 y	ND	17			
		19-30 y	ND	20			
		31-50 y	ND	20			
		Lactation					
		≤18 y	ND	17			
		19-30 y	ND	20			
		31-50 y	ND	20			

Calcium	Essential role in blood clotting, muscle contraction, nerve transmission, and bone and tooth formation		(mg/d)	(mg/d) ND b	Milk, cheese, yogurt, corn tortillas, calcium-set tofu, Chinese cabbage, kale, broccoli	Kidney stones, hyper-calcemia, milk alkali syndrome, and renal insufficiency	Amenorrheic women (exercise- or anorexia nervosa-induced) have reduced net calcium absorption. There is no consistent data to support that a high protein intake increases calcium requirement.
		Infants				High intake might increase risk for prostate cancer	
		0-6 mo	210*	ND			
		7-12 mo	270*	ND			
		Children					
		1-3 y	500*	2,500			
		4-8 y	800*	2,500			
		Males					
		9-13 y	1,300*	2,500			
		14-18 y	1,300*	2,500			
		19-30 y	1,000*	2,500			
		31-50 y	1,000*	2,500			
		51-70 y	1,200*	2,500			
		> 70 y	1,200*	2,500			
		Females					
		9-13 y	1,300*	2,500			
		14-18 y	1,300*	2,500			
		19-30 y	1,000*	2,500			
		31-50 y	1,000*	2,500			
		51-70 y	1,200*	2,500			
		> 70 y	1,200*	2,500			
		Pregnancy					
		≤18 y	1,300*	2,500			
		19-30 y	1,000*	2,500			
		31-50 y	1,000*	2,500			
		Lactation					
		≤18 y	1,300*	2,500			
		19-30 y	1,000*	2,500			
		31-50 y	1,000*	2,500			

Continued

Table D-2 Elements—cont'd

Nutrient	Function	Life Stage Group	RDA/AI*	UL^a	Selected Food Sources	Adverse Effects of Excessive Consumption	Special Considerations
Chromium	Helps to maintain normal blood glucose levels	Infants	(μg/d)		Some cereals, meats, poultry, fish, beer	Chronic renal failure; hepatic dysfunction; cognitive, perceptual, and motor dysfunction	Chromium potentiates the action of insulin
		0-6 mo	0.2*	ND			
		7-12 mo	5.5*	ND			
		Children					
		1-3 y	11*	ND			
		4-8 y	15*	ND			
		Males					
		9-13 y	25*	ND			
		14-18 y	35*	ND			
		19-30 y	35*	ND			
		31-50 y	35*	ND			
		51-70 y	30*	ND			
		> 70 y	30*	ND			
		Females					
		9-13 y	21*	ND			
		14-18 y	24*	ND			
		19-30 y	25*	ND			
		31-50 y	25*	ND			
		51-70 y	20*	ND			
		> 70 y	20*	ND			
		Pregnancy					
		≤18 y	29*	ND			
		19-30 y	30*	ND			
		31-50 y	30*	ND			
		Lactation					
		≤18 y	44*	ND			
		19-30 y	45*	ND			
		31-50 y	45*	ND			

Copper	Component of enzymes in iron metabolism		(µg/d)	(µg/d)ᵇ	Organ meats, seafood, nuts, seeds, wheat bran cereals, whole grain products, cocoa products	Gastro-intestinal distress, liver damage	Individuals with Wilson's disease, Indian childhood cirrhosis and idiopathic copper toxicosis may be at increased risk of adverse effects from excess copper intake.
		Infants					
		0-6 mo	200*	ND ᵇ			
		7-12 mo	220*	ND			
		Children					
		1-3 y	340	1,000			
		4-8 y	440	3,000			
		Males					
		9-13 y	700	5,000			
		14-18 y	890	8,000			
		19-30 y	900	10,000			
		31-50 y	900	10,000			
		51-70 y	900	10,000			
		> 70 y	900	10,000			
		Females					
		9-13 y	700	5,000			
		14-18 y	890	8,000			
		19-30 y	900	10,000			
		31-50 y	900	10,000			
		51-70 y	900	10,000			
		> 70 y	900	10,000			
		Pregnancy					
		≤18 y	1000	8,000			
		19-30 y	1000	10,000			
		31-50 y	1000	10,000			
		Lactation					
		≤18 y	1300	8,000			
		19-30 y	1300	10,000			
		31-50 y	1300	10,000			

Continued

863

Table D-2 Elements—cont'd

Nutrient	Function	Life Stage Group	RDA/AI*	UL[a]	Selected Food Sources	Adverse Effects of Excessive Consumption	Special Considerations
Fluoride	Inhibits the initiation and progression of dental caries and stimulates new bone formation	Infants	(mg/d)	(mg/d)	Fluoridated water, teas, marine fish, fluoridated dental products	Enamel and skeletal fluorosis	None
		0-6 mo	0.01*	0.7			
		7-12 mo	0.5*	0.9			
		Children					
		1-3 y	0.7*	1.3			
		4-8 y	1*	2.2			
		Males					
		9-13 y	2*	10			
		14-18 y	3*	10			
		19-30 y	4*	10			
		31-50 y	4*	10			
		51-70 y	4*	10			
		>70 y	4*	10			
		Females					
		9-13 y	2*	10			
		14-18 y	3*	10			
		19-30 y	3*	10			
		31-50 y	3*	10			
		51-70 y	3*	10			
		>70 y	3*	10			
		Pregnancy					
		≤18 y	3*	10			
		19-30 y	3*	10			
		31-50 y	3*	10			
		Lactation					
		≤18 y	3*	10			
		19-30 y	3*	10			
		31-50 y	3*	10			

Iodine	Life Stage Group	(µg/d) 110* 130*	(µg/d) ND b ND	Marine origin, processed foods, iodized salt	Elevated thyroid stimulating hormone (TSH) concentration	Individuals with autoimmune thyroid disease, previous iodine deficiency, or nodular goiter are distinctly susceptible to the adverse effect of excess iodine intake. Therefore, individuals with these conditions may not be protected by the UL for iodine intake for the general population.
Component of the thyroid hormones; and prevents goiter and cretinism	Infants					
	0-6 mo					
	7-12 mo					
	Children					
	1-3 y	90	200			
	4-8 y	90	300			
	Males					
	9-13 y	120	600			
	14-18 y	150	900			
	19-30 y	150	1,100			
	31-50 y	150	1,100			
	51-70 y	150	1,100			
	>70 y	150	1,100			
	Females					
	9-13 y	120	600			
	14-18 y	150	900			
	19-30 y	150	1,100			
	31-50 y	150	1,100			
	51-70 y	150	1,100			
	>70 y	150	1,100			
	Pregnancy					
	≤18 y	220	900			
	19-30 y	220	1,100			
	31-50 y	220	1,100			
	Lactation					
	≤18 y	290	900			
	19-30 y	290	1,100			
	31-50 y	290	1,100			

Continued

865

Table D-2 Elements—cont'd

Nutrient	Function	Life Stage Group	RDA/AI*	UL[a]	Selected Food Sources	Adverse Effects of Excessive Consumption	Special Considerations
Iron	Component of hemoglobin and numerous enzymes; prevents microcytic hypochromic anemia		(mg/d)	(mg/d)	Fruits, vegetables and fortified bread and grain products such as cereal (non-heme iron sources), meat and poultry (heme iron sources)	Gastrointestinal distress; severe iron poisoning results in damage to intestinal lining of liver. Excess iron can cause hemosiderosis.	Non-heme iron absorption is lower for those consuming vegetarian diets than for those eating nonvegetarian diets. Therefore, it has been suggested that the iron requirement for those consuming a vegetarian diet is approximately 2-fold greater than for those consuming a nonvegetarian diet. Recommended intake assumes 75% of iron is from heme iron sources. Keep all iron supplements out of reach of children.
		Infants					
		0-6 mo	0.27*	40			
		7-12 mo	11	40			
		Children					
		1-3 y	7	40			
		4-8 y	10	40			
		Males					
		9-13 y	8	40			
		14-18 y	11	45			
		19-30 y	8	45			
		31-50 y	8	45			
		51-70 y	8	45			
		>70 y	8	45			
		Females					
		9-13 y	8	40			
		14-18 y	15	45			
		19-30 y	18	45			
		31-50 y	18	45			
		51-70 y	8	45			
		>70 y	8	45			
		Pregnancy					
		≤18 y	27	45			
		19-30y	27	45			
		31-50 y	27	45			
		Lactation					
		≤18 y	10	45			
		19-30 y	9	45			
		31-50 y	9	45			

Nutrient / Function	Life Stage Group	(mg/d)	(mg/d) b	Food Sources		Special Considerations
Magnesium Cofactor for enzyme systems	Infants		ND	Green leafy vegetables, unpolished grains, nuts, meat, starches, milk	There is no evidence of adverse effects from the consumption of naturally occurring magnesium in foods. Adverse effects from magnesium containing supplements may include osmotic diarrhea. The UL for magnesium represents intake from a pharmacological agent only and does not include intake from food and water.	Contraindicated in people with heart block. Use caution with renal dysfunction.
	0-6 mo	30*	ND			
	7-12 mo	75*				
	Children					
	1-3 y	80	65			
	4-8 y	130	110			
	Males					
	9-13 y	240	350			
	14-18 y	410	350			
	19-30 y	400	350			
	31-50 y	420	350			
	51-70 y	420	350			
	> 70 y	420	350			
	Females					
	9-13 y	240	350			
	14-18 y	360	350			
	19-30 y	310	350			
	31-50 y	320	350			
	51-70 y	320	350			
	> 70 y	320	350			
	Pregnancy					
	≤18 y	400	350			
	19-30y	350	350			
	31-50 y	360	350			
	Lactation					
	≤18 y	360	350			
	19-30 y	310	350			
	31-50 y	320	350			

Continued

Table D-2 Elements—cont'd

Nutrient	Function	Life Stage Group	RDA/AI* (mg/d)	UL[a] (mg/d)	Selected Food Sources	Adverse Effects of Excessive Consumption	Special Considerations
Manganese	Involved in the formation of bone, as well as in enzymes involved in amino acid, cholesterol, and carbohydrate metabolism	Infants			Nuts, legumes, tea, and whole grains	Elevated blood concentration and neurotoxicity	Because manganese in drinking water and supplements may be more bioavailable than manganese from food, caution should be taken when using manganese supplements especially among those persons already consuming large amounts of manganese from diets high in plant products. In addition, individuals with liver disease may be distinctly susceptible to the adverse effects of excess manganese intake.
		0-6 mo	0.003*	ND			
		7-12 mo	0.6*	ND			
		Children					
		1-3 y	1.2*	2			
		4-8 y	1.5*	3			
		Males					
		9-13 y	1.9*	6			
		14-18 y	2.2*	9			
		19-30 y	2.3*	11			
		31-50 y	2.3*	11			
		51-70 y	2.3*	11			
		>70 y	2.3*	11			
		Females					
		9-13 y	1.6*	6			
		14-18 y	1.6*	9			
		19-30 y	1.8*	11			
		31-50 y	1.8*	11			
		51-70 y	1.8*	11			
		>70 y	1.8*	11			
		Pregnancy					
		≤18 y	2.0*	9			
		19-30y	2.0*	11			
		31-50 y	2.0*	11			
		Lactation					
		≤18 y	2.6*	9			
		19-30 y	2.6*	11			
		31-50 y	2.6*	11			

		(µg/d)	(µg/d) ND b	Legumes, grain products and nuts	Reproductive effects as observed in animal studies.	Individuals who are deficient in dietary copper intake or have some dysfunction in copper metabolism that makes them copper-deficient could be at increased risk of molybdenum toxicity.
Molybdenum Cofactor for enzymes involved in catabolism of sulfur amino acids, purines and pyridines.	Infants					
	0-6 mo	2*	ND			
	7-12 mo	3*	ND			
	Children					
	1-3 y	**17**	300			
	4-8 y	**22**	600			
	Males					
	9-13 y	**34**	1,100			
	14-18 y	**43**	1,700			
	19-30 y	**45**	2,000			
	31-50 y	**45**	2,000			
	51-70 y	**45**	2,000			
	>70 y	**45**	2,000			
	Females					
	9-13 y	**34**	1,100			
	14-18 y	**43**	1,700			
	19-30 y	**45**	2,000			
	31-50 y	**45**	2,000			
	51-70 y	**45**	2,000			
	>70 y	**45**	2,000			
	Pregnancy					
	≤18 y	**50**	1,700			
	19-30y	**50**	2,000			
	31-50 y	**50**	2,000			
	Lactation					
	≤18 y	**50**	1,700			
	19-30 y	**50**	2,000			
	31-50 y	**50**	2,000			

Continued

Table D-2 Elements—cont'd

Nutrient	Function	Life Stage Group	RDA/AI*	UL[a]	Selected Food Sources	Adverse Effects of Excessive Consumption	Special Considerations
Nickel	No clear biological function in humans has been identified. May serve as a cofactor of metalloenzymes and facilitate iron absorption or metabolism in microorganisms.	Infants		(mg/d)	Nuts, legumes, cereals, sweeteners, chocolate milk powder, chocolate candy	Decreased body weight gain. Note: As observed in animal studies	Individuals with preexisting nickel hypersensitivity (from previous dermal exposure) and kidney dysfunction are distinctly susceptible to the adverse effects of excess nickel intake
		0-6 mo	ND	ND			
		7-12 mo	ND	ND			
		Children					
		1-3 y	ND	0.2			
		4-8 y	ND	0.3			
		Males					
		9-13 y	ND	0.6			
		14-18 y	ND	1.0			
		19-30 y	ND	1.0			
		31-50 y	ND	1.0			
		51-70 y	ND	1.0			
		> 70 y	ND	1.0			
		Females					
		9-13 y	ND	0.6			
		14-18 y	ND	1.0			
		19-30 y	ND	1.0			
		31-50 y	ND	1.0			
		51-70 y	ND	1.0			
		> 70 y	ND	1.0			
		Pregnancy					
		≤18 y	ND	1.0			
		19-30y	ND	1.0			
		31-50 y	ND	1.0			
		Lactation					
		≤18 y	ND	1.0			
		19-30 y	ND	1.0			
		31-50 y	ND	1.0			

Nutrient	Function	Life Stage Group	(mg/d)	(mg/d) ND b	Selected Food Sources	Adverse Effects of Excessive Consumption	Special Considerations
Phosphorus	Maintenance of pH, storage and transfer of energy and nucleotide synthesis	Infants			Milk, yogurt, ice cream, cheese, peas, meat, eggs, some cereals and breads	Metastatic calcification, skeletal porosity, interference with calcium absorption	Athletes and others with high energy expenditure frequently consume amounts from food greater than the UL without apparent effect.
		0-6 mo	100*	ND			
		7-12 mo	275*	ND			
		Children					
		1-3 y	460	3,000			
		4-8 y	500	3,000			
		Males					
		9-13 y	1,250	4,000			
		14-18 y	1,250	4,000			
		19-30 y	700	4,000			
		31-50 y	700	4,000			
		51-70 y	700	4,000			
		>70 y	700	3,000			
		Females					
		9-13 y	1,250	4,000			
		14-18 y	1,250	4,000			
		19-30 y	700	4,000			
		31-50 y	700	4,000			
		51-70 y	700	4,000			
		>70 y	700	3,000			
		Pregnancy					
		≤18 y	1,250	3,500			
		19-30y	700	3,500			
		31-50 y	700	3,500			
		Lactation					
		≤18 y	1,250	4,000			
		19-30 y	700	4,000			
		31-50 y	700	4,000			

Continued

Table D-2 Elements—cont'd

Nutrient	Function	Life Stage Group	RDA/AI*	UL^a	Selected Food Sources	Adverse Effects of Excessive Consumption	Special Considerations
Selenium	Defense against oxidative stress and regulation of thyroid hormone action, and the reduction and oxidation status of vitamin C and other molecules		(µg/d)	(µg/d)	Organ meats, seafood, plants (depending on soil selenium content)	Acute toxicity Hair and nail brittleness and loss, nausea and vomiting, fatigue and irritability Chronic toxicity resembles arsenic toxicity	Use cautiously with renal and hepatic dysfunction.
		Infants					
		0-6 mo	15*	45			
		7-12 mo	20*	60			
		Children					
		1-3 y	20	90			
		4-8 y	30	150			
		Males					
		9-13 y	40	280			
		14-18 y	55	400			
		19-30 y	55	400			
		31-50 y	55	400			
		51-70 y	55	400			
		>70 y	55	400			
		Females					
		9-13 y	40	280			
		14-18 y	55	400			
		19-30 y	55	400			
		31-50 y	55	400			
		51-70 y	55	400			
		>70 y	55	400			
		Pregnancy					
		≤18 y	60	400			
		19-30y	60	400			
		31-50 y	60	400			
		Lactation					
		≤18 y	70	400			
		19-30 y	70	400			
		31-50 y	70	400			

872

Silicon		ND b	ND	Plant-based foods	There is no evidence that silicon that occurs naturally in food and water produces adverse health effects	None
No biological function in humans has been identified. Involved in bone function in animal studies.	Infants					
	0-6 mo	ND b	ND			
	7-12 mo	ND	ND			
	Children					
	1-3 y	ND	ND			
	4-8 y	ND	ND			
	Males					
	9-13 y	ND	ND			
	14-18 y	ND	ND			
	19-30 y	ND	ND			
	31-50 y	ND	ND			
	51-70 y	ND	ND			
	>70 y	ND	ND			
	Females					
	9-13 y	ND	ND			
	14-18 y	ND	ND			
	19-30 y	ND	ND			
	31-50 y	ND	ND			
	51-70 y	ND	ND			
	>70 y	ND	ND			
	Pregnancy					
	≤18 y	ND	ND			
	19-30y	ND	ND			
	31-50 y	ND	ND			
	Lactation					
	≤18 y	ND	ND			
	19-30 y	ND	ND			
	31-50 y	ND	ND			

Continued

873

Nutrient	Function	Life Stage Group	RDA/AI*	UL^a	Selected Food Sources	Adverse Effects of Excessive Consumption	Special Considerations
				(mg/d)			
Vanadium	No biological function in humans has been identified. Appears to be important in normal bone growth and as a co-factor for various enzyme reactions.	Infants			Mushrooms, shellfish, black pepper, parsley, and dill seed.	Renal lesions as observed in animal studies. Might cause nephrotoxicity and lower blood glucose levels.	Use caution with people with diabetes and renal dysfunction.
		0-6 mo	ND	ND			
		7-12 mo	ND	ND			
		Children					
		1-3 y	ND	ND			
		4-8 y	ND	ND			
		Males					
		9-13 y	ND	ND			
		14-18 y	ND	ND			
		19-30 y	ND	1.8			
		31-50 y	ND	1.8			
		51-70 y	ND	1.8			
		> 70 y	ND	1.8			
		Females					
		9-13 y	ND	ND			
		14-18 y	ND	ND			
		19-30 y	ND	1.8			
		31-50 y	ND	1.8			
		51-70 y	ND	1.8			
		> 70 y	ND	1.8			
		Pregnancy					
		≤18 y	ND	ND			
		19-30y	ND	ND			
		31-50 y	ND	ND			
		Lactation					
		≤18 y	ND	ND			
		19-30 y	ND	ND			
		31-50 y	ND	ND			

Zinc	Component of multiple enzymes and proteins; involved in the regulation of gene expression.		(mg/d)	(mg/d)	Fortified cereals, red meats, certain seafood	Reduced copper status, gastrointestinal symptoms, and renal failure	Zinc absorption is lower for those consuming vegetarian diets than for those eating nonvegetarian diets. Therefore, it has been suggested that the zinc requirement for those consuming a vegetarian diet is approximately 2-fold greater than for those consuming a nonvegetarian diet. Caution with renal dysfunction, hemochromatosis, and HIV infection.
		Infants					
		0-6 mo	2*	4			
		7-12 mo	3	5			
		Children					
		1-3 y	3	7			
		4-8 y	5	12			
		Males					
		9-13 y	8	23			
		14-18 y	11	34			
		19-30 y	11	40			
		31-50 y	11	40			
		51-70 y	11	40			
		> 70 y	11	40			
		Females					
		9-13 y	8	23			
		14-18 y	9	34			
		19-30 y	8	40			
		31-50 y	8	40			
		51-70 y	8	40			
		> 70 y	8	40			
		Pregnancy					
		≤18 y	12	34			
		19-30y	11	40			
		31-50 y	11	40			

Continued

Table D-2 Elements—cont'd

Nutrient	Function	Life Stage Group	RDA/AI*	UL[a]	Selected Food Sources	Adverse Effects of Excessive Consumption	Special Considerations
Zinc, cont'd		Lactation					
		≤18 y	**13**	34			
		19-30 y	**12**	40			
		31-50 y	**12**	40			

AI, Adequate intake; DFE, dietary folate equivalents; DHA, dehydroascorbic acid; DRI, dietary reference intake; IU, international units; ND b, not determinable resulting from lack of data of adverse effects in this age group and concern with regard to lack of ability to handle excess amounts. Source of intake should be from food only to prevent high levels of intake; NE, niacin equivalents; PLP, pyridoxal phospate; PMP, pyridoxamine phosphate; PNP, pyridoxine phosphate; RAEs, retinol activity equivalents; RDA, recommended daily allowance; REs, retinol equivalents; UL a, the maximum level of daily nutrient intake that is likely to pose no risk of adverse effects. Unless otherwise specified, the UL represents total intake from food, water, and supplements. Because of the lack of suitable data, ULs could not be established for vitamin K, thiamin, riboflavin, vitamin B12, pantothenic acid, biotin, or carotenoids. In the absence of ULs, extra caution may be warranted in consuming levels above recommended intakes.

Note: The table is adapted from the DRI reports (see www.nap.edu); it represents Recommended Dietary Allowances (RDAs) in **bold type**, Adequate Intakes (AIs) in ordinary type followed by an asterisk (*), and Upper Limits (UL)[a]. RDAs and AIs may both be used as goals for individual intake. RDAs are set to meet the needs of almost all (97% to 98%) individuals in a group. For healthy breast-fed infants, the AI is the mean intake. The AI for other life stage and gender groups is believed to cover the needs of all individuals in the group, but lack of data prevent being able to specify with confidence the percentage of individuals covered by this intake.

Sources: Dietary Reference Intakes for Calcium, Phosphorous, Magnesium, Vitamin D, and Fluoride (1997); Dietary Reference Intakes for Thiamin, Riboflavin, Niacin, Vitamin B6, Folate, Vitamin B12, Pantothenic Acid, Biotin, and Choline (1998); Dietary Reference Intakes for Vitamin C, Vitamin E, Selenium, and Carotenoids (2000); and Dietary Reference Intakes for Vitamin A, Vitamin K, Arsenic, Boron, Chromium, Copper, Iodine, Iron, Manganese, Molybdenum, Nickel, Silicon, Vanadium, and Zinc (2002). These reports may be accessed via www.nap.edu and www4.nationalacademies.org.

PL/PL 2003.

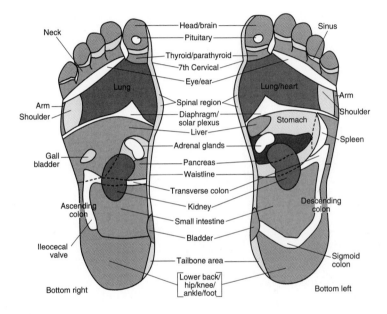

Neck — Head/brain — Sinus
Pituitary
Thyroid/parathyroid
7th Cervical
Eye/ear
Lung — Lung/heart
Arm — Arm
Shoulder — Spinal region — Shoulder
Diaphragm/ solar plexus — Stomach
Liver
Gall bladder — Adrenal glands — Spleen
Pancreas
Waistline
Transverse colon — Descending colon
Ascending colon — Kidney
Small intestine
Ileocecal valve — Bladder — Sigmoid colon
Tailbone area
Bottom right — Lower back/ hip/knee/ ankle/foot — Bottom left

Courtesy Kevin Kunz, Foot Reflexology Project, Albuquerque, NM, 2002.

Index

Note: *t* indicates tables.

879